FIRST AID FOR THE® USMLE STEP 1 2013

TAO LE, MD, MHS
Associate Clinical Professor of Medicine and Pediatrics
Chief, Section of Allergy and Immunology
Department of Medicine
University of Louisville

VIKAS BHUSHAN, MD
Diagnostic Radiologist
Los Angeles

VIVEK T. KULKARNI
Yale School of Medicine
Class of 2014

MATTHEW M. SOCHAT
Warren Alpert Medical School of Brown University
Class of 2013

Mc Graw Hill **Medical**

New York / Chicago / San Francisco / Lisbon / London / Madrid / Mexico City
Milan / New Delhi / San Juan / Seoul / Singapore / Sydney / Toronto

The McGraw·Hill Companies

First Aid for the® USMLE Step 1 2013: A Student-to-Student Guide

1 2 3 4 5 6 7 8 9 0 DOW/DOW 14 13 12

ISBN 978-0-07-180232-1
MHID 0-07-180232-0
ISSN 1532-6020

Notice

Medicine is an ever-changing science. As new research and clinical experience broaden our knowledge, changes in treatment and drug therapy are required. The authors and the publisher of this work have checked with sources believed to be reliable in their efforts to provide information that is complete and generally in accord with the standards accepted at the time of publication. However, in view of the possibility of human error or changes in medical sciences, neither the authors nor the publisher nor any other party who has been involved in the preparation or publication of this work warrants that the information contained herein is in every respect accurate or complete, and they disclaim all responsibility for any errors or omissions or for the results obtained from use of the information contained in this work. Readers are encouraged to confirm the information contained herein with other sources. For example and in particular, readers are advised to check the product information sheet included in the package of each drug they plan to administer to be certain that the information contained in this work is accurate and that changes have not been made in the recommended dose or in the contraindications for administration. This recommendation is of particular importance in connection with new or infrequently used drugs.

This book was set in Electra LH by Rainbow Graphics.
The editors were Catherine A. Johnson and Peter J. Boyle.
Project management was provided by Rainbow Graphics.
The production supervisor was Jeffrey Herzich.
RR Donnelley was printer and binder.

This book is printed on acid-free paper.

Dedication

To the contributors to this and past editions, who took time to share their knowledge, insight, and humor for the benefit of students.

Contents

Contributing Authors

JACOB BARANOSKI
Yale School of Medicine
Class of 2014

VICKI Z. J. BING
Yale School of Medicine
Class of 2014

JEFFREY S. FUTTERLEIB
Yale School of Medicine
Class of 2013

ABHIJEET GUMMADAVELLI
Yale School of Medicine
Class of 2014

LAUREN HIBLER
Yale School of Medicine
Class of 2014

JEFFREY HOFMANN
Warren Alpert Medical School of Brown University
Class of 2016

OLGA LAUR
Yale School of Medicine
Class of 2014

KELSEY B. LOELIGER
Medical Scientist Training Program
Yale School of Medicine

GORAN MICEVIC
Medical Scientist Training Program
Yale School of Medicine

MAX C. PETERSEN
Medical Scientist Training Program
Yale School of Medicine

ROBERT STRETCH
Yale School of Medicine
Class of 2014

GARTH STROHBEHN
Yale School of Medicine
Class of 2014

NICHOLAS THEODOSAKIS
Medical Scientist Training Program
Yale School of Medicine

RICHARD P. USATINE, MD
Dermatology Images Contributor
Professor, Dermatology and Cutaneous Surgery
Professor, Family and Community Medicine
University of Texas Health Science Center San Antonio

CAROLINE A. WALKER
Yale School of Medicine
Class of 2014

SAMANTHA X. Y. WANG
Yale School of Medicine
Class of 2014

WALTER F. WIGGINS, PhD
Editor, firstaidteam.com
Wake Forest School of Medicine
Class of 2014

PETER ZHAO
Yale School of Medicine
Class of 2014

Associate Authors

FADY AKLADIOS
Medical University of the Americas
Class of 2013

ADITYA BARDIA, MD, MPH
Attending Physician, Massachusetts General Hospital Cancer Center
Instructor in Medicine, Harvard Medical School

MICHELLE M. BRAVO
Warren Alpert Medical School of Brown University
Class of 2013

RAFAEL A. BUERBA
Yale School of Medicine
Class of 2014

JONATHAN FU
Yale School of Medicine
Class of 2013

ALEJANDRO RAFAEL GENER
Universidad Central del Caribe
Class of 2015

ASHWANI GORE
St. George's University School of Medicine
Class of 2015

JAMES M. GRAY
University College Dublin School of Medicine and Medical Science
Class of 2014

WILLIAM L. HWANG, MSc
Health Sciences & Technology and Biophysics Programs
Harvard University/Massachusetts Institute of Technology
MD/PhD candidate

KATHARINE JOO
Warren Alpert Medical School of Brown University
Class of 2013

AMY MORENO
Yale School of Medicine
Class of 2014

AYESHA NZERIBE
Warren Alpert Medical School of Brown University
Class of 2013

KEZIA SPENCE
Warren Alpert Medical School of Brown University
Class of 2013

RANY WOO
Yale School of Medicine
Class of 2013

ANDREW HANDI WU
Boston University School of Medicine
Class of 2015

MICHAEL XIONG
Warren Alpert Medical School of Brown University
Class of 2015

PATRICIA ZADNICK
Johns Hopkins School of Medicine
Class of 2014

CHRISTINE ZENDER-PRINCETON, DO
Resident Physician, Lakeland Regional Healthcare
Adjunct Professor, Clinical
Michigan State University College of Medicine

JINYU (JANE) ZHANG
Warren Alpert Medical School of Brown University
Class of 2014

Faculty Reviewers

CHARLES DELA CRUZ, MD
Assistant Professor, Department of Pulmonary and Critical Care Medicine
Yale School of Medicine

EMILY R. ESPOSITO, PhD
Assistant Professor
Sullivan University College of Pharmacy

CONRAD FISCHER, MD
Associate Professor of Physiology, Medicine, and Pharmacology
Touro College of Medicine, New York City

STUART FLYNN, MD
Dean, College of Medicine
The University of Arizona, Phoenix

ANUJ GAGGAR, MD
Clinical Fellow
Department of Infectious Disease
University of San Francisco School of Medicine

MATTHEW GARABEDIAN, MD
Division of Maternal-Fetal Medicine
Department of Obstetrics and Gynecology
Santa Clara Valley Medical Center

ANTHONY GLASER, MD, PhD
Assistant Professor, Department of Family Medicine
Medical University of South Carolina

RYAN C. W. HALL, MD
Assistant Professor, Department of Medical Education
University of Central Florida, Orlando
Affiliate Assistant Professor, Department of Psychiatry
University of South Florida, Tampa

RAJESH JARI, MD, MBA
Spine, Medicine, and Rehabilitation Therapies—SMART Pain Management
Westminster and White Marsh, Maryland

KURT JOHNSON, PhD
Professor, Department of Anatomy and Regenerative Biology and
Department of Obstetrics and Gynecology
George Washington University School of Medicine

SHANTA KAPADIA, MD
Lecturer, Department of Surgery
Yale School of Medicine

BERTRAM KATZUNG, MD, PhD
Professor Emeritus
University of California, San Francisco

GERALD LEE, MD
Assistant Professor, Section of Allergy and Immunology
Department of Internal Medicine
University of Louisville School of Medicine

WARREN LEVINSON, MD, PhD
Professor, Department of Microbiology and Immunology
University of California, San Francisco

NICHOLAS MAHONEY, MD
Assistant Professor, Department of Ophthalmology
Wilmer Eye Institute/Johns Hopkins University

PETER MARKS, MD, PhD
Associate Professor, Department of Internal Medicine
Yale School of Medicine

PATRICIA J. METTING, PhD
Professor of Physiology & Pharmacology and of Medicine
Vice Chancellor and Senior Associate Dean for Student Affairs
The University of Toledo College of Medicine and Life Sciences

AFSOON MOKTAR, PhD
Assistant Professor
Sullivan University College of Pharmacy

ROBERT NOVAK, MD
Chair, Department of Pathology and Laboratory Medicine
Akron Children's Hospital

DAVID PERRY, PhD
Professor, Department of Pharmacology and Physiology
George Washington University School of Medicine

MICHAEL S. RAFII, MD, PhD
Director, Memory Disorders Clinic
Assistant Professor of Neurosciences
University of California San Diego Health System

DANIEL J. RUBIN, MD, MSC
Assistant Professor of Medicine, Division of Endocrinology
Associate Program Director, Endocrinology Fellowship
Temple University School of Medicine

JOSEPH SCHINDLER, MD
Assistant Professor, Department of Neurology and Neurosurgery
Clinical Director, Yale New Haven Stroke Program
Yale School of Medicine

SANJIV SHAH, MD
Assistant Professor, Division of Cardiology
Department of Medicine
Northwestern University

HOWARD STEINMAN, PhD
Professor, Department of Biochemistry
Assistant Dean of Biomedical Science Education
Albert Einstein College of Medicine

STEPHEN THUNG, MD
Associate Professor, Department of Obstetrics/Gynecology
Ohio State University

RICHARD P. USATINE, MD
Professor, Dermatology and Cutaneous Surgery
Professor, Family and Community Medicine
University of Texas Health Science Center San Antonio

HILARY VERNON, MD
Assistant Professor, McKusick-Nathans Institute of Genetic Medicine
Johns Hopkins University

ADAM WEINSTEIN, MD
Assistant Professor, Section of Pediatric Nephrology
Department of Pediatrics
Geisel School of Medicine at Dartmouth

Preface

With this edition of *First Aid for the USMLE Step 1,* we continue our commitment to provide students with the most useful and up-to-date preparation guide for the USMLE Step 1. This edition represents a comprehensive revision in many ways and includes:

- An updated, full-color design with new color photos, enhanced illustrations, and improved formatting of tabular material and mnemonics integrated throughout the text.
- Extensive text and image revisions, clarifications, errata corrections, and new material based on student experience with the 2012 administrations of the USMLE Step 1.
- A revised and updated exam preparation guide for the USMLE Step 1 with updated data from the NBME and NRMP. Includes student feedback as well as study and test-taking strategies for the current exam format.
- Thoroughly revised USMLE advice for international medical graduates and osteopathic medical students.
- More than 1200 frequently tested facts and useful mnemonics, including hundreds of new or revised entries and tables.
- An updated guide to recommended USMLE Step 1 review resources, based on a nationwide survey of randomly selected third-year medical students.
- Bonus Step 1 high-yield facts, cases, video lectures, corrections, and updates can be found exclusively on our blog at **www.firstaidteam.com.**

The improvements in this edition would not have been possible without the help of the thousands of medical students, graduates, and faculty members who contributed their feedback, suggestions, and error corrections. We invite students and faculty to continue sharing their thoughts and ideas to help us improve *First Aid for the USMLE Step 1*. (See How to Contribute, p. xvii.)

Louisville Tao Le
Los Angeles Vikas Bhushan
New Haven Vivek T. Kulkarni
Providence Matthew M. Sochat

Special Acknowledgments

This has been a collaborative project from the start. We gratefully acknowledge the thousands of thoughtful comments, corrections, and advice of the many medical students, international medical graduates, and faculty who have supported the authors in the continuing development of *First Aid for the USMLE Step 1.*

We provide special acknowledgment and thanks to the following students who contributed on many levels: Peter Gayed, Chika Anekwe, Ashleigh Bouchelion, Jack Cossman, Rahul Dalal, Abdelaziz Farhat, Yun Rose Li, Elizabeth Marshall, Sean Martin, and Ajit Rao.

For help on the Web, thanks to Jaysson Brooks, Molly Lewis, Sean Martin, Luke Murray, Sarah-Grace Wesley, and Vamsi Kancherla.

Thanks to the First Aid Step 1 Express team: Jeffrey Hofmann, William Hwang, Stephen A. Allsop, Karolina Brook, Aaron Feinstein, Adrian Haimovich, Katie Lee Hwang, Vivek Kulkarni, Mihan Lee, Nilay Patel, Max Petersen, Nick Theodosakis, and Rany Woo.

For support and encouragement throughout the process, we are grateful to Thao Pham and Jonathan Kirsch, Esq. Thanks to Selina Franklin and Louise Petersen for organizing and supporting the project. Thanks to our publisher, McGraw-Hill, for the valuable assistance of its staff, including Midge Haramis, Jeffrey Herzich, and John Williams. For enthusiasm, support, and commitment for this ongoing and ever-challenging project, thanks to our editor, Catherine Johnson.

For editorial support, enormous thanks to Emma D. Underdown, Linda Bradford, and Linda Davoli. We are also grateful to Tara Price for the interior design of the book and to the medical illustrators, Diana Kryski and Hans Neuhart, for their great work on the new and updated illustrations. Special thanks to Jan Bednarczuk for a greatly improved index. Many thanks to Dr. Richard Usatine of Usatine Media for his outstanding dermatologic image and editorial contributions. We are also very thankful to Fred Howell and Robert Cannon of Textensor for providing access and support to their A.nnotate collaborative platform, which will allow us to more efficiently manage contributions from thousands of medical students and graduates. Lastly, tremendous thanks to Rainbow Graphics, especially David Hommel and Tina Castle, for remarkable ongoing editorial and production work under time pressure.

Louisville Tao Le
Los Angeles Vikas Bhushan
New Haven Vivek T. Kulkarni
Providence Matthew M. Sochat

Acknowledgments for Online Contributors

This year we were fortunate to receive the input of thousands of medical students and graduates who provided new material, clarifications, and potential corrections through our Web site and our new collaborative editing platform. This has been a tremendous help in clarifying difficult concepts, correcting errata from the previous edition, and minimizing new errata during the revision of the current edition. This reflects our long-standing vision of a true student-to-student publication. We have done our best to thank each person individually below, but we recognize that errors and omissions are likely. Therefore, we will post an updated list of acknowledgments at our Web site **www.firstaidteam.com** under the Errata and Updates tab. We will gladly make corrections if they are brought to our attention.

For submitting contributions and corrections, many thanks to Solomon Abay, Hussein Abbas, Ramzi Abboud, Assya Abdallah, Mohamad Abdelfattah, George Abdelmessieh, Salwan Abdullah, Yazan Abou-Ismail, Khalil Abusabha, Stacy Achdjian, Ebele Achebe, James Ackerman, Nivia Acosta, Lance Adams, Robert Adams, Carson Adams, Adebanke Adebayo, Jessica Adefusika, Mona Adeli, Mishuka Adhikary, Amina Adil, Brandon Adler, David Adler, Sumit Agarwal, Deepak Agarwal, Manik Aggarwal, Neha Agnihotri, Nupur Agrawal, Cynthia Aguirre, Daniel Ahmad, Michele Ahmadi, Tina Ahmadinejad, Rabia Ahmed, Kamran Ahmed, Mushfique Ahmed, Annie Ahn, Sahir Ahsan, Zahab Ahsan, Jared Aida, Carol Akers, Oyinade Akinyede, Fady Akladios, Danso Ako-Adjei, Anil Akoon, Erik Akopian, Oluronke Alafe, Mahdi Alajaj, Mohammad Alam, Ridwaan Albeiruti, Carlos Albrecht, Anas Albrejawi Alhomsi, Austin Albright, Carmen Alcala, Tiara Aldridge, Samia Aleem, Michail Alevizakos, Sheby Alexander, Eirene Alexandrou, Shad Ali, Mohammad Ali, Huzair Ali, Munni Ali, Mariam Ali, Zahra Alibrahim, Evan Alicuben, Narges Alipanah, Atush Alipuria, Niloo Allahyari, Laura Almquist, Raed Alnaji, Brock Alonzo, Omar Al-Qudsi, Zina Al-Sakini, Aileen Alviar, Saif Alzoobaee, Chelsey Amer, Kunal Amin, Alec Amram, Keshav Anand, Kayley Ancy, Carl Andersen, Thomas Anderson, Dallin Anderson, Daniel Anderson, Mark Anderson, David Andrews, Zubair Ansari, Ali Ansary, Chase Ansok, Ahmed Antably, Emeka Anyanwu, Dillon Arando, Chris Arbonies, Saeed Arefanian, Alejandro Arenas, Nkiruka Arinze, Anne Armstrong, Grayson Armstrong, Jonathan Arnold, Mack Arroliga, Praag Arya, Rozana Asfour, Derrick Ashong, Karam Asmaro, Ricardo Aulet, Rik Austin, Meghan Auten, Liezl Avila, Shiri Avraham, Temitope Awosogba, Gabriel Axelrud, Derek Axibal, Reed Ayabe, Giselle Ayala, Ndang Azang-Njaah, Ali Ahsan Azeem, Eisha Azhar, Corneliu Bacauanu, Becca Bacharach, Warren Backman, Karam Badran, Javier Baez, Kandy Bahadur, Sara Bahraini, Mirza Baig, Ursula Bailey, Erin Bailey, Mayank Bajpai, Joshua Bakhsheshian, Maria Bakkal, Asha Balakrishnan, Jill Balala, Rajinder Balasuriya, Zach Balest, Rebekah Baltz, Gaurav Bansal, Aiyush Bansal, Faustino Banuelos, Daniel Bar, Nicholas Barasch, Mike Barca, Nicolas Barcelo, Ayse Dalsu Baris, Anne Barnard, Morgan Barnell, Kyle Bartlett, Joshua Barzilai, Bruce Bassi, Bennett Battle, Marianne Bauer, Mark Bauernfeind, Harinder K. Bawa, Omkar Baxi, Michael Baxter, Ahmad Najdat Bazarbashi, Joel Beachey, Tyler Beals, Ryan Beck, Jessica Beckerman, Nic Beckmann, Angela Beckon, Sumeer Bedi, Rachel Beekman, Ryan Begley, Jordan Bell, Joseph Benedict, Nontawan Benja-Athonsirikul, Krista Bergman, Justin Berkowitz, Elizabeth Berry, Adam Berry, Marina Bessel, Adam Betz, Anita Bharath, Suraj Bhargav, Vijay Bhat, Ankit Bhatia, Nita Bhatt, Sajjad Akbar Bhatti, Osman Bhatty, Nora Biary, Charlotte Bibbee, Alexander Bick, David Bishop, Rohan Biswas, Rachel Blair, Max Blanter, Jessamyn Blau, Greg Bligard, David Bluhm, Sarah Bly, Raymond Boakye, Satish Babu Bodapati, Joanne Boisvert, Craig Bollig, Romin Bonakdar, Jeffrey Bonenfant, Valentina Bonev, Namrita Boparai, Nicholas Bope, Sanket Borgaonkar, Joshua Borsook, Tarrah Bowen, Anthony Bowen, Grace Boynton, Hemal Brahmbhatt, Mike Bramati, James Brann, Steve Braun, Kathryn Breidenbach, Jennifer Bress, Jamie Brett, Betsy Breuker, Elizabeth Brezinski, Valerie Brice, Bryan Broach, Benjamin Brockbank, Frank Brodie, Karolina Brooks, Aaron Brown, Sareena Brown, Blair Brown, Gabrielle Brown, Ronnie Brown, Christopher Brown, Will Brubaker, Nataly Bruk, Tina Bruno, Jason Brustein, Daniel Bryan, Campbell Bryson, Rob Buchanan, Floyd Buen, Antiem Bui, John Bui, Jaclyn Burch, Ross Burge, Katelyn Burgess, Adrian Burgos, Colin Burke, Stephen Burks, Bradley Burmeister, Sharlena Burnett, Lauren Burtz, Cathleen Bury, Aaron Bush, Alex Buss, Steve Butala, Emran Butt, Matt Byun, Armando Cabrera, Melissa Cain, Nora Callinan, Sean Campbell, Andrew Campbell, Melissa Campos, Adam Canion, David Capaldi, Lindsay Capron, Jordan Carl, Tyler Carllee, Silva Carlos, Harris Carmichael, Nathan Carpenter, Leah Carr, Madeline Carroll, Evan Carstensen, Phil Carullo, Priscilla Carvalho, Alan Casciola, Ryan Casserly, Leon Castaneda, Crystal Castaneda, Jonas Castaneda, Brandi Castro, Alexander Cavalea, Garrett Cavanaugh, Thomas Cayce, Alberto Cerra, Esther Cha, Ausim Chaghtai, Gaurab Chakrabarti, Jason Chan, Daniela Chan, Maria Chancay, Anisha Chandiramani, Sidharth Chandra, Mahesh Chandrasekhar, Sunny Chang, Khalid Hamid Changal, David Charles, Mubeen Sultan Cheema, Alice Chen, Thomas Chen, Lu Chen, Joanna Chen, Frank Chen, Eric Chen, Andrew Chen, Daniel Cheng, Jacklyn Cheng, Julie Cheng, Esther Cheng, Chris Chesnut, Monica Cheung, Michael Chevinsky, Sharon Chi, Tiffany Chi, Kelly Chien, Jordan Chinai, Cathy Patricia Lee Ching, Anny Ching, Shideh Chinichian, Allen Chiou, Lironn Chitayat, Megan Chock, Michael Choe, Mohammad Rizwan Choudhary, Ahmad Choudhry, Ryan Choudhury, Mohsin Chowdhury, Laura Christensen, Andrew Christiansen, Amy Chu, Kai Chu, Philip Chu, Jonathan Chun, Jina Chung,

Andrew Cichowski, Anthony Cipriano, Dave Ciufo, Andrew Clair, Michael Clark, Summer Clark, Danielle Clark, Emily Clemetson, Michael Cloud, Sarah Codrea, Steven Cogorno, Alex Cohen, Rachel Cohen-Shohet, Elizabeth Collins, Amy Collins, Xavier Colon, Jennifer Colon, Hadassah Consuegra Anderson, Jonathan Copp, Nikhil Cordeiro, Samuel Cordeiro, Elizabeth Cordie, Sarah Cormie, Amarilis Cornejo, Eva Corona, Matthew Cossack, Ryan Cotter, Jennifer Cottral, Molly Cowdrey, Laurel Cox, Katherine Cox, Gordon Crabtree, Paul Craig, Matthew Craig, Crystal Craig, Elizabeth Cramer, Teela Crecelius, Katherine Crifasi, Brian Cripe, Michael Cronin, Nick Crowley, Niall Crowley, Daniel Croymans, Allison Cruse, John Cummins, William Currie, Eileen Curry, Brian Curry, Carl D, Howard Dai, Jessica Dai, David Dai, Thomas Dailey, Pavan Dalal, Mariaana Dalangin, Erika Daley, Keren Dallalzadeh, Thuan Dang, Avace Dani, Gabrielle Daniel, Ameesh Dara, Tyler Darnell, Ryan Daro, Tony Darrington, Alvin Das, Shayna Dattani, Neil Dattani, Shravan Dave, Joshua Davidson, Kerri Davis, Andrew Davis, Chelsea Davis, Michael Davis, Noor Dawood, Solomon Dawson, Andrew Daya, Daniel Dayan, Charles De Jesus, Hector De Jesus, Ivan De Jesus, Nastassia De Souza, Nakyda Dean, Nakydadean Dean, Malcolm Debaun, Cory Deburghgraeve, Johannes Decker, Jennifer Decoste-Lopez, Alison Dedent, Raj Dedhia, Mhair Dekmezian, Henry Del Rosario, Ritchie Mae Delara, Sara Delarosa, Steven Delbello, James Delgadillo, Joseph Delio, Samantha Demar, Dawit Demissie, Kathryn Demitruk, John Demuth, Kara Denby, Vedant Desai, Danielle Desjardins, Danielle Detelich, Andrew Deutsch, Anjan Devaraj, Ryan Devenyi, David Deyoung, Trisha Dickey, Marine Dididze, Christine Dillingham, Bill Diplas, Ebony Dix, Erin Dizon, Teresa Do, Chris Dobson, Taylor Dodgen, Natasha Dolgin, Sarah Donaldson, Patrick Dooling, Amy Dora, Bradleigh Dornfeld, Heather Douthitt, Dr Munaf, Alex Drake, Mariah Dreisinger, Maggie Driscoll, Ian Dryden, Xi Du, Milap Dubal, Genia Dubrovsky, Brittany Duchene, Matthew Duda, Sarah Duhon, Mark Dukshtein, Rachelle Duquette, Zachary Dureau, Jonathan Dutt, Alison Dzwonczyk, Micah Eades, John Eager, Anas Easa, Christian Eckmann, Colin Edwards, Jared Ee, Nima Eftekhary, Ashley Egan, Badi Eghterafi, Nick Eglitis, Ehren Ekhause, Lindsay Elbaum, Justen Elbayar, Ilyas Eli, Tyler Ellington, Alexis Elliott, Alejandra Ellison-Barnes, Sora Ely, Matthew Emerich, Drew Emge, Trine Engebretsen, Christopher English, Chris English, Feras Entabi, Esther Enuanwa, Elizabeth Ernst, Rito Escareno, Michael Esparza, Diego Espinoza, Chris Ethridge, Clay Evans, Brendan Everett, Abieyuwa Eweka, Cyril Eyadiel, Nnenna Ezeilo, Abayomi Fabunmi, Eric Faden, Josh Fage, Laura Fagen, Kerolos Fahmi, Falcon Falcon, Kimberly Faldetta, Lu Fan, Hang Fang, Hongfei Fang, Lawrence Fannon, Joseph Farahany, Abdelaziz Farhat, Bilal Farhat, Amy Farkas, Amanda Farris, Michael Fay, Alicia Febles De Lorow, Ido Feferkorn, Rebecca Fega, Leah Feldman, Robert Feng, Jenny Feng, Yaniv Fenig, Elizabeth Fenstermacher, Agha Hassan Feroze, Abdullah Feroze, Michael Ferro, Michael Fickes, Vikram Fielding-Singh, Tucker Fischbeck, Juliya Fisher, Alex Fisher, Mark Fisher, Erin Fitzgerald, Heidi Fjeldstad, Jason Flamendorf, Kenneth Flax, Mario Flores, Katy Flynn-Meketon, Kelly Fong, Christopher Foote, Jon Forbes, Lisa Fosnot, Andrew Fouche, Nyssa Fox, Loren Fox, Sarah Franjoine, Harris Frank, Miguel Frau, Rob Freeman, Monika Freiser, Appolinia Frey, Yev Freyvert, Martin Fried, Robin Friedman, Jamie Friedmanjamief, Melanie Friess, Jason Frischhertz, Nathan Frogge, Simona Frunza-Stefan, Alicia Fuhrman, Tim Fuller, Tracy Fulton, Brian Fung, August Funk, Nicholas Furlani, Bob Furlong, Michael Gabbard, Alex Gaidarski, James Gallagher, Sylvia Bea Galvan, Nikita Ganatra, Anjalika Gandhi, Niral Gandhi, Niket Gandhi, Abby Gandolfi, Milan Ganger, Akshay Ganju, Jared Gans, Ian Gao, Jennifer Gao, Maria Victoria Garcia, Heidy Garcia, Benjamin Garden, Michael Garitty, John Garlich, Michael Gazes, Daniel Gealy, Alison Gegios, Steven Gelb, Scott Gelman, Alejandro Gener, Douglas George, Ramez Ghabour, Marcel Ghanem, Saad Ghazipura, Alexander Ghobadimanesh, Martin Gibbs, David Gill, Harrison Gimbel, Will Gionfriddo, Jacob Gire, Christine Glendon, Steven Glenn, Joshua Glick, Chad Glisch, Catherine Go, Shanette Go, Michelle Go, Nikhil Godbole, Melanie Goebel, Aneesh Goel, George Gold, Andrew Goldman, Whitney Goldsberry, Ian Goldstein, Greg Goldstein, Aaron Goldstein, Nicholas Golinvaux, Anurekha Gollapudi, Jane Golub, Charles Gonzales, Lillian Gonzalez, Wilfredo Gonzalez, Javier Gonzalez, Abigail Goodman, Avi Goodman, Ashwani Gore, Shaun Gould, Morgen Govindan, Indira Gowda, Daniel Grabell, Trevor Grace, Cynthia Grady, Jaykumar Grandhi, Rebecca Graves, James Gray, Emily Gray, Christian Greco, Clifton Green, Ari Greenbaum, Steven Greenstein, Alexander Greenstein, Tobin Greensweig, Char Grif, Gabriel Griffin, Ashley Grigsby, Brian Grisez, Nathan Grohmann, Britt Gros, Bridget Gross, Kelli Gross, Daniel Grosser, Andrea Grosz, Alan Groves, Joanna Grzadziel, Allen Guehl, Arthur Guepe, Jonah Gunalda, Robin Guo, Ling Guo, Jessie Guo, Akash Gupta, Sheena Gupta, Abhishek Gupta, Gita Gupta, Ankur Gupta, Apar Gupta, Kiran Guthikonda, Kai Ha, Inna Hadass, Cathryn Haeffele, Kevin Hageman, Sue Hahn, Moosa Haider, Adrian Haimovich, Angie Hairrell, Mark Hall, Sarah Hall, Charles Hall, Jeremy Hall, Alexander Hallac, Akbar Hamid, Kam Hanamaikai, John Hanks, Jesse Hansen, Stephanie Harbison, Brian Harms, Jessica Harrell, David Harrington, Holly Harris, Frank Harris, Jennifer Harris, Cynthia Hart, Bridget Hartman, Heather Hartman, Becca Hartog, Georgina Hartzell, Zach Harvanek, Connor Hasbrook, Hasnain Hasham, Omar Hashmi, Jordan Haskins, Ammar Hassan, John Hassani, Kai Hata, Mike Hausberger, Andriy Havrylyan, Liz Haworth, Shane Hawthorne, Shakaib Hayat, Lisa Hayman, George Hayward, Sindalisa Hean, Jason Hedge, Elise Heeringa, Jeff Heimiller, Christine Helou, Krista Hemmesch, Martha Henao, Phillip Hendley, Whitney Hendrickson, Rachel Henrickson, Eduardo Hernandez, Matthew Hernandez, Miriam Herschman, Anthony Herzog, Matthew Hess, Amber Hetrick, Jarred Hicks, Andrew Higdon, David Hilburn, Derek Hill, Graham Hill, Julia Hiner, Jonathan Hirshberg, Whitney Hitchcock, Yoona Ho, Marjorie Ho, Alan Hoang, Sandra Hobson, Max Hockstein, Evan Hodell, Aaron Hodes, Erika Hoenke, Zach Hoffman, Martin Hofmann, Kaitlin Holdstein, Charles Hong, Michael Hong, Chris Hong, Austin Horrocks, Wendy Hosin, Elika Hoss, Reza Hosseini Ghomi, Pearl Houghteling, Nicholas Hountras, L. Mclean House Ii, Kara Hoverson, Lee Howard, Ryan Howard, Tifany Hoyne, Ahmed Hozain, Ruth Hsiao, Jennifer Hsu, Wei-Chun Hsu, Anna Hsu, Annie Hsu, Jen Hsu, Derek Hsu, Peifen Hu, Jessie Hu, Cindy Hu, Charles Hua, Linda Huang, Hanwei Huang, Christopher Huelsman, Brandon Huffman, Myriam Hughes, Hayley Hunt, Nakia Hunter, Jennie Huo, Lara Hurlburt, Irene Hurst, Mustafa Husaini, Adnan Hussain, Hanif Hussaini, Monica Huynh, Daniel Hwang, Michael Hwang, Patrick Hyppolite, Adaora Ifeanyi, Kevan Iffrig, Atanas Iliev, Hasan IMANLI, Peter Ip, Neil Issar, Kilali Iyalla, Mangala Iyengar, Lee Jablow, Deidrya Jackson, Lishan Jackson, Robert Jackson, Joshua Jackson, Jacoby Jacobsen, Asif Jafferani, Syed Jaffery, Ariba Jahan, Supriya Jain, Amita Jain, Sechin Jain, Christopher Jakubowski, Asha Jamzadeh, Samantha Janiga, Daniel Javaherian, Matthew Jaykel, Tim Jaykel, Isaac Jenabi, Jack Jeng, Kimberly Jenkins, Kim Jenna, Brett Jensen, Jonathan Jerkins, Forrest Jespersen, Krishan Jethwa, Shiel Jhaveri, Lunan Ji, Rui Jiang, Yike Jiang, Alice Jiang, William Jiang, Ying Jin, Peter Jin, Bennett Johnson, Ben Johnson, Linda Johnson, Wes Johnson, Stacey Johnson, Ireal Johnson, Brianna Johnson-Rabbett, Benjamin Jones, Roger Jones, Tyler Jones, Chelsea Jones, Andrew Jones, Nate Jones, Patrick Jorda, Mary Kate Jordan, Lia Jordano, Walter Joseph, Claire Joseph, Rahul Joy, Alexander Juhn, Jenny Jun, Sarah Jung, Michael Jung, Sam K, Nida K, Payal Kadakia, Cihan Kadipasaoglu, Jessica Kafer, Jodi Kagihara, Rachel Kahn, Adam Kahn, Charissa Kahue, Mehboob Kalani, Mowffaq Kalantan, Shana Kalaria, Mariya Kalashnikova, Sudhir Kalaskar, Zach Kalb, Omar Kallas, Kunal Kambli, Caroline Kan, Pridvi Kandagatla, Sean Kandel, Ravinder Kang, David Kang, Sarv Kannapiran, Roger Kanumuri, Jordan Kapper, Nima Karamooz, Peter Karempelis, Syed Karim, Justin Karlin, Joshua Karlin, Krupa Karnik, Anthony Kasch, Stephen Kasteler, Kenan Katranji, Igor Katsyv, Leah Katta, Monica Katz, Matthew Katz, Benjamin Kaufman, Anatoly Kazakin, Amir Kazerouninia, Matthew Kelley, Sandra Kellum, Jonathan Ken, Dorian

Kenleigh, Daniel Kennedy, Kristen Kent, Kyle Kern, Amanda Kern, Rohit Kesarwani, Briana Ketterer, Ryan Key, Andrew Keyser, Phue Khaing, Mazen Khan, Rabnawaz Khan, Idrees Khan, Aimal Khan, Muhammad Zubair Khan, Shadab Khan, Rabeea Khan, Tamer Khashab, Sameer Khatri, Ben Khazan, Ali Khiabani, Akhil Khosla, Gohar Khosravi, Michal Kidacki, Zachariah Kidman, Crystal Kiewert, Daniel Kil, David Kim, Ellen Kim, Grace Kim, Jenna Kim, Jun Kim, Kristin Kim, Christopher Kim, Soo Jeong Kim, Phillip Kim, Ajin Kim, Julie Kim, Samuel Kim, David Kimball, Jonathan King, Eric King, Nikhar Kinger, Kathleen Kirkland, Annah Kirkley, Drew Kiser, Joshua Kiss, Wissam Kiwan, Maximilian Klein, Nicole Klekowski, Kris Klem, Isaiah Kletenik, Dane Klett, Bradley Kliewer, Michelle Knoll, Pin-Yi Ko, Brett Kodish, Kristin Koenig, Aaron Kofman, Lauren Kohan, Pratistha Koirala, Nadeem Kolia, Franchesca König Toro, Matthew Koo, Hannah Kooperkamp, Yelena Korotkaya, Jacqueline Korpics, Karthik Kota, Uzma Kothawala, Yann-Fuu Kou, Adam Kowalski, David Kraft, Scott Kramer, Landon Krantz, Sarah Krantz, Brad Krasnick, Carl Kraus, Vijay Krishna, Ross Kristal, Malgorzata Krzyszczak, Paul Kuder, Elizabeth Kuilanoff, Nishat Kulkarni, Robret Kulwin, Keerthana Kumar, Anupam Kumar, Sanjay Kumar, Aashish Kumar, Hanesh Kumar, Preethi Kumar, Hiren Kunadia, Joseph Kundukulam, Edward Kuoy, Daniel Kurbanov, Vadim Kurbatov, Ashleigh M. Kussman, Levon Kuypelyan, Melissa Kwan, Rui Kwan, Janet Kwok, Levon Kyupelyan, Tiffany L, Alison La, Jennifer Ladd, Carlos Lago, Hamed Lahijani, Erica Lai, Isabella Lai, Kuan-Chi Lai, Bryan Lai, Rosalind Lai, Charlene Lai, Chandru Jay Lalwani, Lauren Lambeth, Jon Lamee, Rongpei Lan, Megan Land, Kristen Landry, Maria Lapchenko, Marissa Lapedis, Caroline Larosa, Derek Laskar, Joe Lau, Wincie Lau, Samantha Lavergne, John Le, Jessica Lee, Kacia Lee, Paul Lee, Raymond Lee, Dane Lee, Dianne Lee, Yungah Lee, Jisoo Lee, Christina Lee, Katherine Lee, Joo Yeon Lee, Michelle N Lee, Eunjoo Lee, Anna Lee, Michelle Lee, Jason Lee, Jennifer Lee, Katie Lees, Lucas Lenci, Kyle Leneweaver, Mike Leonard, Scott Lester, Stephanie Leung, Peggy Leung, Celine Leung, Steven Leung, Seth Levin, Matthew Levine, Kate Levy, Vivian Levy, Natashia Lewis, Molly Lewis, Lei Li, Luming Li, Yun Li, Li Li, Angela Li, Kai Li, Carol Li, Bin Li, Qiansheng Liang, Emily Liebling, Sofia Ligard, Caitlin Lim, Simon Lim, Lian Lim, Geoffrey Lim, David Lin, Alex Lin, Tsung Hsien Lin, Jennifer Ling, Matthew Listo, Alison Little, Amy Liu, Kevin Liu, Emberlynn Liu, Lars Logdberg, Kevin Loh, Paula Lomba, David Long, Cesar Lopez Angel, Christopher Lops, Jaime Loso, Kristian Loveridge, Dylan Lovin, Michele Luhm Vigor, Jason Luijasonl, Karen Luk, Chris Lunt, Leo Luo, David Luu, Ying Luu, Catherine Ly, Blair M, E M, Nilam M, Andrea Ma, Stephanie Ma, Ashlee Macdonald, Andrew Macquarrie, Mahesh Madhavan, Jai Madhok, Selena Magalotti, Paula Magee, Isha Mahamud, Michael Mahan, Val Maharaj, Mithu Maheswaranathan, Mithunan Maheswaranathan, Hadi Mahmaljy, Mhd Abdallah Mahrous, Herman Mai, Thi Mai, Leann Mainis, Vivian Mai-Tran, Gary Mak, Lindsay Makara, Vyacheslav Makler, Slava Makler, Mona Malakouti, Veshal Malhotra, William Malins, Ilir Manaj, Sarah Mancini, Jason Mandell, Morgan Mandigo, Nicole Mangiboyat, Christopher Manieri, Alexandra Mannix, Abdallah Mansour, Soohan Mansuri, David Mao, Marnonette Marallag, Leanna Marderian, Fernando Mariz, Dan Marks, Benjamin Marsh, Kerry Marshall, Daniel Martig, Kent Martin, Pablo Martinez, Luis Martinez, Ryan Martinez, Jaime Martinez, Pablo F. Martinez, Jessica Mason, Sunil Mathew, Gladcy Mathew, Irène Mathieu, Sandy Mazzoni, Jamie Mazzurco, Ositadinma Mbadugha, Ndi Mbride, Tom Mcbride, Alexis Mccabe, Heather Mccain, Marissa Mccay, Brittani Mcclain, James Mcclurg, Jonathan Mcgovern, Sarah Mcguffin, Caitlin Mcintyre, Nicholas Mckenna, Tina Mckenzie, Tyler Mckinnon, Lance Mcleroy, Jake Mcmillin, Colton Mcnichols, Casey Means, Oren Mechanic, James Medley, Britton Mehr, Hiral Mehta, Komal Mehta, Dillon Meier, Chris Meinzen, Maayan Melamed, Joshua Melito, Clay Merritt, Phoebe Mesiha, Andrew Meyers, Okechukwu Mgbemena, Erik Miguel, Amir Mikhchi, Mark Mikhly, Brian Miller, Moshe Miller, Andrew Miller, Tom Miller, Chris Millhouse, Steven Mills, Daniel Miranda, Leonidas Miras, Anne Misiura, Stuart Mitchell, Kevin Mitchell, Todd Miyake, Takudzwa Mkorombindo, Lauren Moak, Sarah Mohajeri, Abdirahman Mohamed, Girish Mohan, Desh Mohan, Chaitra Mohan, Shifa Mohiuddin, Ghulam Rehman Mohyuddin, Jeffrey Mojica, Richard Moleno, Domingo Molina, Daniel Mollengarden, Ryan Moore, Lindsay Morgenstern, Marina Morie, Andrew Morris, Elizabeth Morris, Gregory Morris, Aimee Morris, Tyler Morrison, Daniel Mortensen, Chris Morton, Shawn Moshrefi, Natalie Mota, Saba Motakef, Moustafa Moustafa, Murali Mukkamala, Benjamin Mullenbach, Katherine Mun, Marlon Munian, Jacob Murphree, Tim Murphy, Praveen Murthy, Raza Mushtaq, John Muzic, Kledia Myrtolli, Jennifer Mytar, Lucy Na, Elizabeth Nadal, Diana Naderi, Hodad Naderi, Navid Nafissi, Jonathan Nahas, Kiran Naidoo, Neil Naik, Yuree Nam, Hiroya Nambu, Yuree Namyureen, Ashwin Narayana, Dustin Nash, Daniel Nassau, Neelima Navuluri, Shariq Nawab, Giseli Nazmi, Ryan Neeley, Steven Neeley, Anoop Nehra, Steven Nelson, Joseph Nelson, Mithun Neral, Craig Ness, Kevin Nethers, Jordan Newman, Natalie Ngai, Quoc Ngo, Julius Ngu, Bao Nguyen, Mai Trang Nguyen, Jennifer Nguyen, Brian Nguyen, Angeline Nguyen, Nga Nguyen, Vy Nguyen, Andrew Nguyen, Christine Nguyen, Phi Nguyen, Peter Nguyen, Ronald Nguyen, Anthony Nguyen, Hung Nguyen, Sheena Nguyen, Alexandre Nguyen, Dan Nguyen, Janie Nguyen, Tram Nguyen, Ruba Nicola, Carl Nieweld, Lena Ning, Isabella Niu, Conway Niu, Leila Njimoluh, Mark Noble, Tomoki Nomakuchi, Adrian Nugent, Drew Nunziat, Aisulu Nurgozha, Tarik Nurkic, Emmanuel Nwelue, Ada Nwozuzu, Ernestina Nyarko, Kunal Oak, Souzana Obretenova, James O'Dowd, Florence Odufalu, Michael Ofori, Ben Oglivie, Oladoyin Ogunbayo, Kyle Oholendt, Kene Okeke, Michelle Okoronkwo, Bunmi Olaloye, John O'laughlin, Elizabeth Oler, Edgar Olivas, Cara Olsen, Joseph Omlor, Sina Salehi Omran, Neil Onizuka, Abimbola Orisamolu, Christopher Orr, Kenneth Ortiz, Vedran Oruc, Lais Osmani, Erik Ostler, Adetola Otesile, Robert Oubre, Xiaoxi Ouyang, Steve Ovada, Jordan Owens, Kolawole Oyewole, Rudy P, Sigmund Paczkowski, Kevin Padrez, Alyssa Pagliere, Allyson Palmer, Jd Palmer, Brian Palmisano, Jason Pan, Qinshi Pan, Saman Panahipour, Prakash Panchani, Gabrielle Paoletti, Amit Parekh, Ruby Parikh, Sneha Parikh, Sonal Parikh, Jong Park, Anthony Park, Braden Parmer, Christian Parobek, James Parris, Scott Pascal, Vanessa Pascoe, Janaki Paskaradevan, Parimal Patel, Ronak Patel, Suketu Patel, Amy Patel, Satya Patel, Sagar Patel, Shyam Patel, Tariq Patel, Hasita Patel, Parin Patel, Devin Patel, Neal Patel, Hiren Patel, Priya Patel, Maharsh Patel, Kinner Patel, Gaurav Patel, Lance Patel, Tejas Patel, Manisha Patel, Vishal Patel, Krupa Patel, Nilam Patel, Mahesh Patel, Mita Patel, Kershaw Patel, Romy Patel, Janus Patel, Tejas Patil, Rajesh Patnaik, Melissa Patterson, Kelly Paulk, Brit Payton, Justin Peacock, Katherine Pederson, Alla Pekareva, Andrew Pelikan, Andrew Peranteau, Alex Perelman, Enmanuel Perez, Rafael Perez, Mari Perez-Rosendahl, Tiffany Perkins, Liz Perkins, Barry Perlman, Michael Perone, David Perry, Asad Pervez, Max Petersen, Ashley Peterson, Sarah Peterson, Camille Petri, Tracy Pham, Andrew Pham, Tiffany Phanhdone, Douglas Phelan, Adam Phillips, Carson Phillips, Nick Piazza, Michael Pierce, Allison Pierce, Sara Pike, Meredith Plant, Alex Podolsky, Marc Polacco, Quiana Pollock, Kathleen Polonchek, Kristina Pontarelli, Francesco Pontoriero, Adrienne Poon, Nicole Pope, Jeremy Porter, Lesley Portugal, Michael Posch, Emily Pospiech, Thomas Powell, Catherine Powell, Jamila Power, Shrestha Prajib, Tyler Prestwood, Andrea Price, Jason Primus, Emilie Prot, Caroline Protin, Liese Pruitt, Kristina Prus, Alena Prystupa, Ramya Punati, Ashvin Punnyamurthi, David Purger, Anthony Purgianto, Raghuveer Puttagunta, H Q, Zuhab Qamar, Seema Qayum, Hazeeb Qazi, Xiaoming Qi, Ann Qiu, Ming Yi Qiu, Nabila Quadri, Cara Quant, Jose Quesada, Nick Quinn, Thomas Quinn, Sidra Qureshi, Jenn Raab, Amanda Rabideau, Ashwinee Ragam, Preethi Raghu, Vikram Raghu, Christina Ragland, Roxana Rahmanian, Samira Rahmanian, Asima Raja, Akriti Raju, Charles Ramkishun, Josean Ramos, Jonathan Ramsey, Neerva Rana, Jessica Randell, Ajit Rao, Justin Raper, Ken Rapp, Rita Raturi, Rebecca Raub, Curtis Read, Alan Reagan, David Rebedew, Joshua Reber, Matthew Rebesco, Thomas Reher,

Daniel Reid, Joshua Reid, Rebecca Reimers, Steven Reinhart, Michael Reinsbach, Brock Reiter, Sonia Replansky, David Retamar, Monica Rettenmier, Joshua Reuss, Wissam Rhayem, Jamie Rhodes, Fady Riad, Andrew Richardson, Aaron Richler, Sabah R'id, John Riester, Catherine Rim, Ryan Rimer, Kathryn Rimmer, Dalianne Rivera, Alicia Rizzo, Kris Roach, Joshua Roark, Michael Robers, Leslie Robin, Michelle Robinette, Monica Roca, Will Roche, Ellis Rochelson, Alejandro Rodriguez, Jesus Rodriguez, Carmen Rodriguez, Javier Rodriguez Kovacs, Jackeline Rodriguez-Smith, Samuel Rogers, Ben Rogers, Eric Rohman, Sarah Rollins, Christine Rollins, Brice Rolston, Vladimir Romannikov, Bobby Rombola, David Roraff, Javier Rosales, Evan Rosenbaum, Matthew Rosenbaum, Elizabeth Rosenberger, Eric Rosenfeld, Jared Ross, Joshua Ross, Lela Ross, Bryan Roth, Ryan Roth, Ben Roth, Kara Rothenberg, Steven Rothenberg, Zach Rottmann, Jonathan Roy, David Roy, David Rubins, Sharmistha Rudra, Chloe Rugut, Eric Rupe, William Rusnak, Meghan Rutgers, Nidia Ryan, Yamaan Saadeh, Janany Sabescumar, Sandeep Sabhlok, Michael Saco, Radha Sadacharan, Ahmed Sadek, Cameron Saffer, Abigail Sage, Atith Saheba, Sachin Sahni, S M Nazmus Sakib, Yusuf Salah, Mohamad Saleh, Ramy Saleh, Dr. Salway, Diana Samberg, Yoni Samocha, Glenn San Agustin, Christopher Sanchez, Juan Sanchez, Evan Sander, Britt Sandler, Kiri Sandler, Kenneth Sands, Jake Sanning, Margarita Santiago, Nishtha Sareen, Joyatee Sarker, Luay Sarsam, Milan Satcher, Alexander Satin, Alexandra Satty, Christopher Schaefer, William Schaffenburg, Jessica Schancupp, Matthew Schear, Sid Schechet, Eli Scher, Kai Schlingmann, Megan Schmidt, Amanda Schmitt, Drew Schmucker, Sam Schroeder, Adam Schwalje, Dan Schwartz, Brandon Schwartz, Kristopher Schwebler, Sarah Scott, Elliot Scott, Eric Seachrist, Derek Seehausen, Nilmaris Segarra, Tracy Seimears, Jackie Selbst, Philip Senger, Gina Sequeira, Nikhil Seth, Sajiv Sethi, Tasneam Shagroni, Raju Shah, Halie Shah, Rusha Shah, Manan Shah, Kinchit Shah, Bijal Shah, Tejal Shah, Ankur Shah, Anna Shah, Arpeet Shah, Vishal Shah, Anand Shah, Archana Shah, Zoheb Shaikh, Berje Shammassian, Angela Shan, Brett Shannon, Ayesha Shariff, Amal Shariff, Anil Sharma, Aarti Sharma, Allison Shatz, Brian Shayota, Mike Shelton, Kartik Shenoy, Rashna Shetty, Johanna Sheu, Eugenia Shevchenko, Sandra Shi, James Shi, Kyle Shibuya, Jessica Shie, Matthew Shiel, Yushane Shih, John Shin, Mackenzie Shindorf, Justine Shum, Thomas Shum, Erik Shwarts, Shan Siddiqi, Ashhad Siddiqui, Eliud Sifonte, Nathan Silvestri, Aaron Sin, Vikal Singh, Shashank Singh, Harmandeep Singh, Amteshwar Singh, Vikram Singh, Melissa Singh, Punit Singh, Arindam Singha, Varsha Sinha, Mark Sittig, Tim Sitton, Stephanie Skala, Ahalya Skandarajah, David Skoglund, Racquel Skold, Ernest Sliwinski, Justin Sloane, Emily Smergel, Nicholas Smith, Amanda Smith, Justin Smith, Kyle Smith, Craig Smith, Kendall Snyder, Kunmi Sobowale, Matthew Sochat, Jae Ho Sohn, Shantanu Solanki, Sanaa Somalya, David Somsen, Raku Son, Daniel Son, Joohyun Song, Yohan Song, Jasen Sood, Sufian Sorathia, Brett Sorge, Juan Sosa, Michael Sotiriou, Mario Soto, Yehuda Julian Spector, Julian Spector, Cory Spicer, Daniel Spiegel, Lauren Spiegel, Adam Spjute, Kathryn Stadeli, Irina Staicu, Michael Stanaek, Anna-Bianca Stashak, Jake Steel, Christopher Steele, Ruth Stefanos, Mike Stengel, Kevin Stephens, Scott Stiles, Blair Stocks, Jon Stoever, Ilana Stol, Timothy Stooksberry, Tony Stover, Michelle Stram, Alyssa Stram, Jehu Strange, Marshall Strother, Daphna Stroumsa, Sean Sturm, Maham Subhani, Mark Suguitan, Matthew Sullivan, Farheen Sultana, Lishi Sun, Cliff Sung, Srinivas Sunkara, Matthew Surdel, Tyler Surma, Ryan Sutherland, Alex Swan, Christopher Sweat, Adam Sweeney, Tyler Swiss, Ali Syed, David Symister, Ariana Tabing, Hannah Taft, Shahein Tajmir, James Tak, Brandon Takase, Malia Takeuchi, Selorm Takyi, Afsaneh Talai, Sejal Tamakuwala, Neal Tambe, Tanya Tan, Amit Tandon, Lynda Tang, Mengyao Tang, Frances Tangherlini, Dantera Tangpisuthipongsa, Jackie Tanios, Kathryn Tapper, Karen Tart, Christine Tat, Elias Taxakis, Rachel Taylor, Scott Taylor, Miguel Teixeira, Kara Teruya, Zach Testo, Mazell Tetruashvily, Yana Thaker, Prakash Thapa, William Thieu, Aaron Thomas, Jerry Thomas, Taryn Thomas, Barrett Thomas, Alexandra Thomas, Ashley Thompson, Jason Thompson, Sibo Tian, Wayne Tie, Tom Tielleman, Thomas Tielleman, Connie Tien, Meghan Tierney, Tonia Tiewul, Andrew Timmons, Corey Tingey, Joanne Tisak, Wissam Tobea, Marko Todorovic, Josef Tofte, Thomas Tolbert, Justin Tomal, Jimmy Ton, Corey Tong, Olivia Tong, Gabriel Tonkin, Nevkeet Toor, Thalia Torres, Bela Toth, Jamie Totman, Lauren Towne, Jorge Trabanco, Albert Train, Patrick Tran, Bao Tran, Sunyu Tran, Darrell Tran, Pat Tran, Norris Tran Duc, Daniel Treister, Hung Trinh, Adrian Tripp, Chelsea Troiano, Ryan Trowbridge, Kim Truong, Cindy Tsai, Valerie Tsang, Brian Tse, Victor Tseng, Pei-Yuan Tsou, Brian Tu, Alex Turin, Sergey Turin, Stefan Turkula, Alison Ullman, Sphoorti Umarjee, Chelsea Dawn Unruh, Krishna Upadhyaya, Oleg Uryasev, Eric Uzoma, Nataly Vadasz, Kimaya Vaidya, Jason Valadao, Erik Valenti, Kippie Valentine, Carla Valenzuela, Tina Varghese, Ross Varma, Matthew Varner, Bradley Varner, Jacob Varney, Ashley Vaughn, Aria Vazirnia, Christine Velazquez, Laura Veras, Christopher Verdick, Saurabh Verma, Marissa Versalle, Benjamin Vidalis, Albert Vien, Anita Vijapura, Liliana Villamil-Nunez, David Villanueva, Tomas Villarreal, Howard Vo, Peter Vu, Charles Vu, John Vu, Elizabeth W, Christianne Wa, Cherisse Wada, Jacob Wagner, Brittany Wagner, John Wainwright, Kevin Walker, Brandon Walker, Sean Wallace, Scott Walter, Joseph Wan, Tony Wang, Bo Wang, Jessica Wang, Jonathan Wang, Vivian Wang, Wendy Wang, Lindsay Warner, James Warren, Joshua Wasmund, Ryan Watson, Dovie Watson, Daniel Watson, Kathleen Weber, Katie Weber, Catherine Wei, Sam Weimer, Frank Weinberg, Candice Weiner, Ken Weinlander, Mark Weinreich, Lindsay Weiss, Claire Welteroth, Nick Wendling, Michael West, Kyle Westerholt, Derek Weyhrauch, Matthew Wheelwright, Natalie White, Ian Whiteside, Rachel Whynott, Jenna Wickersham, Shira Wieder, Renee Wierz, Olivia Wilcox, Nicholas Wilkie, Sara Williams, Elbert Williams, Emily Willner, Erika Wilson, Brant Wilson, Rachael Winchester, Daniel Wingo, Lee Winkler, Paul Winograd, Keith Wirth, Lauren Wiznia, Sean Wo, Lindsey Woeste, William Wojtusiak, Amanda Wolf, Tiana Won, Christina Wong, Anthony Wong, Kimberly Wong, Stephanie Wong, Linda Wong, James Wong, Christopher Wood, Jennifer Wootton, Megan Worthley, Xinyu Wu, Sarah Wu, Gregory Wu, Wayland Wu, Susan Wu, Chester Wu, Daniel Wu, Andrew Wu, Andrew Wuenstel, Rachel Wurmser, Kirk Wyatt, Jonathan Xia, Michael Xiong, Willa Xiong, Baogang Xu, Ron Yalon, Tarek Yamany, Xiaofeng Yan, Jennifer Yan, Debby Yanes, Kimberly Yang, Jonathan Yang, Christine Yang, Jimmy Yao, Gokul Yaratha, Golsa Yazdy, Allen Ye, Brittany Yee, James Yeh, Emily Yeh, John Yeh, Aleksandr Yelenskiy, Amanda Yen, Albert Yen, Johnny Yep, Nury Yim, Kathleen Yip, Michael Yip, Yin Yiu, Stella Yoo, Jane Yoon, Kei Yoshimatsu, Makoto Yoshino, Jae You, Jovante Young, Andrew Young, Michael Youssef, Xin Yu, Connie Yu, Mary Yu, Hana Yu, Cathy Yu, Michael Yuan, Marshall Yuan, Michael Yudelevich, Etana Zack, Muhammad Usman Zafar, Lisansha Zahirsha, Andreina Zambrano, Ferdous Zannat, Helio Zapata, Katherine Zappia, Rolla Zarifa, Debra Zauner, Mariam Zeini, Jennifer Zhan, Jinmeng Zhang, Steven Zhang, Jane Zhang, Yingtao Zhang, Bingnan Zhang, Qian Zhang, Wency Zhao, Shuang Zhao, Betty Zhao, Ludan Zhao, Sherry Zhao, Theresa Zhou, Xun Zhou, Shira Ziegler, Nicole Zimmerman, Mark Zobeck, Adnan Zubair, and Michael Zumwalt.

For submitting book reviews, thanks to Rami Abukamil, Kristen Anderson, Maureen Ayers Looby, Glorilee Balistrieri, Emaad Basith, Matthew Bloom, Pierre Bueser, Elspeth Call, Hector Casiano, Edgie-Mark Co, Loren Colson, Alex Doudt, Clinton Ezekiel, Kendell Felker, Michael Flores, Cynthia Gee, Michael Greff, Lindsay Henderson, Ryan Tyler Hoff, Sebastian Jacobi, Priyanka Jagar, Kunal Kamboj, Harris Khan, Sameer Lakha, Tsung Hsien Lin, Michelle Liu, Lyndon Luk, Neil Majithia, Vanessa Mallol, Shane Mandalia, Gretchen Metzenberg, Naila Mirza, Steven Mong, Yen Nguyen, Fernando Ovalle, Nirav Patel, Jason Pesqueira, Alison Petrie, Hassan Qadir, Yujie Qiao, Faith Quenzer, Monique Roberts, Jasjeet Sekhon, Gabriel Soto, Kazuhiro Takahashi, Richard Tapnio, Jasmine Toor, Trung Tran, Michael Tran, Dana Turker, Sierra Witte, and Betty Zhao.

How to Contribute

This version of *First Aid for the USMLE Step 1* incorporates hundreds of contributions and changes suggested by faculty and student reviewers. We invite you to participate in this process. We also offer **paid internships** in medical education and publishing ranging from three months to one year. Please send us your suggestions for:

- Study and test-taking strategies for the USMLE Step 1
- New facts, mnemonics, diagrams, and illustrations
- High-yield topics that may appear on future Step 1 exams
- Personal ratings and comments on review books, online question banks, videos, and courses

For each new entry incorporated into the next edition, you will receive up to a **$20 Amazon.com gift certificate** per entry from the author group, as well as personal acknowledgment in the next edition. Diagrams, tables, partial entries, updates, corrections, and study hints are also appreciated, and significant contributions will be compensated at the discretion of the authors. Also, let us know about material in this edition that you feel is low yield and should be deleted.

The preferred way to submit new entries, clarifications, mnemonics, or potential corrections with a valid, authoritative reference is via our Web site:

www.firstaidteam.com

This Web site will be continuously updated with validated errata, new high-yield content, and a new online platform to contribute suggestions, mnemonics, diagrams, clinical images, and potential errata.

Alternatively, you can e-mail us at: firstaidteam@yahoo.com.

Contributions submitted by June 15, 2013, receive priority consideration for the 2014 edition of *First Aid for the USMLE Step 1*. We thank you for taking the time to share your experience and apologize in advance that we cannot individually respond to all contributors as we receive hundreds of contributions each year.

▶ NOTE TO CONTRIBUTORS

All contributions become property of the authors and are subject to editing and reviewing. Please verify all data and spellings carefully. In the event that similar or duplicate entries are received, only the first complete entry received with a valid, authoritative reference will be used. Please follow the style, punctuation, and format of this edition as much as possible.

▶ JOIN THE FIRST AID TEAM

The *First Aid* author team is pleased to offer part-time and full-time paid internships in medical education and publishing to motivated medical students and physicians. Internships may range from a few months (e.g., a summer) up to a full year. Participants will have an opportunity to author, edit, and earn academic credit on a wide variety of projects, including the popular *First Aid* series.

In 2013, we are actively seeking passionate medical students and graduates with a specific interest in improving our medical illustrations and expanding our database of medical photographic images. We welcome people with prior experience and talent in this area. Relevant skills include digital photography, digital asset management, information design, medical illustration, and graphic design. Please email us at **firstaidteam@yahoo.com** with a CV and summary of your interest or sample work.

How to Use This Book

Medical students who have used previous editions of this guide have given us feedback on how best to make use of the book.

It is recommended that you begin using this book as early as possible while learning the basic medical sciences. You can use Section IV to select first-year course review books and Internet resources and then use those books for review while taking your medical school classes.

Use different parts of the book at different stages in your preparation for the USMLE Step 1. Before you begin to study for the USMLE Step 1, we suggest that you read Section I: Guide to Efficient Exam Preparation and Section IV: Top-Rated Review Resources. **If you are an international medical graduate student, an osteopathic medical student, a podiatry student, or a student with a disability,** refer to the appropriate Section I supplement for additional advice. Devise a study plan and decide what resources to buy. We strongly recommend that you invest in the latest edition of at least one or two top-rated review books on each subject.

First Aid is not a comprehensive review book, and it is not a panacea for inadequate preparation during the first two years of medical school. Scanning Sections II and III will give you an initial idea of the diverse range of topics covered on the USMLE Step 1.

As you study each discipline, **use the corresponding high-yield-fact section in *First Aid for the USMLE Step 1* as a means of consolidating the material and testing yourself** to see if you have mastered some of the frequently tested items. Actively work within the book to integrate important facts into your fund of knowledge. Using *First Aid for the USMLE Step 1* as a review can serve as both a self-test of your knowledge and a repetition of important facts to learn. The Rapid Review section includes high-yield topics and vignettes are abstracted from recent exams to help guide your preparation.

To **broaden** your learning strategy, you can **integrate** your *First Aid* study with *First Aid Cases for the USMLE Step 1*, *First Aid Q&A for the USMLE Step 1*, and the USMLE-Rx Qmax Step 1 test bank. *First Aid Cases* and *First Aid Q&A* are organized to match *First Aid for the USMLE Step 1* **chapter for chapter.** After reviewing a discipline or organ system chapter within *First Aid*, you can **review cases** on the same topics and then **test your knowledge** in the corresponding chapters of *First Aid Cases* and *First Aid Q&A* and with USMLE-Rx Qmax Step 1. If you want a **deeper review** of the high-yield topics, consider adding *First Aid for the Basic Sciences: General Principles* and *Organ Systems* and the First Aid Express or Ultimate video courses (www.usmle-rx.com) to your study plan.

Return to Sections II and III frequently during your preparation and fill your short-term memory with remaining high-yield facts a few days before the USMLE Step 1. The book can serve as a useful way of retaining key associations and keeping high-yield facts fresh in your memory just prior to the examination. Reviewing the book immediately after the exam is probably the best way to **help us improve the next edition.** Decide what was truly high and low yield and **send in your comments, post them on our Web site, or send us a scanned copy of your entire annotated book. Remember that you cannot disclose any exam material from the USMLE.**

Common USMLE Laboratory Values

* = Included in the Biochemical Profile (SMA-12)

Blood, Plasma, Serum	Reference Range	SI Reference Intervals
*Alanine aminotransferase (ALT, GPT at 30°C)	8–20 U/L	8–20 U/L
Amylase, serum	25–125 U/L	25–125 U/L
*Aspartate aminotransferase (AST, GOT at 30°C)	8–20 U/L	8–20 U/L
Bilirubin, serum (adult)		
Total // Direct	0.1–1.0 mg/dL // 0.0–0.3 mg/dL	2–17 μmol/L // 0–5 μmol/L
*Calcium, serum (Total)	8.4–10.2 mg/dL	2.1–2.8 mmol/L
*Cholesterol, serum (Total)	140–200 mg/dL	3.6–6.5 mmol/L
*Creatinine, serum (Total)	0.6–1.2 mg/dL	53–106 μmol/L
Electrolytes, serum		
Sodium	135–147 mEq/L	135–147 mmol/L
Chloride	95–105 mEq/L	95–105 mmol/L
* Potassium	3.5–5.0 mEq/L	3.5–5.0 mmol/L
Bicarbonate	22–28 mEq/L	22–28 mmol/L
Gases, arterial blood (room air)		
P_{O_2}	75–105 mmHg	10.0–14.0 kPa
P_{CO_2}	33–44 mmHg	4.4–5.9 kPa
pH	7.35–7.45	$[H^+]$ 36–44 nmol/L
*Glucose, serum	Fasting: 70–110 mg/dL 2-h postprandial: < 120 mg/dL	3.8–6.1 mmol/L < 6.6 mmol/L
Growth hormone – arginine stimulation	Fasting: < 5 ng/mL provocative stimuli: > 7 ng/mL	< 5 μg/L > 7 μg/L
Osmolality, serum	275–295 mOsm/kg	275–295 mOsm/kg
*Phosphatase (alkaline), serum (p-NPP at 30°C)	20–70 U/L	20–70 U/L
*Phosphorus (inorganic), serum	3.0–4.5 mg/dL	1.0–1.5 mmol/L
*Proteins, serum		
Total (recumbent)	6.0–7.8 g/dL	60–78 g/L
Albumin	3.5–5.5 g/dL	35–55 g/L
Globulins	2.3–3.5 g/dL	23–35 g/L
*Urea nitrogen, serum (BUN)	7–18 mg/dL	1.2–3.0 mmol/L
*Uric acid, serum	3.0–8.2 mg/dL	0.18–0.48 mmol/L
Cerebrospinal Fluid		
Glucose	40–70 mg/dL	2.2–3.9 mmol/L

(continues)

Hematologic		
Erythrocyte count	Male: 4.3–5.9 million/mm^3 Female: 3.5–5.5 million/mm^3	$4.3–5.9 \times 10^{12}$/L $3.5–5.5 \times 10^{12}$/L
Hematocrit	Male: 41–53% Female: 36–46%	0.41–0.53 0.36–0.46
Hemoglobin, blood	Male: 13.5–17.5 g/dL Female: 12.0–16.0 g/dL	2.09–2.71 mmol/L 1.86–2.48 mmol/L
Reticulocyte count	0.5–1.5% of red cells	0.005–0.015
Hemoglobin, plasma	1–4 mg/dL	0.16–0.62 μmol/L
Leukocyte count and differential		
Leukocyte count	4500–11,000/mm^3	$4.5–11.0 \times 10^9$/L
Segmented neutrophils	54–62%	0.54–0.62
Band forms	3–5%	0.03–0.05
Eosinophils	1–3%	0.01–0.03
Basophils	0–0.75%	0–0.0075
Lymphocytes	25–33%	0.25–0.33
Monocytes	3–7%	0.03–0.07
Mean corpuscular hemoglobin	25.4–34.6 pg/cell	0.39–0.54 fmol/cell
Mean corpuscular volume	80–100 μm^3	80–100 fL
Platelet count	150,000–400,000/mm^3	$150–400 \times 10^9$/L
Prothrombin time	11–15 seconds	11–15 seconds
Activated partial thromboplastin time	25–40 seconds	25–40 seconds
Sedimentation rate, erythrocyte (Westergren)	Male: 0–15 mm/h Female: 0–20 mm/h	0–15 mm/h 0–20 mm/h
Proteins in urine, total	< 150 mg/24 h	< 0.15 g/24 h

Basic Science Discipline Cross-Reference Table for High-Yield Facts

	Cardio-vascular	Endocri-nology	Gastro-intestinal	Hema-tology/ Oncology	Immu-nology	Musculo-skeletal	Neurology	Psychiatry	Renal	Repro-ductive	Respira-tory
Behavioral Science							61–62	60, 62		59–60	
Embryology	250–252	286	308–309	251			408–410		478	504–514	
Anatomy	253	286–289	309–318	344–347		378–386	411–442		479	514–517	544–546
Biochemistry		110	110–111, 115			77–79, 86, 114				82–89	
Microbiology			124, 135–137, 147, 151–152, 167–168	149	201–202	144, 169, 172, 174	148, 162, 166–167, 169, 174		169–170	138–141, 150, 156, 171, 173	131–132, 168, 174
Pathology	265–278	223, 296–304	324–340	218–224, 350–366	200, 203–208	387–403	416–417, 419–420, 422–448	459–472	488–498	524–537	553–561
Pharmacology	279–284	305–306	340–342	367–375	209–210	404–406	449–456	472–476	499–502	538–541	562–564
Physiology	253–265	289–295	319–323	347–349		378–386	411–442		480–488	518–523	546–552

First Aid Checklist for the USMLE Step 1

This is an example of how you might use the information in Section I to prepare for the USMLE Step 1. Refer to corresponding topics in Section I for more details.

Years Prior

- ☐ Select top-rated review books as study guides for first-year medical school courses.
- ☐ Ask for advice from those who have recently taken the USMLE Step 1.

Months Prior

- ☐ Review computer test format and registration information.
- ☐ Register six months in advance. Carefully verify name and address printed on scheduling permit. Call Prometric or go online for test date ASAP.
- ☐ Define goals for the USMLE Step 1 (e.g., comfortably pass, beat the mean, ace the test).
- ☐ Set up a realistic timeline for study. Cover less crammable subjects first. Review subject-by-subject emphasis and clinical vignette format.
- ☐ Simulate the USMLE Step 1 to pinpoint strengths and weaknesses in knowledge and test-taking skills.
- ☐ Evaluate and choose study methods and materials (e.g., review books, practice tests, software).

Weeks Prior

- ☐ Simulate the USMLE Step 1 again. Assess how close you are to your goal.
- ☐ Pinpoint remaining weaknesses. Stay healthy (exercise, sleep).
- ☐ Verify information on admission ticket (e.g., location, date).

One Week Prior

- ☐ Remember comfort measures (loose clothing, earplugs, etc.).
- ☐ Work out test site logistics such as location, transportation, parking, and lunch.
- ☐ Call Prometric and confirm your exam appointment.

One Day Prior

- ☐ Relax.
- ☐ Lightly review short-term material if necessary. Skim high-yield facts.
- ☐ Get a good night's sleep.
- ☐ Make sure the name printed on your photo ID appears EXACTLY the same as the name printed on your scheduling permit.

Day of Exam

- ☐ Relax. Eat breakfast. Minimize bathroom breaks during the exam by avoiding excessive morning caffeine.
- ☐ Analyze and make adjustments in test-taking technique. You are allowed to review notes/study material during breaks on exam day.

After the Exam

- ☐ Celebrate, regardless.
- ☐ Send feedback to us on our Web site at **www.firstaidteam.com.**

SECTION I

Guide to Efficient Exam Preparation

▶ INTRODUCTION

Relax.

This section is intended to make your exam preparation easier, not harder. Our goal is to reduce your level of anxiety and help you make the most of your efforts by helping you understand more about the United States Medical Licensing Examination, Step 1 (USMLE Step 1). As a medical student, you are no doubt familiar with taking standardized examinations and quickly absorbing large amounts of material. When you first confront the USMLE Step 1, however, you may find it all too easy to become sidetracked from your goal of studying with maximal effectiveness. Common mistakes that students make when studying for Step 1 include the following:

- Not understanding how scoring is performed or what the score means
- Starting to study (including *First Aid*) too late
- Starting to study intensely too early and burning out
- Using inefficient or inappropriate study methods
- Buying the wrong books or buying more books than you can ever use
- Buying only one publisher's review series for all subjects
- Not using practice examinations to maximum benefit
- Not using review books along with your classes
- Not analyzing and improving your test-taking strategies
- Getting bogged down by reviewing difficult topics excessively
- Studying material that is rarely tested on the USMLE Step 1
- Failing to master certain high-yield subjects owing to overconfidence
- Using *First Aid* as your sole study resource
- Trying to do it all alone

In this section, we offer advice to help you avoid these pitfalls and be more productive in your studies.

▶ *The test at a glance:*

- *8-hour exam*
- *Total of 322 multiple choice items*
- *7 test blocks (60 min/block)*
- *46 test items per block*
- *45 minutes of break time, plus another 15 if you skip the tutorial*

▶ USMLE STEP 1—THE BASICS

The USMLE Step 1 is the first of three examinations that you must pass in order to become a licensed physician in the United States. The USMLE is a joint endeavor of the National Board of Medical Examiners (NBME) and the Federation of State Medical Boards (FSMB). The USMLE serves as the single examination system for U.S. medical students and international medical graduates (IMGs) seeking medical licensure in the United States.

The Step 1 exam includes test items drawn from the following content areas:

- Anatomy
- Behavioral sciences
- Biochemistry
- Microbiology and immunology
- Pathology

- Pharmacology
- Physiology
- Interdisciplinary topics such as nutrition, genetics, and aging

How Is the Computer-Based Test (CBT) Structured?

The CBT Step 1 exam consists of one "optional" tutorial/simulation block and seven "real" question blocks of 46 questions each (see Figure 1) for a total of 322 questions, timed at 60 minutes per block. A short 11-question survey follows the last question block. The computer begins the survey with a prompt to proceed to the next block of questions.

Once an examinee finishes a particular question block on the CBT, he or she must click on a screen icon to continue to the next block. Examinees **cannot** go back and change their answers to questions from any previously completed block. However, changing answers is allowed **within** a block of questions as long as time permits—**unless** the questions are part of a sequential item test set (see p. 4).

What Is the CBT Like?

Given the unique environment of the CBT, it's important that you become familiar ahead of time with what your test-day conditions will be like. In fact, you can easily add 15 minutes to your break time! This is because the 15-minute tutorial offered on exam day may be skipped if you are already familiar with the exam procedures and the testing interface. The 15 minutes is then added to your allotted break time of 45 minutes for a total of 1 hour of potential break time. You can download the tutorial from the USMLE Web site and do it before test day. This tutorial is the exact same interface you will use in the exam; learn it now and you can skip taking it during the exam, giving you 15 extra minutes of break time. You can also gain experience with the CBT format by taking the 150 practice questions available online or by

> ▸ *If you know the format, you can skip the tutorial and add 15 minutes to your break time!*

FIGURE 1. Schematic of CBT Exam.

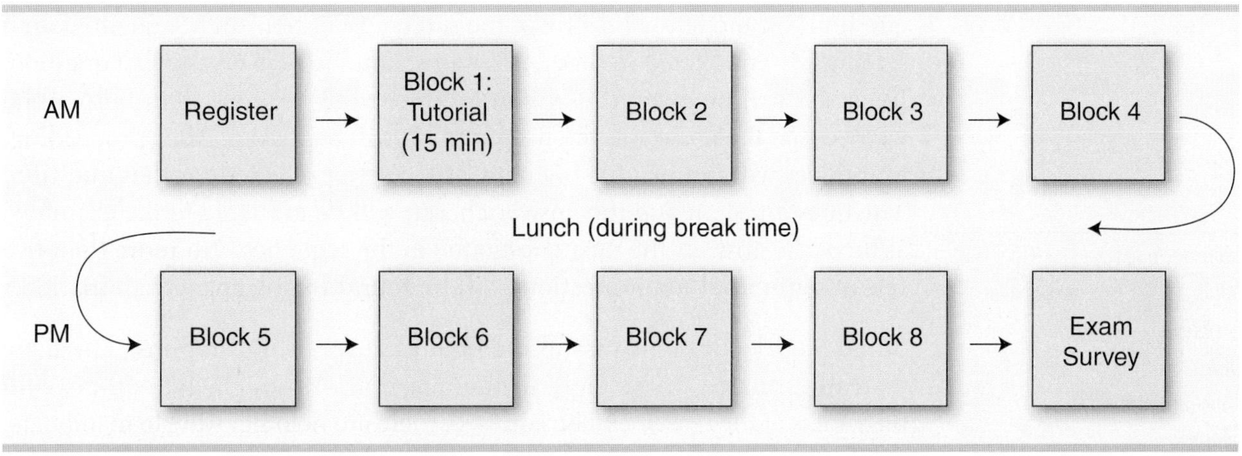

signing up for a practice session at a test center (for details, see What Does the CBT Format Mean to Me?).

For security reasons, examinees are not allowed to bring any personal electronic equipment into the testing area. This includes both digital and analog watches, cellular telephones, and electronic paging devices. Food and beverages are also prohibited. The testing centers are monitored by audio and video surveillance equipment. However, most testing centers allot each examinee a small locker outside the testing area in which he or she can store snacks, beverages, and personal items.

- *Keyboard shortcuts:*
  - *A, B, etc.–letter choices*
  - *Enter or spacebar–move to next question*
  - *Esc–exit pop-up Lab and Exhibit windows*
  - *Alt-T–countdown timers for current session and overall test*

The typical question screen in the CBT consists of a question followed by a number of choices on which an examinee can click, together with several navigational buttons on the top of the screen. There is a countdown timer on the upper left-hand corner of the screen as well. There is also a button that allows the examinee to mark a question for review. If a given question happens to be longer than the screen (which occurs very rarely), a scroll bar will appear on the right, allowing the examinee to see the rest of the question. Regardless of whether the examinee clicks on an answer choice or leaves it blank, he or she must click the "Next" button to advance to the next question.

- *Heart sounds are tested via media questions. Make sure you know how different heart diseases sound on auscultation.*

The USMLE features a small number of media clips in the form of audio and/or video. There may even be a question with a multimedia heart sound simulation. In these questions, a digital image of a torso appears on the screen, and the examinee directs a digital stethoscope to various auscultation points to listen for heart and breath sounds. **No more than five media questions will be found on any given examination,** and the USMLE orientation materials now include several practice questions in these new formats. During the exam tutorial, examinees are given an opportunity to ensure that both the audio headphones and the volume are functioning properly. If you are already familiar with the tutorial and planning on skipping it, first skip ahead to the section where you can test your headphones. After you are sure the headphones are working properly, proceed to the exam.

Recently the USMLE introduced a sequential item test format for some questions. Sequential item questions are grouped together in the list of questions on the left-hand side of the screen. Questions in a sequential item set must be completed in order. After an examinee answers the first question, he or she will be given the option to proceed to the next item but will be warned that the answer to the first question will be locked. **After proceeding, examinees will not be able to change the answer selected for that question.** The question stem and the answer chosen will be available to the examinee as he or she answers the next question(s) in the sequence. **No more than five sets of sequential item questions will be found in any given examination.**

- *Test illustrations include:*
  - *Gross photos*
  - *Histology slides*
  - *Radiographs*
  - *Electron micrographs*
  - *Line drawings*

Some Step 1 questions may also contain figures or illustrations. These are typically situated to the right of the question. Although the contrast and brightness of the screen can be adjusted, there are no other ways to manipulate the picture (e.g., there is no zooming or panning).

The examinee can call up a window displaying normal laboratory values. In order to do so, he or she must click the "Lab" icon on the top part of the screen. Afterward, the examinee will have the option to choose between "Blood," "Cerebrospinal," "Hematologic," or "Sweat and Urine." The normal-values screen may obscure the question if it is expanded. The examinee may have to scroll down to search for the needed lab values. You might want to memorize some common lab values so you spend less time on questions that require you to analyze these.

▸ *Familiarize yourself with the commonly tested lab values.*

The CBT interface provides a running list of questions on the left part of the screen at all times. The software also permits examinees to highlight or cross out information by using their mouse. Finally, there is an "Annotate" icon on the top part of the screen that allows students to write notes to themselves for review at a later time. Being familiar with these features can save time and may help you better organize the information you need to answer a question.

▸ *Ctrl-Alt-Delete are the keys of death during the exam. Don't touch them!*

What Does the CBT Format Mean to Me?

The significance of the CBT to you depends on the requirements of your school and your level of computer knowledge. If you are a Mac user, you might want to spend some time using a Windows-based system and pointing and clicking icons or buttons with a mouse.

For those who feel they might benefit, the USMLE offers an opportunity to take a simulated test, or "CBT Practice Session at a Prometric center." Students are eligible to register for this three-and-one-half-hour practice session after they have received their scheduling permit.

The same USMLE Step 1 sample test items (150 questions) available on the USMLE Web site, www.usmle.org, are used at these sessions. **No new items will be presented.** The session is divided into three one-hour blocks of 50 test items each and costs about $42. Students receive a printed percent-correct score after completing the session. **No explanations of questions are provided.**

▸ *You can take a shortened CBT practice test at a Prometric center.*

You may register for a practice session online at www.usmle.org. A separate scheduling permit is issued for the practice session. Students should allow two weeks for receipt of this permit.

How Do I Register to Take the Exam?

Prometric test centers offer Step 1 on a year-round basis, except for the first two weeks in January and major holidays. The exam is given every day except Sunday at most centers. Some schools administer the exam on their own campuses. Check with the test center you want to use before making your exam plans.

U.S. students can apply to take Step 1 at the NBME Web site. This application allows you to select one of 12 overlapping three-month blocks in which to be tested (e.g., April–May–June, June–July–August). Choose your three-month eligibility period wisely. If you need to reschedule outside your initial three-month period, you can request a one-time extension of eligibility for the next contiguous three-month period, and pay a rescheduling fee. The application also includes a photo ID form that must be certified by an official at your medical school to verify your enrollment. After the NBME processes your application, it will send you a scheduling permit.

> *The Prometric Web site will display a calendar with open test dates.*

The scheduling permit you receive from the NBME will contain your USMLE identification number, the eligibility period in which you may take the exam, and two additional numbers. The first of these is known as your "scheduling number." You must have this number in order to make your exam appointment with Prometric. The second number is known as the "candidate identification number," or CIN. Examinees must enter their CINs at the Prometric workstation in order to access their exams. Prometric has no access to the codes. **Do not lose your permit!** You will not be allowed to take the exam unless you present this permit along with an unexpired, government-issued photo ID that includes your signature (such as a driver's license or passport). Make sure the name on your photo ID exactly matches the name that appears on your scheduling permit.

> *The confirmation emails that Prometric and NBME send are not the same as the scheduling permit.*

> *Test scheduling is done on a "first-come, first-served" basis. It's important to call and schedule an exam date as soon as you receive your scheduling permit.*

Once you receive your scheduling permit, you may access the Prometric Web site or call Prometric's toll-free number to arrange a time to take the exam. You may contact Prometric two weeks before the test date if you want to confirm identification requirements. Although requests for taking the exam may be completed more than six months before the test date, examinees will not receive their scheduling permits earlier than six months before the eligibility period. The eligibility period is the three-month period you have chosen to take the exam. Most medical students choose the April–June or June–August period. Because exams are scheduled on a "first-come, first-served" basis, it is recommended that you contact Prometric as soon as you receive your permit. After you've scheduled your exam, it's a good idea to confirm your exam appointment with Prometric at least one week before your test date. Prometric does not provide written confirmation of exam date, time, or location. Be sure to read the *2013 USMLE Bulletin of Information* for further details.

What If I Need to Reschedule the Exam?

You can change your test date and/or center by contacting Prometric at 1-800-MED-EXAM (1-800-633-3926) or www.prometric.com. Make sure to have your CIN when rescheduling. If you are rescheduling by phone, you must speak with a Prometric representative; leaving a voice-mail message will not suffice. To avoid a rescheduling fee, you will need to request a change at least 31 calendar days before your appointment. Please note that your rescheduled test date must fall within your assigned three-month eligibility period.

When Should I Register for the Exam?

Although there are no deadlines for registering for Step 1, you should plan to register at least six months ahead of your desired test date. This will guarantee that you will get either your test center of choice or one within a 50-mile radius of your first choice. For most U.S. medical students, the desired testing window is in June, since most medical school curricula for the second year end in May or June. Thus, U.S. medical students should plan to register before January in anticipation of a June test date. The timing of the exam is more flexible for IMGs, as it is related only to when they finish exam preparation. Talk with upperclassmen who have already taken the test so you have real-life experience from students who went through a similar curriculum, then formulate your own strategy.

> *Register six months in advance for seating and scheduling preference.*

Where Can I Take the Exam?

Your testing location is arranged with Prometric when you call for your test date (after you receive your scheduling permit). For a list of Prometric locations nearest you, visit www.prometric.com.

How Long Will I Have to Wait Before I Get My Scores?

The USMLE reports scores three to four weeks, unless there are delays in score processing. Examinees will be notified via email when their scores are available. By following the online instructions, examinees will be able to view, download, and print their score report. Additional information about score timetables and accessibility is available on the official USMLE Web site.

What About Time?

Time is of special interest on the CBT exam. Here's a breakdown of the exam schedule:

> *Gain extra break time by skipping the tutorial or finishing a block early.*

15 minutes	Tutorial (skip if familiar with test format and features)
7 hours	Seven 60-minute question blocks
45 minutes	Break time (includes time for lunch)

The computer will keep track of how much time has elapsed on the exam. However, the computer will show you only how much time you have remaining in a given block. Therefore, it is up to you to determine if you are pacing yourself properly (at a rate of approximately one question per 77 seconds).

The computer will not warn you if you are spending more than your allotted time for a break. You should therefore budget your time so that you can take a short break when you need one and have time to eat. You must be especially careful not to spend too much time in between blocks (you should keep track of how much time elapses from the time you finish a block of questions to the time you start the next block). After you finish one question block, you'll need to click on a button to proceed to the next block of questions. If you do not click to proceed to the next question block, you will automatically be entered into a break period.

Forty-five minutes is the minimum break time for the day, but you are not required to use all of it, nor are you required to use any of it. You can gain extra break time (but not time for the question blocks) by skipping the tutorial or by finishing a block ahead of the allotted time. Any time remaining on the clock when you finish a block gets added to your remaining break time. Once a new question block has been started, you may not take a break until you have reached the end of that block. If you do so, this will be recorded as an "unauthorized break" and will be reported on your final score report.

▶ *Be careful to watch the clock on your break time.*

Finally, be aware that it may take a few minutes of your break time to "check out" of the secure resting room and then "check in" again to resume testing, so plan accordingly. The "check-in" process may include fingerprints and pocket checks. Some students recommend pocketless clothing on exam day to streamline the process.

If I Freak Out and Leave, What Happens to My Score?

Your scheduling permit shows a CIN that you will enter onto your computer screen to start your exam. Entering the CIN is the same as breaking the seal on a test book, and you are considered to have started the exam when you do so. However, no score will be reported if you do not complete the exam. In fact, if you leave at any time from the start of the test to the last block, no score will be reported. The fact that you started but did not complete the exam, however, will appear on your USMLE score transcript. Even though a score is not posted for incomplete tests, examinees can still request that their scores be calculated and reported if they desire; unanswered questions will be scored as incorrect.

The exam ends when all question blocks have been completed or when their time has expired. As you leave the testing center, you will receive a printed test-completion notice to document your completion of the exam. To receive an official score, you must finish the entire exam.

What Types of Questions Are Asked?

▶ *Nearly three-fourths of Step 1 questions begin with a description of a patient.*

One-best-answer multiple-choice items (either singly or as part of a sequential item set) are the only question type on the exam. Most questions consist of a clinical scenario or a direct question followed by a list of five or more options. You are required to select the single best answer among the options given. There are no "except," "not," or matching questions on the exam. A number of options may be partially correct, in which case you must select the option that best answers the question or completes the statement. Additionally, keep in mind that experimental questions may appear on the exam, which do not affect your score (see Difficult Questions, p. 20).

How Is the Test Scored?

Each Step 1 examinee receives an electronic score report that includes the examinee's pass/fail status, two test scores, and a graphic depiction of the examinee's performance by discipline and organ system or subject area. The actual organ system profiles reported may depend on the statistical characteristics of a given administration of the examination.

The NBME provides two overall test scores based on the total number of items answered correctly on the examination (see Figure 2). The first score, the three-digit score, is reported as a scaled score in which the mean is 225 and the standard deviation is approximately 21. This is the only score that gets reported to residency program directors. The second score scale, the two-digit score, defines 75 as the minimum passing score (equivalent to a score of 188 on the first scale). This score is only reported to state licensing boards that may have statutory requirements that the score scale have 75 as the minimum passing score. In 2011, the USMLE stopped reporting the two-digit score to score users (e.g., residency programs) and now reports only the three-digit score. Throughout this book we refer to scores using the three-digit scale only.

▸ *The mean Step 1 score for U.S. medical students continues to rise, from 200 in 1991 to 225 in 2011.*

A score of 188 or higher is required to pass Step 1. The NBME does not report the minimum number of correct responses needed to pass, but estimates that it is roughly 60–70%. The NBME may adjust the minimum passing score in the future, so please check the USMLE Web site or www.firstaidteam.com for updates.

According to the USMLE, medical schools receive a listing of total scores and pass/fail results plus group summaries by discipline and organ system. Students can withhold their scores from their medical school if they wish. Official USMLE transcripts, which can be sent on request to residency programs, include only total scores, not performance profiles.

Consult the USMLE Web site or your medical school for the most current and accurate information regarding the examination.

FIGURE 2. 2011 Scoring Scales for the USMLE Step 1.

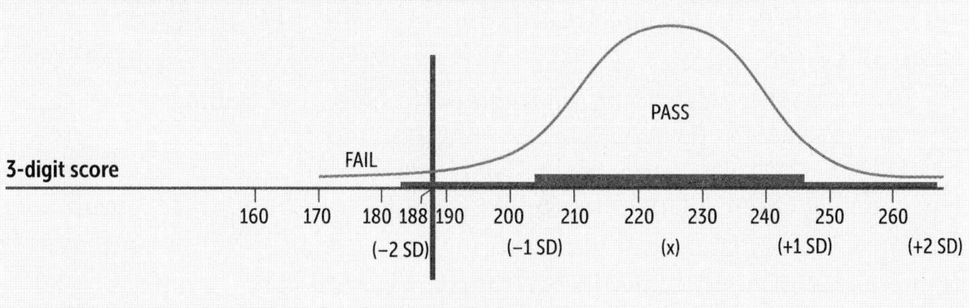

TABLE 1. Passing Rates for the 2010-2011 USMLE Step 1.

	2010		2011	
	No. Tested	% Passing	No. Tested	% Passing
Allopathic 1st takers	18,116	92%	18,312	94%
Repeaters	1,726	61%	1,498	70%
Allopathic total	19,842	90%	19,810	93%
Osteopathic 1st takers	1,964	82%	2,145	89%
Repeaters	75	41%	66	65%
Osteopathic total	2,039	80%	2,211	88%
Total U.S./Canadian	**21,881**	**89%**	**22,021**	**92%**
IMG 1st takers	14,203	70%	14,855	73%
Repeaters	4,656	33%	4,621	36%
IMG total	18,859	61%	19,476	64%
Total Step 1 examinees	**40,740**	**76%**	**41,497**	**79%**

What Does My Score Mean?

The most important point with the Step 1 score is passing versus failing. Passing essentially means, "Hey, you're on your way to becoming a fully licensed doc." As Table 1 shows, the majority of students pass the exam, so remember, we told you to relax.

Beyond that, the main point of having a quantitative score is to give you a sense of how well you've done on the exam and to help schools and residencies rank their students and applicants, respectively.

Official NBME/USMLE Resources

We strongly encourage students to use the materials provided by the testing agencies (see p. 23) and to study in detail the following NBME resources, all of which are available at the USMLE Web site, www.usmle.org:

- *USMLE Step 1 Computer-based Content and Sample Test Questions* (free to all examinees)
- *2013 USMLE Bulletin of Information* (free to all examinees)
- Comprehensive Basic Science Self-Assessment

▸ *Practice questions may be easier than the actual exam.*

The *USMLE Step 1 Computer-based Content and Sample Test Questions* contains approximately 150 questions that are similar in format and content to the questions on the actual USMLE Step 1 exam. This practice test offers one of the best means of assessing your test-taking skills. However, it does not contain enough questions to simulate the full length of the examination, and its content represents a limited sampling of the basic science material that may be covered on Step 1. Moreover, most students felt that the questions on the actual 2012 exam were more challenging than those contained in that year's sample questions. Interestingly, some students reported that they had encountered a few near-duplicates of these sample questions on the actual Step 1 exam. Presumably, these are "experimental" questions, but who knows? So the bottom line is, know these questions!

The extremely detailed *Step 1 Content Outline* provided by the USMLE has not proved useful for students studying for the exam. The USMLE even states that ". . . the content outline is not intended as a curriculum development or study guide."[1] We concur with this assessment.

The *2013 USMLE Bulletin of Information* contains detailed procedural and policy information regarding the CBT, including descriptions of all three Steps, scoring of the exams, reporting of scores to medical schools and residency programs, procedures for score rechecks and other inquiries, policies for irregular behavior, and test dates.

The NBME also offers the Comprehensive Basic Science Self-Assessment (CBSSA), which tests users on topics covered during basic science courses in a format similar to that of the USMLE Step 1 examination. Students who prepared for the examination using this Web-based tool reported that they found the format and content highly indicative of questions tested on the Step 1 examination. In addition, the CBSSA is a fair predictor of USMLE performance (see Table 2).

TABLE 2. CBSSA to USMLE Score Prediction.

CBSSA Score	Approximate USMLE Step 1 Score
200	151
250	163
300	175
350	186
400	198
450	210
500	221
550	233
600	245
650	257
700	268
750	280
800	292

The CBSSA exists in two forms: a standard-paced and a self-paced format, both of which consist of four sections of 50 questions each (for a total of 200 multiple-choice items). The standard-paced format allows the user up to one hour to complete each section, reflecting the time limits of the actual exam. By contrast, the self-paced format places a four-hour time limit on answering the multiple-choice questions. Keep in mind that this bank of questions is available only on the Web. The NBME requires that users log on, register, and start the test within 30 days of registration. Once the assessment has begun, users are required to complete the sections within 20 days. Following completion of the questions, the CBSSA will provide a performance profile indicating each user's relative strengths and weaknesses, much like the report profile for the USMLE Step 1 exam. It is scaled with an average score of 500 and a standard deviation of 100. Please note that CBSSAs do not provide correct answers to the questions at the end of the session. However, some forms can be purchased with an extended feedback option; these tests show you which questions you answered incorrectly, but do not show you the correct answer or explain why your choice was wrong. Feedback from the self-assessment takes the form of a performance profile and nothing more. The NBME charges $50 for assessments without feedback and $60 for assessments with feedback. The fees are payable by credit card or money order. For more information regarding the CBSSA, please visit the NBME's Web site at www.nbme.org and click on the link labeled "NBME Self-Assessment Services."

▶ DEFINING YOUR GOAL

▶ *Fourth-year medical students have the best feel for how Step 1 scores factor into the residency application process.*

It is useful to define your own personal performance goal when approaching the USMLE Step 1. Your style and intensity of preparation can then be matched to your goal. Furthermore, your goal may depend on your school's requirements, your specialty choice, your grades to date, and your personal assessment of the test's importance. Do your best to define your goals early so that you can prepare accordingly.

▶ *Some competitive residency programs place more weight on Step 1 scores in their selection process.*

Certain highly competitive residency programs, such as those in plastic surgery and orthopedic surgery, have acknowledged their use of Step 1 scores in the selection process. In such residency programs, greater emphasis may be placed on attaining a high score, so students who seek to enter these programs may wish to consider aiming for a very high score on the Step 1 exam (see Figure 3). At the same time, your Step 1 score is only one of a number of factors that are assessed when you apply for residency. In fact, many residency programs value other criteria such as letters of recommendation, third-year clerkship grades, honors, and research experience more than a high score on Step 1. Fourth-year medical students who have recently completed the residency application process can be a valuable resource in this regard.

▶ TIMELINE FOR STUDY

Before Starting

Your preparation for the USMLE Step 1 starts with entering medical school. Organize your studying so that when the time comes to prepare for the USMLE, you will be ready with a strong background.

FIGURE 3. Median USMLE Step 1 Score by Specialty for Matched U.S. Seniors.[a]

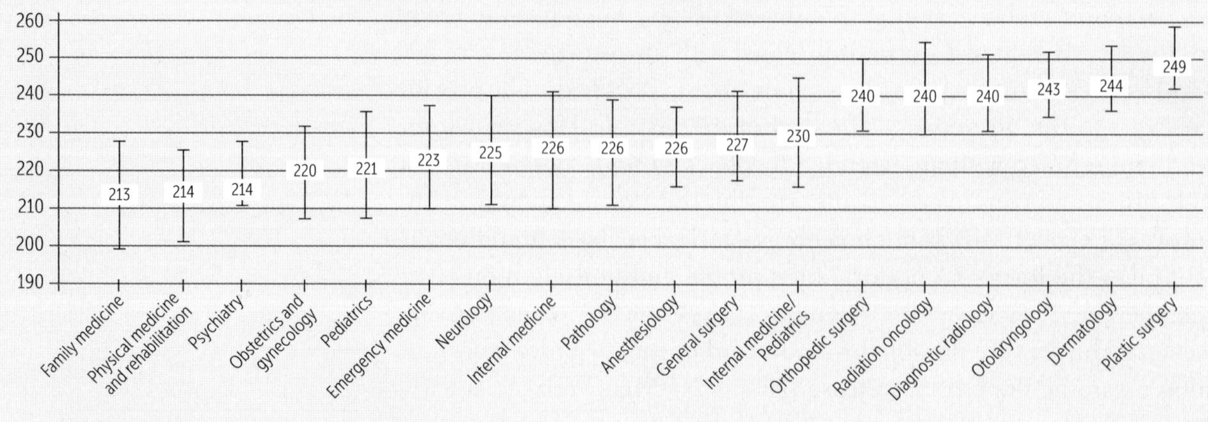

[a] Vertical lines show interquartile range. Source: www.nrmp.org.

Make a Schedule

After you have defined your goals, map out a study schedule that is consistent with your objectives, your vacation time, the difficulty of your ongoing coursework, and your family and social commitments (see Figure 4). Determine whether you want to spread out your study time or concentrate it into 14-hour study days in the final weeks. Then factor in your own history in preparing for standardized examinations (e.g., SAT, MCAT). Talk to students at your school who have recently taken Step 1. Ask them for their study schedules, especially those who have study habits and goals similar to yours.

Typically, U.S. medical students allot between five and seven weeks for dedicated preparation for Step 1. The time you dedicate to exam preparation will depend on your target score as well as your success in preparing yourself during the first two years of medical school. Some students reserve about a week at the end of their study period for final review; others save just a few days. When you have scheduled your exam date, do your best to adhere to it. Studies show that a later testing date does not translate into a higher score, so avoid pushing back your test date without good reason.[2]

▸ *Customize your schedule. Tackle your weakest section first.*

Another important consideration is when you will study each subject. Some subjects lend themselves to cramming, whereas others demand a substantial long-term commitment. The "crammable" subjects for Step 1 are those for which concise yet relatively complete review books are available. (See Section

FIGURE 4. Typical Timeline for the USMLE Step 1.

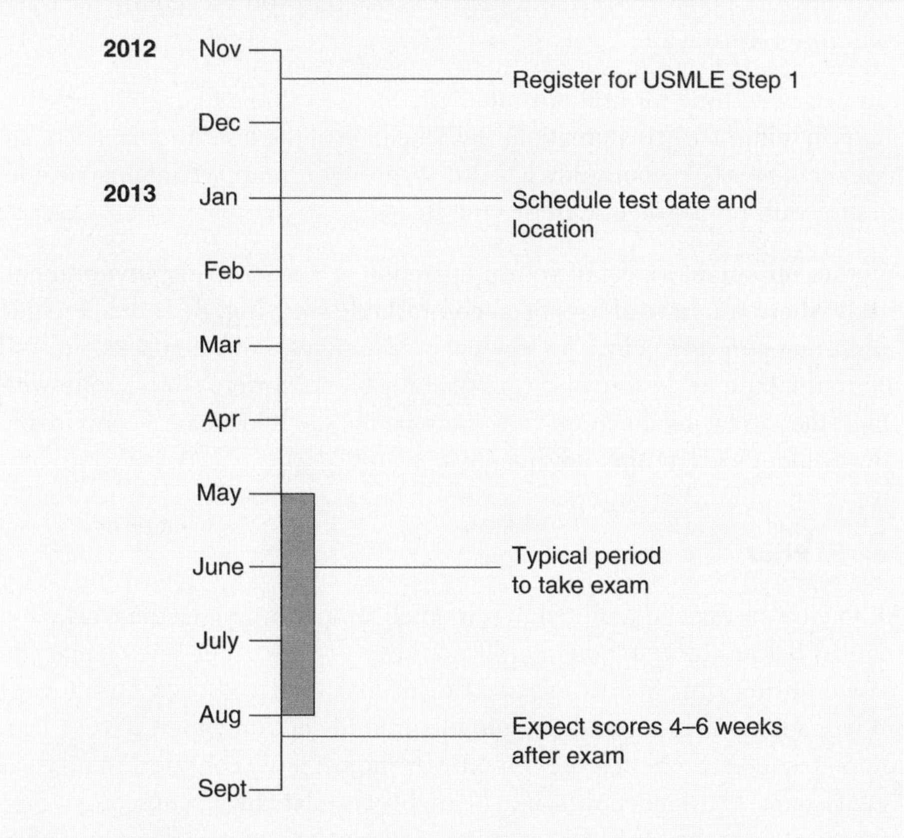

IV for highly rated review and sample examination materials.) Behavioral science and physiology are two subjects with concise review books. Three subjects with longer but quite comprehensive review books are microbiology, pharmacology, and biochemistry. Thus, these subjects could be covered toward the end of your schedule, whereas other subjects (anatomy and pathology) require a longer time commitment and could be studied earlier. Many students prefer using a "systems-based" approach (e.g., GI, renal, cardiovascular) to integrate the material across basic science subjects. See Section III to study anatomy, pathology, physiology, and pharmacology facts by organ system. Each subject may make up a different percentage of the test. For example, although anatomy may require a longer time commitment to review, you may encounter fewer anatomy questions on the test than questions on pharmacology. You can find more details of the breakdown of the test at the NBME's Web site.

▸ *"Crammable" subjects should be covered later and less crammable subjects earlier.*

Make your schedule realistic, and set achievable goals. Many students make the mistake of studying at a level of detail that requires too much time for a comprehensive review—reading *Gray's Anatomy* in a couple of days is not a realistic goal! Have at least two catch-up days in your schedule. No matter how well you stick to your schedule, unexpected events happen. But don't let yourself procrastinate because you have catch-up days; stick to your schedule as closely as possible and revise it regularly on the basis of your actual progress. Be careful not to lose focus. Beware of feelings of inadequacy when comparing study schedules and progress with your peers. **Avoid others who stress you out.** Focus on a few top-rated resources that suit your learning style—not on some obscure books your friends may pass down to you. Accept the fact that you cannot learn it all.

▸ *Avoid burnout. Maintain proper diet, exercise, and sleep habits.*

You will need time for uninterrupted and focused study. Plan your personal affairs to minimize crisis situations near the date of the test. Allot an adequate number of breaks in your study schedule to avoid burnout. Maintain a healthy lifestyle with proper diet, exercise, and sleep.

Another important aspect of your preparation is your studying environment. **Study where you have always been comfortable studying.** Be sure to include everything you need close by (review books, notes, coffee, snacks, etc.). If you're the kind of person who cannot study alone, form a study group with other students taking the exam. The main point here is to create a comfortable environment with minimal distractions.

Year(s) Prior

Although you may be tempted to rely solely on cramming in the weeks and months before the test, you should not have to do so. The knowledge you gained during your first two years of medical school and even during your undergraduate years should provide the groundwork on which to base your test preparation. Student scores on NBME subject tests (commonly known as "shelf exams") have been shown to be highly correlated with subsequent Step

1 scores.[3] Moreover, undergraduate science GPAs as well as MCAT scores are strong predictors of performance on the Step 1 exam.[4]

▸ *Buy review books early (first year) and use while studying for courses.*

We also recommend that you buy highly rated review books early in your first year of medical school and use them as you study throughout the two years. When Step 1 comes along, these books will be familiar and personalized to the way in which you learn. It is risky and intimidating to use unfamiliar review books in the final two or three weeks preceding the exam. Some students find it helpful to personalize and annotate *First Aid* throughout the curriculum.

Months Prior

Review test dates and the application procedure. Testing for the USMLE Step 1 is done on a year-round basis. If you have any disabilities or "special circumstances," contact the NBME as early as possible to discuss test accommodations (see p. 43, First Aid for the Student with a Disability).

▸ *Simulate the USMLE Step 1 under "real" conditions before beginning your studies.*

Before you begin to study earnestly, **simulate the USMLE Step 1 under "real" conditions** to pinpoint strengths and weaknesses in your knowledge, test endurance, and test-taking skills. Be sure that you are well informed about the examination and that you have planned your strategy for studying. Consider what study methods you will use, the study materials you will need, and how you will obtain your materials. Plan ahead. Do a lot of practice questions. Get advice from third- and fourth-year medical students who have recently taken the USMLE Step 1. There might be strengths and weaknesses in your school's curriculum that you should take into account in deciding where to focus your efforts. You might also choose to share books, notes, and study hints with classmates. That is how this book began.

Three Weeks Prior

Two to four weeks before the examination is a good time to resimulate the USMLE Step 1. You may want to do this earlier depending on the progress of your review, but be sure not to do it later, when there will be little time to remedy gaps in your knowledge or test-taking skills. Make use of any remaining good-quality sample USMLE test questions, and try to simulate the computerized test conditions so that you can adequately assess your test performance. One way to simulate a full-length exam is doing a full, timed NBME CBSSA followed by three 46-question blocks from your question bank or the free 150 questions from the USMLE Web site. Recognize, too, that time pressure is increasing as more and more questions are framed as clinical vignettes. Most sample exam questions are shorter than the real thing. Focus on reviewing the high-yield facts, your own notes, clinical images, and very short review books. Do not fall into the trap of reviewing your strengths repeatedly; spend time on your weaknesses.

▸ *In the final two weeks, focus on review, practice questions, and endurance. Stay confident!*

One Week Prior

Make sure you have your CIN (found on your scheduling permit) as well as other items necessary for the day of the examination, including a current driver's license or another form of photo ID with your signature (make sure the name on your **ID exactly** matches that on your scheduling permit). Confirm the Prometric testing center location and test time. Work out how you will get to the testing center and what parking and traffic problems you might encounter. If possible, visit the testing site to get a better idea of the testing conditions you will face. Determine what you will do for lunch. Make sure you have everything you need to ensure that you will be comfortable and alert at the test site. It may be beneficial to adjust your schedule to start waking up at the same time that you will on your test day. And of course, make sure to maintain a healthy lifestyle and get enough sleep.

- *One week before the test:*
  - *Sleep according to the same schedule you'll use on test day*
  - *Review the CBT tutorial one last time*
  - *Call Prometric to confirm test date and time*

One Day Prior

Try your best to relax and rest the night before the test. Double-check your admissions and test-taking materials as well as the comfort measures discussed earlier so that you will not have to deal with such details on the morning of the exam. At this point it will be more effective to review short-term memory material that you're already familiar with than to try to learn new material. The Rapid Review section at the end of this book is high yield for last-minute studying. Remember that regardless of how hard you have studied, you cannot know everything. There will be things on the exam that you have never even seen before, so do not panic. Do not underestimate your abilities.

Many students report difficulty sleeping the night prior to the exam. This is often exacerbated by going to bed much earlier than usual. Do whatever it takes to ensure a good night's sleep (e.g., massage, exercise, warm milk, no back-lit screens at night). Do not change your daily routine prior to the exam. Exam day is not the day for a caffeine-withdrawal headache.

- *No notes, books, calculators, pagers, cell phones, recording devices, or watches of any kind are allowed in the testing area, but they are allowed in lockers.*

Morning of the Exam

On the morning of the Step 1 exam, wake up at your regular time and eat a normal breakfast. If you think it will help you, have a close friend or family member check to make sure you get out of bed. Make sure you have your scheduling permit admission ticket, test-taking materials, and comfort measures as discussed earlier. Wear loose, comfortable clothing. Plan for a variable temperature in the testing center. Arrive at the test site 30 minutes before the time designated on the admission ticket; however, do not come too early, as doing so may intensify your anxiety. When you arrive at the test site, the proctor should give you a USMLE information sheet that will explain critical factors such as the proper use of break time. The USMLE uses the Biometric Identity Management System (BIMS) at some test center locations. BIMS converts a fingerprint, taken on test day, to a digital image used for identification of examinees during the testing process. Seating may be assigned, but ask to be reseated if necessary; you need to be seated in an area that will allow you to remain comfortable and to concentrate. Get to know your testing station, especially if you have never been in a Prometric testing center before. Listen to your proctors regarding any changes in instructions or testing procedures that may apply to your test site.

Finally, remember that it is natural (and even beneficial) to be a little nervous. Focus on being mentally clear and alert. Avoid panic. Avoid panic. Avoid panic. When you are asked to begin the exam, take a deep breath, focus on the screen, and then begin. Keep an eye on the timer. Take advantage of breaks between blocks to stretch, maybe do some jumping jacks, and relax for a moment with deep breathing or stretching.

> *Arrive at the testing center 30 minutes before your scheduled exam time. If you arrive more than half an hour late, you will not be allowed to take the test.*

After the Test

After you have completed the exam, be sure to have fun and relax regardless of how you may feel. Taking the test is an achievement in itself. Remember, you are much more likely to have passed than not. Enjoy the free time you have before your clerkships. Expect to experience some "reentry" phenomena as you try to regain a real life. Once you have recovered sufficiently from the test (or from partying), we invite you to send us your feedback, corrections, and suggestions for entries, facts, mnemonics, strategies, resource ratings, and the like (see p. xvii, How to Contribute). Sharing your experience will benefit fellow medical students and IMGs.

STUDY MATERIALS

Quality and Cost Considerations

Although an ever-increasing number of review books and software are now available on the market, the quality of such material is highly variable. Some common problems are as follows:

- Certain review books are too detailed to allow for review in a reasonable amount of time or cover subtopics that are not emphasized on the exam.
- Many sample question books were originally written years ago and have not been adequately updated to reflect recent trends.
- Many sample question books use poorly written questions or contain factual errors in their explanations.
- Explanations for sample questions vary in quality.

> *If a given review book is not working for you, stop using it no matter how highly rated it may be or how much it costs.*

Basic Science Review Books

In selecting review books, be sure to weigh different opinions against each other, read the reviews and ratings in Section IV of this guide, examine the books closely in the bookstore, and choose carefully. You are investing not only money but also your limited study time. Do not worry about finding the "perfect" book, as many subjects simply do not have one, and different students prefer different formats. Supplement your chosen books with personal notes from other sources, including what you learn from question banks.

There are two types of review books: those that are stand-alone titles and those that are part of a series. Books in a series generally have the same style, and you must decide if that style works for you. However, a given style is not optimal for every subject.

> *Charts and diagrams may be the best approach for physiology and biochemistry, whereas tables and outlines may be preferable for microbiology.*

You should also find out which books are up to date. Some recent editions reflect major improvements, whereas others contain only cursory changes. Take into consideration how a book reflects the format of the USMLE Step 1.

Practice Tests

Taking practice tests provides valuable information about potential strengths and weaknesses in your fund of knowledge and test-taking skills. Some students use practice examinations simply as a means of breaking up the monotony of studying and adding variety to their study schedule, whereas other students rely almost solely on practice tests. Your best preview of the computerized exam can be found in the practice exams on the USMLE Web site. Some students also recommend using computerized test simulation programs. In addition, students report that many current practice-exam books have questions that are, on average, shorter and less clinically oriented than those on the current USMLE Step 1.

> *Most practice exams are shorter and less clinical than the real thing.*

After taking a practice test, try to identify concepts and areas of weakness, not just the facts that you missed. Do not panic if you miss a lot of questions on a practice examination; instead, use the experience you have gained to motivate your study and prioritize those areas in which you need the most work. Use quality practice examinations to improve your test-taking skills. Analyze your ability to pace yourself.

> *Use practice tests to identify concepts and areas of weakness, not just facts that you missed.*

Clinical Review Books

Keep your eye out for more clinically oriented review books; purchase them early and begin to use them. A number of students are turning to Step 2 books, pathophysiology books, and case-based reviews to prepare for the clinical vignettes. Examples of such books include:

- *First Aid Cases for the USMLE Step 1* (McGraw-Hill)
- *First Aid for the Wards* (McGraw-Hill)
- *First Aid Clerkship* series (McGraw-Hill)
- *Blueprints* clinical series (Lippincott Williams & Wilkins)
- *PreTest Physical Diagnosis* (McGraw-Hill)
- *Washington Manual* (Lippincott Williams & Wilkins)
- Various USMLE Step 2 review books

Texts, Syllabi, and Notes

Limit your use of textbooks and course syllabi for Step 1 review. Many textbooks are too detailed for high-yield review and include material that is generally not tested on the USMLE Step 1 (e.g., drug dosages, complex chemical structures). Syllabi, although familiar, are inconsistent across medical schools and frequently reflect the emphasis of individual faculty, which often does not correspond to that of the USMLE Step 1. Syllabi also tend to be less organized than top-rated books and generally contain fewer diagrams and study questions.

▶ TEST-TAKING STRATEGIES

Your test performance will be influenced by both your knowledge and your test-taking skills. You can strengthen your performance by considering each of these factors. Test-taking skills and strategies should be developed and perfected well in advance of the test date so that you can concentrate on the test itself. We suggest that you try the following strategies to see if they might work for you.

▶ *Practice and perfect test-taking skills and strategies well before the test date.*

Pacing

You have seven hours to complete 322 questions. Note that each one-hour block contains 46 questions. This works out to about 77 seconds per question. If you find yourself spending too much time on a question, mark the question, make an educated guess, and move on. If time permits, come back to the question later. In the past, pacing errors have been detrimental to the performance of even highly prepared examinees. The bottom line is to keep one eye on the clock at all times!

▶ *Time management is an important skill for exam success.*

Dealing with Each Question

There are several established techniques for efficiently approaching multiple-choice questions; find what works for you. One technique begins with identifying each question as easy, workable, or impossible. Your goal should be to answer all easy questions, resolve all workable questions in a reasonable amount of time, and make quick and intelligent guesses on all impossible questions. Most students read the stem, think of the answer, and turn immediately to the choices. A second technique is to first skim the answer choices and the **last sentence of the question** and then read through the passage quickly, extracting only relevant information to answer the question. Try a variety of techniques on practice exams and see what works best for you.

Difficult Questions

Because of the exam's clinical emphasis, you may find that many of the questions on the Step 1 exam appear workable but take more time than is available to you. It can be tempting to dwell on such questions because you feel you are on the verge of "figuring it out," but resist this temptation and budget your time. Answer difficult questions with your best guess, mark them for review, and come back to them only if you have time after you have completed the rest of the questions in the block. This will keep you from inadvertently leaving any questions blank in your efforts to "beat the clock."

- *Do not dwell excessively on questions that you are on the verge of "figuring out." Make your best guess and move on.*

Another reason for not dwelling too long on any one question is that certain questions may be **experimental** or may be **incorrectly phrased**. Moreover, not all questions are scored. Some questions serve as "embedded pretest items" that do not count toward your overall score. In fact, anywhere from 10% to 20% of exam questions have been designated as experimental on past exams.

- *Remember that some questions may be experimental.*

Guessing

There is **no penalty** for wrong answers. Thus, **no test block should be left with unanswered questions.** A hunch is probably better than a random guess. If you have to guess, we suggest selecting an answer you recognize over one with which you are totally unfamiliar.

Changing Your Answer

The conventional wisdom is not to change answers that you have already marked unless there is a convincing and logical reason to do so—in other words, go with your "first hunch." However, studies show that if you change your answer, you are twice as likely to change it from an incorrect answer to a correct one than vice versa. So if you have a strong "second hunch," go for it!

- *Your first hunch is not always correct.*

Fourth-Quarter Effect (Avoiding Burnout)

Pacing and endurance are important. Practice helps develop both. Fewer and fewer examinees are leaving the examination session early. Use any extra time you might have at the end of each block to return to marked questions or to recheck your answers; you cannot add the extra time to any remaining blocks of questions. Do not be too casual in your review or you may overlook serious mistakes. Remember your goals, and keep in mind the effort you have devoted to studying compared with the small additional effort you will need to maintain focus and concentration throughout the examination. **Never give up.** If you begin to feel frustrated, try taking a 30-second breather.

- *Do not terminate a question block too early. Carefully review your answers if possible.*

▶ CLINICAL VIGNETTE STRATEGIES

In recent years, the USMLE Step 1 has become increasingly clinically oriented. This change mirrors the trend in medical education toward introducing students to clinical problem solving during the basic science years. The increasing clinical emphasis on Step 1 may be challenging to those students who attend schools with a more traditional curriculum.

> ▶ *Be prepared to read fast and think on your feet!*

What Is a Clinical Vignette?

A clinical vignette is a short (usually paragraph-long) description of a patient, including demographics, presenting symptoms, signs, and other information concerning the patient. Sometimes this paragraph is followed by a brief listing of important physical findings and/or laboratory results. The task of assimilating all this information and answering the associated question in the span of one minute can be intimidating. So be prepared to read quickly and think on your feet. Remember that the question is often indirectly asking something you already know.

> ▶ *Practice questions that include case histories or descriptive vignettes are critical for Step 1 preparation.*

Strategy

Remember that Step 1 vignettes usually describe diseases or disorders in their most classic presentation. So look for buzzwords or cardinal signs (e.g., malar rash for SLE or nuchal rigidity for meningitis) in the narrative history. Be aware, however, that the question may contain classic signs and symptoms instead of mere buzzwords. Sometimes the data from labs and the physical exam will help you confirm or reject possible diagnoses, thereby helping you rule answer choices in or out. In some cases, they will be a dead giveaway for the diagnosis.

> ▶ *Step 1 vignettes usually describe diseases or disorders in their most classic presentation.*

Making a diagnosis from the history and data is often not the final answer. Not infrequently, the diagnosis is divulged at the end of the vignette, after you have just struggled through the narrative to come up with a diagnosis of your own. The question might then ask about a related aspect of the diagnosed disease.

> ▶ *Sometimes making a diagnosis is not necessary at all.*

One strategy that many students suggest is to skim the questions and answer choices before reading a vignette, especially if the vignette is lengthy. This focuses your attention on the relevant information and reduces the time spent on that vignette. Sometimes you may not need much of the information in the vignette to answer the question. However, be careful with skimming the answer choices; going too fast may warp your perception of what the vignette is asking.

▶ IF YOU THINK YOU FAILED

After the test, many examinees feel that they have failed, and most are at the very least unsure of their pass/fail status. There are several sensible steps you can take to plan for the future in the event that you do not achieve a passing score. First, save and organize all your study materials, including review books, practice tests, and notes. Familiarize yourself with the reapplication procedures for Step 1, including application deadlines and upcoming test dates. The CBT format allows an examinee who has failed the exam to retake it no earlier than the first day of the month after 60 days have elapsed since the last test date. Examinees will, however, be allowed to take the Step 1 exam no more than four times within a 12-month period should they repeatedly fail.

▶ *If you pass Step 1, you are not allowed to retake the exam.*

The performance profiles on the back of the USMLE Step 1 score report provide valuable feedback concerning your relative strengths and weaknesses. Study these profiles closely. Set up a study timeline to strengthen gaps in your knowledge as well as to maintain and improve what you already know. Do not neglect high-yield subjects. It is normal to feel somewhat anxious about retaking the test, but if anxiety becomes a problem, seek appropriate counseling.

Although the NBME allows an unlimited number of attempts to pass Step 1, they recommend that licensing authorities allow a maximum of six attempts for each Step examination.[5] Again, review your school's policy regarding retakes.

▶ IF YOU FAILED

Even if you came out of the exam room feeling that you failed, seeing that failing grade can be traumatic, and it is natural to feel upset. Different people react in different ways: For some it is a stimulus to buckle down and study harder; for others it may "take the wind out of their sails" for a few days; and it may even lead to a reassessment of individual goals and abilities. In some instances, however, failure may trigger weeks or months of sadness, feelings of hopelessness, social withdrawal, and inability to concentrate—in other words, true clinical depression. If you think you are depressed, please seek help.

▶ *Near the failure threshold, each point on the three-digit scale is equivalent to about 1.5 questions answered correctly.[6]*

▶ TESTING AGENCIES

- **National Board of Medical Examiners (NBME)**
  Department of Licensing Examination Services
  3750 Market Street
  Philadelphia, PA 19104-3102
  (215) 590-9700
  Fax: (215) 590-9457
  Email: webmail@nbme.org
  www.nbme.org
- **Educational Commission for Foreign Medical Graduates (ECFMG)**
  3624 Market Street
  Philadelphia, PA 19104-2685
  (215) 386-5900
  Fax: (215) 386-9196
  Email: info@ecfmg.org
  www.ecfmg.org
- **Federation of State Medical Boards (FSMB)**
  400 Fuller Wiser Road, Suite 300
  Euless, TX 76039-3856
  (817) 868-4000
  Fax: (817) 868-4099
  Email: usmle@fsmb.org
  www.fsmb.org
- **USMLE Secretariat**
  3750 Market Street
  Philadelphia, PA 19104-3190
  (215) 590-9700
  Fax: (215) 590-9457
  Email: webmail@nbme.org
  www.usmle.org

▶ REFERENCES

1. United States Medical Licensing Examination. Step 1 Content Description Online. Available at: http://www.usmle.org/pdfs/step-1/2012content_step1.pdf. Accessed September 26, 2012.
2. Pohl, Charles A., Robeson, Mary R., Hojat, Mohammadreza, and Veloski, J. Jon, "Sooner or Later? USMLE Step 1 Performance and Test Administration Date at the End of the Second Year," *Academic Medicine*, 2002, Vol. 77, No. 10, pp. S17–S19.
3. Holtman, Matthew C., Swanson, David B., Ripkey, Douglas R., and Case, Susan M., "Using Basic Science Subject Tests to Identify Students at Risk for Failing Step 1," *Academic Medicine*, 2001, Vol. 76, No. 10, pp. S48–S51.

4. Basco, William T., Jr., Way, David P., Gilbert, Gregory E., and Hudson, Andy, "Undergraduate Institutional MCAT Scores as Predictors of USMLE Step 1 Performance," *Academic Medicine*, 2002, Vol. 77, No. 10, pp. S13–S16.
5. United States Medical Licensing Examination. 2013 USMLE Bulletin: Eligibibiilty. Available at: http://www.usmle.org/bulletin/eligibility. Accessed September 26, 2012.
6. O'Donnell, M. J., Obenshain, S. Scott, and Erdmann, James B., "I: Background Essential to the Proper Use of Results of Step 1 and Step 2 of the USMLE," *Academic Medicine*, October 1993, Vol. 68, No. 10, pp. 734–739.

SECTION I SUPPLEMENT

Special Situations

FIRST AID FOR THE INTERNATIONAL MEDICAL GRADUATE

> *IMGs make up approximately 25% of the U.S. physician population.*

"International medical graduate" (IMG) is the accepted term now used to describe any student or graduate of a non-U.S., non-Canadian, non–Puerto Rican medical school, regardless of whether he or she is a U.S. citizen or resident. Technically the term IMG encompasses FMGs (foreign medical graduates; i.e., medical graduates from medical schools outside the United States who are not residents of the United States—that is, U.S. citizens or green-card holders), although the terms IMG and FMG are often used interchangeably.

IMG's Steps to Licensure in the United States

> *More detailed information can be found in the ECFMG* Information Booklet, *available at www.ecfmg.org/pubshome.html.*

To be eligible to take the USMLE Steps, you (the applicant) must be officially enrolled in a medical school located outside the United States and Canada that is listed in the International Medical Education Directory (IMED; http://www.faimer.org/resources/imed.html), both at the time you apply for examination and on your test day. In addition, your "Graduation Year" must be listed as "Current" at the time you apply and on your test day.

If you are an IMG, you must go through the following steps (not necessarily in this order) to apply for residency programs and become licensed to practice in the United States. You must complete these steps even if you are already a practicing physician and have completed a residency program in your own country.

> *Applicants may apply online for USMLE Step 1, Step 2 CK, or Step 2 CS at www.ecfmg.org.*

- Pass USMLE Step 1, Step 2 CK, and Step 2 CS, as well as obtain a medical school diploma (not necessarily in this order). All three exams can be taken during medical school.
- Apply for certification from the Educational Commission for Foreign Medical Graduates (ECFMG) after above steps are successfully completed. There will be a delay of 4–8 weeks between your ECFMG application and your receipt of the ECFMG certificate; the ECFMG will not issue a certificate (even if all the USMLE scores are submitted) until it verifies your medical diploma with your medical school.
- You must have a valid ECFMG certificate before entering an accredited residency program in the United States, although you can begin the Electronic Residency Application Service (ERAS) application and interviews before you receive the certificate. However, many programs prefer to interview IMGs who have an ECFMG certificate, so obtaining it by the time you submit your ERAS application is ideal.
- Apply for residency positions in your fields of interest, either directly or through the ERAS and the National Residency Matching Program (NRMP), otherwise known as "the Match." To be entered into the Match, you need to have passed all the examinations necessary for ECFMG certification (i.e., Step 1, Step 2 CK, and Step 2 CS) by the rank order list deadline (usually in late February before the Match). If you do not pass these exams by the deadline, you will be withdrawn from the Match.

- If you are not a U.S. citizen or green-card holder (permanent resident), obtain a visa that will allow you to enter and work in the United States.
- Sign up to receive the ECFMG and ERAS email newsletter to keep up to date with their most current policies and deadlines.
- If required by the state in which your residency program is located, obtain an educational/training/limited medical license. Your residency program may assist you with this application. Note that medical licensing is the prerogative of each individual state, not of the federal government, and that states vary with respect to their laws about licensing.
- Once you have the ECFMG certification, take the USMLE Step 3 during your residency, and then obtain a full medical license. Once you have a state-issued license, you are permitted to practice in federal institutions such as Veterans Affairs (VA) hospitals and Indian Health Service facilities in any state. This can open the door to "moonlighting" opportunities and possibilities for an H1B visa application if relevant. For details on individual state rules, write to the licensing board in the state in question or contact the Federation of State Medical Boards (FSMB). If you need to apply for an H1B visa for starting residency, you will need to take and pass the USMLE Step 3 exam, preferably before you Match.
- Complete your residency and then take the appropriate specialty board exams if you wish to become board certified (e.g., in internal medicine or surgery). If you already have a specialty certification in another country, some specialty boards may grant you six months' or one year's credit toward your total residency time.
- Currently, most residency programs are accepting applications through ERAS. For more information, see *First Aid for the Match* or contact:

  ECFMG/ERAS Program
  3624 Market Street
  Philadelphia, PA 19104-2685 USA
  (215) 386-5900
  Email: eras-support@ecfmg.org
  www.ecfmg.org/eras

- For detailed information on the USMLE Steps, visit the USMLE Web site at http://www.usmle.org.

The USMLE and the IMG

The USMLE is a series of standardized exams that give IMGs and U.S. medical graduates a level playing field. The passing marks for IMGs for Step 1, Step 2 CK, and Step 2 CS are determined by a statistical distribution that is based on the scores of U.S. medical school students. For example, to pass Step 1, you will probably have to score higher than the bottom 8–10% of U.S. and Canadian graduates.

> *IMGs have a maximum of six attempts to pass any USMLE Step, and must pass the USMLE Steps required for ECFMG certification within a seven-year period.*

Under new USMLE program rules, a maximum of six attempts will be permitted to pass any USMLE Step or component exam starting January 1, 2012 for new examinees, and January 1, 2013 for previous examinees. There is a limit of three attempts within a 12-month period for any of the USMLE Steps.

Timing of the USMLE

For an IMG, the timing of a complete application is critical. It is extremely important that you send in your application early if you are to obtain the maximum number of interviews. Complete all exam requirements by August of the year in which you wish to apply. Check the ECFMG Web site for deadlines to take and pass the various Step exams to be eligible for the NRMP Match.

IMG applicants must pass the USMLE Steps required for ECFMG certification within a seven-year period. The USMLE program recommends, although not all jurisdictions impose, a seven-year limit for completion of the three-step USMLE program.

> *If your clinical experience is recent, consider taking the Step 2 CK first, followed by the Step 1.*

In terms of USMLE exam order, arguments can be made for taking the Step 1 or the Step 2 CK exam first. For example, you may consider taking the Step 2 CK exam first if you have just graduated from medical school and the clinical topics are still fresh in your mind. However, keep in mind that there is substantial overlap between Step 1 and Step 2 CK topics in areas such as pharmacology, pathophysiology, and biostatistics. You might therefore consider taking the Step 1 and Step 2 CK exams close together to take advantage of this overlap in your test preparation.

USMLE Step 1 and the IMG

Significance of the Test. Step 1 is required for the ECFMG certificate as well as for registration for the Step 2 CS. Since most U.S. graduates apply to residency with their Step 1 scores only, it may be the only objective tool available with which to compare IMGs with U.S. graduates.

Eligibility Period. A three-month period of your choice.

Fee. The fee for Step 1 is $790 plus an international test delivery surcharge (if you choose a testing region other than the United States or Canada).

Statistics. In 2011–2012, 73% of IMG examinees passed Step 1 on their first attempt, compared with 94% of those from the United States and Canada.

> *A higher Step 1 score will improve your chances of getting into a highly competitive specialty.*

Tips. Although few if any students feel totally prepared to take Step 1, IMGs in particular require serious study and preparation in order to reach their full potential on this exam. It is also imperative that IMGs do their best on Step 1, as a poor score on Step 1 is a distinct disadvantage in applying for most residencies. Remember that if you pass Step 1, you cannot retake it in an attempt to improve your score. Your goal should thus be to beat the mean, because you can then assert with confidence that you have done better than average for U.S. students. Higher Step 1 scores will also lend credibility to your residency application and help you get into highly competitive specialties such as radiology, orthopedics, and dermatology.

Commercial Review Courses. Do commercial review courses help improve your scores? Reports vary, and such courses can be expensive. For some students these programs can provide a more structured learning environment with professional support. However, review courses consume a significant chunk of time away from independent study. Many IMGs decide to prepare for Step 1 on their own and then consider a review course only if they fail. (For more information on review courses, see Section IV.)

USMLE Step 2 CK and the IMG

What Is the Step 2 CK? It is a computerized test of the clinical sciences consisting of up to 355 multiple-choice questions divided into eight blocks. It can be taken at Prometric centers in the United States and several other countries.

Content. The Step 2 CK includes test items in the following content areas:

- Internal medicine
- Obstetrics and gynecology
- Pediatrics
- Preventive medicine
- Psychiatry
- Surgery
- Other areas relevant to the provision of care under supervision

> *The areas tested on the Step 2 CK relate to the clerkships provided at U.S. medical schools.*

Significance of the Test. The Step 2 CK is required for the ECFMG certificate. It reflects the level of clinical knowledge of the applicant. It tests clinical subjects, primarily internal medicine. Other areas that are tested are surgery, obstetrics and gynecology, pediatrics, orthopedics, psychiatry, ENT, ophthalmology, and medical ethics.

Eligibility. Students and graduates from medical schools that are listed in IMED are eligible to take the Step 2 CK. Students must have completed at least two years of medical school. This means that students must have completed the basic medical science component of the medical school curriculum by the beginning of the eligibility period selected.

Eligibility Period. A three-month period of your choice.

Fee. The fee for the Step 2 CK is $790 plus an international test delivery surcharge (if you choose a testing region other than the United States or Canada).

Statistics. In 2011–2012, 84% of ECFMG candidates passed the Step 2 CK on their first attempt, compared with 96% of U.S. and Canadian candidates.

▸ *Be familiar with topics that are heavily emphasized in U.S. medicine, such as cholesterol screening.*

Tips. It's better to take the Step 2 CK after your internal medicine rotation because most of the questions on the exam give clinical scenarios and ask you to make medical diagnoses and clinical decisions. In addition, because this is a clinical sciences exam, cultural and geographic considerations play a greater role than is the case with Step 1. For example, if your medical education gave you ample exposure to malaria, brucellosis, and malnutrition but little to alcohol withdrawal, child abuse, and cholesterol screening, you must work to familiarize yourself with topics that are more heavily emphasized in U.S. medicine. You must also have a basic understanding of the legal and social aspects of U.S. medicine, because you will be asked questions about communicating with and advising patients.

USMLE Step 2 CS and the IMG

What Is the Step 2 CS? The Step 2 CS is a test of clinical and communication skills administered as a one-day, eight-hour exam. It includes 10 to 12 encounters with standardized patients (15 minutes each, with 10 minutes to write a note after each encounter).

Content. The Step 2 CS tests the ability to communicate in English as well as interpersonal skills, data-gathering skills, the ability to perform a physical exam, and the ability to formulate a brief note, a differential diagnosis, and a list of diagnostic tests. The areas that are covered in the exam are as follows:

- Internal medicine
- Surgery
- Obstetrics and gynecology
- Pediatrics
- Psychiatry
- Family medicine

▸ *The Step 2 CS is graded as pass/fail.*

Unlike the USMLE Step 1, Step 2 CK, or Step 3, **there are no numerical grades for the Step 2 CS**—it's simply either a "pass" or a "fail." To pass, a candidate must attain a passing performance in **each** of the following three components:

- Integrated Clinical Encounter (ICE): includes Data Gathering, Physical Exam, and the Patient Note
- Spoken English Proficiency (SEP)
- Communication and Interpersonal Skills (CIS)

According to the NBME, the most commonly failed component for IMGs is the CIS.

Significance of the Test. The Step 2 CS assesses spoken English language proficiency and is required for the ECFMG certificate. The Test of English as a Foreign Language (TOEFL) is no longer required.

Eligibility. Students must have completed at least two years of medical school in order to take the test. That means students must have completed the basic medical science component of the medical school curriculum at the time they apply for the exam.

Fee. The fee for the Step 2 CS is $1375.

Scheduling. You must schedule the Step 2 CS within **four months** of the date indicated on your notification of registration. You must take the exam within 12 months of the date indicated on your notification of registration. It is generally advisable to take the Step 2 CS as soon as possible in the year before your Match, as often the results either come in late or arrive too late to allow you to retake the test and pass it before the Match.

> *Try to take the Step 2 CS the year before you plan to Match.*

Test Site Locations. The Step 2 CS is currently administered at the following five locations:

- Philadelphia, PA
- Atlanta, GA
- Los Angeles, CA
- Chicago, IL
- Houston, TX

For more information about the Step 2 CS exam, please refer to *First Aid for the Step 2 CS*.

USMLE Step 3 and the IMG

What Is the USMLE Step 3? It is a two-day computerized test in clinical medicine consisting of 480 multiple-choice questions and nine computer-based case simulations (CCS). The exam aims at testing your knowledge and its application to patient care and clinical decision making (i.e., this exam tests if you can safely practice medicine independently and without supervision).

Significance of the Test. Taking Step 3 before residency is critical for IMGs seeking an H1B visa and is also a bonus that can be added to the residency application. Step 3 is also required to obtain a full medical license in the United States and can be taken during residency for this purpose.

> *Complete the Step 3 exam before you apply for an H1B visa.*

Fee. The fee for Step 3 is $780 in all states except Iowa ($830), South Dakota ($930), and Vermont ($815).

Eligibility. Most states require that applicants have completed one, two, or three years of postgraduate training (residency) before they apply for Step 3 and permanent state licensure. The exceptions are the 13 states mentioned below, which allow IMGs to take Step 3 at the beginning of or even before residency. So if you don't fulfill the prerequisites to taking Step 3 in your state of choice, simply use the name of one of the 13 states in your Step 3 application. You can take the exam in any state you choose regardless of the state that you mentioned on your application. Once you pass Step 3, it will be recognized by all states. Basic eligibility requirements for the USMLE Step 3 are as follows:

- Obtaining an MD or DO degree (or its equivalent) by the application deadline.
- Obtaining an ECFMG certificate if you are a graduate of a foreign medical school or are successfully completing a "fifth pathway" program (at a date no later than the application deadline).
- Meeting the requirements imposed by the individual state licensing authority to which you are applying to take Step 3. Please refer to www.fsmb.org for more information.

The following states do not have postgraduate training as an eligibility requirement to apply for Step 3:

- Arkansas
- California
- Connecticut
- Florida
- Louisiana
- Maryland
- Nebraska*
- New York
- South Dakota
- Texas
- Utah*
- Washington
- West Virginia

* Requires that IMGs obtain a "valid indefinite" ECFMG certificate.

The Step 3 exam is not available outside the United States. Applications can be found online at www.fsmb.org and must be submitted to the FSMB.

In 2011–2012, 84% of IMG candidates passed the Step 3 on their first attempt, compared with 97% of U.S. and Canadian candidates.

Residencies and the IMG

In the Match, the number of U.S.-citizen IMG applications has grown over the past few years, while the percentage accepted has remained constant (see Table 4). More information about residency programs can be obtained at www.ama-assn.org.

The Match and the IMG

Given the growing number of IMG candidates with strong applications, you should bear in mind that good USMLE scores are not the only way to gain a competitive edge. However, USMLE Step 1 and Step 2 CK scores continue to be used as the initial screening mechanism when candidates are being considered for interviews.

TABLE 4. IMGs in the Match.

Applicants	2010	2011	2012
U.S.-citizen IMGs	3,695	3,769	4,279
% U.S.-citizen IMGs accepted	47	50	49
Non-U.S.-citizen IMGs	7,246	6,659	6,828
% non-U.S.-citizen IMGs accepted	40	41	41
U.S. seniors (non-IMGs)	16,070	16,559	16,527
% U.S. seniors accepted	93	94	95

Source: www.nrmp.org.

Based on accumulated IMG Match experiences over recent years, here are a few pointers to help IMGs maximize their chances for a residency interview:

- **Apply early.** Programs offer a limited number of interviews and often select candidates on a first-come, first-served basis. Because of this, you should aim to complete the entire process of applying for the ERAS token, registering with the Association of American Medical Colleges (AAMC), mailing necessary documents to ERAS, and completing the ERAS application before September (see Figure 5). Community programs usually send out interview offers earlier than do university and university-affiliated programs.
- **U.S. clinical experience helps.** Externships and observerships in a U.S. hospital setting have emerged as an important credential on an IMG application. Externships are like short-term medical school internships and offer hands-on clinical experience. Observerships, also called "shadowing," involve following a physician and observing how he or she manages patients. Some programs require students to have participated in an externship or observership before applying. It is best to gain such an experience before or at the time you apply to various programs so that you can mention it on your ERAS application. If such an experience or opportunity comes up after you apply, be sure to inform the programs accordingly.

▸ *Most U.S. hospitals allow externship only when the applicant is actively enrolled in a medical school, so plan ahead.*

- **Clinical research helps.** University programs are attracted to candidates who show a strong interest in clinical research and academics. They may even relax their application criteria for individuals with unique backgrounds and strong research experience. Publications in well-known journals are an added bonus.
- **Time the Step 2 CS well.** ECFMG has published the new Step 2 CS score-reporting schedule for 2012–2013 at http://www.ecfmg.org/news/category/step-2-cs. Most program directors would like to see a passing score on the Step 1, Step 2 CK, and Step 2 CS exams before they rank an IMG on their rank order list in mid-February. There have been many instances in which candidates have lost a potential Match—either because of delayed CS results or because they have been unable to retake the

FIGURE 5. IMG Timeline for Application.

June	Obtain ERAS token and obtain AAMC ID If USMLE Steps 1, 2 CS, and 2CK completed: request ECFMG certification
July	Send documents to ERAS Request letters of recommendation be uploaded Complete CAF and personal statement on MyERAS
August	
September	Select and apply to programs through MyERAS
October	Schedule and attend interviews Complete any pending USMLE Step exams
November	
December	
January	Obtain ECFMG certification (if not done earlier)
February	Submit rank order list Complete USMLE Step 3 (if interested in H1B)
March	Match results (day 1) SOAP (days 3–5) Matched program results (day 5)

exam on time following a failure. It is difficult to predict a result on the Step 2 CS, since the grading process is not very transparent. Therefore, it is advisable to take the Step 2 CS as early as possible in the application year.

- **U.S. letters of recommendation help.** Letters of recommendation from clinicians practicing in the United States carry more weight than recommendations from home countries.

> *A good score on the Step 3 may help offset poorer scores on the Step 1 or 2 CK exams.*

- **Step up the Step 3.** If H1B visa sponsorship is desired, aim to have Step 3 results by January of the Match year. In addition to the visa advantage you will gain, an early and good Step 3 score may benefit IMGs who have been away from clinical medicine for a while as well as those who have low scores on Step 1 and the Step 2 CK.

- **Verify medical credentials in a timely manner.** Do not overlook the medical school credential verification process. The ECFMG certificate arrives only after credentials have been verified and after you have passed

Step 1, the Step 2 CK, and the Step 2 CS, so you should keep track of the process and check with the ECFMG from time to time about your status.

- **Don't count on a pre-Match.** Of note, as of the 2013 Match, programs participating in NRMP Match can no longer offer a pre-Match.

What if You Do Not Match?

For applicants who do not Match into a residency program, there's SOAP (Supplemental Offer and Acceptance Program). Under SOAP, unmatched applicants will have access to the list of unfilled programs at noon Eastern time on the Monday of Match week. The unfilled programs electing to participate in SOAP will offer positions to unmatched applicants through the Registration, Ranking, and Results (R3) system. A series of "rounds" will begin at noon Eastern time on Wednesday of Match week until 5:00 P.M. Eastern time on Friday of Match week. Detailed information about SOAP can be found at the NRMP Web site at http://www.nrmp.org/res_match/policies/map_main.html.

> *The Scramble has been replaced by SOAP (Supplemental Offer and Acceptance Program).*

Resources for the IMG

- **ECFMG**
  3624 Market Street
  Philadelphia, PA 19104-2685
  (215) 386-5900
  Fax: (215) 386-9196
  www.ecfmg.org

  The ECFMG telephone number is answered only between 9:00 A.M. and 12:30 P.M. and between 1:30 P.M. and 5:00 P.M. Monday through Friday EST. The ECFMG often takes a long time to answer the phone, which is frequently busy at peak times of the year, and then gives you a long voice-mail message—so it is better to write or fax early than to rely on a last-minute phone call. Do not contact the NBME, as all IMG exam matters are conducted by the ECFMG. The ECFMG also publishes an information booklet on ECFMG certification and the USMLE program, which gives details on the dates and locations of forthcoming Step tests for IMGs together with application forms. It is free of charge and is also available from the public affairs offices of U.S. embassies and consulates worldwide as well as from Overseas Educational Advisory Centers. You may order single copies of the handbook by calling (215) 386-5900, preferably on weekends or between 6 P.M. and 6 A.M. Philadelphia time, or by faxing to (215) 386-9196. Requests for multiple copies must be made by fax or mail on organizational letterhead. The full text of the booklet is also available on the ECFMG's Web site at www.ecfmg.org.

- **FSMB**
  400 Fuller Wiser Road, Suite 300
  Euless, TX 76039
  (817) 868-4000
  Fax: (817) 868-4099
  www.fsmb.org

  The FSMB has a number of publications available, including free policy documents. To obtain these publications, print and mail the order form on the Web site listed above. Alternatively, write to Federation Publications at the above address. All orders must be prepaid with a personal check drawn on a U.S. bank, a cashier's check, or a money order payable to the FSMB. Foreign orders must be accompanied by an international money order or the equivalent, payable in U.S. dollars through a U.S. bank or a U.S. affiliate of a foreign bank. For Step 3 inquiries, the telephone number is (817) 868-4041. You may e-mail the FSMB at usmle@fsmb.org or write to Examination Services at the address above.

The AMA has dedicated a portion of its Web site to information on IMG demographics, residencies, immigration, and the like. This information can be found at www.ama-assn.org/ama/pub/about-ama/our-people/member-groups-sections/international-medical-graduates.shtml.

Other resources that may be useful and of interest to IMGs include the following:

- *The International Medical Graduate's Guide to US Medicine and Residency Training*, by Patrick C. Alquire, Gerald P. Whelan, and Vijay Rajput (2009; ISBN 9781934465080).
- *The International Medical Graduate's Best Hope*, by Franck Belibi and Suzanne Belibi (2009; ISBN 9780979877308).

▶ FIRST AID FOR THE OSTEOPATHIC MEDICAL STUDENT

What Is the COMLEX-USA Level 1?

The National Board of Osteopathic Medical Examiners (NBOME) administers the Comprehensive Osteopathic Medical Licensing Examination, or COMLEX-USA. Like the USMLE, the COMLEX-USA is administered over three levels.

The COMLEX-USA series assesses osteopathic medical knowledge and clinical skills using clinical presentations and physician tasks. A description of the COMLEX-USA Written Examination Blueprints for each level, which outline the various clinical presentations and physician tasks that examinees will encounter, is given on the NBOME Web site. Another stated goal of the COMLEX-USA Level 1 is to create a more primary care–oriented exam that integrates osteopathic principles into clinical situations.

To be eligible to take the COMLEX-USA Level 1, you must have satisfactorily completed your first year in an American Osteopathic Association (AOA)–approved medical school. The office of the dean at each school informs the NBOME that a student has completed his or her first year of school and is in good standing. At this point, the NBOME sends out an email with detailed instructions on how to register for the exam.

For all three levels of the COMLEX-USA, raw scores are converted to a percentile score and a score ranging from 5 to 800. For Levels 1 and 2, a score of 400 is required to pass; for Level 3, a score of 350 is needed. COMLEX-USA scores are posted at the NBOME Web site 4–6 weeks after the test and usually mailed within 8 weeks after the test. The mean score is always 500.

If you pass a COMLEX-USA examination, you are not allowed to retake it to improve your grade. If you fail, there is no specific limit to the number of times you can retake it in order to pass. However, a student may not take the exam more than four times in one year. Levels 2 and 3 exams must be passed in sequential order within seven years of passing Level 1.

What Is the Structure of the COMLEX-USA Level 1?

The COMLEX-USA Level 1 is a computer-based examination consisting of 400 questions over an eight-hour period in a single day (nine hours if you count breaks). Most of the questions are in one-best-answer format, but a small number are matching-type questions. Some one-best-answer questions are bundled together around a common question stem that usually takes the form of a clinical scenario. Every section of the COMLEX-USA Level 1 ends with either matching questions, multiple questions around a single stem, or both. New question formats may gradually be introduced, but candidates will be notified if this occurs. In 2012, the NBOME introduced multimedia questions and have stated that multimedia questions will continue to be a larger part of the exam.

Questions are grouped into eight sections of 50 questions each in a manner similar to the USMLE. Reviewing and changing answers may be done only in the current section. A "review page" is presented for each block in order to advise test takers of questions completed, questions marked for further review, and incomplete questions for which no answer has been given.

Breaks are even more structured with COMLEX-USA than they are with the USMLE. Students are allowed to take a 10-minute break at the end of the second and sixth sections. Students who do not take these 10-minute breaks can apply the time toward their test time. After section 4, students are given a 40-minute lunch break. These are the only times a student is permitted a break. More information about the computer-based COMLEX-USA examinations can be obtained from www.nbome.org.

What Is the Difference Between the USMLE and the COMLEX-USA?

According to the NBOME, the COMLEX-USA Level 1 focuses broadly on the following categories, with osteopathic principles and practices integrated into each section:

- Health promotion and disease prevention
- The history and physical
- Diagnostic technologies
- Management
- Scientific understanding of mechanisms
- Health care delivery

> *The test interface for the COMLEX-USA Level 1 is not the same as the USMLE Step 1 interface.*

Although the COMLEX-USA and the USMLE are similar in scope, content, and emphasis, some differences are worth noting. For example, the interface is different; you cannot search for lab values. The expectation is that you can make a diagnosis without having performed testing. Fewer details are given about a patient's condition, so a savvy student needs to know how to differentiate between similar pathologies. Also, age, gender, and race are key factors for diagnosis on the COMLEX-USA. Images are embedded in the question stem and the examinee has to click an attachment button to see the image. If you don't read the question carefully, the attachment buttons are very easy to miss.

COMLEX-USA Level 1 tests osteopathic principles in addition to basic science materials but does not emphasize lab techniques. Although both exams often require that you apply and integrate knowledge over several areas of basic science to answer a given question, many students who took both tests reported that the questions differed somewhat in style. Students reported, for example, that USMLE questions generally required that the test taker reason and draw from the information given (often a two-step process), whereas those on the COMLEX-USA exam tended to be more straightforward. Furthermore, USMLE questions were on average found to be considerably longer than those on the COMLEX-USA.

COMLEX-USA test takers can expect to have only a few questions on biochemistry, molecular biology, or lab technique. On the other hand, microbiology is very heavily tested by clinical presentation and by lab identification. Another main difference is that the COMLEX-USA exam stresses osteopathic manipulative medicine. Therefore, question banks specific to the USMLE will not be adequate, and supplementation with a question bank specific to the COMLEX-USA is highly recommended.

Students also commented that the COMLEX-USA utilized "buzzwords," although limited in their use (e.g., "rose spots" in typhoid fever), whereas the USMLE avoided buzzwords in favor of descriptions of clinical findings or symptoms (e.g., rose-colored papules on the abdomen rather than rose spots). Finally, USMLE appeared to have more photographs than did the COMLEX-USA. In general, the overall impression was that the USMLE was a more "thought-provoking" exam, while the COMLEX-USA was more of a "knowledge-based" exam.

Who Should Take Both the USMLE and the COMLEX-USA?

Aside from facing the COMLEX-USA Level 1, you must decide if you will also take the USMLE Step 1. We recommend that you consider taking both the USMLE and the COMLEX-USA under the following circumstances:

- **If you are applying to allopathic residencies.** Although there is growing acceptance of COMLEX-USA certification on the part of allopathic residencies, some allopathic programs prefer or even require passage of the USMLE Step 1. These include many academic programs, programs in competitive specialties (e.g., orthopedics, ophthalmology, or dermatology), and programs in competitive geographic areas (such as Vermont, Utah, and California). Fourth-year doctor of osteopathy (DO) students who have already Matched may be a good source of information about which programs and specialties look for USMLE scores. It is also a good idea to contact program directors at the institutions you are interested in to ask about their policy regarding the COMLEX-USA versus the USMLE.
- **If you are unsure about your postgraduate training plans.** Successful passage of both the COMLEX-USA Level 1 and the USMLE Step 1 is certain to provide you with the greatest possible range of options when you are applying for internship and residency training.

> ▶ *If you're not sure whether you need to take either the COMLEX-USA Level 1 or the USMLE Step 1, consider taking both to keep your Match options open.*

In addition, the COMLEX-USA Level 1 has in recent years placed increasing emphasis on questions related to primary care medicine and prevention. Having a strong background in family or primary care medicine can help test takers when they face questions on prevention.

How Do I Prepare for the COMLEX-USA Level 1?

Student experience suggests that you should start studying for the COMLEX-USA four to six months before the test is given, as an early start will allow you to spend up to a month on each subject. The recommendations made in Section I regarding study and testing methods, strategies, and resources, as well as the books suggested in Section IV for the USMLE Step 1, hold true for the COMLEX-USA as well.

Another important source of information is in the *Examination Guidelines and Sample Exam*, a booklet that discusses the breakdown of each subject while also providing sample questions and corresponding answers. Many students, however, felt that this breakdown provided only a general guideline and was not representative of the level of difficulty of the actual COMLEX-USA. The sample questions did not provide examples of clinical vignettes, which made up approximately 25% of the exam. You will receive this publication with registration materials for the COMLEX-USA Level 1, but you can also receive a copy and additional information by writing:

NBOME
8765 W. Higgins Road, Suite 200
Chicago, IL 60631-4174
(773) 714-0622
Fax: (773) 714-0631

or by visiting the NBOME Web page at www.nbome.org.

The NBOME developed the Comprehensive Osteopathic Medical Self-Assessment Examination (COMSAE) series to fill the need for self-assessment on the part of osteopathic medical students. Many students take the COMSAE exam before the COMLEX-USA in addition to using test-bank questions and board review books. Students can purchase a copy of this exam at www.nbome.org/comsae.asp.

In recent years, students have reported an emphasis in certain areas. For example:

- There was an increased emphasis on upper limb anatomy/brachial plexus.
- Specific topics were repeatedly tested on the exam. These included cardiovascular physiology and pathology, acid-base physiology, diabetes, benign prostatic hyperplasia, sexually transmitted diseases, measles, and rubella. Thyroid and adrenal function, neurology (head injury), specific drug treatments for bacterial infection, migraines/cluster headaches, and drug mechanisms also received heavy emphasis.
- Behavioral science questions were based on psychiatry.
- High-yield osteopathic manipulative technique (OMT) topics included an emphasis on the sympathetic and parasympathetic innervations of viscera and nerve roots, rib mechanics/diagnosis, and basic craniosacral theory. Students who spend time reviewing basic anatomy, studying nerve and dermatome innervations, and understanding how to perform basic OMT techniques (e.g., muscle energy or counterstrain) can improve their scores.

> *You must know the Chapman reflex points and the obscure names of physical exam signs.*

The COMLEX-USA Level 1 also includes multimedia-based questions. Such questions test the student's ability to perform a good physical exam and to elicit various physical diagnostic signs (e.g., Murphy's sign).

Since topics that were repeatedly tested appeared in all four booklets, students found it useful to review them in between the two test days. It is important to understand that the topics emphasized on the current exam may not be stressed on future exams. However, some topics are heavily tested each year, so it may be beneficial to have a solid foundation in the above-mentioned topics.

▶ FIRST AID FOR THE PODIATRIC MEDICAL STUDENT

The National Board of Podiatric Medical Examiners (NBPME) tests are designed to assess whether a candidate possesses the knowledge required to practice as a minimally competent entry-level podiatrist. The NBPME examinations are used as part of the licensing process governing the practice of podiatric medicine. The NBPME exam is recognized by all 50 states and the District of Columbia, the U.S. Army, the U.S. Navy, and the Canadian provinces of Alberta, British Columbia, and Ontario. Individual states use the examination scores differently; therefore, doctor of podiatric medicine (DPM) candidates should refer to the *NBPME Bulletin of Information: 2012 Examinations.*

The NBPME Part I is generally taken after the completion of the second year of podiatric medical education. Unlike the USMLE Step 1, there is no behavioral science section, nor is biomechanics tested. The exam samples seven basic science disciplines: general anatomy (10%); lower extremity anatomy (22%); biochemistry (10%); physiology (12%); medical microbiology and immunology (15%); pathology (15%); and pharmacology (16%). A detailed outline of topics and subtopics covered on the exam can be found in the NBPME Bulletin of Information, available on the NBPME Web site.

> ▶ *Areas tested on the NBPME Part I:*
> - *General anatomy*
> - *Lower extremity anatomy*
> - *Biochemistry*
> - *Physiology*
> - *Medical microbiology & immunology*
> - *Pathology*
> - *Pharmacology*

Your NBPME Appointment

In early spring, your college registrar will have you fill out an application for the NBPME Part I. After your application and registration fees are received, you will be mailed the *NBPME Bulletin of Information: 2012 Examinations.* The exam will be offered at an independent location in each city with a podiatric medical school (New York, Philadelphia, Miami, Cleveland, Chicago, Des Moines, Phoenix, and San Francisco). You may take the exam at any of these locations regardless of which school you attend. However, you must designate on your application which testing location you desire. Specific instructions about exam dates and registration deadlines can be found in the *NBPME Bulletin.*

Exam Format

The NBPME Part I is a written exam consisting of 205 questions. The test consists entirely of multiple-choice questions with four answer choices. Examinees have three hours in which to take the exam and are given scratch paper and a calculator, both of which must be turned in at the end of the exam. Some questions on the exam will be "trial questions." These questions are evaluated as future board questions but are not counted in your score.

Interpreting Your Score

Three to four weeks following the exam date, test takers will receive their scores by mail. NBPME scores are reported as pass/fail, with a scaled score of at least 75 needed to pass. Eighty-five percent of first-time test takers pass the NBPME Part I. Failing candidates receive a report with one score between 55 and 74 in addition to diagnostic messages intended to help identify strengths or weaknesses in specific content areas. If you fail the NBPME Part I, you must retake the entire examination at a later date. There is no limit to the number of times you can retake the exam.

Preparation for the NBPME Part I

Students suggest that you begin studying for the NBPME Part I at least three months prior to the test date. The suggestions made in Section I regarding study and testing methods for the USMLE Step 1 can be applied to the NBPME as well. This book should, however, be used as a supplement and not as the sole source of information. Keep in mind that you need only a passing score. Neither you nor your school or future residency will ever see your actual numerical score. Competing with colleagues should not be an issue, and study groups are beneficial to many.

- *Know the anatomy of the lower extremity!*

A potential study method that helps many students is to copy the outline of the material to be tested from the *NBPME Bulletin*. Check off each topic during your study, because doing so will ensure that you have engaged each topic. If you are pressed for time, prioritize subjects on the basis of their weight on the exam. Approximately 22% of the NBPME Part I focuses on lower extremity anatomy. In this area, students should rely on the notes and material that they received from their class. Remember, lower extremity anatomy is the podiatric physician's specialty—so everything about it is important. Do not forget to study osteology. Keep your old tests and look through old lower extremity class exams, since each of the podiatric colleges submits questions from its own exams. This strategy will give you an understanding of the types of questions that may be asked. On the NBPME Part I, you will see some of the same classic lower extremity anatomy questions you were tested on in school.

The NBPME, like the USMLE, requires that you apply and integrate knowledge over several areas of basic science in order to answer exam questions. Students report that many questions emphasize clinical presentations; however, the facts in this book are very useful in helping students recall the various diseases and organisms. DPM candidates should expand on the high-yield pharmacology section and study antifungal drugs and treatments for *Pseudomonas*, methicillin-resistant *S. aureus*, candidiasis, and erythrasma. The high-yield section focusing on pathology is very useful; however, additional emphasis on diabetes mellitus and all its secondary manifestations, particularly peripheral neuropathy, should not be overlooked. Students should also focus on renal physiology and drug elimination, the biochemistry of gout, and neurophysiology, all of which have been noted to be important topics on the NBPME Part I exam.

A sample set of questions is found in the *NBPME Bulletin of Information: 2012 Examinations*. These samples are similar in difficulty to actual board questions. If you do not receive an *NBPME Bulletin* or if you have any questions regarding registration, fees, test centers, authorization forms, or score reports, please contact your college registrar or:

NBPME
P.O. Box 510
Bellefonte, PA 16823
(814) 357-0487
Email: NBPMEOfc@aol.com

or visit the NBPME Web page at www.nbpme.info.

▶ FIRST AID FOR THE STUDENT WITH A DISABILITY

The USMLE provides accommodations for students with documented disabilities. The basis for such accommodations is the Americans with Disabilities Act (ADA) of 1990. The ADA defines a disability as "a significant limitation in one or more major life activities." This includes both "observable/physical" disabilities (e.g., blindness, hearing loss, narcolepsy) and "hidden/mental disabilities" (e.g., attention-deficit hyperactivity disorder, chronic fatigue syndrome, learning disabilities).

To provide appropriate support, the administrators of the USMLE must be informed of both the nature and the severity of an examinee's disability. Such documentation is required for an examinee to receive testing accommodations. Accommodations include extra time on tests, low-stimulation environments, extra or extended breaks, and zoom text.

> ▶ *U.S. students seeking ADA-compliant accommodations must contact the NBME directly; IMGs, contact the ECFMG.*

Who Can Apply for Accommodations?

Students or graduates of a school in the United States or Canada that is accredited by the Liaison Committee on Medical Education (LCME) or the AOA may apply for test accommodations directly from the NBME. Requests are granted only if they meet the ADA definition of a disability. If you are a disabled student or a disabled graduate of a foreign medical school, you must contact the ECFMG (see below).

Who Is Not Eligible for Accommodations?

Individuals who do not meet the ADA definition of disabled are not eligible for test accommodations. Difficulties not eligible for test accommodations include test anxiety, slow reading without an identified underlying cognitive deficit, English as a second language, and learning difficulties that have not been diagnosed as a medically recognized disability.

Understanding the Need for Documentation

Although most learning-disabled medical students are all too familiar with the often exhausting process of providing documentation of their disability, you should realize that **applying for USMLE accommodation is different from these previous experiences.** This is because the NBME determines whether an individual is disabled solely on the basis of the guidelines set by the ADA. **Previous accommodation does not in itself justify provision of an accommodation,** so be sure to review the NBME guidelines carefully.

Getting the Information

The first step in applying for USMLE special accommodations is to contact the NBME and obtain a guidelines and questionnaire booklet. This can be obtained by calling or writing to:

Testing Coordinator
Office of Test Accommodations
National Board of Medical Examiners
3750 Market Street
Philadelphia, PA 19104-3102
(215) 590-9509

Internet access to this information is also available at www.nbme.org. This information is also relevant for IMGs, since the information is the same as that sent by the ECFMG.

Foreign graduates should contact the ECFMG to obtain information on special accommodations by calling or writing to:

ECFMG
3624 Market Street
Philadelphia, PA 19104-2685
(215) 386-5900

When you get this information, take some time to read it carefully. The guidelines are clear and explicit about what you need to do to obtain accommodations.

SECTION II

High-Yield General Principles

"There comes a time when for every addition of knowledge you forget something that you knew before. It is of the highest importance, therefore, not to have useless facts elbowing out the useful ones."

—Sir Arthur Conan Doyle, A *Study in Scarlet*

"Never regard study as a duty, but as the enviable opportunity to learn."

—Albert Einstein

"Live as if you were to die tomorrow. Learn as if you were to live forever."

—Gandhi

▶ HOW TO USE THE DATABASE

The 2013 edition of *First Aid for the USMLE Step 1* contains a revised and expanded database of basic science material that student authors and faculty have identified as high yield for board review. The information is presented in a partially organ-based format. Hence, Section II is devoted to pathology and the foundational principles of behavioral science, biochemistry, microbiology, immunology, and pharmacology. Section III focuses on organ systems, with subsections covering the embryology, anatomy and histology, physiology, pathology, and pharmacology relevant to each. Each subsection is then divided into smaller topic areas containing related facts. Individual facts are generally presented in a three-column format, with the **Title** of the fact in the first column, the **Description** of the fact in the second column, and the **Mnemonic** or **Special Note** in the third column. Some facts do not have a mnemonic and are presented in a two-column format. Others are presented in list or tabular form in order to emphasize key associations.

The database structure used in Sections II and III is useful for reviewing material already learned. These sections are **not** ideal for learning complex or highly conceptual material for the first time.

The database of high-yield facts is not comprehensive. Use it to complement your core study material and not as your primary study source. The facts and notes have been condensed and edited to emphasize the essential material, and as a result, each entry is "incomplete" and arguably "over-simplified." Often the more you research a topic, the more complex it gets, and certain topics resist simplification. Work with the material, add your own notes and mnemonics, and recognize that not all memory techniques work for all students.

We update the database of high-yield facts annually to keep current with new trends in boards content as well as to expand our database of information. However, we must note that inevitably many other very high-yield entries and topics are not yet included in our database.

We actively encourage medical students and faculty to submit entries and mnemonics so that we may enhance the database for future students. We also solicit recommendations of alternate tools for study that may be useful in preparing for the examination, such as diagrams, charts, and computer-based tutorials (see How to Contribute, p. xvii).

Image Acknowledgments

Images marked with ☒ are reproduced with permission of USMLE-Rx.com. Images marked with RU are reproduced with permission of Dr. Richard P. Usatine and the *Color Atlas of Family Medicine* (www.usatinemedia.com). Images marked with ☒ are reproduced with permission of other sources. Citations are listed on page 633.

Disclaimer

The entries in this section reflect student opinions of what is high yield. Because of the diverse sources of material, no attempt has been made to trace or reference the origins of entries individually. We have regarded mnemonics as essentially in the public domain. Errors and important omissions will gladly be corrected if brought to the attention of the authors, either through our online errata process or directly by e-mail.

NOTES

HIGH-YIELD PRINCIPLES IN

Behavioral Science

"It's psychosomatic. You need a lobotomy. I'll get a saw."

—Calvin, "Calvin & Hobbes"

A heterogeneous mix of epidemiology, biostatistics, ethics, psychology, sociology, and more falls under the heading of behavioral science. Many medical students do not study this discipline diligently because the material is felt to be easy or a matter of common sense. In our opinion, this is a missed opportunity.

Behavioral science questions may seem less concrete than questions from other disciplines, requiring an awareness of the social aspects of medicine. For example, if a patient does or says something, what should you do or say in response? These so-called quote questions now constitute much of the behavioral science section. Medical ethics and medical law are also appearing with increasing frequency. In addition, the key aspects of the doctor-patient relationship (e.g., communication skills, open-ended questions, facilitation, silence) are high yield, as are biostatistics and epidemiology. Make sure you can apply biostatistical concepts such as specificity and predictive values in a problem-solving format.

▸ BEHAVIORAL SCIENCE–EPIDEMIOLOGY/BIOSTATISTICS

Types of studies

STUDY TYPE	DESIGN	MEASURES/EXAMPLE
Case-control study Observational and retrospective	Compares a group of people with disease to a group without disease. Looks for prior exposure or risk factor. Asks, "What happened?"	Odds ratio (OR). "Patients with COPD had higher odds of a history of smoking than those without COPD had."
Cohort study Observational and prospective or retrospective	Compares a group with a given exposure or risk factor to a group without such exposure. Looks to see if exposure ↑ the likelihood of disease. Can be prospective (asks, "Who will develop disease?") or retrospective (asks, "Who developed the disease [exposed vs. nonexposed]?").	Relative risk (RR). "Smokers had a higher risk of developing COPD than nonsmokers had."
Cross-sectional study Observational	Collects data from a group of people to assess frequency of disease (and related risk factors) at a particular point in time. Asks, "What is happening?"	Disease prevalence. Can show risk factor association with disease, but does not establish causality.
Twin concordance study	Compares the frequency with which both monozygotic twins or both dizygotic twins develop same disease.	Measures heritability.
Adoption study	Compares siblings raised by biological vs. adoptive parents.	Measures heritability and influence of environmental factors.

Clinical trial

Experimental study involving humans. Compares therapeutic benefits of 2 or more treatments, or of treatment and placebo. Study quality improves when study is randomized, controlled, and double-blinded (i.e., neither patient nor doctor knows whether the patient is in the treatment or control group). Triple-blind refers to the additional blinding of the researchers analyzing the data.

	STUDY SAMPLE	PURPOSE
Phase I	Small number of healthy volunteers.	Assesses safety, toxicity, and pharmacokinetics.
Phase II	Small number of patients with disease of interest.	Assesses treatment efficacy, optimal dosing, and adverse effects.
Phase III	Large number of patients randomly assigned either to the treatment under investigation or to the best available treatment (or placebo).	Compares the new treatment to the current standard of care.
Phase IV	Postmarketing surveillance trial of patients after approval.	Detects rare or long-term adverse effects.

Evaluation of diagnostic tests

Uses 2 × 2 table comparing test results with the actual presence of disease. TP = true positive; FP = false positive; TN = true negative; FN = false negative.

Sensitivity and specificity are fixed properties of test; however, PPV and NPV vary with prevalence or pretest probability.

Test \ Disease	⊕	⊖
⊕	TP	FP
⊖	FN	TN

Sensitivity (true-positive rate)

Proportion of all people with disease who test positive, or the probability that a test detects disease when disease is present.

Value approaching 100% is desirable for **ruling out** disease and indicates a low false-negative rate. Used for screening in diseases with low prevalence.

= TP / (TP + FN)
= 1 – false-negative rate
PID = **P**ositive **I**n **D**isease
SNOUT = **S**e**N**sitivity rules **OUT**
If 100% sensitivity, TP / (TP + FN) = 1, FN = 0, and all negatives must be TNs

Specificity (true-negative rate)

Proportion of all people without disease who test negative, or the probability that a test indicates non-disease when disease is absent.

Value approaching 100% is desirable for **ruling in** disease and indicates a low false-positive rate. Used as a confirmatory test after a positive screening test.

Example: HIV testing. Screen with ELISA (sensitive, high false-positive rate, low threshold); confirm with Western blot (specific, high false-negative rate, high threshold).

= TN / (TN + FP)
= 1 – false-positive rate
NIH = **N**egative **I**n **H**ealth
SPIN = **SP**ecificity rules **IN**
If 100% specificity, TN / (TN + FP) = 1, FP = 0, and all positives must be TPs

Positive predictive value (PPV)

Proportion of positive test results that are true positive.

Probability that person actually has the disease given a positive test result.

= TP / (TP + FP)
PPV varies directly with prevalence or pretest probability: high pretest probability → high PPV

Negative predictive value (NPV)

Proportion of negative test results that are true negative.

Probability that person actually is disease free given a negative test result.

= TN / (FN + TN)
NPV varies inversely with prevalence or pretest probability: high pretest probability → low NPV

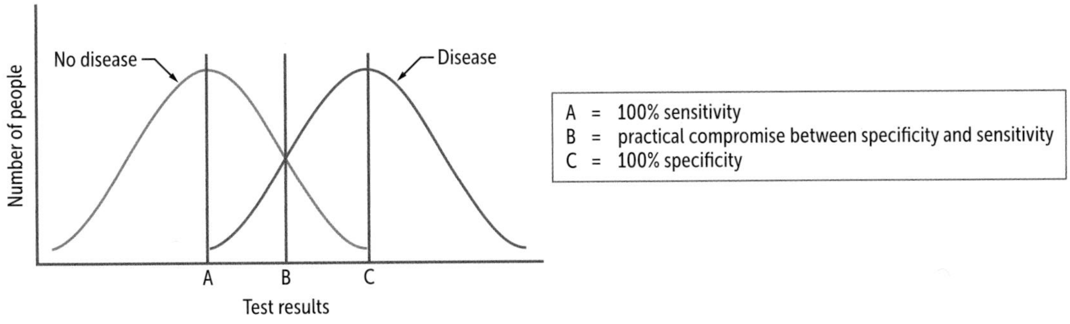
No disease
Disease
Number of people
A
B
C
Test results
A = 100% sensitivity
B = practical compromise between specificity and sensitivity
C = 100% specificity

Incidence vs. prevalence	$\text{Incidence rate} = \dfrac{\text{\# of new cases in a specified time period}}{\text{Population at risk during same time period}}$	**Incidence** looks at new **incidents**.
	$\text{Prevalence} = \dfrac{\text{\# of existing cases}}{\text{Population at risk}}$ Prevalence ≈ incidence rate × average disease duration. Prevalence > incidence for chronic diseases (e.g., diabetes).	Prevalence looks at **all** current cases.

Quantifying risk

Odds ratio (OR)	Typically used in case-control studies. Odds that the group with the disease (cases) was exposed to a risk factor (a/c) divided by the odds that the group without the disease (controls) was exposed (b/d).	$\text{Odds ratio} = \dfrac{a/c}{b/d} = \dfrac{ad}{bc}$
Relative risk (RR)	Typically used in cohort studies. Risk of developing disease in the exposed group divided by risk in the unexposed group (e.g., if 21% of smokers develop lung cancer vs. 1% of nonsmokers, RR = 21/1 = 21). If prevalence is low, RR ≈ OR.	$\text{Relative risk} = \dfrac{a/(a+b)}{c/(c+d)}$
Attributable risk	The difference in risk between exposed and unexposed groups, or the proportion of disease occurrences that are attributable to the exposure (e.g., if risk of lung cancer in smokers is 21% and risk in nonsmokers is 1%, then 20% of the 21% risk of lung cancer in smokers is attributable to smoking).	$\text{Attributable risk} = \dfrac{a}{a+b} - \dfrac{c}{c+d}$
Absolute risk reduction (ARR)	Absolute reduction in risk associated with a treatment as compared to a control (e.g., if 8% of people who receive a placebo vaccine develop flu vs. 2% of people who receive a flu vaccine, then ARR = 8% – 2% = 6%).	(see 2×2 table below)
Number needed to treat	Number of patients who need to be treated for 1 patient to benefit. Calculated as 1/absolute risk reduction.	
Number needed to harm	Number of patients who need to be exposed to a risk factor for 1 patient to be harmed. Calculated as 1/attributable risk.	

Risk factor	Disease ⊕	Disease ⊖
⊕	a	b
⊖	c	d

Precision vs. accuracy

Precision	The consistency and reproducibility of a test (reliability). The absence of random variation in a test.	Random error—reduces precision in a test. ↑ precision → ↓ standard deviation.
Accuracy	The trueness of test measurements (validity). The absence of systematic error or bias in a test.	Systematic error—reduces accuracy in a test.

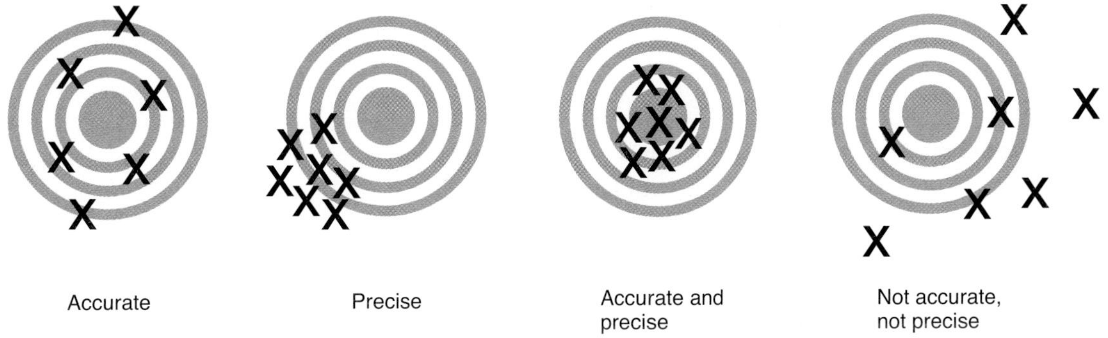
Accurate
Precise
Accurate and precise
Not accurate, not precise

Bias

Occurs when there is systematic error or favor in a particular direction.

Selection bias	Nonrandom assignment to participation in a study group (e.g., Berkson's bias, loss to follow-up)	Ways to reduce bias: ▪ Blind studies to limit influence of participants and researchers on interpretation of outcomes ▪ Placebo control groups ▪ Crossover studies (each subject acts as own control) to limit confounding bias ▪ Randomization to limit selection bias and confounding bias ▪ Matching to reduce confounding bias
Recall bias	Knowledge of presence of disorder alters recall by subjects; common in retrospective studies	
Sampling bias	Subjects are not representative of the general population; therefore, results are not generalizable. A type of selection bias.	
Late-look bias	Information gathered at an inappropriate time—e.g., using a survey to study a fatal disease (only those patients still alive will be able to answer survey)	
Procedure bias	Subjects in different groups are not treated the same—e.g., more attention is paid to treatment group, stimulating greater adherence	
Confounding bias	Occurs when factor is related to both exposure and outcome, but is not on the causal pathway; factor distorts or confuses effect of exposure on outcome	
Lead-time bias	Early detection confused with ↑ survival; seen with improved screening (natural history of disease is not changed, but early detection makes it seem as though survival ↑)	
Observer-expectancy effect	Occurs when a researcher's belief in the efficacy of a treatment changes the outcome of that treatment	
Hawthorne effect	Occurs when the group being studied changes its behavior owing to the knowledge of being studied	Dr. **Hawthorne** is watching you

Statistical distribution	Measures of central tendency = mean, median, mode. Measures of dispersion = standard deviation (SD), standard error of the mean (SEM), Z-score, confidence interval.
Normal distribution	Gaussian, also called bell-shaped. Mean = median = mode.
SD and SEM	σ = SD; n = sample size. SEM = $\sigma/\sqrt{n}$. SEM ↓ as n ↑.

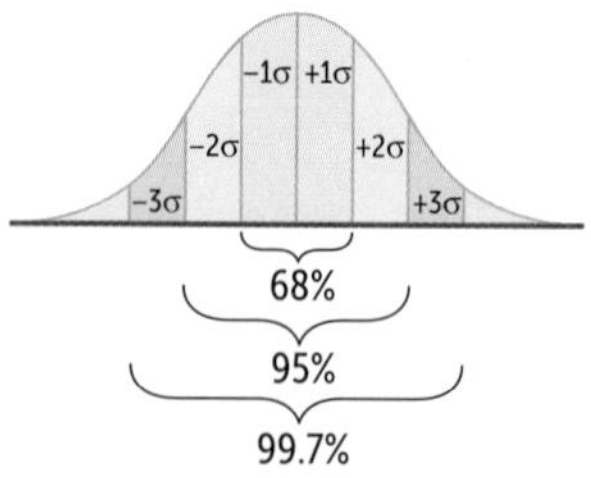

Positive skew	Typically, mean > median > mode. Asymmetry with longer tail on right. Mode is least affected by outliers in the sample.

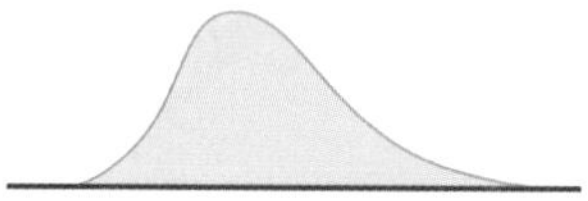

Negative skew	Typically, mean < median < mode. Asymmetry with longer tail on left.

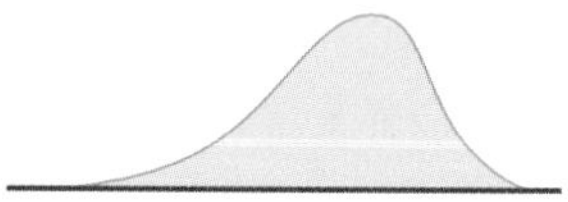

Statistical hypotheses

Null (H_0)	Hypothesis of no difference (e.g., there is no association between the disease and the risk factor in the population).
Alternative (H_1)	Hypothesis of some difference (e.g., there is some association between the disease and the risk factor in the population).

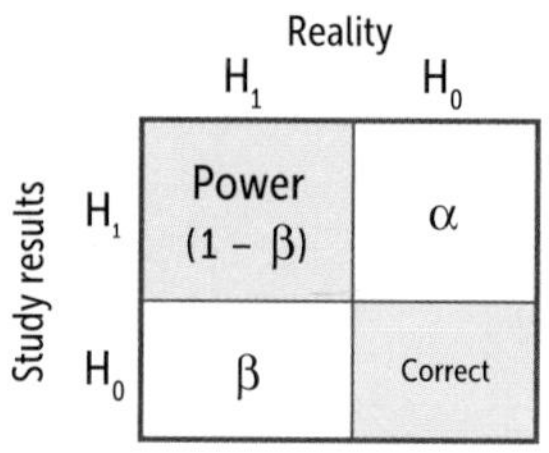

Statistical error types

Type I error (α)	Stating that there **is** an effect or difference when none exists (to mistakenly accept the alternative hypothesis and reject the null hypothesis). α is the probability of making a type I error. p is judged against a preset α level of significance (usually < .05).	Also known as false-positive error. If $p < .05$, then there is less than a 5% chance that the data will show something that is not really there. α = you saw a difference that did not exist—e.g., convicting an innocent man.
Type II error (β)	Stating that there **is not** an effect or difference when one exists (to fail to reject the null hypothesis when it is in fact false). β is the probability of making a type II error.	Also known as false-negative error. β = you were **b**lind to a difference that did exist—e.g., setting a guilty man free.

Power (1 − β)	Probability of rejecting null hypothesis when it is in fact false, or the likelihood of finding a difference if one in fact exists. It increases with: ▪ ↑ sample size ▪ ↑ expected effect size ▪ ↑ precision of measurement	If you ↑ sample size, you ↑ power. There is power in numbers.
Meta-analysis	Pools data and integrates results from several similar studies to reach an overall conclusion. ↑ statistical power.	Limited by quality of individual studies or bias in study selection.
Confidence interval	Range of values in which a specified probability of the means of repeated samples would be expected to fall. CI = confidence interval. CI = range from [mean − Z(SEM)] to [mean + Z(SEM)]. The 95% CI (corresponding to $p = .05$) is often used. For the 95% CI, Z = 1.96. For the 99% CI, Z = 2.58.	If the 95% CI for a mean difference between 2 variables includes 0, then there is no significant difference and H_0 is not rejected. If the 95% CI for odds ratio or relative risk includes 1, H_0 is not rejected. If the CIs between 2 groups do not overlap → significant difference exists. If the CIs between 2 groups overlap → usually no significant difference exists.
t-test vs. ANOVA vs. χ^2		
***t*-test**	Checks difference between the **means** of 2 groups.	Mr. **T** is **mean**.
ANOVA	Checks difference between the means of 3 or more groups.	**ANOVA** = **AN**alysis **O**f **VA**riance of 3 or more groups.
Chi-square (χ^2)	Test checks difference between 2 or more percentages or proportions of categorical outcomes (not mean values).	χ^2 = compare percentages (%) or proportions.
Pearson's correlation coefficient (*r*)	*r* is always between −1 and +1. The closer the absolute value of *r* is to 1, the stronger the linear correlation between the 2 variables. Coefficient of determination = r^2 (value that is usually reported).	
Disease prevention		
Primary	Prevent disease occurrence (e.g., HPV vaccination).	PDR: Prevent Detect Reduce disability
Secondary	Early detection of disease (e.g., Pap smear).	
Tertiary	Reduce disability from disease (e.g., chemotherapy).	

Medicare and Medicaid

Medicare and Medicaid—federal programs that originated from amendments to the Social Security Act.

Medicare is available to patients ≥ 65 years of age, < 65 with certain disabilities, and those with end-stage renal disease.

Medicaid is joint federal and state health assistance for people with very low income.

MedicarE is for Elderly.
MedicaiD is for Destitute.

▸ BEHAVIORAL SCIENCE–ETHICS

Core ethical principles

Patient autonomy	Obligation to respect patients as individuals and to honor their preferences in medical care.
Beneficence	Physicians have a special ethical (fiduciary) duty to act in the patient's best interest. May conflict with autonomy. If the patient can make an informed decision, ultimately the patient has the right to decide.
Nonmaleficence	"Do no harm." However, if the benefits of an intervention outweigh the risks, a patient may make an informed decision to proceed (most surgeries and medications fall into this category).
Justice	To treat persons fairly.

Informed consent

Legally requires:

- Discussion of pertinent information
- Patient's voluntary agreement to the plan of care
- Freedom from coercion

Exceptions to informed consent:

- Patient lacks decision-making capacity or is legally incompetent
- Implied consent in an emergency
- Therapeutic privilege—withholding information when disclosure would severely harm the patient or undermine informed decision-making capacity
- Waiver—patient waives the right of informed consent

Patients must have an intelligent understanding of the risks, benefits, and alternatives, which include no intervention

Written consent can be revoked by the patient at any time, even orally.

Consent for minors

A minor is generally any person < 18 years of age. Parental consent laws in relation to health care vary state by state. Generally, consent must be obtained unless minor is emancipated (e.g., is married, is self-supporting, has children, or is in the military). Parental consent is **not** required in (1) emergency situations, (2) prescribing contraceptives, (3) treating STDs, (4) medical care of pregnancy, and (5) treatment of drug addiction.

Decision-making capacity	Physician must determine whether the patient is psychologically and legally capable of making a particular health care decision. Components: ▪ Patient makes and communicates a choice ▪ Patient is informed (knows and understands) ▪ Decision remains stable over time ▪ Decision is consistent with patient's values and goals, not clouded by a mood disorder ▪ Decision is not a result of delusions or hallucinations	The patient's family cannot require that a doctor withhold information from the patient if patient demonstrates decision-making capacity.
Advance directives	Instructions given by a patient in anticipation of the need for a medical decision. State-specific.	
Oral advance directive	Incapacitated patient's prior oral statements commonly used as guide. Problems arise from variance in interpretation. If patient was informed, directive was specific, patient made a choice, and decision was repeated over time to multiple people, the oral directive is more valid.	
Living will (written advance directive)	Describes treatments the patient wishes to receive or not receive if he/she loses decision-making capacity. Usually, patient directs physician to withhold or withdraw life-sustaining treatment if he/she develops a terminal disease or enters a persistent vegetative state.	
Medical power of attorney	Patient designates an agent to make medical decisions in the event that he/she loses decision-making capacity. Patient may also specify decisions in clinical situations. Patient can revoke anytime patient wishes (regardless of competence). More flexible than a living will.	
Surrogate decision-maker	If an incompetent patient has not prepared an advance directive, individuals (surrogates) who know the patient must determine what the patient would have done if he/she were competent. Priority of surrogates: spouse, adult children, parents, adult siblings, other relatives.	
Confidentiality	Confidentiality respects patient privacy and autonomy. If patient is not present or is incapacitated, disclosing information to family and friends should be guided by professional judgment of patient's best interest. The patient may waive the right to confidentiality (e.g., insurance companies). General principles for exceptions to confidentiality: ▪ Potential harm to others is serious ▪ Likelihood of harm to self is great ▪ No alternative means exists to warn or to protect those at risk ▪ Physicians can take steps to prevent harm Examples of exceptions (many are state-specific) include: ▪ Reportable diseases (STDs, TB, hepatitis, food poisoning)—physicians may have a duty to warn public officials, who will then notify people at risk ▪ The Tarasoff decision—California Supreme Court decision requiring physician to directly inform and protect potential victim from harm; may involve breach of confidentiality ▪ Child and/or elder abuse ▪ Impaired automobile drivers ▪ Suicidal/homicidal patients	

Ethical situations

SITUATION	APPROPRIATE RESPONSE
Patient is not adherent.	Attempt to identify the patient's reason for nonadherence and determine his/her willingness to change; do not attempt to coerce the patient into adhering or refer the patient to another physician.
Patient desires an unnecessary procedure.	Attempt to understand why the patient wants the procedure and address underlying concerns. Do not refuse to see the patient or refer him/her to another physician. Avoid performing unnecessary procedures.
Patient has difficulty taking medications.	Provide written instructions; attempt to simplify treatment regimens; use teach-back method (ask patient to repeat medication regimen back to physician) to ensure patient comprehension.
Family members ask for information about patient's prognosis.	Avoid discussing issues with relatives without the permission of the patient.
A child wishes to know more about his/her illness.	Ask what the parents have told the child about his/her illness. Parents of a child decide what information can be relayed about the illness.
A 17-year-old girl is pregnant and requests an abortion.	Many states require parental notification or consent for minors for an abortion. Unless she is at medical risk, do not advise a patient to have an abortion regardless of her age or the condition of the fetus.
A 15-year-old girl is pregnant and wants to keep the child. Her parents want you to tell her to give the child up for adoption.	The patient retains the right to make decisions regarding her child, even if her parents disagree. Provide information to the teenager about the practical issues of caring for a baby. Discuss the options, if requested. Encourage discussion between the teenager and her parents to reach the best decision.
A terminally ill patient requests physician assistance in ending own life.	In the overwhelming majority of states, refuse involvement in any form of physician-assisted suicide. Physicians may, however, prescribe medically appropriate analgesics that coincidentally shorten the patient's life.
Patient is suicidal.	Assess the seriousness of the threat; if it is serious, suggest that the patient remain in the hospital voluntarily; patient can be hospitalized involuntarily if he/she refuses.
Patient states that he/she finds you attractive.	Ask direct, closed-ended questions and use a chaperone if necessary. Romantic relationships with patients are never appropriate. Never say, "There can be no relationship while you are a patient," because this implies that a relationship may be possible if the individual is no longer a patient.
A woman who had a mastectomy says she feels "ugly" when she undresses.	Find out why the patient feels this way. Do not offer falsely reassuring statements (e.g., "You still look good.").
Patient is angry about the amount of time he/she spent in the waiting room.	Acknowledge the patient's anger, but do not take a patient's anger personally. Apologize for any inconvenience. Stay away from efforts to explain the delay.
Patient is upset with the way he/she was treated by another doctor.	Suggest that the patient speak directly to that physician regarding the patient's concerns. If the problem is with a member of the office staff, tell the patient you will speak to that individual.
A drug company offers a "referral fee" for every patient a physician enrolls in a study.	Eligible patients who may benefit from the study may be enrolled, but it is never acceptable for a physician to receive compensation from a drug company. Patients must be told about the existence of a referral fee.
A physician orders an invasive test for the wrong patient.	No matter how serious or trivial a medical error, a physician is ethically obligated to inform a patient that a mistake has been made.
A patient requires a treatment not covered by his/her insurance.	Never limit or deny care because of the expense in time or money. Discuss all treatment options with patients, even if some are not covered by their insurance companies.

▸ BEHAVIORAL SCIENCE–DEVELOPMENT

Apgar score

Assessment of newborn vital signs following labor via a 10-point scale evaluated at 1 minute and 5 minutes. **Apgar** score is based on **A**ppearance, **P**ulse, **G**rimace, **A**ctivity, and **R**espiration ($\geq$ 7 = good; 4–6 = assist and stimulate; < 4 = resuscitate). If Apgar score remains < 4 at later time points, there is ↑ risk that the child will develop long-term neurological damage.

Low birth weight

Defined as < 2500 g. Caused by prematurity or intrauterine growth retardation. Associated with ↑ risk of SIDS, and with ↑ overall mortality. Other problems include impaired thermoregulation and immune function, hypoglycemia, polycythemia, and impaired neurocognitive/emotional development. Complications include infections, respiratory distress syndrome, necrotizing enterocolitis, intraventricular hemorrhage, and persistent fetal circulation.

Early developmental milestones

AGE	MOTOR	SOCIAL	VERBAL/COGNITIVE
Infant			
Birth–3 mo	Rooting reflex, holds head up, Moro reflex disappears	Social smile	Orients and responds to voice
7–9 mo	Sits alone, crawls, transfers toys from hand to hand	Stranger anxiety	Responds to name and simple instructions, uses gestures, plays peek-a-boo
12–15 mo	Walks, Babinski sign disappears	Separation anxiety	Few words
Toddler			
12–24 mo	Climbs stairs; stacks 3 blocks at 1 yr, 6 blocks at 2 yr (**age × 3 = no. of blocks**)	Rapprochement (moves away from and then returns to mother)	200 words and 2-word phrases at age **2**
24–36 mo	Feeds self with fork and spoon, kicks ball	Core gender identity, parallel play	Toilet training ("**pee** at age **3**")
Preschool			
3 yr	Rides tricycle (rides **3**-cycle at age **3**); copies line or circle drawings	Comfortably spends part of day away from mother	900 words and complete sentences
4 yr	Uses buttons and zippers, grooms self (brushes teeth), hops on 1 foot, makes simple drawings (stick figures)	Cooperative play, imaginary friends	Can tell detailed stories and use prepositions

Changes in the elderly	Sexual changes: ▪ Men—slower erection/ejaculation, longer refractory period ▪ Women—vaginal shortening, thinning, and dryness Sleep patterns: ↓ REM and slow-wave sleep; ↑ latency and awakenings ↑ suicide rate (men 65–74 years of age have the highest suicide rate in the United States) ↓ vision, hearing, immune response, bladder control ↓ renal, pulmonary, GI function ↓ muscle mass, ↑ fat	Sexual interest does not ↓. Intelligence does not ↓.
Grief	Normal bereavement characterized by shock, denial, guilt, and somatic symptoms. Can last up to 1 year. May experience illusions. Pathologic grief includes excessively intense grief; prolonged grief lasting > 2–6 months; or grief that is delayed, inhibited, or denied. May experience depressive symptoms, delusions, and hallucinations.	

▸ BEHAVIORAL SCIENCE–PHYSIOLOGY

Sexual dysfunction	Includes sexual desire disorders (hypoactive sexual desire or sexual aversion), sexual arousal disorders (erectile dysfunction), orgasmic disorders (anorgasmia and premature ejaculation), and sexual pain disorders (dyspareunia and vaginismus). Differential diagnosis includes: ▪ Drugs (e.g., antihypertensives, neuroleptics, SSRIs, ethanol) ▪ Diseases (e.g., depression, diabetes) ▪ Psychological (e.g., performance anxiety)	
Body-mass index (BMI)	BMI is a measure of weight adjusted for height. $\text{BMI} = \frac{\text{weight in kg}}{(\text{height in meters})^2}$	< 18.5 underweight 18.5–24.9 normal weight 25.0–29.9 overweight > 30.0 obesity > 35.0 severe obesity > 40.0 morbid obesity > 45.0 super obesity

Sleep stages

STAGE (% OF TOTAL SLEEP TIME IN YOUNG ADULTS)	DESCRIPTION	EEG WAVEFORM
Awake (eyes open)	Alert, active mental concentration	Beta (highest frequency, lowest amplitude)
Awake (eyes closed)		Alpha
Stage N1 (5%)	Light sleep	Theta
Stage N2 (45%)	Deeper sleep; bruxism	Sleep spindles and K complexes
Stage N3 (25%)	Deepest, non-REM sleep (slow-wave sleep); sleepwalking; night terrors; bedwetting	Delta (lowest frequency, highest amplitude)
REM (25%)	Dreaming, loss of motor tone, possibly a memory processing function, erections, ↑ brain O_2 use	Beta
	Serotonergic predominance of raphe nucleus is key to initiating sleep. Sleep enuresis is treated with oral desmopressin acetate (DDAVP), which mimics vasopressin (ADH, antidiuretic hormone); preferred over imipramine because of the latter's adverse effects. Alcohol, benzodiazepines, and barbiturates are associated with reduced REM and delta sleep. Benzodiazepines are useful for night terrors and sleepwalking.	At night, **BATS Drink Blood**

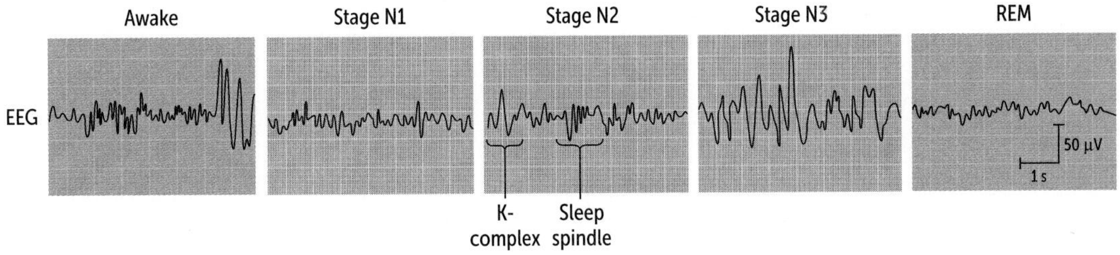

(Adapted, with permission, from Barrett KE et al. *Ganong's Review of Medical Physiology,* 23rd ed. New York: McGraw-Hill, 2010, Fig. 15–7.)

REM sleep

Occurs every 90 minutes; duration ↑ through the night. ACh is the principal neurotransmitter in REM sleep. NE reduces REM sleep.

Findings: ↑ and variable pulse and blood pressure. Extraocular movements during REM sleep due to activity of PPRF (paramedian pontine reticular formation/conjugate gaze center). Penile/clitoral tumescence.

REM sleep is like sex: ↑ pulse, penile/clitoral tumescence, ↓ frequency with age.

Because REM sleep has the same EEG patterns as wakefulness, it has been termed "paradoxical sleep" and "desynchronized sleep."

Sleep patterns of depressed patients	Patients with depression typically have the following changes in their sleep stages: ▪ ↓ slow-wave sleep ▪ ↓ REM latency ▪ ↑ REM early in sleep cycle ▪ ↑ total REM sleep ▪ Repeated nighttime awakenings ▪ Early-morning awakening (important screening question)
Narcolepsy	Disordered regulation of sleep-wake cycles; primary characteristic is excessive daytime sleepiness. May include hypnagogic (just before sleep) or hypnopompic (just before awakening) hallucinations. The patient's nocturnal and narcoleptic sleep episodes start off with REM sleep. Cataplexy (loss of all muscle tone following a strong emotional stimulus) in some patients. Strong genetic component. Treated with daytime stimulants (e.g., amphetamines, modafinil) and nighttime sodium oxybate (GHB).
Circadian rhythm	Driven by suprachiasmatic nucleus (SCN) of hypothalamus. Controls ACTH, prolactin, melatonin, nocturnal NE release. SCN → NE release → pineal gland → melatonin. SCN is regulated by environment (i.e., light).
Sleep terror disorder	Periods of terror with screaming in the middle of the night; occurs during slow-wave sleep. Most common in children. Occurs during non-REM sleep (no memory of arousal) as opposed to nightmares that occur during REM sleep (memory of a scary dream). Cause unknown, but triggers may include emotional stress during the previous day, fever, or lack of sleep. Usually self limited.

HIGH-YIELD PRINCIPLES IN

Biochemistry

"Biochemistry is the study of carbon compounds that crawl."

—Mike Adams

"We think we have found the basic mechanism by which life comes from life."

—Francis H. C. Crick

This high-yield material includes molecular biology, genetics, cell biology, and principles of metabolism (especially vitamins, cofactors, minerals, and single-enzyme-deficiency diseases). When studying metabolic pathways, emphasize important regulatory steps and enzyme deficiencies that result in disease, as well as reactions targeted by pharmacologic interventions. For example, understanding the defect in Lesch-Nyhan syndrome and its clinical consequences is higher yield than memorizing every intermediate in the purine salvage pathway. Do not spend time on hard-core organic chemistry, mechanisms, or physical chemistry. Detailed chemical structures are infrequently tested; however, many structures have been included here to help students learn reactions and the important enzymes involved. Familiarity with the biochemical techniques that have medical relevance—such as enzyme-linked immunosorbent assay (ELISA), immunoelectrophoresis, Southern blotting, and PCR—is useful. Beware if you placed out of your medical school's biochemistry class, as the emphasis of the test differs from that of many undergraduate courses. Review the related biochemistry when studying pharmacology or genetic diseases as a way to reinforce and integrate the material.

▸ BIOCHEMISTRY–MOLECULAR

Chromatin structure	DNA exists in the condensed, chromatin form in order to fit into the nucleus. Negatively charged DNA loops twice around positively charged histone octamer to form nucleosome "**bead**." Histones are rich in the amino acids lysine and arginine. H1 ties nucleosome beads together in a string. In mitosis, DNA condenses to form chromosomes.	Think of "**beads on a string.**" 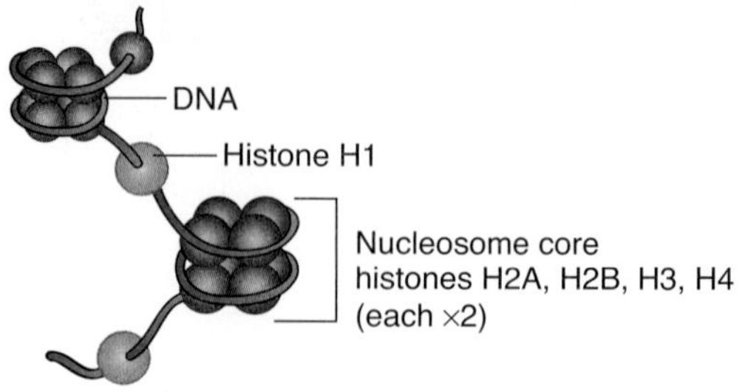 H1 is the only histone that is not in the nucleosome core.
Heterochromatin	Condensed, transcriptionally inactive, sterically inaccessible.	**H**etero**C**hromatin = **H**ighly **C**ondensed.
Euchromatin	Less condensed, transcriptionally active, sterically accessible.	*Eu* = true, "truly transcribed."
DNA methylation	Template strand cytosine and adenine are methylated in DNA replication, which allows mismatch repair enzymes to distinguish between old and new strands in prokaryotes.	
Histone methylation	Inactivates transcription of DNA.	**M**ethylation makes DNA **M**ute.
Histone acetylation	Relaxes DNA coiling, allowing for transcription.	**A**cetylation makes DNA **A**ctive.

Nucleotides

PURines (A, G)—2 rings.
PYrimidines (C, T, U)—1 ring.
Guanine has a ketone. Thymine has a methyl. Deamination of cytosine makes uracil.
Uracil found in RNA; thymine in DNA.
G-C bond (3 H bonds) stronger than A-T bond (2 H bonds). ↑ G-C content → ↑ melting temperature.

PURe **A**s **G**old.
CUT the **PY** (pie).
Thymine has a me**thy**l.

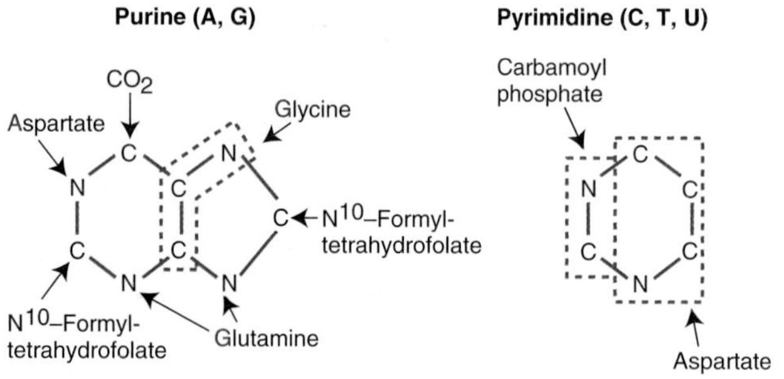

GAG—Amino acids necessary for purine synthesis:
Glycine
Aspartate
Glutamine
Nucleo**S**ide = base + ribose (**S**ugar).
Nucleo**T**ides = base + ribose + phospha**T**e; linked by 3′-5′ phosphodiester bond.

De novo pyrimidine and purine synthesis

Purines	Pyrimidines
	Make temporary base (orotic acid)
Start with sugar + phosphate (PRPP)	Add sugar + phosphate (PRPP)
Add base	Modify base

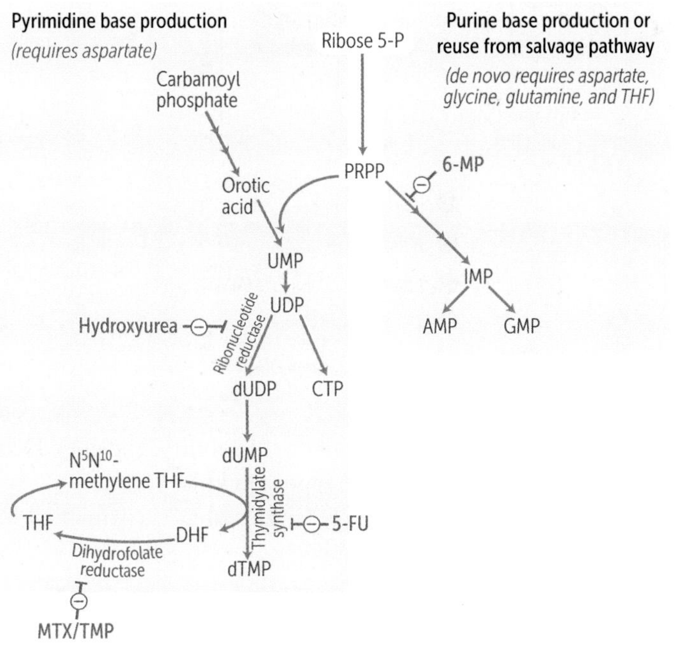

Ribonucleotides are synthesized first and are converted to deoxyribonucleotides by ribonucleotide reductase.

Carbamoyl phosphate is involved in 2 metabolic pathways: de novo pyrimidine synthesis and the urea cycle. Ornithine transcarbamoylase deficiency (OTC, key enzyme in the urea cycle) leads to an accumulation of carbamoyl phosphate, which is then converted to orotic acid.

Various antineoplastic and antibiotic drugs function by interfering with purine synthesis:

- Hydroxyurea inhibits ribonucleotide reductase
- 6-mercaptopurine (6-MP) blocks de novo purine synthesis
- 5-fluorouracil (5-FU) inhibits thymidylate synthase (↓ deoxythymidine monophosphate [dTMP])
- Methotrexate (MTX) inhibits dihydrofolate reductase (↓ dTMP)
- Trimethoprim (TMP) inhibits bacterial dihydrofolate reductase (↓ dTMP)

Orotic aciduria

Inability to convert orotic acid to UMP (de novo pyrimidine synthesis pathway) because of defect in UMP synthase (a bifunctional enzyme). Autosomal recessive.

FINDINGS	↑ orotic acid in urine, megaloblastic anemia (does not improve with administration of vitamin B_{12} or folic acid), failure to thrive. No hyperammonemia (vs. OTC deficiency—↑ orotic acid with hyperammonemia).
TREATMENT	Oral uridine administration.

Purine salvage deficiencies

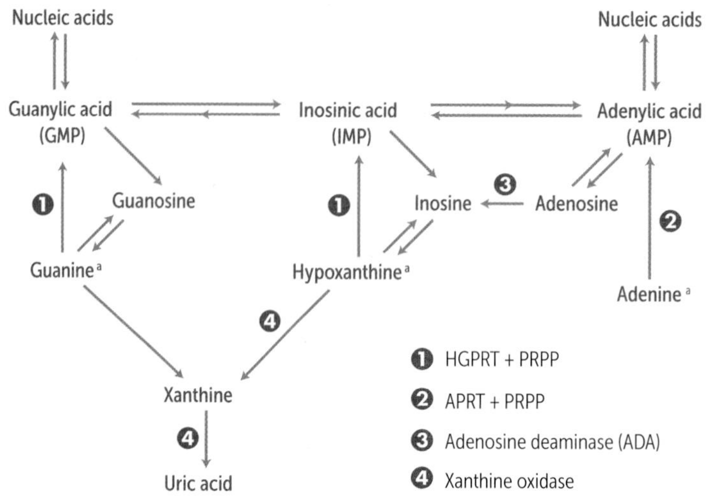
Nucleic acids
Nucleic acids
Guanylic acid (GMP)
Inosinic acid (IMP)
Adenylic acid (AMP)
Guanosine
Inosine
Adenosine
Guanine[a]
Hypoxanthine[a]
Adenine[a]
Xanthine
Uric acid
1 HGPRT + PRPP
2 APRT + PRPP
3 Adenosine deaminase (ADA)
4 Xanthine oxidase
[a] Base from degraded DNA/RNA

Adenosine deaminase deficiency	Excess ATP and dATP imbalances nucleotide pool via feedback inhibition of ribonucleotide reductase → prevents DNA synthesis and thus ↓ lymphocyte count. One of the major causes of SCID. Autosomal recessive.	**S**evere **C**ombined **I**mmuno**d**eficiency **D**isease (**SCID**) happens to **kids**. 1st disease to be treated by experimental human gene therapy.
Lesch-Nyhan syndrome	Defective purine salvage owing to absence of **HGPRT**, which converts hypoxanthine to IMP and guanine to GMP. Results in excess uric acid production and de novo purine synthesis. X-linked recessive. Findings: retardation, self-mutilation, aggression, hyperuricemia, gout, choreoathetosis.	**H**e's **G**ot **P**urine **R**ecovery **T**rouble.

Genetic code features

Unambiguous	Each codon specifies only 1 amino acid.	
Degenerate/ redundant	Most amino acids are coded by multiple codons.	Exceptions: methionine and tryptophan encoded by only 1 codon (AUG and UGG, respectively).
Commaless, nonoverlapping	Read from a fixed starting point as a continuous sequence of bases.	Exceptions: some viruses.
Universal	Genetic code is conserved throughout evolution.	Exception in humans: mitochondria.

Point mutations in DNA	Severity of damage: silent < missense < nonsense < frameshift.	
Silent	Same amino acid, often base change in 3rd position of codon (tRNA wobble).	
Missense	Changed amino acid (conservative—new amino acid is similar in chemical structure).	
Nonsense	Change resulting in early **stop** codon.	**Stop** the **nonsense**!
Frameshift	Change resulting in misreading of all nucleotides downstream, usually resulting in a truncated, nonfunctional protein.	

DNA replication	Eukaryotic DNA replication is more complex than the prokaryotic process but uses many enzymes analogous to those listed below. In both prokaryotes and eukaryotes, DNA replication is semiconservative and involves both continuous and discontinuous (Okazaki fragment) synthesis.	
Origin of replication	Particular consensus sequence of base pairs in genome where DNA replication begins. May be single (prokaryotes) or multiple (eukaryotes).	
Replication fork	Y-shaped region along DNA template where leading and lagging strands are synthesized.	
Helicase	Unwinds DNA template at replication fork.	
Single-stranded binding proteins	Prevent strands from reannealing.	
DNA topoisomerases	Create a nick in the helix to relieve supercoils created during replication.	Fluoroquinolones—inhibit DNA gyrase (prokaryotic topoisomerase II).
Primase	Makes an RNA primer on which DNA polymerase III can initiate replication.	
DNA polymerase III	Prokaryotic only. Elongates leading strand by adding deoxynucleotides to the 3′ end. Elongates lagging strand until it reaches primer of preceding fragment. 3′ → 5′ exonuclease activity "proofreads" each added nucleotide.	DNA polymerase III has 5′ → 3′ synthesis and proofreads with 3′ → 5′ exonuclease.
DNA polymerase I	Prokaryotic only. Degrades RNA primer; replaces it with DNA.	Has same functions as DNA polymerase III but also excises RNA primer with 5′ → 3′ exonuclease.
DNA ligase	Catalyzes the formation of phosphodiesterase bond within a strand of double-stranded DNA (i.e., joins Okazaki fragments).	Seals.
Telomerase	Enzyme adds DNA to 3' ends of chromosomes to avoid loss of genetic material with every duplication.	

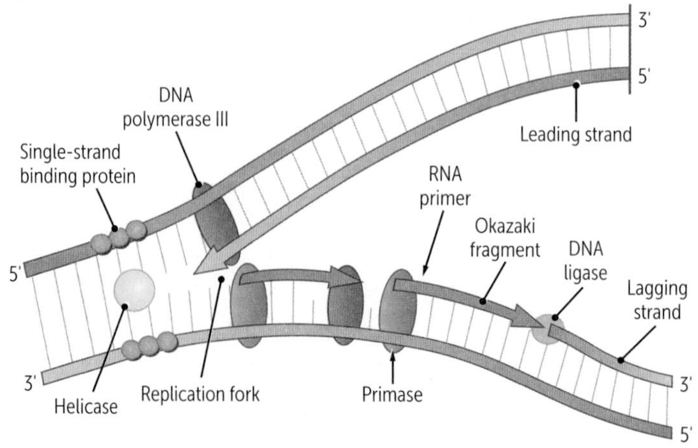

DNA repair

Single strand		
Nucleotide excision repair	Specific endonucleases release the oligonucleotide-containing damaged bases; DNA polymerase and ligase fill and reseal the gap, respectively. Repairs bulky helix-distorting lesions.	Mutated in xeroderma pigmentosum, which prevents repair of pyrimidine dimers because of ultraviolet light exposure.
Base excision repair	Specific glycosylases recognize and remove damaged bases, apurinic/apyrimidinic endonuclease cuts DNA at both apurinic and apyrimidinic sites, empty sugar is removed, and the gap is filled and resealed.	Important in repair of spontaneous/toxic deamination.
Mismatch repair	Newly synthesized strand is recognized, mismatched nucleotides are removed, and the gap is filled and resealed.	Mutated in hereditary nonpolyposis colorectal cancer (HNPCC).
Double strand		
Nonhomologous end joining	Brings together 2 ends of DNA fragments to repair double-stranded breaks. No requirement for homology.	Mutated in ataxia telangiectasia.

DNA/RNA/protein synthesis direction

DNA and RNA are both synthesized 5′ → 3′. Remember that the 5′ of the incoming nucleotide bears the triphosphate (energy source for bond).

The triphosphate bond is the target of the 3′ hydroxyl attack. Drugs blocking DNA replication often have modified 3′ OH, preventing addition of the next nucleotide ("chain termination").

mRNA is read 5′ to 3′.

Protein synthesis is N-terminus to C-terminus.

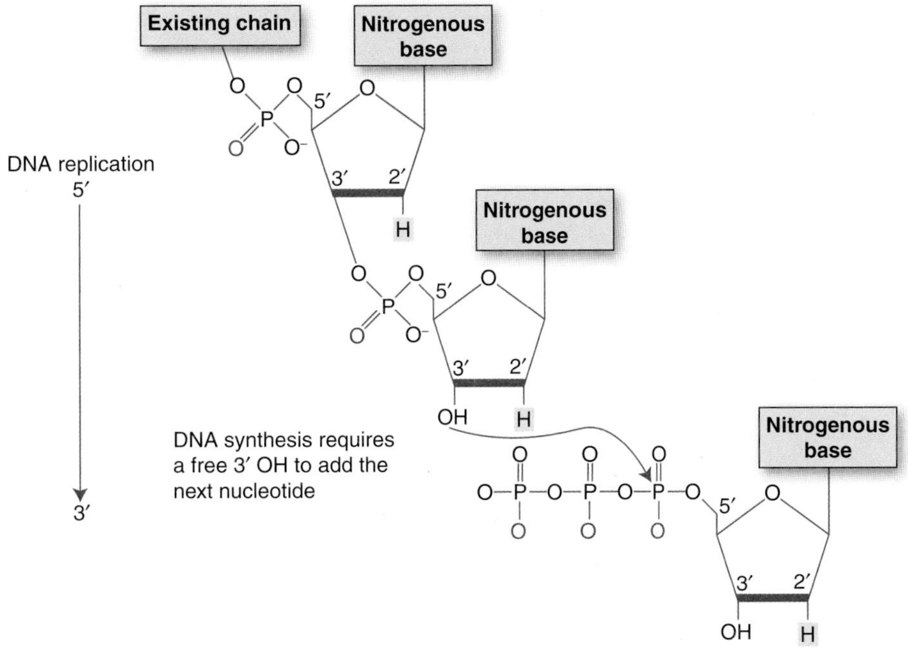

Types of RNA	rRNA is the most abundant type. mRNA is the longest type. tRNA is the smallest type.	rampant, massive, tiny.

Start and stop codons

mRNA start codons	AUG (or rarely GUG).	AUG inAUGurates protein synthesis.
Eukaryotes	Codes for methionine, which may be removed before translation is completed.	
Prokaryotes	Codes for formylmethionine (f-met).	
mRNA stop codons	UGA, UAA, UAG.	UGA = U Go Away. UAA = U Are Away. UAG = U Are Gone.

Functional organization of the gene

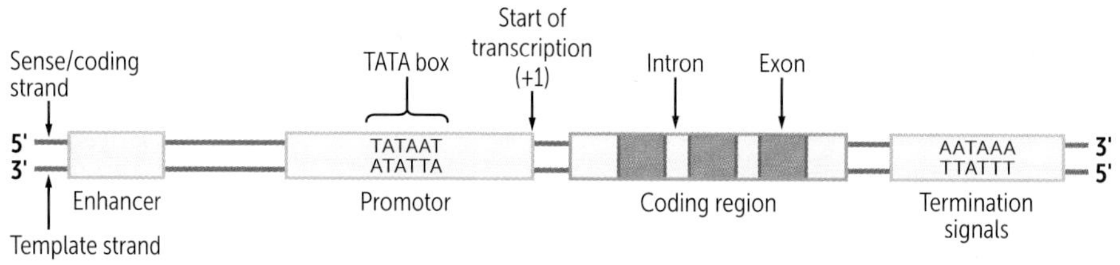

Regulation of gene expression

Promoter	Site where RNA polymerase and multiple other transcription factors bind to DNA upstream from gene locus (AT-rich upstream sequence with TATA and CAAT boxes).	Promoter mutation commonly results in dramatic ↓ in amount of gene transcribed.
Enhancer	Stretch of DNA that alters gene expression by binding transcription factors.	Enhancers and silencers may be located close to, far from, or even within (in an intron) the gene whose expression it regulates.
Silencer	Site where negative regulators (repressors) bind.	

RNA polymerases

Eukaryotes	RNA polymerase I makes rRNA (most numerous RNA, rampant). RNA polymerase II makes mRNA (largest RNA, massive). RNA polymerase III makes tRNA (smallest RNA, tiny). No proofreading function, but can initiate chains. RNA polymerase II opens DNA at promotor site.	I, II, and III are numbered as their products are used in protein synthesis. α-amanitin, found in *Amanita phalloides* (death cap mushrooms), inhibits RNA polymerase II. Causes severe hepatotoxicity if ingested.
Prokaryotes	1 RNA polymerase (multisubunit complex) makes all 3 kinds of RNA.	

RNA processing (eukaryotes)

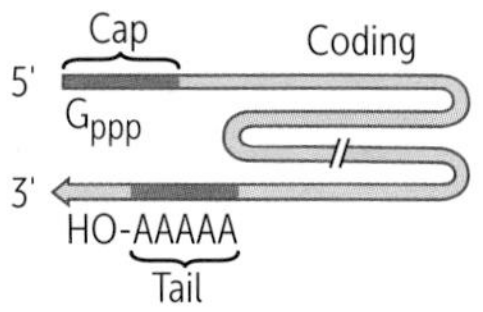

Initial transcript is called heterogeneous nuclear RNA (hnRNA). hnRNA destined for translation is called pre-mRNA.

Processing occurs in nucleus. After transcription:

- Capping on 5′ end (addition of 7-methylguanosine cap)
- Polyadenylation on 3′ end (≈ 200 A's)
- Splicing out of introns

Capped, tailed, and spliced transcript is called mRNA.

Only processed RNA is transported out of the nucleus.

Poly-A polymerase does not require a template. AAUAAA = polyadenylation signal.

Splicing of pre-mRNA

❶ Primary transcript combines with snRNPs and other proteins to form spliceosome.
❷ Lariat-shaped (looped) intermediate is generated.
❸ Lariat is released to remove intron precisely and join 2 exons.

Patients with lupus make antibodies to spliceosomal snRNPs.

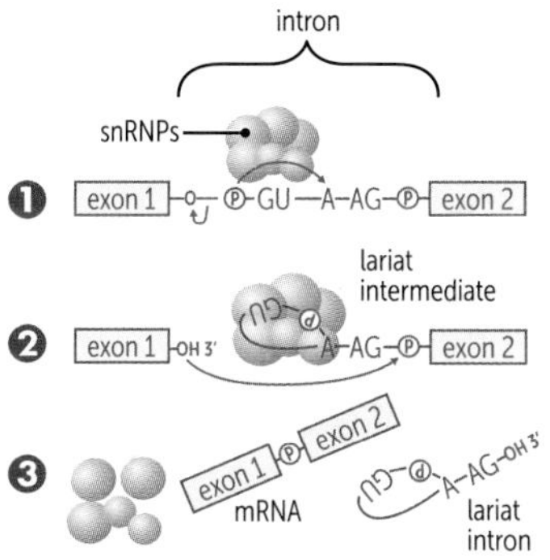

Introns vs. exons

Exons contain the actual genetic information coding for protein.

Introns are intervening noncoding segments of DNA.

Introns are **in**tervening sequences and stay **in** the nucleus, whereas **ex**ons **ex**it and are **ex**pressed.

Different exons can be combined by alternative splicing to make unique proteins in different tissues (e.g., β-thalassemia mutations).

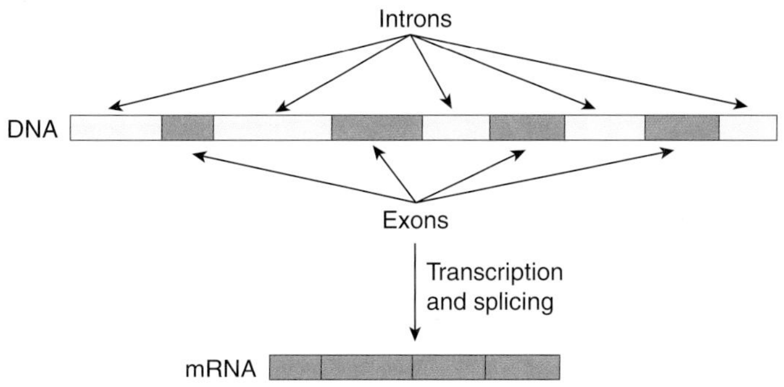

tRNA

Structure	75–90 nucleotides, 2° structure, cloverleaf form, anticodon end is opposite 3′ aminoacyl end. All tRNAs, both eukaryotic and prokaryotic, have **CCA** at 3′ end along with a high percentage of chemically modified bases. The amino acid is covalently bound to the 3′ end of the tRNA.	**CCA: C**an **C**arry **A**mino acids.
Charging	Aminoacyl-tRNA synthetase (1 per amino acid, "matchmaker," uses ATP) scrutinizes amino acid before and after it binds to tRNA. If incorrect, bond is hydrolyzed. The amino acid-tRNA bond has energy for formation of peptide bond. A mischarged tRNA reads usual codon but inserts wrong amino acid.	Aminoacyl-tRNA synthetase and binding of charged tRNA to the codon are responsible for accuracy of amino acid selection. Tetracyclines bind 30S subunit, preventing attachment of aminoacyl-tRNA.

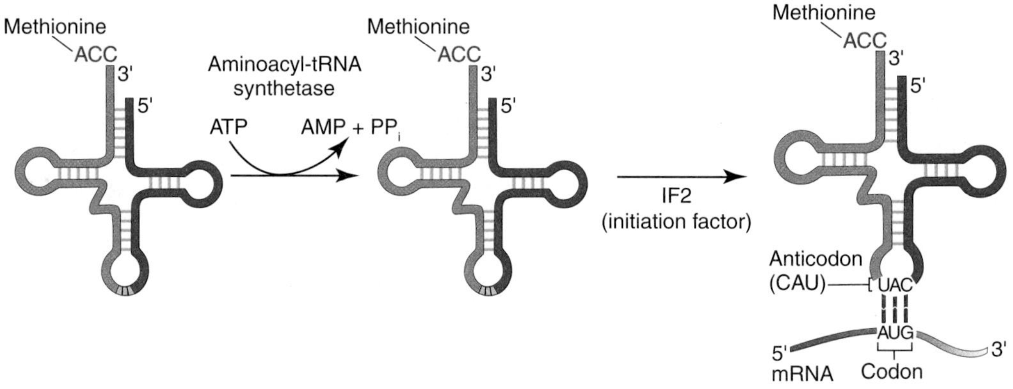

tRNA wobble	Accurate base pairing is required only in the first 2 nucleotide positions of an mRNA codon, so codons differing in the 3rd "wobble" position may code for the same tRNA/amino acid (as a result of degeneracy of genetic code).

Protein synthesis

Initiation	Activated by GTP hydrolysis, initiation factors (eukaryotic IFs) help assemble the 40S ribosomal subunit with the initiator tRNA and are released when the mRNA and the ribosomal subunit assemble with the complex.	Eukaryotes: 40S + 60S → 80S (Even). PrOkaryotes: 30S + 50S → 70S (Odd). ATP—tRNA Activation (charging). GTP—tRNA Gripping and Going places (translocation).
Elongation	1. Aminoacyl-tRNA binds to A site (except for initiator methionine) 2. Ribosomal rRNA ("ribozyme") catalyzes peptide bond formation, transfers growing polypeptide to amino acid in A site 3. Ribosome advances 3 nucleotides toward 3′ end of mRNA, moving peptidyl tRNA to P site (translocation)	Think of "going **APE**": **A** site = incoming **A**minoacyl-tRNA. **P** site = accommodates growing **P**eptide. **E** site = holds **E**mpty tRNA as it **E**xits.
Termination	Stop codon is recognized by release factor, and completed protein is released from ribosome.	

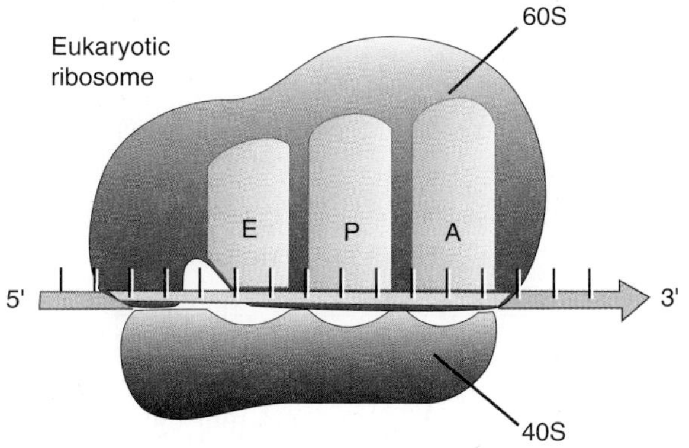

Many antibiotics act as protein synthesis inhibitors:
- Aminoglycosides bind 30S and inhibit formation of initiation complex and cause misreading of mRNA
- Tetracyclines bind 30S and block aminoacyl tRNA from entering the acceptor site
- Chloramphenicol binds 50S and inhibits peptidyl transferase
- Macrolides bind 50S and prevent release of uncharged tRNA after it has donated its amino acid

Posttranslational modifications

Trimming	Removal of N- or C-terminal propeptides from zymogens to generate mature proteins.
Covalent alterations	Phosphorylation, glycosylation, hydroxylation, methylation, and acetylation.
Proteasomal degradation	Attachment of ubiquitin to defective proteins to tag them for breakdown.

▸ BIOCHEMISTRY–CELLULAR

Cell cycle phases Checkpoints control transitions between phases of cell cycle. This process is regulated by cyclins, CDKs, and tumor suppressors. Mitosis (shortest phase): prophase-metaphase-anaphase-telophase. G_1 and G_0 are of variable duration.

REGULATION OF CELL CYCLE		
CDKs	Cyclin-dependent kinases; constitutive and inactive.	G = Gap or Growth. S = Synthesis.
Cyclins	Regulatory proteins that control cell cycle events; phase specific; activate CDKs.	
Cyclin-CDK complexes	Must be both activated and inactivated for cell cycle to progress.	
Tumor suppressors	p53 and hypophosphorylated Rb normally inhibit G_1-to-S progression; mutations in these genes result in unrestrained cell division.	

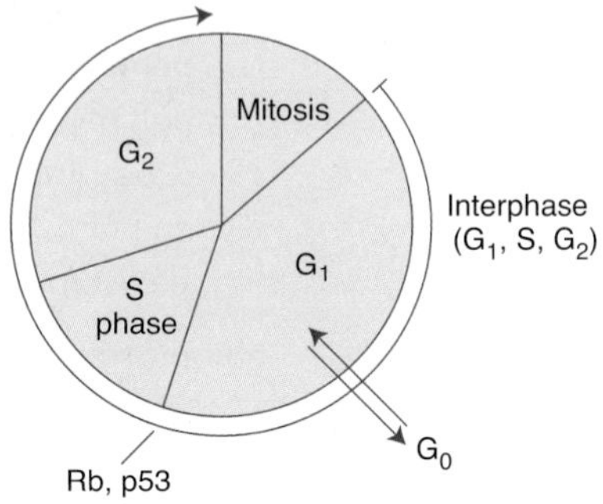

CELL TYPES		
Permanent	Remain in G_0, regenerate from stem cells.	Neurons, skeletal and cardiac muscle, RBCs.
Stable (quiescent)	Enter G_1 from G_0 when stimulated.	Hepatocytes, lymphocytes.
Labile	Never go to G_0, divide rapidly with a short G_1.	Bone marrow, gut epithelium, skin, hair follicles, germ cells.

Rough endoplasmic reticulum	Site of synthesis of secretory (exported) proteins and of N-linked oligosaccharide addition to many proteins. Nissl bodies (RER in neurons)—synthesize enzymes (e.g., ChAT [choline acetyltransferase] makes ACh) and peptide neurotransmitters. Free ribosomes—unattached to any membrane; site of synthesis of cytosolic and organellar proteins.	Mucus-secreting goblet cells of the small intestine and antibody-secreting plasma cells are rich in RER.
Smooth endoplasmic reticulum	Site of steroid synthesis and detoxification of drugs and poisons.	Liver hepatocytes and steroid hormone–producing cells of the adrenal cortex are rich in SER.

Cell trafficking

Golgi is the distribution center for proteins and lipids from the ER to the vesicles and plasma membrane. Modifies N-oligosaccharides on asparagine. Adds O-oligosaccharides on serine and threonine. Adds mannose-6-phosphate to proteins for trafficking to lysosomes.

Endosomes are sorting centers for material from outside the cell or from the Golgi, sending it to lysosomes for destruction or back to the membrane/Golgi for further use.

I-cell disease (inclusion cell disease)—inherited lysosomal storage disorder; failure of addition of mannose-6-phosphate to lysosome proteins (enzymes are secreted outside the cell instead of being targeted to the lysosome). Results in coarse facial features, clouded corneas, restricted joint movement, and high plasma levels of lysosomal enzymes. Often fatal in childhood.

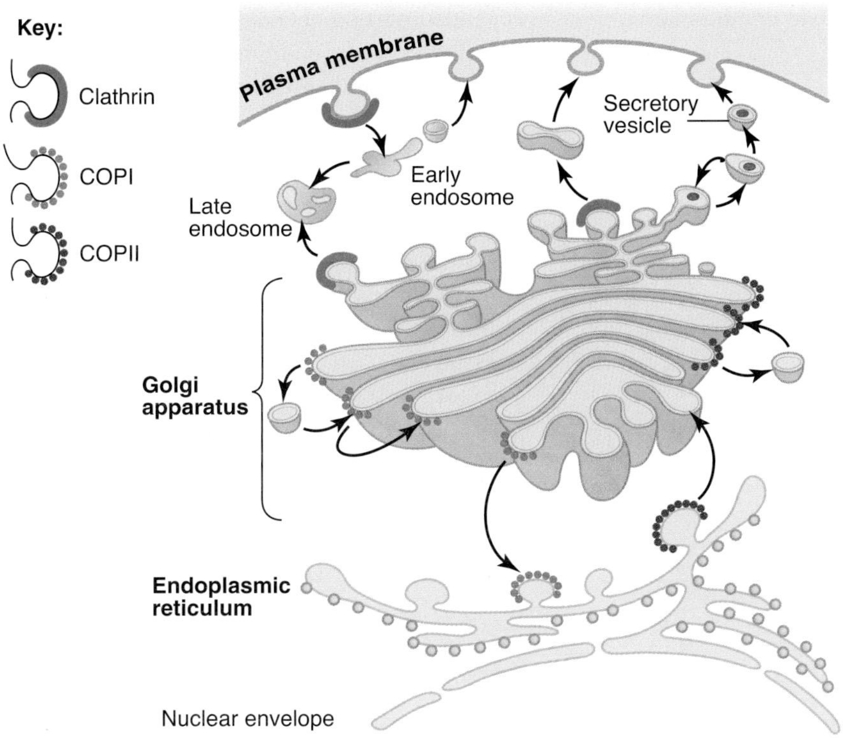
Key:
Clathrin
COPI
COPII
Plasma membrane
Secretory vesicle
Early endosome
Late endosome
Golgi apparatus
Endoplasmic reticulum
Nuclear envelope

Vesicular trafficking proteins

COPI: Golgi → Golgi (retrograde); Golgi → ER.

COPII: Golgi → Golgi (anterograde); ER → Golgi.

Clathrin: *trans*-Golgi → lysosomes; plasma membrane → endosomes (receptor-mediated endocytosis).

Peroxisome

Membrane-enclosed organelle involved in catabolism of very long fatty acids and amino acids.

Proteasome

Barrel-shaped protein complex that degrades damaged or unnecessary proteins tagged for destruction with ubiquitin.

Microtubule

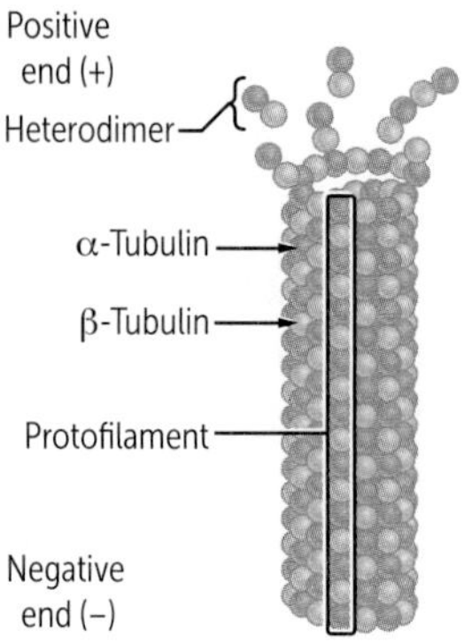
Positive end (+)
Heterodimer
α-Tubulin
β-Tubulin
Protofilament
Negative end (–)

Cylindrical structure composed of a helical array of polymerized dimers of α- and β-tubulin. Each dimer has 2 GTP bound. Incorporated into flagella, cilia, mitotic spindles. Grows slowly, collapses quickly. Also involved in slow axoplasmic transport in neurons.

Molecular motor proteins—transport cellular cargo toward opposite ends of microtubule tracks.

- Dynein = retrograde to microtubule (+ → –).
- Kinesin = anterograde to microtubule (– → +).

Drugs that act on microtubules:

- Mebendazole/thiabendazole (antihelminthic)
- Griseofulvin (antifungal)
- Vincristine/vinblastine (anti-cancer)
- Paclitaxel (anti–breast cancer)
- Colchicine (anti-gout)

Chédiak-Higashi syndrome—mutation in the lysosomal trafficking regulator gene (*LYST*), whose product is required for the microtubule-dependent sorting of endosomal proteins into late multivesicular endosomes. Results in recurrent pyogenic infections, partial albinism, and peripheral neuropathy.

Cilia structure

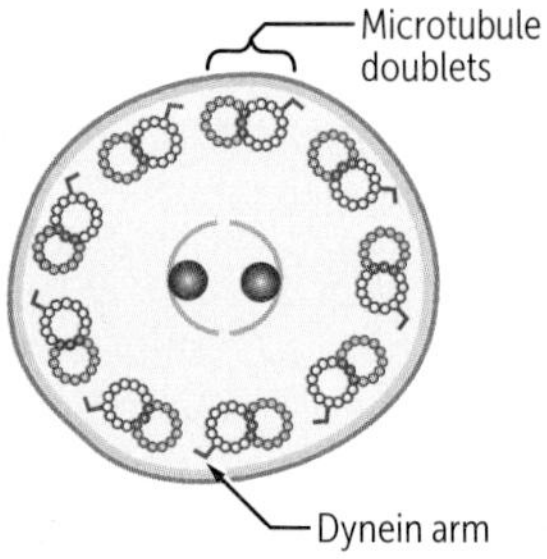
Microtubule doublets
Dynein arm

9 + 2 arrangement of microtubules.

Axonemal dynein—ATPase that links peripheral 9 doublets and causes bending of cilium by differential sliding of doublets.

Kartagener's syndrome (primary ciliary dyskinesia)—immotile cilia due to a dynein arm defect. Results in male infertility (immotile sperm) and ↓ female fertility, bronchiectasis, and recurrent sinusitis (bacteria and particles not pushed out); associated with situs inversus.

Cytoskeletal elements

Actin and myosin	Microvilli, muscle contraction, cytokinesis, adherens junctions.
Microtubule	Movement. Cilia, flagella, mitotic spindle, axonal trafficking, centrioles.
Intermediate filaments	Structure. Vimentin, desmin, cytokeratin, lamins, glial fibrillary acid proteins (GFAP), neurofilaments.

Plasma membrane composition

Asymmetric lipid bilayer.

Contains cholesterol, phospholipids, sphingolipids, glycolipids, and proteins.

Immunohistochemical stains for intermediate filaments

STAIN	CELL TYPE
Vimentin	Connective tissue
Desmin	Muscle
Cytokeratin	Epithelial cells
GFAP	NeuroGlia
Neurofilaments	Neurons

Sodium-potassium pump	Na^+-K^+ ATPase is located in the plasma membrane with ATP site on cytosolic side. For each ATP consumed, 3 Na^+ go out and 2 K^+ come in. During cycle, pump is phosphorylated.	Ouabain inhibits by binding to K^+ site. Cardiac glycosides (digoxin and digitoxin) directly inhibit the Na^+-K^+ ATPase, which leads to indirect inhibition of Na^+/Ca^{2+} exchange → ↑ $[Ca^{2+}]_i$ → ↑ cardiac contractility.

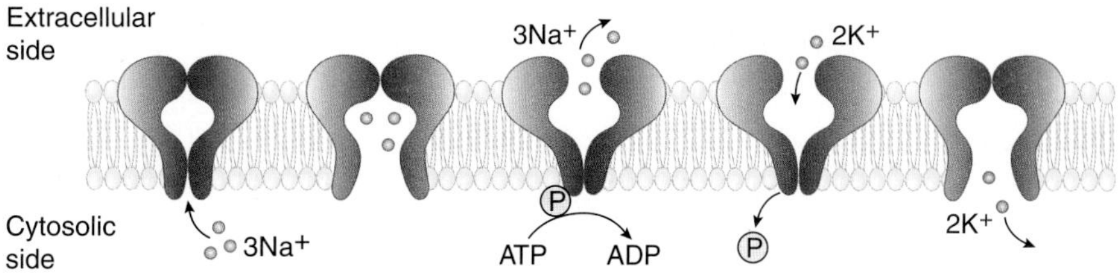

Collagen	Most abundant protein in the human body. Extensively modified by posttranslational modification. Organizes and strengthens extracellular matrix.	**B**e (**S**o **T**otally) **C**ool, **R**ead **B**ooks.
Type I	Most common (90%)—**B**one, **S**kin, **T**endon, dentin, fascia, cornea, late wound repair.	Type **I**: b**one**. Defective in osteogenesis imperfecta.
Type II	**C**artilage (including hyaline), vitreous body, nucleus pulposus.	Type **II**: car**two**lage.
Type III	**R**eticulin—skin, blood vessels, uterus, fetal tissue, granulation tissue.	Type **III**: defective in Ehlers-Danlos (**Thre**E **D**).
Type IV	**B**asement membrane or basal lamina.	Type **IV**: under the **floor** (basement membrane). Defective in Alport syndrome.

Collagen synthesis and structure

Inside fibroblasts	
1. Synthesis (RER)	Translation of collagen α chains (preprocollagen)—usually Gly-X-Y (X and Y are proline or lysine).
2. Hydroxylation (ER)	Hydroxylation of specific proline and lysine residues (requires vitamin C; deficiency → scurvy).
3. Glycosylation (ER)	Glycosylation of pro-α-chain hydroxylysine residues and formation of procollagen via hydrogen and disulfide bonds (triple helix of 3 collagen α chains). Problems forming triple helix → osteogenesis imperfecta.
4. Exocytosis	Exocytosis of procollagen into extracellular space.
Outside fibroblasts	
5. Proteolytic processing	Cleavage of disulfide-rich terminal regions of procollagen, transforming it into insoluble tropocollagen.
6. Cross-linking	Reinforcement of many staggered tropocollagen molecules by covalent lysine-hydroxylysine cross-linkage (by Cu^{2+}-containing lysyl oxidase) to make collagen fibrils. Problems with cross-linking → Ehlers-Danlos.

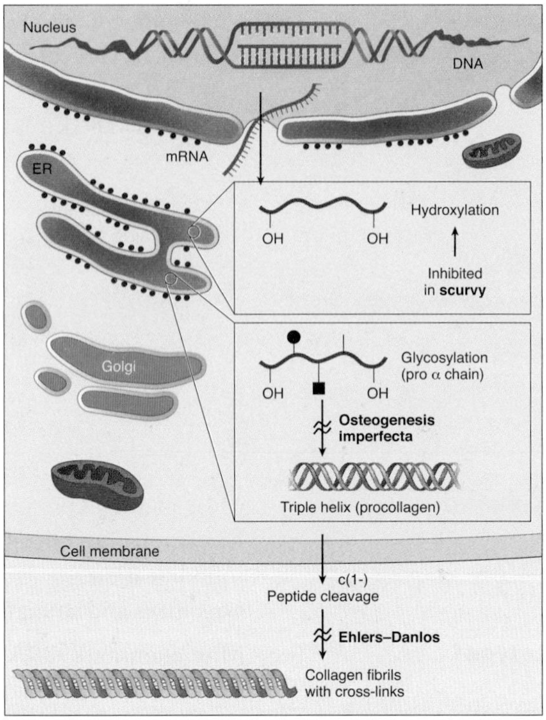

Osteogenesis imperfecta

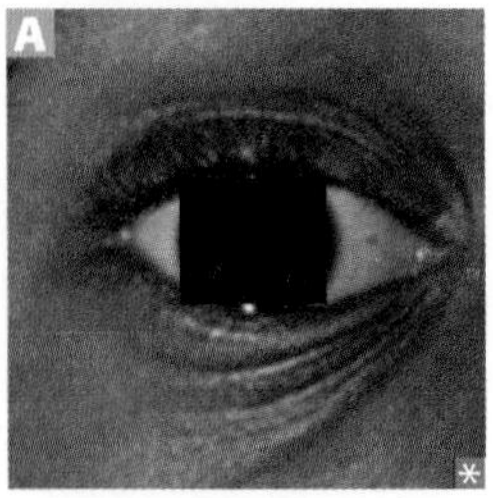

Genetic bone disorder (brittle bone disease) caused by a variety of gene defects.

Most common form is autosomal dominant with abnormal type I collagen, causing:

- Multiple fractures with minimal trauma; may occur during the birth process
- Blue sclerae A due to the translucency of the connective tissue over the choroidal veins
- Hearing loss (abnormal middle ear bones)
- Dental imperfections due to lack of dentin

May be confused with child abuse. Incidence is 1:10,000.

Ehlers-Danlos syndrome

Faulty collagen synthesis causing hyperextensible skin, tendency to bleed (easy bruising), and hypermobile joints.

6 types. Inheritance and severity vary. Can be autosomal dominant or recessive. May be associated with joint dislocation, berry aneurysms, organ rupture.

Type I or Type V collagen most frequently affected in severe classic Ehlers-Danlos syndrome.

Alport syndrome	Due to a variety of gene defects resulting in abnormal type IV collagen. Most common form is X-linked recessive. Characterized by progressive hereditary nephritis and deafness. May be associated with ocular disturbances.	Type IV collagen is an important structural component of the basement membrane of the kidney, ears, and eyes.
Elastin	Stretchy protein within skin, lungs, large arteries, elastic ligaments, vocal cords, ligamenta flava (connect vertebrae → relaxed and stretched conformations). Rich in proline and glycine, nonhydroxylated forms. Tropoelastin with fibrillin scaffolding. Cross-linking takes place extracellularly and gives elastin its elastic properties. Broken down by elastase, which is normally inhibited by α_1-antitrypsin.	Marfan's syndrome—caused by a defect in fibrillin. Emphysema—can be caused by α_1-antitrypsin deficiency, resulting in excess elastase activity. Wrinkles of aging are due to reduced collagen and elastin production.

▶ BIOCHEMISTRY—LABORATORY TECHNIQUES

Polymerase chain reaction

Molecular biology laboratory procedure used to amplify a desired fragment of DNA.

Steps:

1. Denaturation—DNA is denatured by heating to generate 2 separate strands
2. Annealing—during cooling, excess premade DNA primers anneal to a specific sequence on each strand to be amplified.
3. Elongation—heat-stable DNA polymerase replicates the DNA sequence following each primer.

These steps are repeated multiple times for DNA sequence amplification.

Agarose gel electrophoresis—used for size separation of PCR products (smaller molecules travel further); compared against DNA ladder.

Blotting procedures

Southern blot	A **DNA** sample is electrophoresed on a gel and then transferred to a filter. The filter is then soaked in a denaturant and subsequently exposed to a radiolabeled DNA probe that recognizes and anneals to its complementary strand. The resulting double-stranded, labeled piece of DNA is visualized when the filter is exposed to film.	SNoW DRoP: Southern = DNA Northern = RNA Western = Protein
Northern blot	Similar to Southern blot, except that an **RNA** sample is electrophoresed. Useful for studying mRNA levels.	
Western blot	Sample protein is separated via gel electrophoresis and transferred to a filter. Labeled antibody is used to bind to relevant **protein.**	
Southwestern blot	Identifies **DNA-binding proteins** (e.g., transcription factors) using labeled oligonucleotide probes.	

Microarrays

Thousands of nucleic acid sequences are arranged in grids on glass or silicon. DNA or RNA probes are hybridized to the chip, and a scanner detects the relative amounts of complementary binding.

Used to profile gene expression levels of thousands of genes simultaneously to study certain diseases and treatments. Able to detect single nucleotide polymorphisms (SNPs) for a variety of applications including genotyping, forensic analysis, predisposition to disease, cancer mutations, and genetic linkage analysis.

Enzyme-linked immunosorbent assay

A rapid immunologic technique testing for antigen-antibody reactivity.

Patient's blood sample is probed with either

1. Indirect ELISA: uses a test **antigen** to see if a specific antibody is present in the patient's blood; a secondary antibody coupled to a color-generating enzyme is added to detect the first antibody; or
2. Direct ELISA: uses a test **antibody** coupled to a color-generating enzyme to see if a specific antigen is present in the patient's blood.

If the target substance is present in the sample, the test solution will have an intense color reaction, indicating a positive test result.

Used in many laboratories to determine whether a particular antibody (e.g., anti-HIV) is present in a patient's blood sample. Both the sensitivity and the specificity of ELISA approach 100%, but both false-positive and false-negative results do occur.

Fluorescence in situ hybridization (FISH)

Fluorescent DNA or RNA probe binds to specific gene site of interest on chromosomes.
Used for specific localization of genes and direct visualization of anomalies (e.g., microdeletions) at molecular level (when deletion is too small to be visualized by karyotype).
Fluorescence = gene is present; no fluorescence = gene has been deleted.

Cloning methods

Cloning is the production of a recombinant DNA molecule that is self-perpetuating.
Steps:
1. Isolate eukaryotic mRNA (post-RNA processing steps) of interest.
2. Expose mRNA to reverse transcriptase to produce cDNA.
3. Insert cDNA fragments into bacterial plasmids containing antibiotic resistance genes.
4. Surviving bacteria on antibiotic medium produce cDNA library.

Gene expression modifications

Transgenic strategies in mice involve:
- Random insertion of gene into mouse genome
- Targeted insertion or deletion of gene through homologous recombination with mouse gene

Cre-lox system—Can inducibly manipulate genes at specific developmental points using an antibiotic-controlled promoter (e.g., to study a gene whose deletion causes embryonic death).
RNA interference (RNAi)—dsRNA is synthesized that is complementary to the mRNA sequence of interest. When transfected into human cells, dsRNA separates and promotes degradation of target mRNA, knocking down gene expression.

Knock-**out** = removing a gene, taking it **out**.
Knock-**in** = **in**serting a gene.

Karyotyping

A process in which metaphase chromosomes are stained, ordered, and numbered according to morphology, size, arm-length ratio, and banding pattern. Can be performed on a sample of blood, bone marrow, amniotic fluid, or placental tissue. Used to diagnose chromosomal imbalances (e.g., autosomal trisomies, sex chromosome disorders).

▶ BIOCHEMISTRY–GENETICS

Genetic terms

TERM	DEFINITION	EXAMPLE
Codominance	Both alleles contribute to the phenotype of the heterozygote.	Blood groups A, B, AB.
Variable expressivity	Phenotype varies among individuals with same genotype.	2 patients with neurofibromatosis type 1 (NF1) may have varying disease severity.
Incomplete penetrance	Not all individuals with a mutant genotype show the mutant phenotype.	*BRCA1* gene mutations do not always result in breast or ovarian cancer.
Pleiotropy	One gene contributes to multiple phenotypic effects.	PKU causes many seemingly unrelated symptoms, ranging from mental retardation to hair/skin changes.
Imprinting	Differences in gene expression depend on whether the mutation is of maternal or paternal origin.	Prader-Willi and Angelman's syndromes.
Anticipation	Increased severity or earlier onset of disease in succeeding generations.	Huntington's disease.
Loss of heterozygosity	If a patient inherits or develops a mutation in a tumor suppressor gene, the complementary allele must be deleted/mutated before cancer develops. This is not true of oncogenes.	Retinoblastoma and the "two-hit hypothesis."
Dominant negative mutation	Exerts a dominant effect. A heterozygote produces a nonfunctional altered protein that also prevents the normal gene product from functioning.	Mutation of a transcription factor in its allosteric site. Nonfunctioning mutant can still bind DNA, preventing wild-type transcription factor from binding.
Linkage disequilibrium	Tendency for certain alleles at 2 linked loci to occur together more often than expected by chance. Measured in a population, not in a family, and often varies in different populations.	
Mosaicism	Occurs when cells in the body differ in genetic makeup due to postfertilization loss or change of genetic information during mitosis. Can be a germ-line mosaic (gonadal mosaicism), which may produce disease that is not carried by parent's somatic cells.	Mutation in the embryonic precursor of the bone marrow stem cell → a hematologic mosaic individual. A chimeric individual is derived from 2 zygotes that subsequently fuse.
Locus heterogeneity	Mutations at different loci can produce the same phenotype.	Marfan's syndrome, MEN 2B, and homocystinuria; all cause marfanoid habitus. Albinism.
Heteroplasmy	Presence of both normal and mutated mtDNA, resulting in variable expression in mitochondrial inherited disease.	

Genetic terms *(continued)*

TERM	DEFINITION	EXAMPLE
Uniparental disomy	Offspring receives 2 copies of a chromosome from 1 parent and no copies from the other parent. Heterodisomy (heterozygous) indicates a meiosis I error. Isodisomy (homozygous) indicates a meiosis II error or postzygotic chromosomal duplication of one of a pair of chromosomes, and loss of the other of the original pair.	Uniparental is eUploid (correct number of chromosomes), not aneuploid. Most occurrences of UPD → normal phenotype. Consider UPD in an individual manifesting a recessive disorder when only one parent is a carrier.
Hardy-Weinberg population genetics	If a population is in Hardy-Weinberg equilibrium and if p and q are the frequencies of separate alleles, then: $p^2 + 2pq + q^2 = 1$ and $p + q = 1$, which implies that: p^2 = frequency of homozygosity for allele p q^2 = frequency of homozygosity for allele q $2pq$ = frequency of heterozygosity (carrier frequency, if an autosomal recessive disease). The frequency of an X-linked recessive disease in males = q and in females = q^2.	Hardy-Weinberg law assumes: ▪ No mutation occurring at the locus ▪ No selection for any of the genotypes at the locus ▪ Completely random mating ▪ No net migration
Imprinting	At some loci, only 1 allele is active; the other is inactive (imprinted/inactivated by methylation). With 1 allele inactivated, deletion of the active allele → disease.	Both Prader-Willi and Angelman's syndromes due to inactivation or deletion of genes on chromosome 15. Can also occur as a result of uniparental disomy.
Prader-Willi syndrome	Paternal allele is not expressed.	Mental retardation, hyperphagia, obesity, hypogonadism, hypotonia.
AngelMan's syndrome	Maternal allele is not expressed.	Mental retardation, seizures, ataxia, inappropriate laughter.

Modes of inheritance

Autosomal dominant 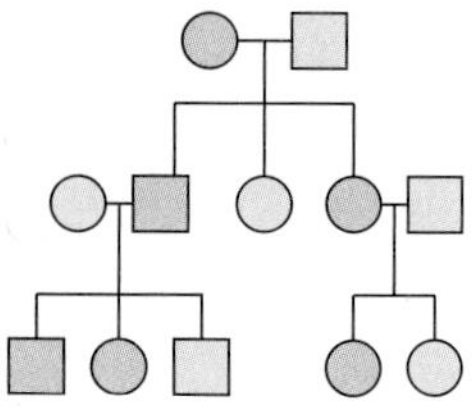	Often due to defects in structural genes. Many generations, both male and female, affected.	Often pleiotropic. Family history crucial to diagnosis.
Autosomal recessive 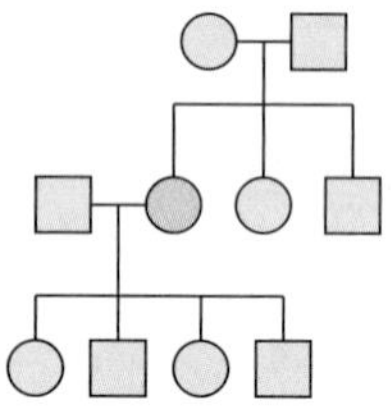	25% of offspring from 2 carrier parents are affected. Often due to enzyme deficiencies. Usually seen in only 1 generation.	Commonly more severe than dominant disorders; patients often present in childhood.
X-linked recessive 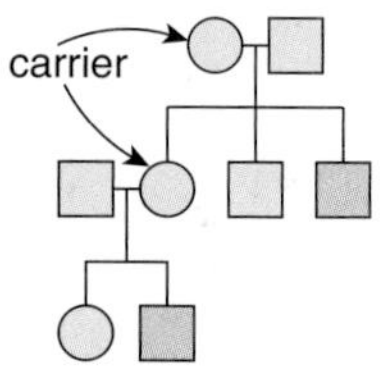	Sons of heterozygous mothers have a 50% chance of being affected. No male-to-male transmission.	Commonly more severe in males. Females usually must be homozygous to be affected.
X-linked dominant 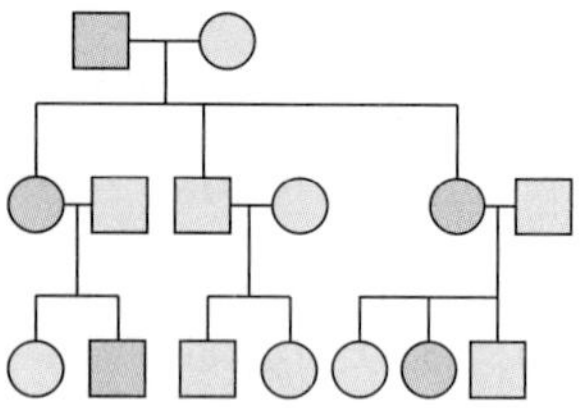	Transmitted through both parents. Either male or female offspring of the affected mother may be affected, whereas all female offspring of the affected father are affected.	**Hypophosphatemic rickets**—formerly known as vitamin D–resistant rickets. Inherited disorder resulting in ↑ phosphate wasting at proximal tubule. Results in rickets-like presentation.
Mitochondrial inheritance 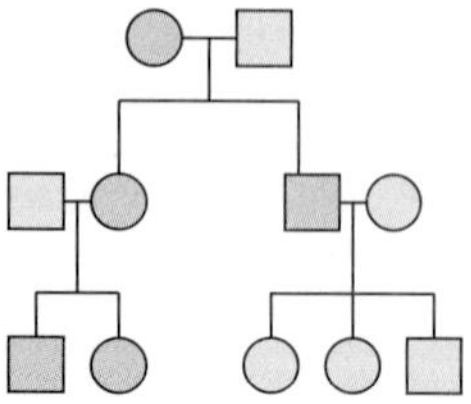	Transmitted only through mother. All offspring of affected females may show signs of disease. Often due to failures in oxidative phosphorylation.	Variable expression in population due to heteroplasmy. **Mitochondrial myopathies**—group of rare disorders resulting from mutations affecting mitochondrial function. Often present with myopathy and CNS disease. Muscle biopsy often shows "ragged red fibers."

Autosomal-dominant diseases

Achondroplasia	Cell-signaling defect of fibroblast growth factor (FGF) receptor 3. Results in dwarfism; short limbs, larger head, but trunk size is normal. Associated with advanced paternal age.
Autosomal-dominant polycystic kidney disease (ADPKD)	Formerly known as adult polycystic kidney disease. Always bilateral, massive enlargement of kidneys due to multiple large cysts. Patients present with flank pain, hematuria, hypertension, progressive renal failure. 85% of cases are due to mutation in *PKD1* (chromosome **16**; **16** letters in "polycystic kidney"). Associated with polycystic liver disease, berry aneurysms, mitral valve prolapse. Infantile form is recessive.
Familial adenomatous polyposis	Colon becomes covered with adenomatous polyps after puberty. Progresses to colon cancer unless colon is resected. Mutations on chromosome **5** (*APC* gene); **5** letters in "polyp."
Familial hypercholesterolemia (hyperlipidemia type IIA)	Elevated LDL due to defective or absent LDL receptor. Heterozygotes (1:500) have cholesterol ≈ 300 mg/dL. Homozygotes (very rare) have cholesterol ≈ 700+ mg/dL, severe atherosclerotic disease early in life, and tendon xanthomas (classically in the Achilles tendon); MI may develop before age 20.
Hereditary hemorrhagic telangiectasia (Osler-Weber-Rendu syndrome)	Inherited disorder of blood vessels. Findings: telangiectasia, recurrent epistaxis, skin discolorations, arteriovenous malformations (AVMs).
Hereditary spherocytosis	Spheroid erythrocytes due to spectrin or ankyrin defect; hemolytic anemia; ↑ MCHC. Splenectomy is curative.
Huntington's disease	Findings: depression, progressive dementia, choreiform movements, caudate atrophy, and ↓ levels of GABA and ACh in the brain. Symptoms manifest in affected individuals between the ages of 20 and 50. Gene located on chromosome **4**; trinucleotide repeat disorder: $(CAG)_n$. "**Hunting 4** food."
Marfan's syndrome	Fibrillin-1 gene mutation → connective tissue disorder affecting skeleton, heart, and eyes. Findings: tall with long extremities, pectus excavatum, hypermobile joints, and long, tapering fingers and toes (arachnodactyly); cystic medial necrosis of aorta → aortic incompetence and dissecting aortic aneurysms; floppy mitral valve. Subluxation of lenses.
Multiple endocrine neoplasias (MEN)	Several distinct syndromes (1, 2A, 2B) characterized by familial tumors of endocrine glands, including those of the pancreas, parathyroid, pituitary, thyroid, and adrenal medulla. MEN 2A and 2B are associated with *ret* gene.
Neurofibromatosis type 1 (von Recklinghausen's disease)	Findings: café-au-lait spots, neural tumors, Lisch nodules (pigmented iris hamartomas). Also marked by skeletal disorders (e.g., scoliosis) and optic pathway gliomas. On long arm of chromosome **17**; **17** letters in "von Recklinghausen."
Neurofibromatosis type 2	Bilateral acoustic schwannomas, juvenile cataracts. *NF2* gene on chromosome **22**; type **2** = **22**.
Tuberous sclerosis	Findings: facial lesions (adenoma sebaceum), hypopigmented "ash leaf spots" on skin, cortical and retinal hamartomas, seizures, mental retardation, renal cysts and renal angiomyolipomas, cardiac rhabdomyomas, ↑ incidence of astrocytomas. Incomplete penetrance, variable presentation.
von Hippel–Lindau disease	Findings: hemangioblastomas of retina/cerebellum/medulla; the majority of affected individuals develop multiple bilateral renal cell carcinomas and other tumors. Associated with deletion of *VHL* gene (tumor suppressor) on chromosome **3** (3p). Results in constitutive expression of HIF (transcription factor) and activation of angiogenic growth factors. Von Hippel–Lindau = **3** words for chromosome **3**.

Autosomal-recessive diseases	Albinism, ARPKD (formerly known as infantile polycystic kidney disease), cystic fibrosis, glycogen storage diseases, hemochromatosis, mucopolysaccharidoses (except Hunter's), phenylketonuria, sickle cell anemias, sphingolipidoses (except Fabry's), thalassemias.	
Cystic fibrosis	Autosomal-recessive defect in *CFTR* gene on chromosome 7, commonly deletion of Phe 508. CFTR channel actively secretes Cl^- in lungs and GI tract and actively reabsorbs Cl^- from sweat. Defective Cl^- channel → secretion of abnormally thick mucus that plugs lungs, pancreas, and liver → recurrent pulmonary infections (*Pseudomonas* species and *S. aureus*), chronic bronchitis, bronchiectasis, pancreatic insufficiency (malabsorption and steatorrhea), nasal polyps, and meconium ileus in newborns. Mutation often causes abnormal protein folding, resulting in degradation of channel before reaching cell surface.	Infertility in males due to bilateral absence of vas deferens. Fat-soluble vitamin deficiencies (A, D, E, K). Can present as failure to thrive in infancy. Most common lethal genetic disease of white population. ↑ concentration of Cl^- ions in sweat test is diagnostic. Treatment: N-acetylcysteine to loosen mucous plugs (cleaves disulfide bonds within mucous glycoproteins).
X-linked recessive disorders	**B**ruton's agammaglobulinemia, **W**iskott-Aldrich syndrome, **F**abry's disease, **G**6PD deficiency, **O**cular albinism, **L**esch-Nyhan syndrome, **D**uchenne's (and Becker's) muscular dystrophy, **H**unter's **S**yndrome, **H**emophilia A and B, **O**rnithine transcarbamoylase deficiency. Female carriers may be affected, and may have less severe symptoms due to random X chromosome inactivation in each cell.	**B**e **W**ise, **F**ool's **GOLD** **H**eeds **S**illy **HO**pe.
Muscular dystrophies		
Duchenne's	X-linked frameshift mutation → deletion of dystrophin gene → accelerated muscle breakdown. Weakness begins in pelvic girdle muscles and progresses superiorly. Pseudohypertrophy of calf muscles due to fibrofatty replacement of muscle; cardiac myopathy. Use of Gowers' maneuver, requiring assistance of the upper extremities to stand up, is characteristic. Onset before 5 years of age.	**D**uchenne's = **d**eleted **d**ystrophin. Dystrophin gene (*DMD*) is the longest known human gene → ↑ rate of spontaneous mutation. Dystrophin helps anchor muscle fibers, primarily in skeletal and cardiac muscle. Diagnose muscular dystrophies by ↑ CPK and muscle biopsy.
Becker's	X-linked mutated dystrophin gene. Less severe than Duchenne's. Onset in adolescence or early adulthood.	

Fragile X syndrome	X-linked defect affecting the methylation and expression of the *FMR1* gene. The 2nd most common cause of genetic mental retardation (after Down syndrome). Findings: macro-orchidism (enlarged testes), long face with a large jaw, large everted ears, autism, mitral valve prolapse.	Trinucleotide repeat disorder $(CGG)_n$. Fragile **X** = e**X**tra large testes, jaw, ears.
Trinucleotide repeat expansion diseases	**Hunting**ton's disease, **my**otonic dystrophy, **Fried**reich's ataxia, fragile **X** syndrome. Fragile **X** syndrome = $(CGG)_n$. Friedreich's ataxia = $(GAA)_n$. **H**untington's disease = $(CAG)_n$. **M**yotonic dystrophy = $(CTG)_n$.	**Try** (trinucleotide) **hunting** for **my fried eggs** (X). **X**-**G**irlfriend's **F**irst **A**id **H**elped **A**ce **M**y **T**est. May show genetic anticipation (disease severity ↑ and age of onset ↓ in successive generations).

Autosomal trisomies

Down syndrome (trisomy 21), 1:700	Findings: mental retardation, flat facies, prominent epicanthal folds, simian crease, gap between 1st 2 toes, duodenal atresia, congenital heart disease (most commonly ostium primum–type ASD). Associated with ↑ risk of ALL and Alzheimer's disease (> 35 years of age). 95% of cases due to meiotic nondisjunction of homologous chromosomes (associated with advanced maternal age; from 1:1500 in women < 20 to 1:25 in women > 45). 4% of cases due to Robertsonian translocation. 1% of cases due to Down mosaicism (no maternal association).	Drinking age (21). Most common viable chromosomal disorder and most common cause of genetic mental retardation. Results of pregnancy quad screen: ↓ α-fetoprotein, ↑ β-hCG, ↓ estriol, ↑ inhibin A. Ultrasound shows ↑ nuchal in first trimester translucency.
Edwards' syndrome (trisomy 18), 1:8000	Findings: severe mental retardation, rocker-bottom feet, micrognathia (small jaw), low-set Ears, clenched hands, prominent occiput, congenital heart disease. Death usually occurs within 1 year of birth.	Election age (18). Most common trisomy resulting in live birth after Down syndrome. Results of pregnancy quad screen: ↓ α-fetoprotein, ↓ β-hCG, ↓ estriol, normal inhibin A.
Patau's syndrome (trisomy 13), 1:15,000	Findings: severe mental retardation, rocker-bottom feet, microphthalmia, microcephaly, cleft liP/Palate, holoProsencephaly, Polydactyly, congenital heart disease. Death usually occurs within 1 year of birth.	Puberty (13). Results of first-trimester pregnancy screen: ↓ free β-hCG, ↓ PAPP-A, and ↑ nuchal translucency.

Meiotic nondisjunction

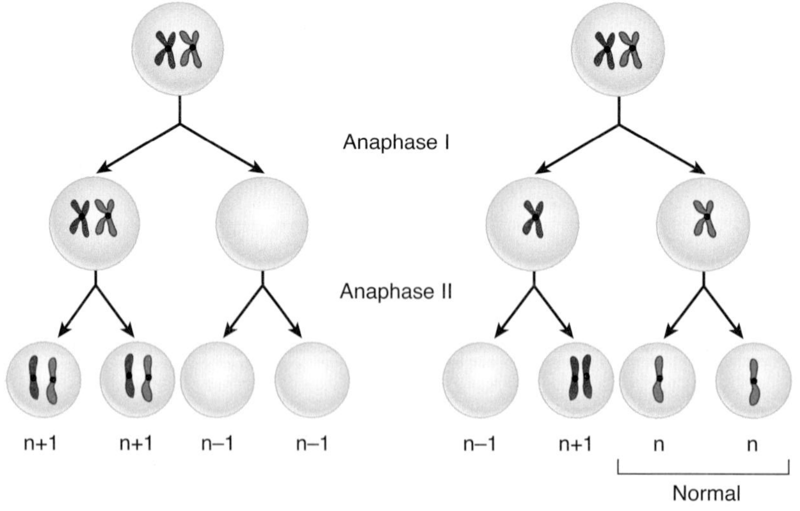

Robertsonian translocation	Nonreciprocal chromosomal translocation that commonly involves chromosome pairs 13, 14, 15, 21, and 22. One of the most common types of translocation. Occurs when the long arms of 2 acrocentric chromosomes (chromosomes with centromeres near their ends) fuse at the centromere and the 2 short arms are lost. Balanced translocations normally do not cause any abnormal phenotype. Unbalanced translocations can result in miscarriage, stillbirth, and chromosomal imbalance (e.g., Down syndrome, Patau's syndrome).

Cri-du-chat syndrome	Congenital microdeletion of short arm of chromosome 5 (46,XX or XY, 5p−). Findings: microcephaly, moderate to severe mental retardation, high-pitched crying/**mewing**, epicanthal folds, cardiac abnormalities (VSD).	*Cri du chat* = cry of the **cat**.
Williams syndrome	Congenital microdeletion of long arm of chromosome 7 (deleted region includes elastin gene). Findings: distinctive "elfin" facies, intellectual disability, hypercalcemia (↑ sensitivity to vitamin D), well-developed verbal skills, extreme friendliness with strangers, cardiovascular problems.	
22q11 deletion syndromes	Variable presentation, including **C**left palate, **A**bnormal facies, **T**hymic aplasia → T-cell deficiency, **C**ardiac defects, **H**ypocalcemia 2° to parathyroid aplasia, due to microdeletion at chromosome **22**q11. DiGeorge syndrome—thymic, parathyroid, and cardiac defects. Velocardiofacial syndrome—palate, facial, and cardiac defects.	CATCH-22. Due to aberrant development of 3rd and 4th branchial pouches.

▶ BIOCHEMISTRY–NUTRITION

Vitamins: fat soluble	A, D, E, K. Absorption dependent on gut (ileum) and pancreas. Toxicity more common than for water-soluble vitamins, because these accumulate in fat.	Malabsorption syndromes (steatorrhea), such as cystic fibrosis and sprue, or mineral oil intake can cause fat-soluble vitamin deficiencies.
Vitamins: water soluble	B_1 (thiamine: TPP) B_2 (riboflavin: FAD, FMN) B_3 (niacin: NAD^+) B_5 (pantothenic acid: CoA) B_6 (pyridoxine: PLP) B_7 (biotin) B_9 (folate) B_{12} (cobalamin) C (ascorbic acid)	All wash out easily from body except B_{12} and folate (stored in liver). B-complex deficiencies often result in dermatitis, glossitis, and diarrhea.

Vitamin A (retinol)

FUNCTION	Antioxidant; constituent of visual pigments (retinal); essential for normal differentiation of epithelial cells into specialized tissue (pancreatic cells, mucus-secreting cells); prevents squamous metaplasia. Used to treat measles and AML, subtype M3.	**Retin**ol is vitamin **A**, so think **retin-A** (used topically for wrinkles and acne). Found in liver and leafy vegetables.
DEFICIENCY	Night blindness, dry skin.	
EXCESS	Arthralgias, fatigue, headaches, skin changes, sore throat, alopecia. Teratogenic (cleft palate, cardiac abnormalities), so a negative pregnancy test and reliable contraception are needed before isotretinoin is prescribed for severe acne.	

Vitamin B_1 (thiamine)

FUNCTION	In thiamine pyrophosphate (TPP), a cofactor for several enzymes in decarboxylation reactions: ▪ Pyruvate dehydrogenase (links glycolysis to TCA cycle) ▪ α-ketoglutarate dehydrogenase (TCA cycle) ▪ Transketolase (HMP shunt) ▪ Branched-chain amino acid dehydrogenase	**α**-ketoglutarate DH, **T**ransketolase, and **P**yruvate DH required for **ATP** synthesis. Spell beriberi as **BerIBerI** to remember vitamin **B_1**. Wernicke-Korsakoff—confusion, ophthalmoplegia, ataxia (classic triad) + confabulation, personality change, memory loss (permanent). Damage to medial dorsal nucleus of thalamus, mammillary bodies. Dry beriberi—polyneuritis, symmetrical muscle wasting. Wet beriberi—high-output cardiac failure (dilated cardiomyopathy), edema.
DEFICIENCY	Impaired glucose breakdown → ATP depletion worsened by glucose infusion; highly aerobic tissues (brain and heart) are affected first. Wernicke-Korsakoff syndrome and beriberi. Seen in malnutrition as well as alcoholism (2° to malnutrition and malabsorption).	

Vitamin B_2 (riboflavin)

FUNCTION	Cofactor in oxidation and reduction (e.g., $FADH_2$).	FAD and FMN are derived from riboFlavin (B_2 = 2 ATP).
DEFICIENCY	Cheilosis (inflammation of lips, scaling and fissures at the corners of the mouth), Corneal vascularization.	The **2 C's** of B_2.

Vitamin B_3 (niacin)

FUNCTION	Constituent of NAD^+, $NADP^+$ (used in redox reactions). Derived from tryptophan. Synthesis requires vitamin B_6.	NAD derived from **N**iacin (B_3 = 3 ATP).
DEFICIENCY	Glossitis. Severe deficiency leads to pellagra, which can be caused by Hartnup disease (↓ tryptophan absorption), malignant carcinoid syndrome (↑ tryptophan metabolism), and INH (↓ vitamin B_6). Symptoms of pellagra: **D**iarrhea, **D**ementia, and **D**ermatitis.	The **3 D's** of B_3: **D**iarrhea, **D**ermatitis, **D**ementia.
EXCESS	Facial flushing (due to pharmacologic doses for treatment of hyperlipidemia).	

Vitamin B_5 (pantothenate)

FUNCTION	Essential component of CoA (a cofactor for acyl transfers) and fatty acid synthase.	B_5 is "**pento**"thenate.
DEFICIENCY	Dermatitis, enteritis, alopecia, adrenal insufficiency.	

Vitamin B_6 (pyridoxine)

FUNCTION	Converted to pyridoxal phosphate, a cofactor used in transamination (e.g., ALT and AST), decarboxylation reactions, glycogen phosphorylase. Synthesis of cystathionine, heme, niacin, histamine, and neurotransmitters including serotonin, epinephrine, norepinephrine, and GABA.
DEFICIENCY	Convulsions, hyperirritability, peripheral neuropathy (deficiency inducible by INH and oral contraceptives), sideroblastic anemias due to impaired hemoglobin synthesis and iron excess.

Vitamin B_7 (biotin)

FUNCTION	Cofactor for carboxylation enzymes (which add a 1-carbon group): ▪ Pyruvate carboxylase: pyruvate (3C) → oxaloacetate (4C) ▪ Acetyl-CoA carboxylase: acetyl-CoA (2C) → malonyl-CoA (3C) ▪ Propionyl-CoA carboxylase: propionyl-CoA (3C) → methylmalonyl-CoA (4C)	"**Avid**in in egg whites **avid**ly binds biotin."
DEFICIENCY	Relatively rare. Dermatitis, alopecia, enteritis. Caused by antibiotic use or excessive ingestion of raw eggs.	

Vitamin B_9 (folic acid)

FUNCTION	Converted to tetrahydrofolate (THF), a coenzyme for 1-carbon transfer/methylation reactions. Important for the synthesis of nitrogenous bases in DNA and RNA.	Found in leafy green vegetables. **Fol**ate from **fol**iage. Small reserve pool stored primarily in the liver.
DEFICIENCY	Macrocytic, megaloblastic anemia; no neurologic symptoms (as opposed to vitamin B_{12} deficiency). Most common vitamin deficiency in the United States. Seen in alcoholism and pregnancy.	Deficiency can be caused by several drugs (e.g., phenytoin, sulfonamides, MTX). Supplemental folic acid in early pregnancy reduces neural tube defects.

Vitamin B_{12} (cobalamin)

FUNCTION	Cofactor for homocysteine methyltransferase (transfers CH_3 groups as methylcobalamin) and methylmalonyl-CoA mutase.	Found in animal products. Synthesized only by microorganisms. Very large reserve pool (several years) stored primarily in the liver. Deficiency is usually caused by malabsorption (sprue, enteritis, *Diphyllobothrium latum*), lack of intrinsic factor (pernicious anemia, gastric bypass surgery), or absence of terminal ileum (Crohn's disease). Use Schilling test to detect the etiology of the deficiency.
DEFICIENCY	Macrocytic, megaloblastic anemia, hypersegmented PMNs, neurologic symptoms (paresthesias, subacute combined degeneration) due to abnormal myelin. Prolonged deficiency leads to irreversible nervous system damage.	

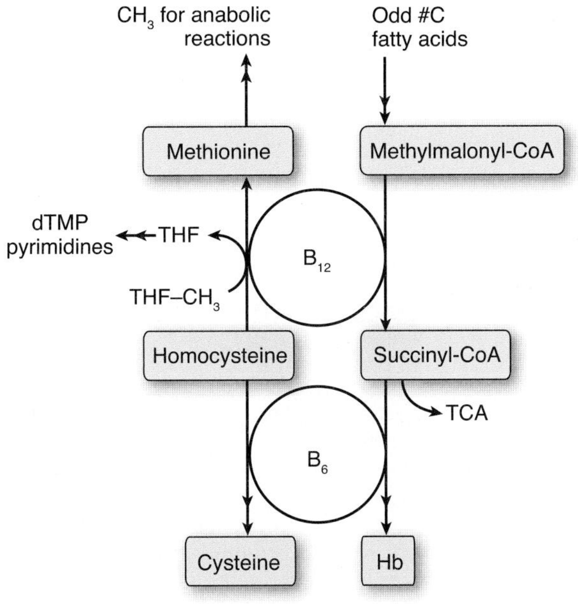

S-adenosyl-methionine

ATP + methionine → **SAM.**
SAM transfers methyl units.
Regeneration of methionine (and thus SAM) is dependent on vitamin B_{12} and folate.

SAM the methyl donor man.
Required for the conversion of NE to epinephrine.

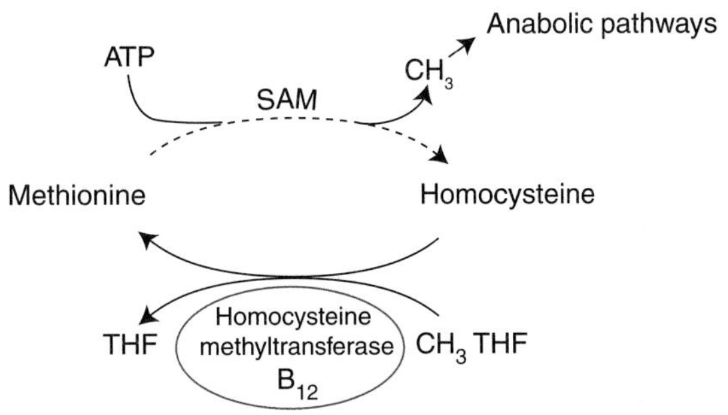

Vitamin C (ascorbic acid)

FUNCTION	Antioxidant. Also facilitates iron absorption by keeping iron in Fe^{2+} reduced state. Necessary for hydroxylation of proline and lysine in collagen synthesis. Necessary for dopamine β-hydroxylase, which converts dopamine to NE.	Found in fruits and vegetables. Pronounce "**absorbic**" acid.
DEFICIENCY	Scurvy—swollen gums, bruising, hemarthrosis, anemia, poor wound healing. Weakened immune response.	Vitamin C deficiency causes sCurvy due to a Collagen synthesis defect.
EXCESS	Nausea, vomiting, diarrhea, fatigue, sleep problems. Can ↑ risk of iron toxicity in predisposed individuals (e.g., those with transfusions, hereditary hemochromatosis).	

Vitamin D

	D_2 = ergocalciferol—ingested from plants. D_3 = cholecalciferol—consumed in milk, formed in sun-exposed skin. 25-OH D_3 = storage form. 1,25-$(OH)_2$ D_3 (calcitriol) = active form.	Drinking milk (fortified with vitamin D) is good for bones.
FUNCTION	↑ intestinal absorption of calcium and phosphate, ↑ bone mineralization.	
DEFICIENCY	Rickets A in children (bone pain and deformity), osteomalacia in adults (bone pain and muscle weakness), hypocalcemic tetany. Breast milk has ↓ vitamin D (supplement in dark-skinned patients).	
EXCESS	Hypercalcemia, hypercalciuria, loss of appetite, stupor. Seen in sarcoidosis (↑ activation of vitamin D by epithelioid macrophages).	

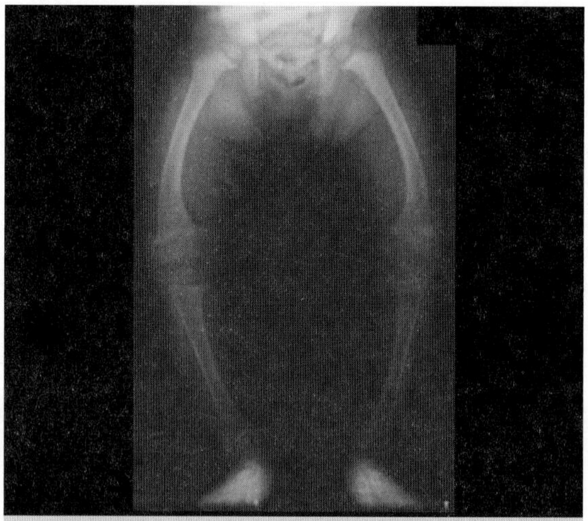

A **Rickets.** X-ray of legs in toddler shows bowing of femurs (genu varum).

Vitamin E

FUNCTION	Antioxidant (protects erythrocytes and membranes from free-radical damage).	E is for Erythrocytes.
DEFICIENCY	↑ fragility of erythrocytes (hemolytic anemia), muscle weakness, posterior column and spinocerebellar tract demyelination.	

Vitamin K

FUNCTION	Catalyzes γ-carboxylation of glutamic acid residues on various proteins concerned with blood clotting. Synthesized by intestinal flora.	**K** is for **K**oagulation. Necessary for the synthesis of clotting factors II, VII, IX, X, and proteins C and S. Warfarin—vitamin K antagonist.
DEFICIENCY	Neonatal hemorrhage with ↑ PT and ↑ aPTT but normal bleeding time (neonates have sterile intestines and are unable to synthesize vitamin K). Can also occur after prolonged use of broad-spectrum antibiotics.	Not in breast milk; neonates are given vitamin K injection at birth to prevent hemorrhage.

Zinc

FUNCTION	Essential for the activity of 100+ enzymes. Important in the formation of zinc fingers (transcription factor motif).
DEFICIENCY	Delayed wound healing, hypogonadism, ↓ adult hair (axillary, facial, pubic), dysgeusia, anosmia. May predispose to alcoholic cirrhosis.

Ethanol metabolism

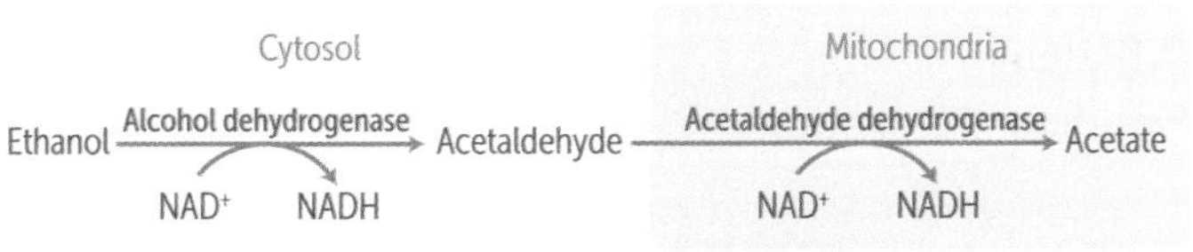
Cytosol
Mitochondria
Ethanol
Alcohol dehydrogenase
Acetaldehyde
Acetaldehyde dehydrogenase
Acetate
NAD⁺
NADH
NAD⁺
NADH

NAD^+ is the limiting reagent.

Alcohol dehydrogenase operates via zero-order kinetics.

Fomepizole—inhibits alcohol dehydrogenase and is an antidote for methanol or ethylene glycol poisoning.

Disulfiram (Antabuse)—inhibits acetaldehyde dehydrogenase (acetaldehyde accumulates, contributing to hangover symptoms).

Ethanol hypoglycemia

Ethanol metabolism ↑ NADH/NAD^+ ratio in liver, causing diversion of pyruvate to lactate and OAA to malate, thereby inhibiting gluconeogenesis and stimulating fatty acid synthesis. → hypoglycemia and hepatic fatty change (hepatocellular steatosis) seen in chronic alcoholics. Overproduction of lactate → acidosis. Depletion of oxaloacetate shuts down the TCA cycle, shunting acetyl-CoA into ketone production. Breakdown of excess malate ↑ NADPH and thus fatty acid synthesis.

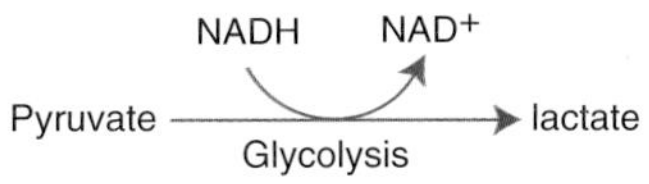
NADH
NAD+
Pyruvate
lactate
Glycolysis

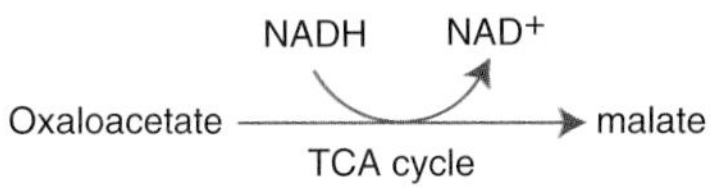
NADH
NAD+
Oxaloacetate
malate
TCA cycle

Malnutrition

Kwashiorkor	Protein malnutrition resulting in skin lesions, edema, liver malfunction (fatty change due to ↓ apolipoprotein synthesis). Clinical picture is small child with swollen belly.	Kwashiorkor results from a protein-deficient **MEAL**: **M**alnutrition **E**dema **A**nemia **L**iver (fatty)
Marasmus	Energy malnutrition resulting in tissue and muscle wasting, loss of subcutaneous fat, and variable edema.	**M**arasmus results in **M**uscle wasting.

▸ BIOCHEMISTRY–METABOLISM

Metabolism sites

Mitochondria	Fatty acid oxidation (β-oxidation), acetyl-CoA production, TCA cycle, oxidative phosphorylation.	
Cytoplasm	Glycolysis, fatty acid synthesis, HMP shunt, protein synthesis (RER), steroid synthesis (SER), cholesterol synthesis.	
Both	**H**eme synthesis, **U**rea cycle, **G**luconeogenesis.	**HUGs** take **two** (i.e., both).

Enzyme terminology

An enzyme's name often describes its function. For example, glucokinase is an enzyme that catalyzes the phosphorylation of glucose using a molecule of ATP. The following are commonly used enzyme descriptors.

Kinase	Uses ATP to add high-energy phosphate group onto substrate (e.g., phosphofructokinase)
Phosphorylase	Adds inorganic phosphate onto substrate without using ATP (e.g., glycogen phosphorylase)
Phosphatase	Removes phosphate group from substrate (e.g., fructose-1,6-bisphosphatase)
Dehydrogenase	Catalyzes oxidation-reduction reactions (e.g., pyruvate dehydrogenase)
Carboxylase	Transfers CO_2 groups with the help of biotin (e.g., pyruvate carboxylase)

Rate-determining enzymes of metabolic processes

PROCESS	ENZYME	REGULATORS
Glycolysis	Phosphofructokinase-1 (PFK-1)	AMP ⊕, fructose-2,6-BP ⊕, ATP ⊖, citrate ⊖
Gluconeogenesis	Fructose-1,6-bisphosphatase	ATP ⊕, AMP ⊖, fructose-2,6-BP ⊖
TCA cycle	Isocitrate dehydrogenase	ADP ⊕, ATP ⊖, NADH ⊖
Glycogen synthesis	Glycogen synthase	Glucose ⊕, insulin ⊕, epinephrine ⊖, glucagon ⊖
Glycogenolysis	Glycogen phosphorylase	AMP ⊕, epinephrine ⊕, glucagon ⊕, insulin ⊖, ATP ⊖
HMP shunt	Glucose-6-phosphate dehydrogenase (G6PD)	$NADP^+$ ⊕, NADPH ⊖
De novo pyrimidine synthesis	Carbamoyl phosphate synthetase II	
De novo purine synthesis	Glutamine-PRPP amidotransferase	AMP ⊖, IMP ⊖, GMP ⊖
Urea cycle	Carbamoyl phosphate synthetase I	N-acetylglutamate ⊕
Fatty acid synthesis	Acetyl-CoA carboxylase (ACC)	Insulin ⊕, citrate ⊕, glucagon ⊖, palmitoyl-CoA ⊖
Fatty acid oxidation	Carnitine acyltransferase I	Malonyl-CoA ⊖
Ketogenesis	HMG-CoA synthase	
Cholesterol synthesis	HMG-CoA reductase	Insulin ⊕, thyroxine ⊕, glucagon ⊖, cholesterol ⊖

Summary of pathways

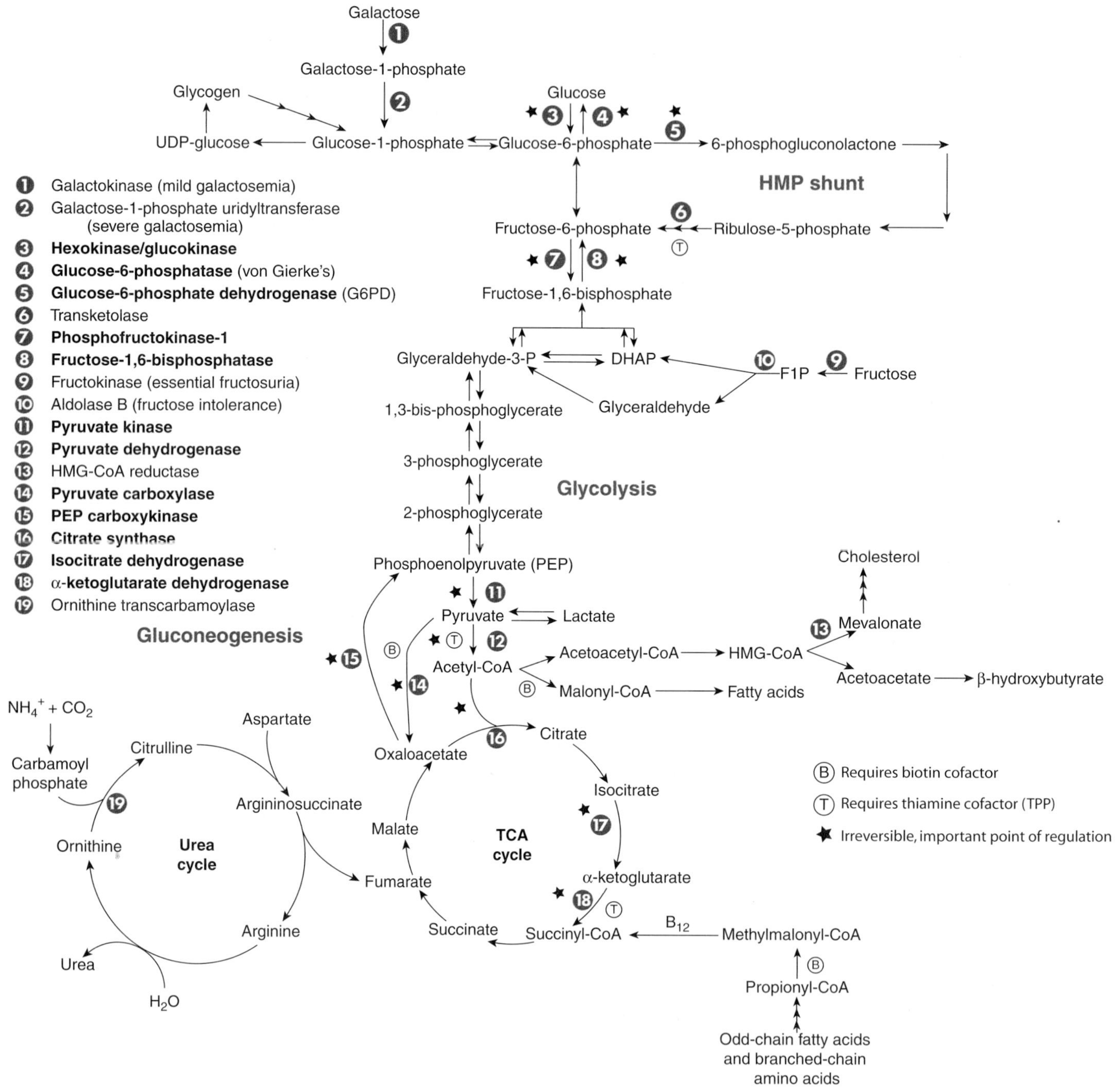
Galactose
Galactose-1-phosphate
Glycogen
UDP-glucose
Glucose-1-phosphate
Glucose
Glucose-6-phosphate
6-phosphogluconolactone
HMP shunt
Fructose-6-phosphate
Ribulose-5-phosphate
Fructose-1,6-bisphosphate
Glyceraldehyde-3-P
DHAP
F1P
Fructose
Glyceraldehyde
1,3-bis-phosphoglycerate
3-phosphoglycerate
Glycolysis
2-phosphoglycerate
Phosphoenolpyruvate (PEP)
Pyruvate
Lactate
Acetyl-CoA
Acetoacetyl-CoA
HMG-CoA
Mevalonate
Cholesterol
Acetoacetate
β-hydroxybutyrate
Malonyl-CoA
Fatty acids
Gluconeogenesis
Oxaloacetate
Citrate
Isocitrate
α-ketoglutarate
Succinyl-CoA
Succinate
Fumarate
Malate
TCA cycle
B12
Methylmalonyl-CoA
Propionyl-CoA
Odd-chain fatty acids and branched-chain amino acids
$NH_4^+ + CO_2$
Carbamoyl phosphate
Citrulline
Aspartate
Argininosuccinate
Ornithine
Urea cycle
Arginine
Urea
H_2O
1 Galactokinase (mild galactosemia)
2 Galactose-1-phosphate uridyltransferase (severe galactosemia)
3 Hexokinase/glucokinase
4 Glucose-6-phosphatase (von Gierke's)
5 Glucose-6-phosphate dehydrogenase (G6PD)
6 Transketolase
7 Phosphofructokinase-1
8 Fructose-1,6-bisphosphatase
9 Fructokinase (essential fructosuria)
10 Aldolase B (fructose intolerance)
11 Pyruvate kinase
12 Pyruvate dehydrogenase
13 HMG-CoA reductase
14 Pyruvate carboxylase
15 PEP carboxykinase
16 Citrate synthase
17 Isocitrate dehydrogenase
18 α-ketoglutarate dehydrogenase
19 Ornithine transcarbamoylase
B Requires biotin cofactor
T Requires thiamine cofactor (TPP)
★ Irreversible, important point of regulation

ATP production

Aerobic metabolism of glucose produces 32 ATP via malate-aspartate shuttle (heart and liver), 30 ATP via glycerol-3-phosphate shuttle (muscle).
Anaerobic glycolysis produces only 2 net ATP per glucose molecule.
ATP hydrolysis can be coupled to energetically unfavorable reactions.

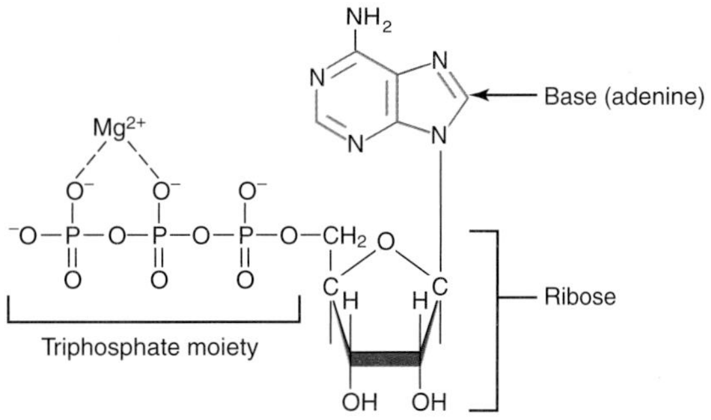

Activated carriers

CARRIER MOLECULE	CARRIED IN ACTIVATED FORM
ATP	Phosphoryl groups
NADH, NADPH, $FADH_2$	Electrons
Coenzyme A, lipoamide	Acyl groups
Biotin	CO_2
Tetrahydrofolates	1-carbon units
SAM	CH_3 groups
TPP	Aldehydes

Universal electron acceptors

Nicotinamides (NAD^+ from vitamin B_3, $NADP^+$) and flavin nucleotides (FAD^+ from vitamin B_2).
NAD^+ is generally used in **catabolic** processes to carry reducing equivalents away as NADH.
NADPH is used in **anabolic** processes (steroid and fatty acid synthesis) as a supply of reducing equivalents.

NADPH is a product of the HMP shunt.
NADPH is used in:
- Anabolic processes
- Respiratory burst
- P-450
- Glutathione reductase

Hexokinase vs. glucokinase

Phosphorylation of glucose to yield glucose-6-phosphate serves as the 1st step of glycolysis (also serves as the 1st step of glycogen synthesis in the liver). Reaction is catalyzed by either hexokinase or glucokinase, depending on the tissue.

Hexokinase	Ubiquitous. High affinity (low K_m), low capacity (low V_{max}), uninduced by insulin.	Feedback inhibited by glucose-6-phosphate.
Glucokinase	Liver and β cells of pancreas. Low affinity (high K_m), high capacity (high V_{max}), induced by insulin. (**glu**cokinase is a **glu**tton. It has a high V_{max} because it cannot be satisfied.)	At low glucose concentrations, hexokinase sequesters glucose in the tissue. At high glucose concentrations, excess glucose is stored in the liver.

Glycolysis regulation, key enzymes

Net glycolysis (cytoplasm):
Glucose + 2 P_i + 2 ADP + 2 NAD^+ → 2 pyruvate + 2 ATP + 2 NADH + 2 H^+ + 2 H_2O.

Equation not balanced chemically, and exact balanced equation depends on ionization state of reactants and products.

REQUIRE ATP

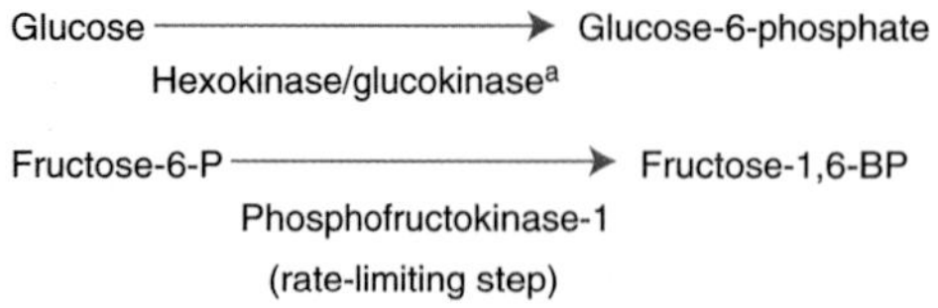
Glucose
Glucose-6-phosphate
Hexokinase/glucokinase[a]
Fructose-6-P
Fructose-1,6-BP
Phosphofructokinase-1
(rate-limiting step)

[a]Glucokinase in liver; hexokinase in all other tissues.

Glucose-6-P ⊖ hexokinase.
Fructose-6-P ⊖ glucokinase.
ATP ⊖, AMP ⊕, citrate ⊖, fructose-2,6-BP ⊕.

PRODUCE ATP

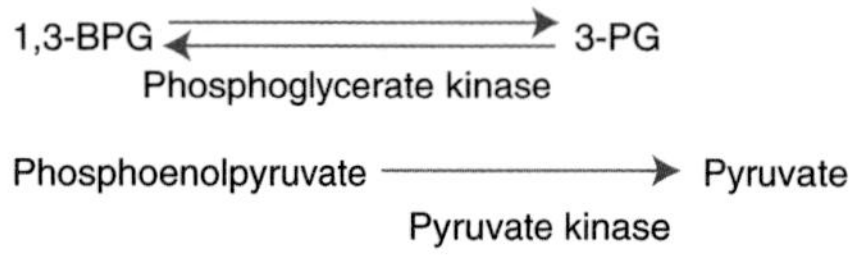
1,3-BPG
3-PG
Phosphoglycerate kinase
Phosphoenolpyruvate
Pyruvate
Pyruvate kinase

ATP ⊖, alanine ⊖, fructose-1,6-BP ⊕.

Regulation by F2,6BP

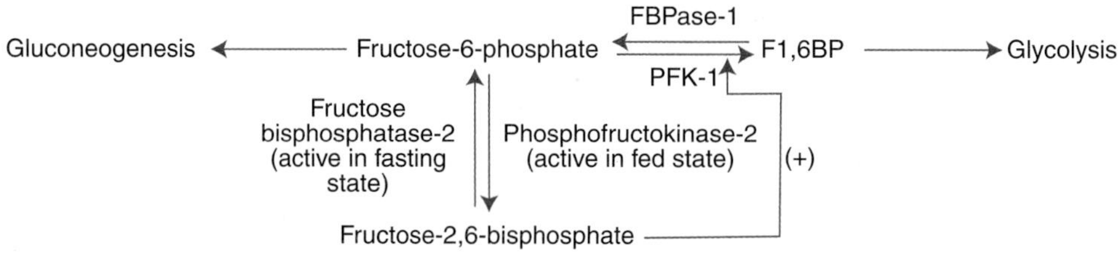
FBPase-1
Gluconeogenesis
Fructose-6-phosphate
F1,6BP
Glycolysis
PFK-1
Fructose bisphosphatase-2 (active in fasting state)
Phosphofructokinase-2 (active in fed state)
(+)
Fructose-2,6-bisphosphate

FBPase-2 and PFK-2 are part of the same complex but respond in opposite manners to phosphorylation by protein kinase A.
Fasting state: ↑ glucagon → ↑ cAMP → ↑ protein kinase A → ↑ FBPase-2, ↓ PFK-2, less glycolysis.
Fed state: ↑ insulin → ↓ cAMP → ↓ protein kinase A → ↓ FBPase-2, ↑ PFK-2, more glycolysis.

Pyruvate dehydrogenase complex

Reaction: pyruvate + NAD^+ + CoA → acetyl-CoA + CO_2 + NADH.
The complex contains 3 enzymes that require 5 cofactors:
1. Pyrophosphate (B_1, thiamine; TPP)
2. FAD (B_2, riboflavin)
3. NAD (B_3, niacin)
4. CoA (B_5, pantothenate)
5. Lipoic acid

Activated by exercise:
- ↑ NAD^+/NADH ratio
- ↑ ADP
- ↑ Ca^{2+}

The complex is similar to the α-ketoglutarate dehydrogenase complex (same cofactors, similar substrate and action), which converts α-ketoglutarate → succinyl-CoA (TCA cycle).
Arsenic inhibits lipoic acid. Findings: vomiting, rice water stools, garlic breath.

Pyruvate dehydrogenase complex deficiency

Causes backup of substrate (pyruvate and alanine) resulting in lactic acidosis. Most cases are due to mutations in X-linked gene for E1-α subunit of PDC.
Findings: neurologic defects, usually starting in infancy.
Treatment: ↑ intake of ketogenic nutrients (e.g., high fat content or ↑ lysine and leucine).

Lysine and Leucine—the onLy pureLy ketogenic amino acids.

Pyruvate metabolism

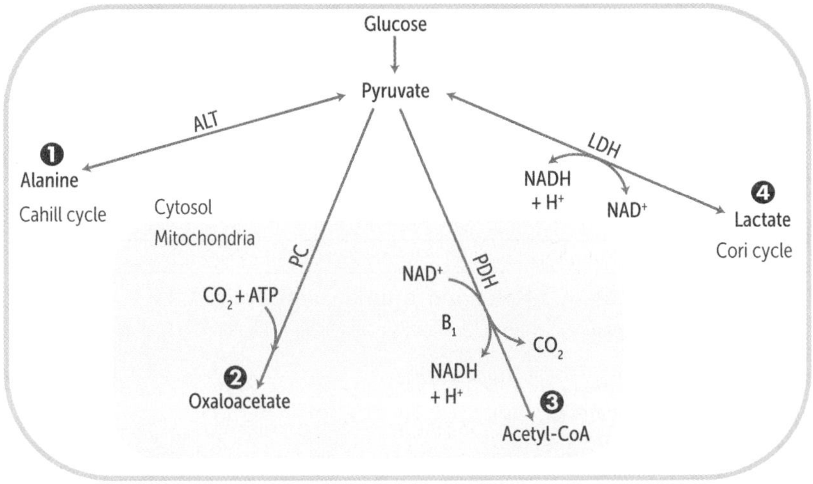

Functions of different pyruvate metabolic pathways:
❶ Alanine aminotransferase (B_6): alanine carries amino groups to the liver from muscle
❷ Pyruvate carboxylase (biotin): oxaloacetate can replenish TCA cycle or be used in gluconeogenesis
❸ Pyruvate dehydrogenase (B_1, B_2, B_3, B_5, lipoic acid): transition from glycolysis to the TCA cycle
❹ Lactic acid dehydrogenase (B_3): end of anaerobic glycolysis (major pathway in RBCs, leukocytes, kidney medulla, lens, testes, and cornea)

TCA cycle (Krebs cycle)

Pyruvate → acetyl-CoA produces 1 NADH, 1 CO_2.

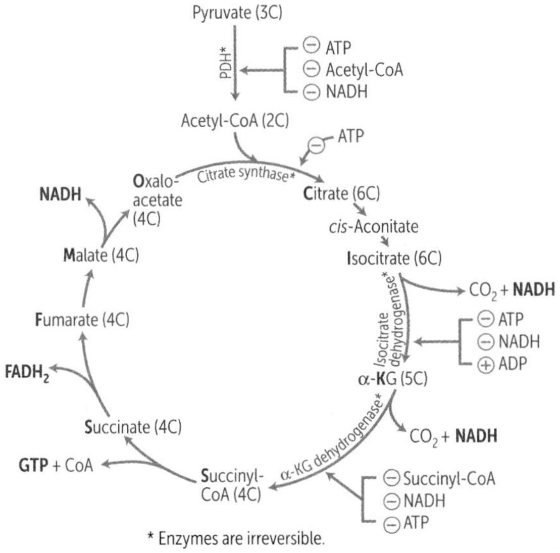

The TCA cycle produces 3 NADH, 1 $FADH_2$, 2 CO_2, 1 GTP per acetyl-CoA = 10 ATP/acetyl-CoA (2× everything per glucose). TCA cycle reactions occur in the mitochondria.
α-ketoglutarate dehydrogenase complex requires the same cofactors as the pyruvate dehydrogenase complex (B_1, B_2, B_3, B_5, lipoic acid).
Citrate Is Krebs' Starting Substrate For Making Oxaloacetate.

Electron transport chain and oxidative phosphorylation

NADH electrons from glycolysis enter mitochondria via the malate-aspartate or glycerol-3-phosphate shuttle. $FADH_2$ electrons are transferred to complex II (at a lower energy level than NADH). The passage of electrons results in the formation of a proton gradient that, coupled to oxidative phosphorylation, drives the production of ATP.

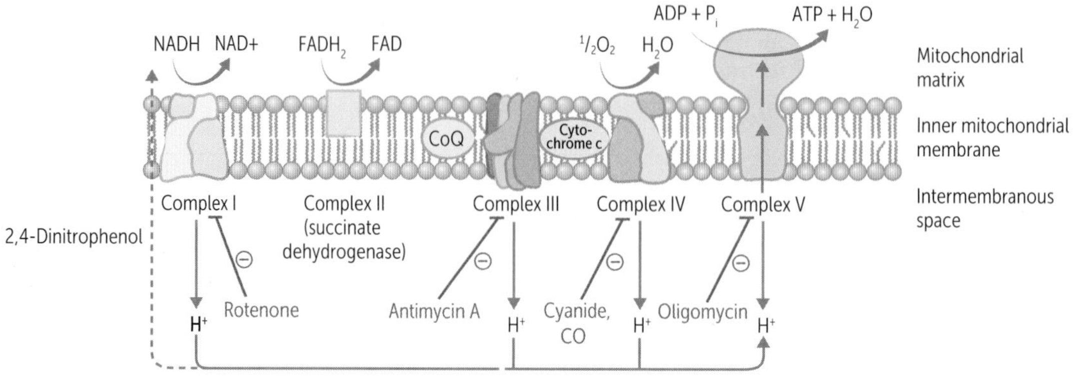

ATP PRODUCED VIA ATP SYNTHASE		
	1 NADH → 3 ATP; 1 $FADH_2$ → 2 ATP.	
OXIDATIVE PHOSPHORYLATION POISONS		
Electron transport inhibitors	Directly inhibit electron transport, causing a ↓ proton gradient and block of ATP synthesis.	Rotenone, cyanide, antimycin A, CO.
ATP synthase inhibitors	Directly inhibit mitochondrial ATPsynthase, causing an ↑ proton gradient. No ATP is produced because electron transport stops.	Oligomycin.
Uncoupling agents	↑ permeability of membrane, causing a ↓ proton gradient and ↑ O_2 consumption. ATP synthesis stops, but electron transport continues. Produces heat.	2,4-DNP, aspirin (fevers often occur after aspirin overdose), thermogenin in brown fat.

Gluconeogenesis, irreversible enzymes		Pathway Produces Fresh Glucose.
Pyruvate carboxylase	In mitochondria. Pyruvate → oxaloacetate.	Requires biotin, ATP. Activated by acetyl-CoA.
PEP carboxykinase	In cytosol. Oxaloacetate → phosphoenolpyruvate.	Requires GTP.
Fructose-1,6-bisphosphatase	In cytosol. Fructose-1,6-bisphosphate → fructose-6-P.	
Glucose-6-phosphatase	In ER. Glucose-6-P → glucose.	

Occurs primarily in liver. Enzymes also found in kidney, intestinal epithelium. Deficiency of the key gluconeogenic enzymes causes hypoglycemia. (Muscle cannot participate in gluconeogenesis because it lacks glucose-6-phosphatase).

Odd-chain fatty acids yield 1 propionyl-CoA during metabolism, which can enter the TCA cycle (as succinyl-CoA), undergo gluconeogenesis, and serve as a glucose source. Even-chain fatty acids cannot produce new glucose, since they yield only acetyl-CoA equivalents.

HMP shunt (pentose phosphate pathway)

Provides a source of NADPH from an abundantly available glucose-6-phosphate (NADPH is required for reductive reactions, e.g., glutathione reduction inside RBCs). Additionally, this pathway yields ribose for nucleotide synthesis and glycolytic intermediates. 2 distinct phases (oxidative and nonoxidative), both of which occur in the cytoplasm. No ATP is used or produced.

Sites: lactating mammary glands, liver, adrenal cortex (sites of fatty acid or steroid synthesis), RBCs.

REACTIONS	KEY ENZYMES	PRODUCTS
Oxidative (irreversible)	Glucose-6-P_i → (NADP$^+$ → NADPH) **Glucose-6-P dehydrogenase**, Rate-limiting step (inhibited by NADPH)	CO_2, 2 NADPH, Ribulose-5-P_i
Nonoxidative (reversible)	Ribulose-5-P_i → **Phosphopentose isomerase, transketolases**, Requires B_1	Ribose-5-P_i, G3P, F6P

Respiratory burst (oxidative burst)

Involves the activation of membrane-bound NADPH oxidase (e.g., in neutrophils, monocytes). Plays an important role in the immune response → rapid release of reactive oxygen intermediates (ROIs). Note that NADPH plays a role in the creation of ROIs and in their neutralization.

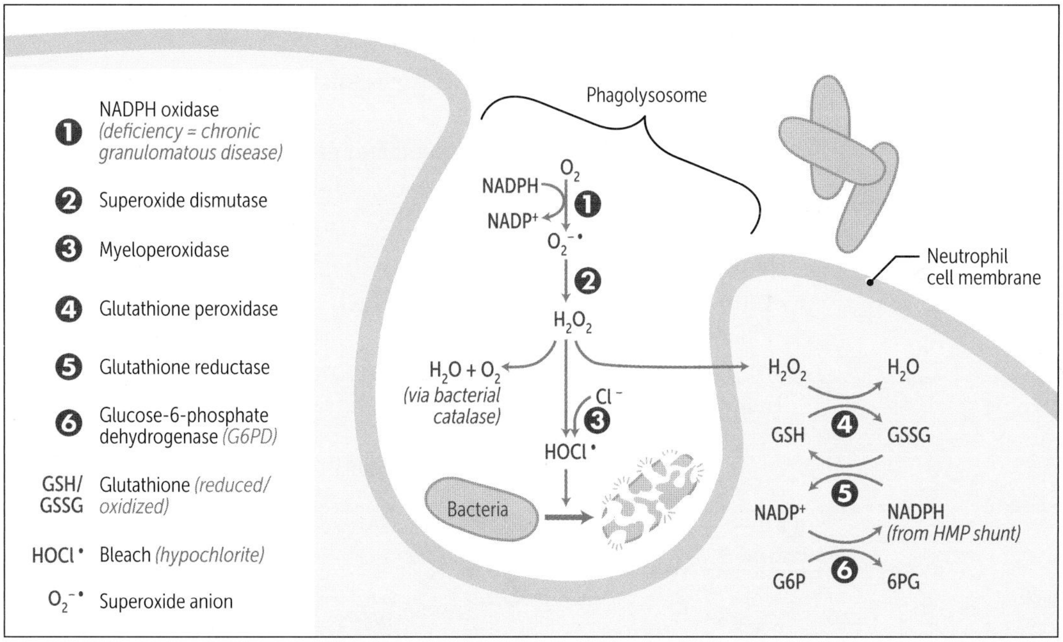

WBCs of patients with CGD can utilize H_2O_2 generated by invading organisms and convert it to ROIs. Patients are at ↑ risk for infection by catalase-positive species (e.g., *S. aureus*, *Aspergillus*) because they neutralize their own H_2O_2, leaving WBCs without ROIs for fighting infections.

Glucose-6-phosphate dehydrogenase deficiency

NADPH is necessary to keep glutathione reduced, which in turn detoxifies free radicals and peroxides. ↓ NADPH in RBCs leads to hemolytic anemia due to poor RBC defense against oxidizing agents (e.g., fava beans, sulfonamides, primaquine, antituberculosis drugs). Infection can also precipitate hemolysis (free radicals generated via inflammatory response can diffuse into RBCs and cause oxidative damage).

X-linked recessive disorder; most common human enzyme deficiency; more prevalent among blacks. ↑ malarial resistance.

Heinz bodies—oxidized **H**emoglobin precipitated within RBCs.

Bite cells—result from the phagocytic removal of **Heinz** bodies by splenic macrophages. Think, "**Bite** into some **Heinz** ketchup."

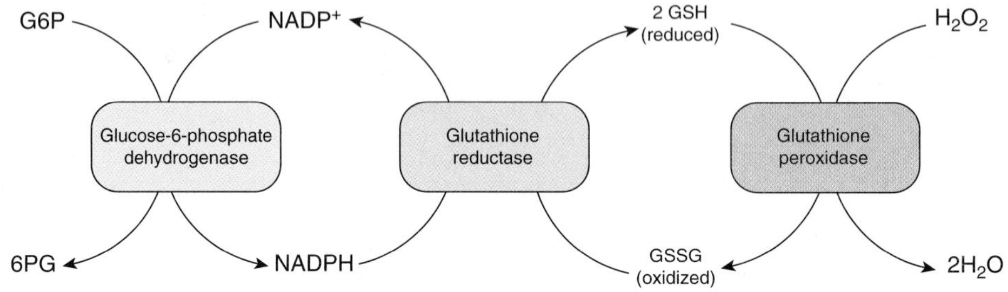

Disorders of fructose metabolism

Essential fructosuria

Involves a defect in **fructokinase.** Autosomal recessive. A benign, asymptomatic condition, since fructose is not trapped in cells.

Symptoms: fructose appears in blood and urine.

Disorders of fructose metabolism cause milder symptoms than analogous disorders of galactose metabolism.

Fructose intolerance

Hereditary deficiency of **aldolase B.** Autosomal recessive. Fructose-1-phosphate accumulates, causing a ↓ in available phosphate, which results in inhibition of glycogenolysis and gluconeogenesis.

Symptoms: hypoglycemia, jaundice, cirrhosis, vomiting.

Treatment: ↓ intake of both fructose and sucrose (glucose + fructose).

Fructose metabolism (liver)

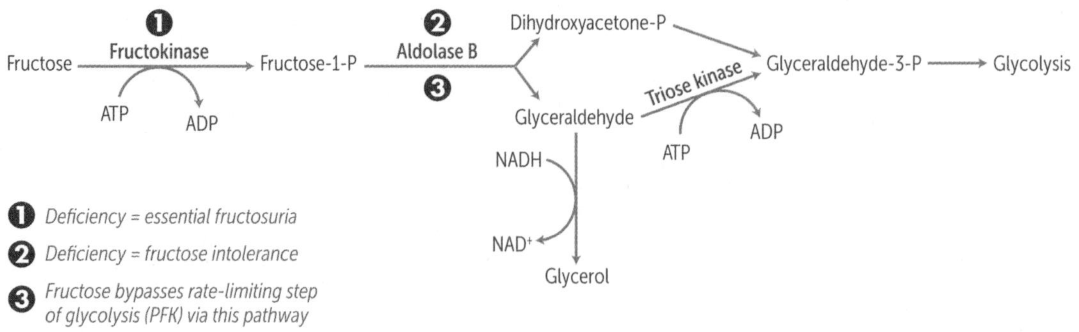

Disorders of galactose metabolism

Galactokinase deficiency

Hereditary deficiency of **galactokinase.** Galactitol accumulates if galactose is present in diet. Relatively mild condition. Autosomal recessive.

Symptoms: galactose appears in blood and urine, infantile cataracts. May initially present as failure to track objects or to develop a social smile.

Classic galactosemia

Absence of **galactose-1-phosphate uridyltransferase.** Autosomal recessive. Damage is caused by accumulation of toxic substances (including galactitol, which accumulates in the lens of the eye).

Symptoms: failure to thrive, jaundice, hepatomegaly, infantile cataracts, mental retardation.

Treatment: exclude galactose and lactose (galactose + glucose) from diet.

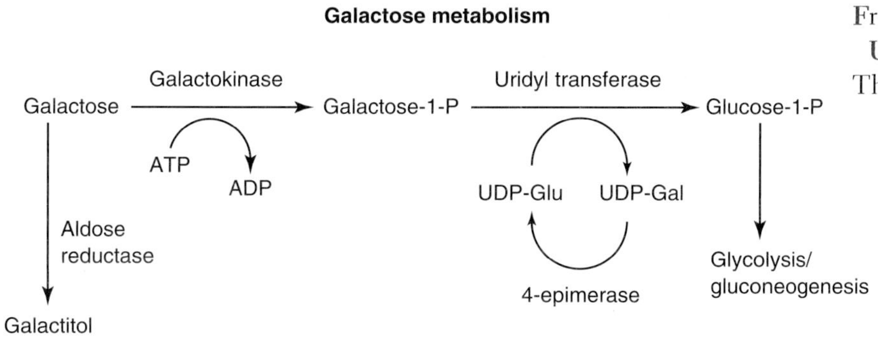

Fructose is to Aldolase B as Galactose is to UridylTransferase (**FAB GUT**).

The more serious defects lead to PO_4 depletion.

Sorbitol

An alternative method of trapping glucose in the cell is to convert it to its alcohol counterpart, called sorbitol, via aldose reductase. Some tissues then convert sorbitol to fructose using sorbitol dehydrogenase; tissues with an insufficient amount of this enzyme are at risk for intracellular sorbitol accumulation, causing osmotic damage (e.g., cataracts, retinopathy, and peripheral neuropathy seen with chronic hyperglycemia in diabetes).

High blood levels of galactose also result in conversion to osmotically active alcohol forms via aldose reductase.

Liver, lens, ovaries, and seminal vesicles have both enzymes.

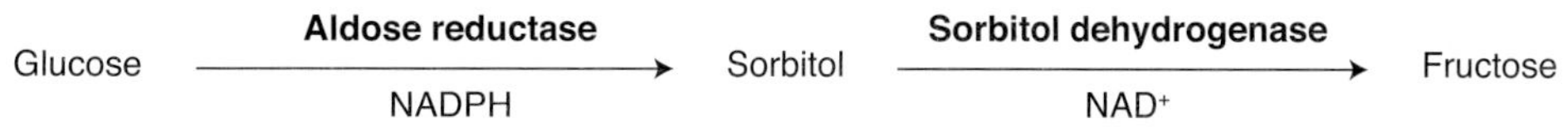

Schwann cells, retina, and kidneys have only aldose reductase.

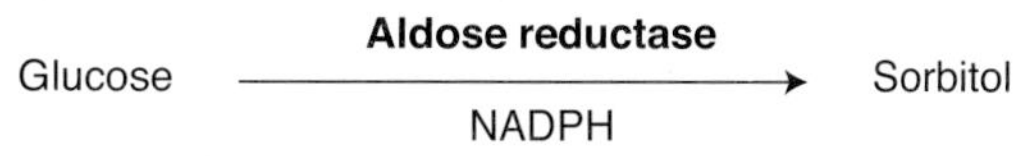

Lactase deficiency

Age-dependent and/or hereditary lactose intolerance (African Americans, Asians) due to loss of brush-border enzyme. May also follow gastroenteritis.

Symptoms: bloating, cramps, osmotic diarrhea.

Treatment: avoid dairy products or add lactase pills to diet.

Amino acids	Only L-form amino acids are found in proteins.	
Essential	Glucogenic: Met, Val, His. Glucogenic/ketogenic: Ile, Phe, Thr, Trp. Ketogenic: Leu, Lys.	All essential amino acids need to be supplied in the diet.
Acidic	Asp and Glu (negatively charged at body pH).	
Basic	Arg, Lys, and His. Arg is most basic. His has no charge at body pH.	Arg and His are required during periods of growth. Arg and Lys are ↑ in histones, which bind negatively charged DNA.

Urea cycle	Amino acid catabolism results in the formation of common metabolites (e.g., pyruvate, acetyl-CoA), which serve as metabolic fuels. Excess nitrogen (NH_4^+) generated by this process is converted to urea and excreted by the kidneys.	**O**rdinarily, **C**areless **C**rappers **A**re **A**lso **F**rivolous **A**bout **U**rination.

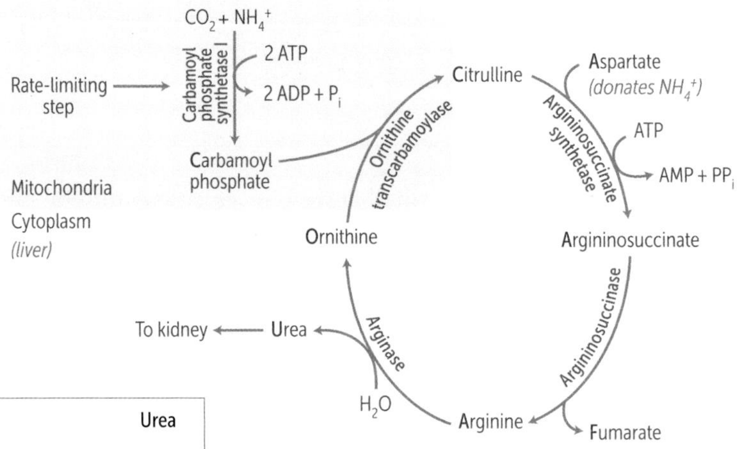

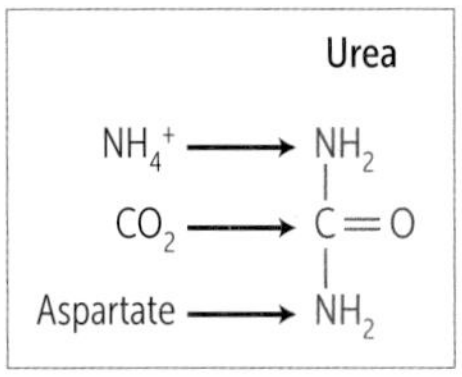

Transport of ammonium by alanine and glutamate

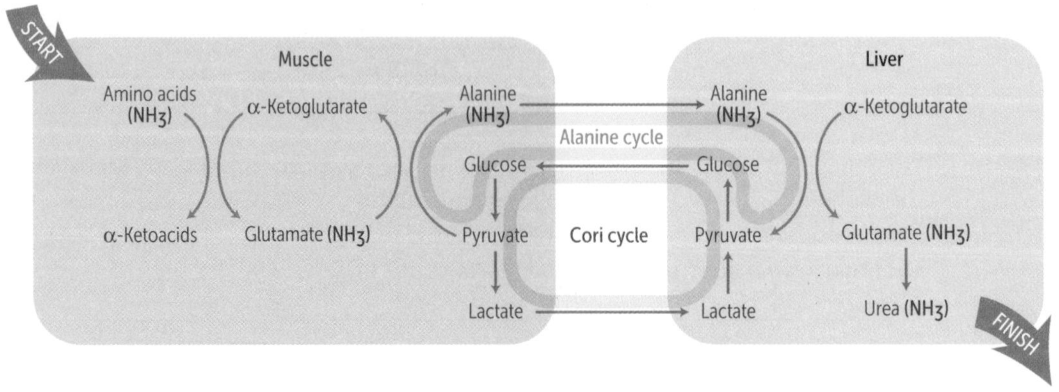

Hyperammonemia

Can be acquired (e.g., liver disease) or hereditary (e.g., urea cycle enzyme deficiencies).

Results in excess NH_4^+, which depletes α-ketoglutarate, leading to inhibition of TCA cycle.

Treatment: limit protein in diet. Benzoate or phenylbutyrate (both of which bind amino acid and lead to excretion) may be given to ↓ ammonia levels. Lactulose to acidify the GI tract and trap NH_4^+ for excretion.

Ammonia intoxication—tremor (asterixis), slurring of speech, somnolence, vomiting, cerebral edema, blurring of vision.

Ornithine transcarbamoylase deficiency

Most common urea cycle disorder. X-linked recessive (vs. other urea cycle enzyme deficiencies, which are autosomal recessive). Interferes with the body's ability to eliminate ammonia. Often evident in the first few days of life, but may present with late onset. Excess carbamoyl phosphate is converted to orotic acid (part of the pyrimidine synthesis pathway).

Findings: ↑ orotic acid in blood and urine, ↓ BUN, symptoms of hyperammonemia.

Amino acid derivatives

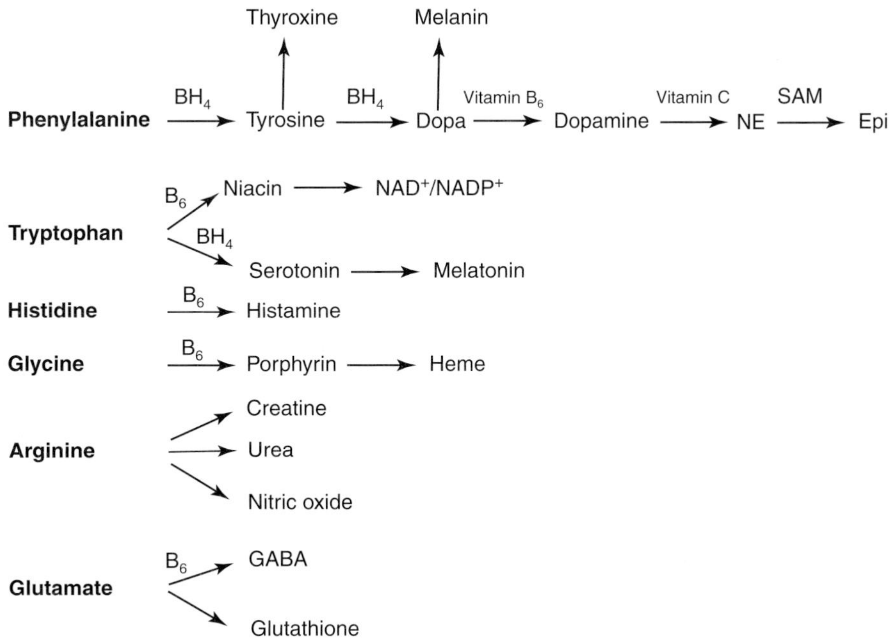

Catecholamine synthesis/tyrosine catabolism

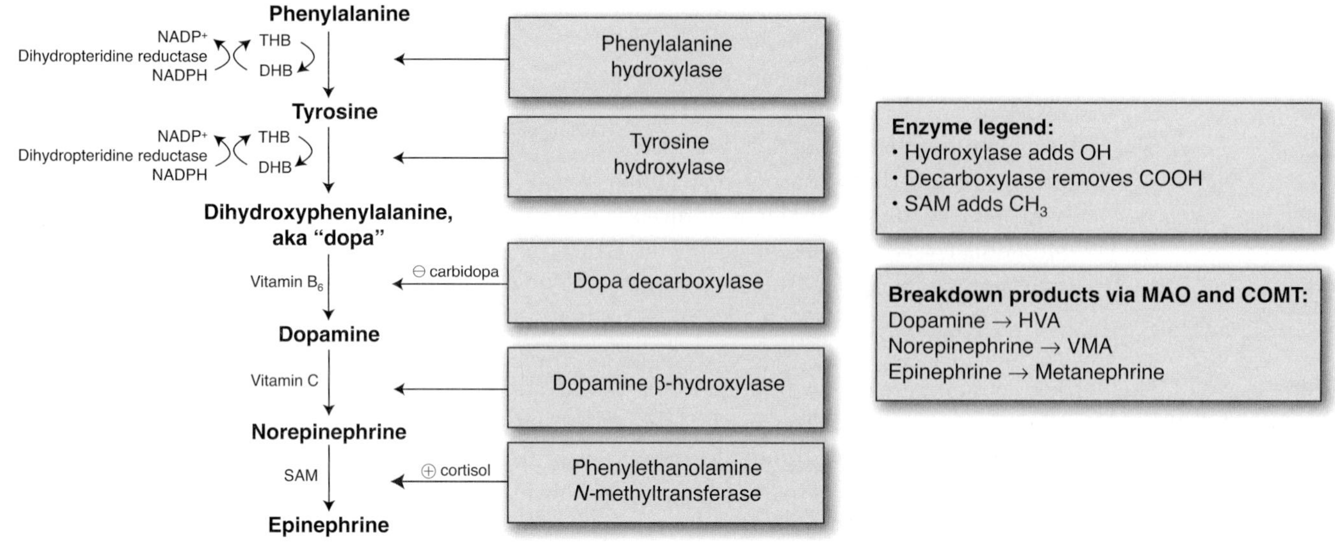
Phenylalanine
NADP+
Dihydropteridine reductase
NADPH
THB
DHB
Phenylalanine hydroxylase
Tyrosine
NADP+
Dihydropteridine reductase
NADPH
THB
DHB
Tyrosine hydroxylase
Dihydroxyphenylalanine, aka "dopa"
Vitamin B_6
⊖ carbidopa
Dopa decarboxylase
Dopamine
Vitamin C
Dopamine β-hydroxylase
Norepinephrine
SAM
⊕ cortisol
Phenylethanolamine *N*-methyltransferase
Epinephrine
Enzyme legend:
• Hydroxylase adds OH
• Decarboxylase removes COOH
• SAM adds CH_3
Breakdown products via MAO and COMT:
Dopamine → HVA
Norepinephrine → VMA
Epinephrine → Metanephrine

Phenylketonuria

Due to ↓ phenylalanine hydroxylase or ↓ tetrahydrobiopterin cofactor (malignant phenylketonuria). Tyrosine becomes essential. ↑ phenylalanine leads to excess phenylketones in urine.

Findings: mental retardation, growth retardation, seizures, fair skin, eczema, musty body odor.

Treatment: ↓ phenylalanine (contained in aspartame [e.g., NutraSweet]) and ↑ tyrosine in diet.

Maternal PKU—lack of proper dietary therapy during pregnancy. Findings in infant: microcephaly, mental retardation, growth retardation, congenital heart defects.

Autosomal recessive. Incidence ≈ 1:10,000.

Screened for 2–3 days after birth (normal at birth because of maternal enzyme during fetal life).

Phenylketones—phenylacetate, phenyllactate, and phenylpyruvate.

Disorder of **aromatic** amino acid metabolism → musty body **odor.**

Alkaptonuria (ochronosis)

Congenital deficiency of homogentisic acid oxidase in the degradative pathway of tyrosine to fumarate. Autosomal recessive. Benign disease.

Findings: dark connective tissue, brown pigmented sclera, urine turns black on prolonged exposure to air. May have debilitating arthralgias (homogentisic acid toxic to cartilage).

Albinism

Congenital deficiency of either of the following:
- Tyrosinase (inability to synthesize melanin from tyrosine)—autosomal recessive
- Defective tyrosine transporters (↓ amounts of tyrosine and thus melanin)

Can result from a lack of migration of neural crest cells.

Lack of melanin results in an ↑ risk of skin cancer.

Variable inheritance due to locus heterogeneity (vs. ocular albinism—X-linked recessive).

Homocystinuria

3 forms (all autosomal recessive):

- Cystathionine synthase deficiency (treatment: ↓ Met and ↑ Cys, and ↑ B_{12} and folate in diet)
- ↓ affinity of cystathionine synthase for pyridoxal phosphate (treatment: ↑↑ vitamin B_6 in diet)
- Homocysteine methyltransferase (requires B_{12}) deficiency

All forms result in excess homocysteine. Cysteine becomes essential.

Findings: ↑↑ homocysteine in urine, mental retardation, osteoporosis, tall stature, kyphosis, lens subluxation (downward and inward), and atherosclerosis (stroke and MI).

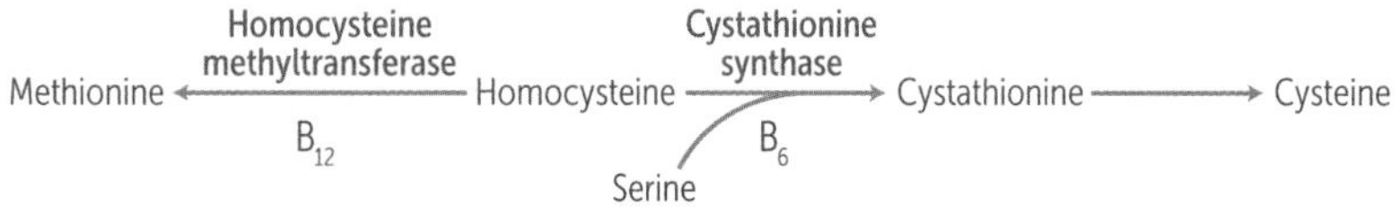

Cystinuria

Hereditary defect of renal tubular amino acid transporter for cysteine, ornithine, lysine, and arginine in the PCT of the kidneys.

Excess cystine in the urine can lead to precipitation of hexagonal crystals and renal staghorn calculi.

Autosomal recessive. Common (1:7000). Treatment: good hydration and urinary alkalinization.

Cystine is made of 2 cysteines connected by a disulfide bond.

Maple syrup urine disease

Blocked degradation of **branched** amino acids (Ile, Leu, Val) due to ↓ α-ketoacid dehydrogenase (B_1). Causes ↑ α-ketoacids in the blood, especially Leu.

Causes severe CNS defects, mental retardation, and death.

Autosomal recessive.

Urine smells like maple syrup.

I Love Vermont maple syrup from maple trees (with **branches**).

Hartnup disease

An autosomal-recessive disorder characterized by defective neutral amino acid transporter on renal and intestinal epithelial cells.

Causes tryptophan excretion in urine and ↓ absorption from the gut. Leads to pellagra.

Glycogen regulation by insulin and glucagon/epinephrine

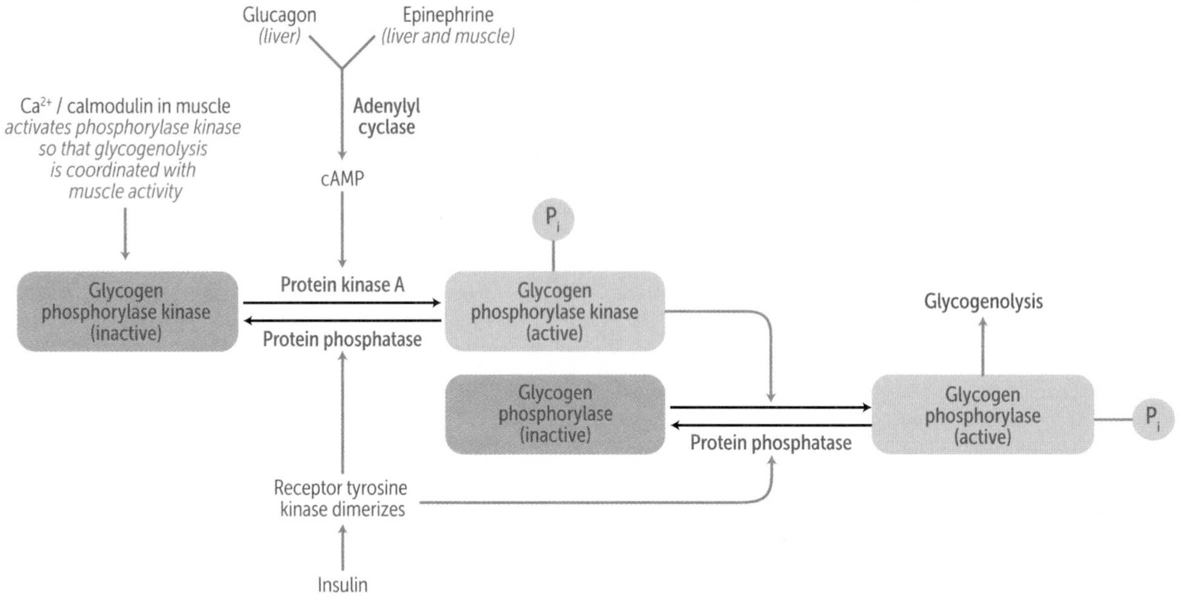

Glycogen	Branches have α (1,6) bonds; linkages have α (1,4) bonds.
Skeletal muscle	Glycogen undergoes glycogenolysis → glucose-1-phosphate → glucose-6-phosphate, which is rapidly metabolized during exercise.
Hepatocytes	Glycogen is stored and undergoes glycogenolysis to maintain blood sugar at appropriate levels.

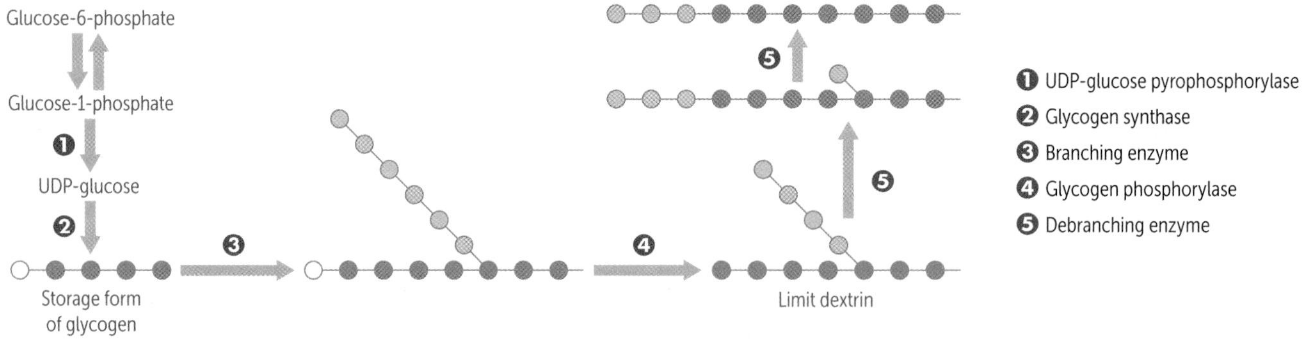

Note: A small amount of glycogen is degraded in lysosomes by α-1,4-glucosidase.

Glycogenolysis/glycogen synthesis

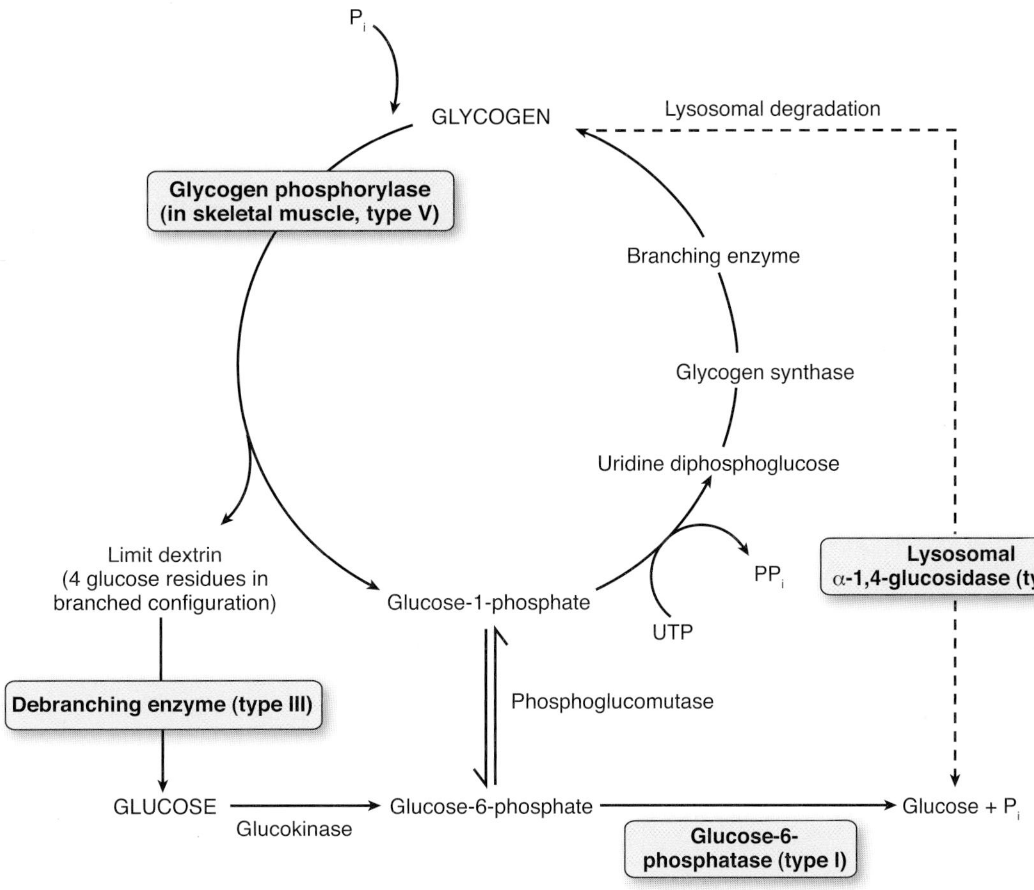

Glycogen storage diseases	12 types, all resulting in abnormal glycogen metabolism and an accumulation of glycogen within cells.	Very Poor Carbohydrate Metabolism.

DISEASE	FINDINGS	DEFICIENT ENZYME	COMMENTS
Von Gierke's disease (type I)	Severe fasting hypoglycemia, ↑↑ glycogen in liver, ↑ blood lactate, hepatomegaly	Glucose-6-phosphatase	Autosomal recessive.
Pompe's disease (type II)	Cardiomegaly and systemic findings leading to early death	Lysosomal α-1,4-glucosidase (acid maltase)	Autosomal recessive. Pompe's trashes the Pump (heart, liver, and muscle).
Cori's disease (type III)	Milder form of type I with normal blood lactate levels	Debranching enzyme (α-1,6-glucosidase)	Autosomal recessive. Gluconeogenesis is intact.
McArdle's disease (type V)	↑ glycogen in muscle, but cannot break it down, leading to painful muscle cramps, myoglobinuria with strenuous exercise	Skeletal muscle glycogen phosphorylase	Autosomal recessive. McArdle's = Muscle.

Lysosomal storage diseases — Each is caused by a deficiency in one of the many lysosomal enzymes. Results in an accumulation of abnormal metabolic products.

DISEASE	FINDINGS	DEFICIENT ENZYME	ACCUMULATED SUBSTRATE	INHERITANCE
Sphingolipidoses				
Fabry's disease	Peripheral neuropathy of hands/feet, angiokeratomas, cardiovascular/renal disease	α-galactosidase A	Ceramide trihexoside	XR
Gaucher's disease A 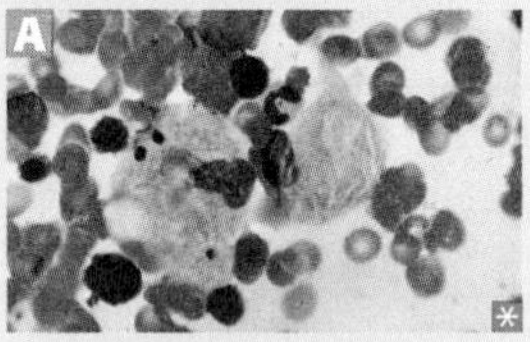	Most common. Hepatosplenomegaly, aseptic necrosis of femur, bone crises, Gaucher's cells A (macrophages that look like crumpled tissue paper)	Glucocerebrosidase	Glucocerebroside	AR
Niemann-Pick disease B 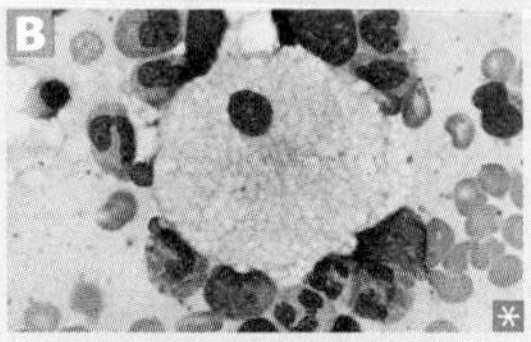	Progressive neurodegeneration, hepatosplenomegaly, cherry-red spot on macula, foam cells B	Sphingomyelinase	Sphingomyelin	AR
Tay-Sachs disease	Progressive neurodegeneration, developmental delay, cherry-red spot on macula, lysosomes with onion skin, no hepatosplenomegaly (vs. Niemann-Pick)	Hexosaminidase A	GM_2 ganglioside	AR
Krabbe's disease	Peripheral neuropathy, developmental delay, optic atrophy, globoid cells	Galactocerebrosidase	Galactocerebroside	AR
Metachromatic leukodystrophy	Central and peripheral demyelination with ataxia, dementia	Arylsulfatase A	Cerebroside sulfate	AR
Mucopolysaccharidoses				
Hurler's syndrome	Developmental delay, gargoylism, airway obstruction, corneal clouding, hepatosplenomegaly	α-L-iduronidase	Heparan sulfate, dermatan sulfate	AR
Hunter's syndrome	Mild Hurler's + aggressive behavior, no corneal clouding	Iduronate sulfatase	Heparan sulfate, dermatan sulfate	XR

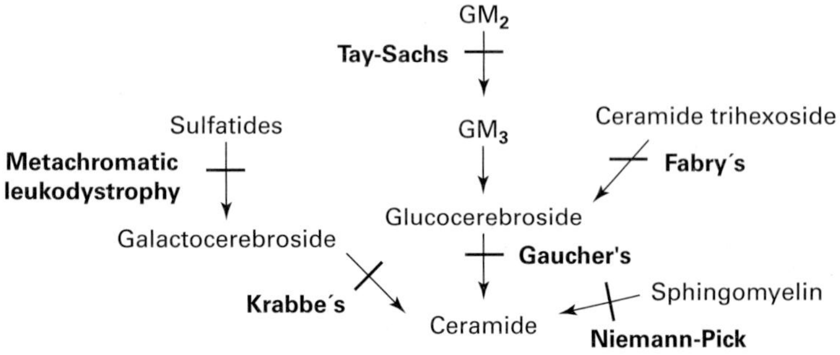

No man picks (Niemann-Pick) his nose with his **sphinger** (**sphing**omyelinase).
Tay-Sa**X** lacks he**X**osaminidase.
Hunters see clearly (no corneal clouding) and aim for the **X** (**X**-linked recessive).
↑ incidence of Tay-Sachs, Niemann-Pick, and some forms of Gaucher's disease in Ashkenazi Jews.

Fatty acid metabolism

Fatty acid degradation occurs where its products will be consumed—in the mitochondrion.

Carnitine deficiency: inability to transport LCFAs into the mitochondria, resulting in toxic accumulation. Causes weakness, hypotonia, and hypoketotic hypoglycemia.

Acyl-CoA dehydrogenase deficiency: ↑ dicarboxylic acids, ↓ glucose and ketones.

"**SY**trate" = **SY**nthesis.
CARnitine = **CAR**nage of fatty acids.

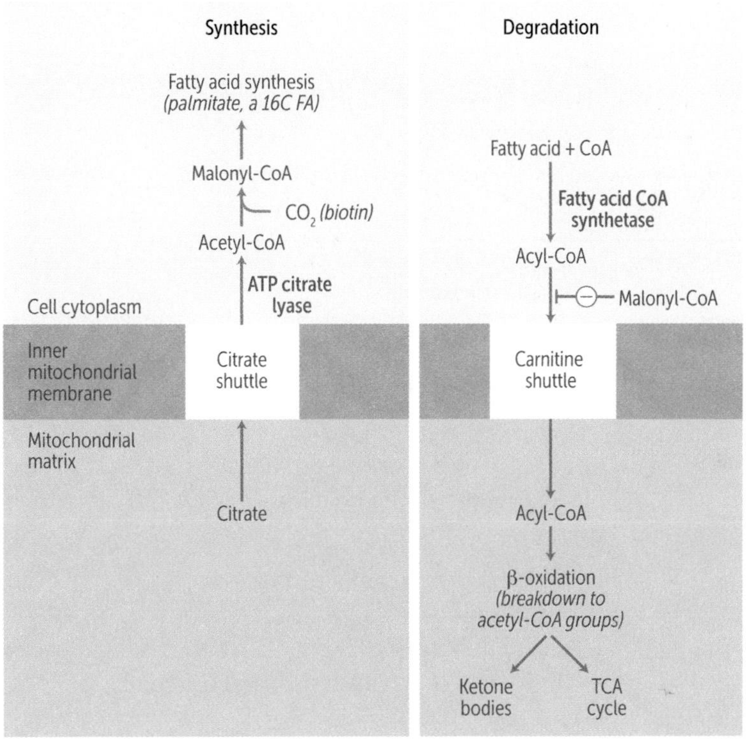

Ketone bodies

In the liver, fatty acids and amino acids are metabolized to acetoacetate and β-hydroxybutyrate (to be used in muscle and brain).

In prolonged starvation and diabetic ketoacidosis, oxaloacetate is depleted for gluconeogenesis. In alcoholism, excess NADH shunts oxaloacetate to malate. Both processes stall the TCA cycle, which shunts glucose and FFA toward the production of ketone bodies.

Made from HMG-CoA. Metabolized by the brain to 2 molecules of acetyl-CoA. Excreted in urine.

Breath smells like acetone (fruity odor).

Urine test for ketones does not detect β-hydroxybutyrate (favored by high redox state).

Metabolic fuel use

Exercise

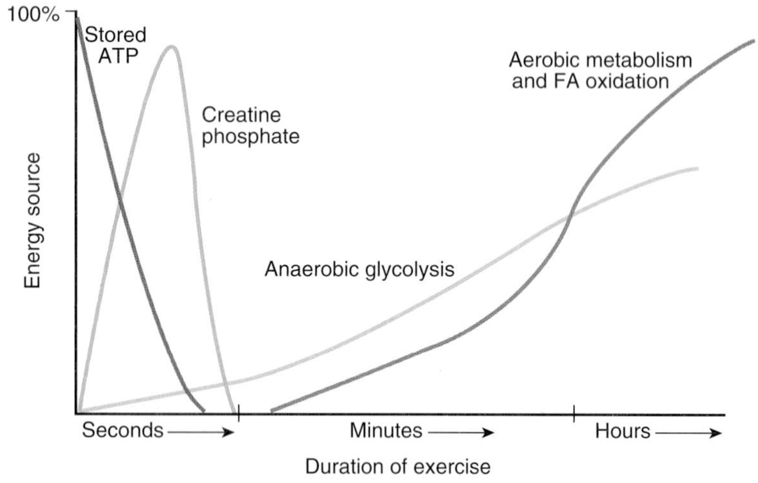

1 g protein or carbohydrate = 4 kcal.
1 g fat = 9 kcal.

Fasting and starvation	Priorities are to supply sufficient glucose to the brain and RBCs and to preserve protein.	
Fed state (after a meal)	Glycolysis and aerobic respiration.	Insulin stimulates storage of lipids, proteins, glycogen.
Fasting (between meals)	Hepatic glycogenolysis (major); hepatic gluconeogenesis, adipose release of FFA (minor).	Glucagon, adrenaline stimulate use of fuel reserves.
Starvation days 1–3	Blood glucose level maintained by: ▪ Hepatic glycogenolysis ▪ Adipose release of FFA ▪ Muscle and liver, which shift fuel use from glucose to FFA ▪ Hepatic gluconeogenesis from peripheral tissue lactate and alanine, and from adipose tissue glycerol and propionyl-CoA (from odd-chain FFA—the only triacylglycerol components that contribute to gluconeogenesis)	Glycogen reserves depleted after day 1. RBCs lack mitochondria and so cannot use ketones.
Starvation after day 3	Adipose stores (ketone bodies become the main source of energy for the brain and heart). After these are depleted, vital protein degradation accelerates, leading to organ failure and death.	Amount of adipose stores determines survival time.

Cholesterol synthesis	Rate-limiting step is catalyzed by HMG-CoA reductase, which converts HMG-CoA to mevalonate. ⅔ of plasma cholesterol is esterified by lecithin-cholesterol acyltransferase (LCAT).	Statins (e.g., lovastatin) inhibit HMG-CoA reductase.

Lipid transport, key enzymes

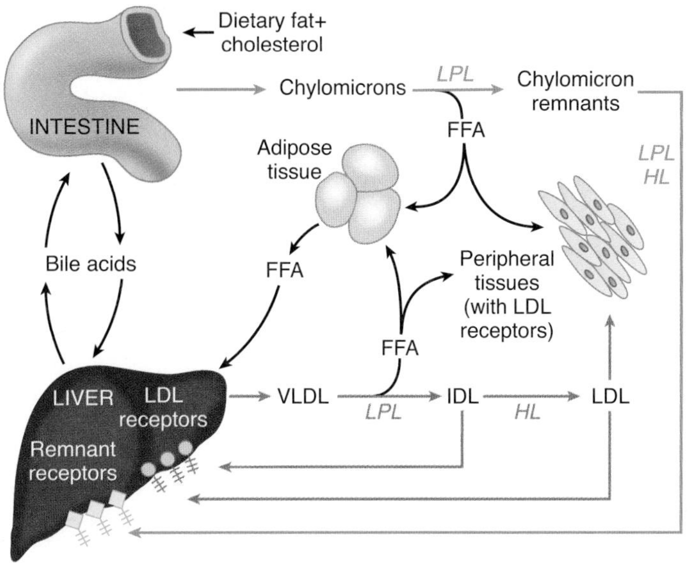

Pancreatic lipase—degradation of dietary TG in small intestine.
Lipoprotein lipase (LPL)—degradation of TG circulating in chylomicrons and VLDLs.
Hepatic TG lipase (HL)—degradation of TG remaining in IDL.
Hormone-sensitive lipase—degradation of TG stored in adipocytes.

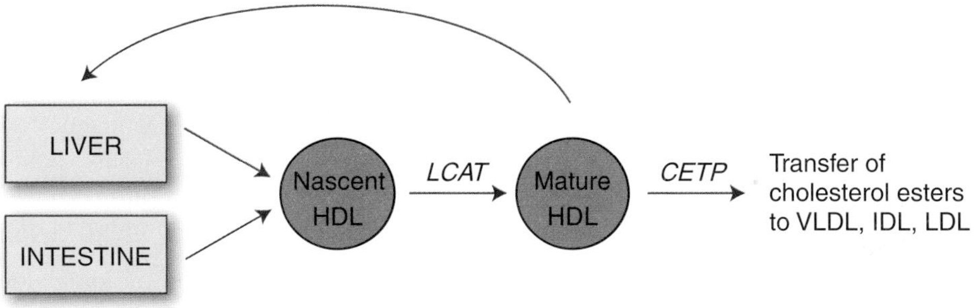

Lecithin-cholesterol acyltransferase (LCAT)—catalyzes esterification of cholesterol.
Cholesterol ester transfer protein (CETP)—mediates transfer of cholesterol esters to other lipoprotein particles.

Major apolipoproteins

Apolipoprotein	Function	Chylomicron	Chylomicron remnant	VLDL	IDL	LDL	HDL
E	Mediates remnant uptake	X	X	X	X		X
A-I	Activates LCAT						X
C-II	Lipoprotein lipase cofactor	X		X			X
B-48	Mediates chylomicron secretion	X	X				
B-100	Binds LDL receptor			X	X	X	

Lipoprotein functions	Lipoproteins are composed of varying proportions of cholesterol, triglycerides (TGs), and phospholipids. LDL and HDL carry most cholesterol. LDL transports cholesterol from liver to tissues. HDL transports cholesterol from periphery to liver.	 LDL is Lousy. HDL is Healthy.
Chylomicron	Delivers dietary TGs to peripheral tissue. Delivers cholesterol to liver in the form of chylomicron remnants, which are mostly depleted of their triacylglycerols. Secreted by intestinal epithelial cells.	
VLDL	Delivers hepatic TGs to peripheral tissue. Secreted by liver.	
IDL	Formed in the degradation of VLDL. Delivers triglycerides and cholesterol to liver.	
LDL	Delivers hepatic cholesterol to peripheral tissues. Formed by hepatic lipase modification of IDL in the peripheral tissue. Taken up by target cells via receptor-mediated endocytosis.	
HDL	Mediates reverse cholesterol transport from periphery to liver. Acts as a repository for apoC and apoE (which are needed for chylomicron and VLDL metabolism). Secreted from both liver and intestine.	

Familial dyslipidemias

TYPE	INCREASED BLOOD LEVEL	PATHOPHYSIOLOGY
I—hyper-chylomicronemia	Chylomicrons, TG, cholesterol	Autosomal recessive. Lipoprotein lipase deficiency or altered apolipoprotein C-II. Causes pancreatitis, hepatosplenomegaly, and eruptive/pruritic xanthomas (no ↑ risk for atherosclerosis).
IIa—familial hyper-cholesterolemia	LDL, cholesterol	Autosomal dominant. Absent or ↓ LDL receptors. Causes accelerated atherosclerosis, tendon (Achilles) xanthomas, and corneal arcus.
IV—hyper-triglyceridemia	VLDL, TG	Autosomal dominant. Hepatic overproduction of VLDL. Causes pancreatitis.

Abetalipoproteinemia	Autosomal recessive mutation in microsomal triglyceride transfer protein (MTP) gene → ↓ B-48 and B-100 → ↓ chylomicron and VLDL synthesis and secretion. Symptoms appear in the first few months of life. Intestinal biopsy shows lipid accumulation within enterocytes due to inability to export absorbed lipid as chylomicrons. Findings: failure to thrive, steatorrhea, acanthocytosis, ataxia, night blindness.

HIGH-YIELD PRINCIPLES IN

Microbiology

"Support bacteria. They're the only culture some people have."

—Anonymous

"What lies behind us and what lies ahead of us are tiny matters compared to what lies within us."

—Oliver Wendell Holmes

This high-yield material covers the basic concepts of microbiology. The emphasis in previous examinations has been approximately 40% bacteriology (20% basic, 20% quasi-clinical), 25% immunology, 25% virology (10% basic, 15% quasi-clinical), 5% parasitology, and 5% mycology.

Microbiology questions on the Step 1 exam often require two (or more) steps: Given a certain clinical presentation, you will first need to identify the most likely causative organism, and you will then need to provide an answer regarding some feature of that organism. For example, a description of a child with fever and a petechial rash will be followed by a question that reads, "From what site does the responsible organism usually enter the blood?"

This section therefore presents organisms in two major ways: in individual microbial "profiles" and in the context of the systems they infect and the clinical presentations they produce. You should become familiar with both formats. When reviewing the systems approach, remind yourself of the features of each microbe by returning to the individual profiles. Also be sure to memorize the laboratory characteristics that allow you to identify microbes.

Additional tables that organize infectious diseases and syndromes according to the most commonly affected hosts and the most likely microbes are available on the First Aid team blog at www.firstaidteam.com.

▸ MICROBIOLOGY—BASIC BACTERIOLOGY

Bacterial structures

STRUCTURE	FUNCTION	CHEMICAL COMPOSITION
Peptidoglycan	Gives rigid support, protects against osmotic pressure.	Sugar backbone with peptide side chains cross-linked by transpeptidase.
Cell wall/cell membrane (gram positives)	Major surface antigen.	Peptidoglycan for support. Lipoteichoic acid induces TNF and IL-1.
Outer membrane (gram negatives)	Site of endotoxin (lipopolysaccharide [LPS]); major surface antigen.	Lipid A induces TNF and IL-1; O polysaccharide is the antigen.
Plasma membrane	Site of oxidative and transport enzymes.	Lipoprotein bilayer.
Ribosome	Protein synthesis.	50S and 30S subunits.
Periplasm	Space between the cytoplasmic membrane and outer membrane in gram-negative bacteria.	Contains many hydrolytic enzymes, including β-lactamases.
Capsule	Protects against phagocytosis.	Polysaccharide (except *Bacillus anthracis*, which contains D-glutamate).
Pilus/fimbria	Mediate adherence of bacteria to cell surface; sex pilus forms attachment between 2 bacteria during conjugation.	Glycoprotein.
Flagellum	Motility.	Protein.
Spore	Resistant to dehydration, heat, and chemicals.	Keratin-like coat; dipicolinic acid; peptidoglycan.
Plasmid	Contains a variety of genes for antibiotic resistance, enzymes, and toxins.	DNA.
Glycocalyx	Mediates adherence to surfaces, especially foreign surfaces (e.g., indwelling catheters).	Polysaccharide.

Cell walls

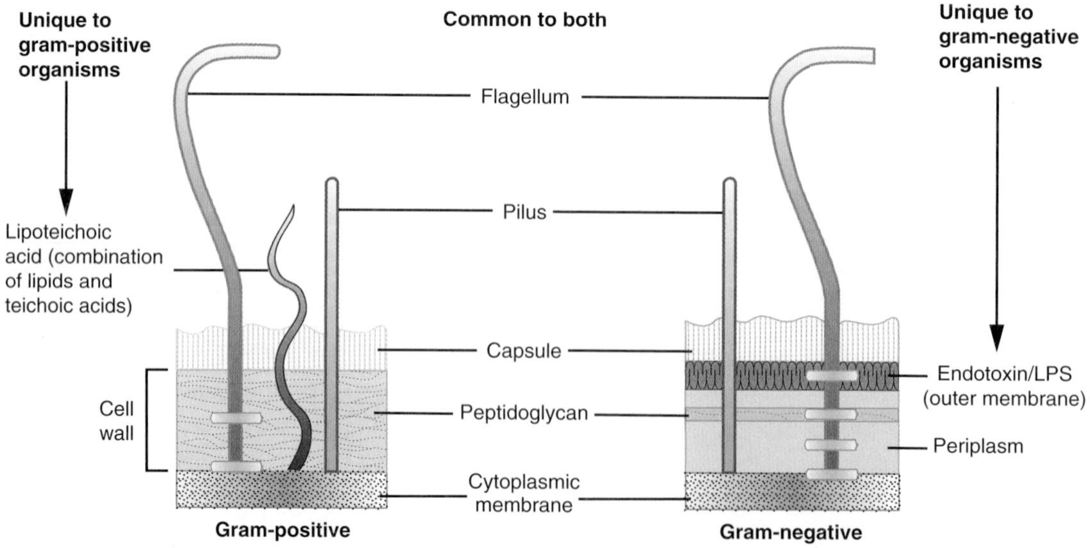

(Adapted, with permission, from Levinson W, Jawetz E. *Medical Microbiology and Immunology: Examination and Board Review, 9th ed.* New York: McGraw-Hill, 2006: 7.)

Bacterial taxonomy

MORPHOLOGY	Gram-positive examples	Gram-negative examples
Circular (coccus)	*Staphylococcus* *Streptococcus*	*Neisseria*
Rod (bacillus)	*Clostridium* *Corynebacterium* *Bacillus* *Listeria* *Mycobacterium* (acid fast) *Gardnerella* (Gram variable)	Enterics: ▪ *E. coli* ▪ *Shigella* ▪ *Salmonella* ▪ *Yersinia* ▪ *Klebsiella* ▪ *Proteus* ▪ *Enterobacter* ▪ *Serratia* ▪ *Vibrio* ▪ *Campylobacter* ▪ *Helicobacter* ▪ *Pseudomonas* ▪ *Bacteroides* Respiratory: ▪ *Haemophilus* (pleomorphic) ▪ *Legionella* (silver) ▪ *Bordetella* Zoonotic: ▪ *Francisella* ▪ *Brucella* ▪ *Pasteurella* ▪ *Bartonella*
Branching filamentous	*Actinomyces* *Nocardia* (weakly acid fast)	
Pleomorphic		Rickettsiae (Giemsa) Chlamydiae (Giemsa)
Spiral		Spirochetes: ▪ *Leptospira* ▪ *Borrelia* (Giemsa) ▪ *Treponema*
No cell wall	*Mycoplasma* (does not Gram stain)	

Bacteria with unusual cell membranes/walls

Mycoplasma	Contain sterols and have no cell wall.
Mycobacteria	Contain mycolic acid. High lipid content.

Gram stain limitations	These bugs do not Gram stain well: *Treponema* (too thin to be visualized). *Rickettsia* (intracellular parasite). Mycobacteria (high lipid content in cell wall detected by carbolfuchsin in acid-fast stain). *Mycoplasma* (no cell wall). *Legionella pneumophila* (primarily intracellular). *Chlamydia* (intracellular parasite; lacks muramic acid in cell wall).	These **R**ascals **M**ay **M**icroscopically **L**ack **C**olor. Treponemes—dark-field microscopy and fluorescent antibody staining. *Legionella*—silver stain.

Stains

Giemsa	*Chlamydia*, *Borrelia*, Rickettsiae, Trypanosomes, *Plasmodium*.	**C**ertain **B**ugs **R**eally **T**ry my **P**atience.
PAS (periodic acid-Schiff)	Stains **glycogen**, mucopolysaccharides; used to diagnose Whipple's disease (*Tropheryma whipplei*).	**PAS**s the **sugar**.
Ziehl-Neelsen (carbol fuchsin)	Acid-fast organisms (*Nocardia*, *Mycobacterium*).	
India ink	*Cryptococcus neoformans* (mucicarmine can also be used to stain thick polysaccharide capsule red).	
Silver stain	Fungi (e.g., *Pneumocystis*), *Legionella*, *Helicobacter pylori*.	

Special culture requirements

BUG	MEDIA USED FOR ISOLATION
H. influenzae	Chocolate agar with factors V (NAD^+) and X (hematin)
N. gonorrhoeae, *N. meningitidis*	Thayer-Martin (or VPN) media—**V**ancomycin (inhibits gram-positive organisms), **P**olymyxin (inhibits gram-negative organisms except *Neisseria*), and **N**ystatin (inhibits fungi); "to connect to *Neisseria*, please use your **VPN** client"
B. pertussis	Bordet-Gengou (potato) agar (**Bordet** for ***Bordet**ella*)
C. diphtheriae	Tellurite plate, Löffler's media
M. tuberculosis	Löwenstein-Jensen agar
M. pneumoniae	Eaton's agar
Lactose-fermenting enterics	Pink colonies on MacConkey's agar (fermentation produces acid, turning colony pink); *E. coli* is also grown on eosin–methylene blue (EMB) agar as colonies with green metallic sheen
Legionella	Charcoal yeast extract agar buffered with cysteine and iron
Fungi	Sabouraud's agar. "Sab's a **fun guy**!"

Obligate aerobes	Use an O_2-dependent system to generate ATP. Examples include *Nocardia*, *Pseudomonas aeruginosa*, *Mycobacterium tuberculosis*, and *Bacillus*. Reactivation of *M. tuberculosis* (e.g., after immune compromise or TNF-α inhibitor use) has a predilection for the apices of the lung, which have the highest P_{O_2}.	Nagging Pests Must Breathe. *P. aeruginosa* is an aerobe seen in burn wounds, complications of diabetes, nosocomial pneumonia, and pneumonias in cystic fibrosis patients.
Obligate anaerobes	Examples include *Clostridium*, *Bacteroides*, and *Actinomyces*. They lack catalase and/or superoxide dismutase and are thus susceptible to oxidative damage. Generally foul smelling (short-chain fatty acids), are difficult to culture, and produce gas in tissue (CO_2 and H_2).	Anaerobes Can't Breathe Air. Anaerobes are normal flora in GI tract, pathogenic elsewhere. AminO_2glycosides are ineffective against anaerobes because these antibiotics require O_2 to enter into bacterial cell.
Intracellular bugs		
Obligate intracellular	*Rickettsia*, *Chlamydia*. Can't make own ATP.	Stay inside (cells) when it is Really Cold.
Facultative intracellular	*Salmonella*, *Neisseria*, *Brucella*, *Mycobacterium*, *Listeria*, *Francisella*, *Legionella*, *Yersinia pestis*.	Some Nasty Bugs May Live FacultativeLY.
Encapsulated bacteria	Positive quellung reaction—if encapsulated bug is present, capsule swells when specific anticapsular antisera are added. Examples are *Streptococcus pneumoniae*, *Haemophilus influenzae* type B, *Neisseria meningitidis*, *Escherichia coli*, *Salmonella*, *Klebsiella pneumoniae*, *and* group B Strep. Their capsules serve as an antiphagocytic virulence factor. Capsule + protein conjugate serve as an antigen in vaccines.	Quellung = capsular "swellung." SHiNE SKiS. Are opsonized, and then cleared by spleen. Asplenics have decreased opsonizing ability and are at risk for severe infections. Give *S. pneumoniae*, *H. influenzae*, *N. meningitidis* vaccines.
Catalase-positive organisms	Catalase degrades H_2O_2 before it can be converted to microbicidal products by the enzyme myeloperoxidase. People with chronic granulomatous disease (NADPH oxidase deficiency) have recurrent infections with these microbes because they degrade the limited H_2O_2. Examples: *Pseudomonas*, *Listeria*, *Aspergillus*, *Candida*, *E. coli*, *S. aureus*, *Serratia*.	You need PLACESS for your cats.

Vaccines	For vaccines containing polysaccharide capsule antigens, a protein is conjugated to the polysaccharide antigen to promote T-cell activation and subsequent class switching. A polysaccharide antigen alone cannot be presented to T cells; therefore, only IgM antibodies would be produced.	Pneumovax (polysaccharide vaccine with no conjugated protein) and Prevnar (conjugated vaccine) *H. influenzae* type B (conjugated vaccine) Meningococcal vaccines (conjugated vaccines)
Urease-positive bugs	*Cryptococcus, **H.** pylori, **P**roteus, **U**reaplasma, **N**ocardia, **K**lebsiella, **S**. epidermidis, **S**. saprophyticus.*	**CH**uck Norris hates **PUNKSS**.
Pigment-producing bacteria	*Actinomyces **israelii***—**yellow** "sulfur" **granules**, which are composed of filaments of bacteria.	**Israel** has **yellow sand**.
	S. aureus—**yellow** pigment.	*aureus* (Latin) = **gold**.
	*Pseudomonas **aeruginosa***—blue-**green** pigment.	**Aerugula** is **green**.
	*Serratia **marcescens***—**red** pigment.	*Serratia marcescens*—think **red maraschino** cherries.
Bacterial virulence factors	These promote evasion of host immune response.	
Protein A	Binds Fc region of Ig. Prevents opsonization and phagocytosis. Expressed by *S. aureus*.	
IgA protease	Enzyme that cleaves IgA. Secreted by *S. pneumoniae*, ***H**. influenzae* type B, and ***N**eisseria* (**SHiN**) in order to colonize respiratory mucosa.	
M protein	Helps prevent phagocytosis. Expressed by group A streptococci.	

Main features of exotoxins and endotoxins

PROPERTY	Exotoxin	Endotoxin
SOURCE	Certain species of some gram-positive and gram-negative bacteria	Outer cell membrane of most gram-negative bacteria
SECRETED FROM CELL	Yes	No
CHEMISTRY	Polypeptide	Lipopolysaccharide (structural part of bacteria; released when lysed)
LOCATION OF GENES	Plasmid or bacteriophage	Bacterial chromosome
TOXICITY	High (fatal dose on the order of 1 µg)	Low (fatal dose on the order of hundreds of micrograms)
CLINICAL EFFECTS	Various effects (see below)	Fever, shock
MODE OF ACTION	Various modes (see below)	Induces TNF and IL-1
ANTIGENICITY	Induces high-titer antibodies called antitoxins	Poorly antigenic
VACCINES	Toxoids used as vaccines	No toxoids formed and no vaccine available
HEAT STABILITY	Destroyed rapidly at 60°C (except staphylococcal enterotoxin)	Stable at 100°C for 1 hour
TYPICAL DISEASES	Tetanus, botulism, diphtheria	Meningococcemia; sepsis by gram-negative rods

Bugs with exotoxins

BACTERIA	TOXIN	MECHANISM	MANIFESTATION
Inhibit protein synthesis			
Corynebacterium diphtheriae	Diphtheria toxin[a]	Inactivate elongation factor (EF-2)	Pharyngitis with pseudomembranes in throat and severe lymphadenopathy (bull neck)
Pseudomonas aeruginosa	Exotoxin A[a]		Host cell death
***Shigella* spp.**	Shiga toxin (ST)	Inactivate 60S ribosome by removing adenine from rRNA	GI mucosal damage → dysentery; ST also enhances cytokine release, causing HUS
Enterohemorrhagic *E. coli* (EHEC), including O157:H7 strain	Shiga-like toxin (SLT)		SLT enhances cytokine release, causing HUS; unlike *Shigella*, EHEC does not invade host cells
Increase fluid secretion			
Enterotoxigenic *E. coli* (ETEC)	Heat-**labile** toxin (LT)[a]	Overactivates adenylate cyclase (↑ cAMP) → ↑ Cl^- secretion in gut and H_2O efflux	Watery diarrhea: **labile** in the **A**ir (**A**denylate cyclase), **stable** on the **G**round (**G**uanylate cyclase).
	Heat-**stable** toxin (ST)	Overactivate guanylate cyclase (↑ cGMP) → ↓ resorption of NaCl and H_2O in gut	
Bacillus anthracis	Edema factor	Mimics the adenylate cyclase enzyme (↑ cAMP)	Likely responsible for characteristic edematous borders of black eschar in cutaneous anthrax
Vibrio cholerae	Cholera toxin[a]	Overactivates adenylate cyclase (↑ cAMP) by permanently activating G_s → ↑ Cl^- secretion in gut and H_2O efflux	Voluminous "rice-water" diarrhea
Inhibit phagocytic ability			
Bordetella pertussis	Pertussis toxin[a]	Overactivates adenylate cyclase (↑ cAMP) by disabling G_i, impairing phagocytosis to permit survival of microbe	**Whooping cough**: child coughs on expiration and "whoops" on inspiration (toxin may not actually be a cause of cough; can cause "100-day cough" in adults)
Inhibit release of neurotransmitter			
Clostridium tetani	Tetanospasmin	Cleave SNARE protein required for neurotransmitter release	Muscle rigidity and "lock jaw"; toxin prevents release of **inhibitory** (GABA and glycine) neurotransmitters in spinal cord
Clostridium botulinum	Botulinum toxin		Flaccid paralysis, floppy baby; toxin prevents release of **stimulatory** (ACh) signals at neuromuscular junctions → flaccid paralysis

[a]Toxin is an ADP ribosylating A-B toxin: B (binding) component binds to host cell surface receptor, enabling endocytosis; A (active) component attaches ADP-ribosyl to disrupt host cell proteins.

Bugs with exotoxins *(continued)*

BACTERIA	TOXIN	MECHANISM	MANIFESTATION
Lyse cell membranes			
Clostridium perfringens	Alpha toxin	Phospholipase that degrades tissue and cell membranes	Degradation of phospholipid C → myonecrosis ("gas gangrene") and hemolysis ("double zone" of hemolysis on blood agar)
Streptococcus pyogenes	Streptolysin O	Protein that degrades cell membrane	Lyses RBCs; contributes to β-hemolysis; host antibodies against toxin (ASO) used to diagnose rheumatic fever (do not confuse with immune complexes of poststreptococcal glomerulonephritis)
Superantigens causing shock			
Staphylococcus aureus	Toxic shock syndrome toxin (TSST-1)	Bring MHC II and TCR in proximity to outside of antigen binding site to cause overwhelming release of IFN-γ and IL-2 → shock	Toxic shock syndrome: fever, rash, shock; other toxins cause scalded skin syndrome (exfoliative toxin) and food poisoning (enterotoxin)
Streptococcus pyogenes	Exotoxin A		Toxic shock syndrome: fever, rash, shock

Endotoxin

A lipopolysaccharide found in outer membrane of gram-negative bacteria.

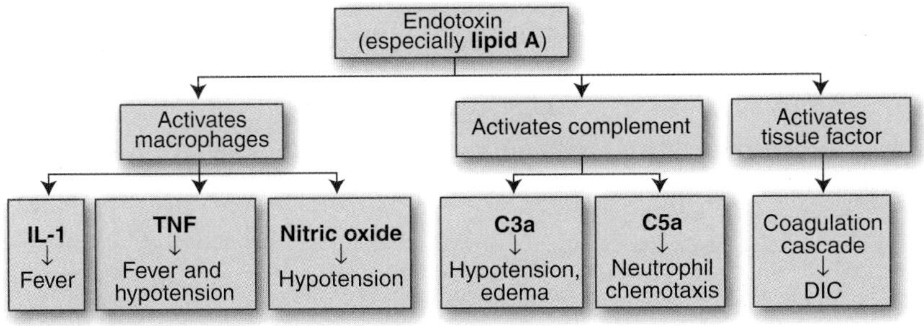

(Adapted, with permission, from Levinson W. *Review of Medical Microbiology and Immunology,* 12th ed. New York: McGraw-Hill, 2012: Fig. 7-4.)

ENDOTOXIN:
- Edema
- Nitric oxide
- DIC/Death
- Outer membrane
- TNF-α
- O-antigen
- eXtremely heat stable
- IL-1
- Neutrophil chemotaxis

Bacterial growth curve

Lag phase	Metabolic activity without division.
Exponential/log phase	Rapid cell division. Penicillins and cephalosporins act here as peptidoglycan is being made.
Stationary phase	Nutrient depletion slows growth. Spore formation in some bacteria.
Death	Prolonged nutrient depletion and buildup of waste products lead to death.

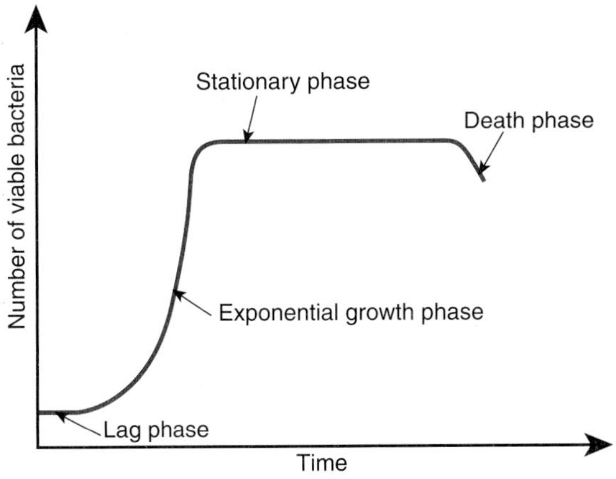

Bacterial genetics

Transformation	Ability to take up naked DNA (i.e., from cell lysis) from environment (also known as "competence"). A feature of many bacteria, especially ***S. pneumoniae***, ***H. influenzae*** type B, and *Neisseria* (**SHiN**). Any DNA can be used. Adding deoxyribonuclease to environment will degrade naked DNA in medium → no transformation seen.
Conjugation	
$F^+ \times F^-$	F^+ plasmid contains genes required for sex pilus and conjugation. Bacteria without this plasmid are termed F^-. Plasmid (dsDNA) is replicated and transferred through pilus from F^+ cell. No transfer of chromosomal genes.
Hfr $\times F^-$	F^+ plasmid can become incorporated into bacterial chromosomal DNA, termed high-frequency recombination (Hfr) cell. Replication of incorporated plasmid DNA may include some flanking chromosomal DNA. Transfer of plasmid and chromosomal genes.
Transposition	Segment of DNA that can "jump" (excision and reintegration) from one location to another, can transfer genes from plasmid to chromosome and vice versa. When excision occurs, may include some flanking chromosomal DNA, which can be incorporated into a plasmid and transferred to another bacterium.
Transduction	
Generalized	A "packaging" event. Lytic phage infects bacterium, leading to cleavage of bacterial DNA. Parts of bacterial chromosomal DNA may become packaged in viral capsid. Phage infects another bacterium, transferring these genes.
Specialized	An "excision" event. Lysogenic phage infects bacterium; viral DNA incorporates into bacterial chromosome. When phage DNA is excised, flanking bacterial genes may be excised with it. DNA is packaged into phage viral capsid and can infect another bacterium.

Lysogeny, specialized transduction

Genes for the following 5 bacterial toxins encoded in a lysogenic phage:

- Shig**A**-like toxin
- **B**otulinum toxin (certain strains)
- **C**holera toxin
- **D**iphtheria toxin
- **E**rythrogenic toxin of *Streptococcus pyogenes*

ABCDE

▶ MICROBIOLOGY—CLINICAL BACTERIOLOGY

Gram-positive lab algorithm

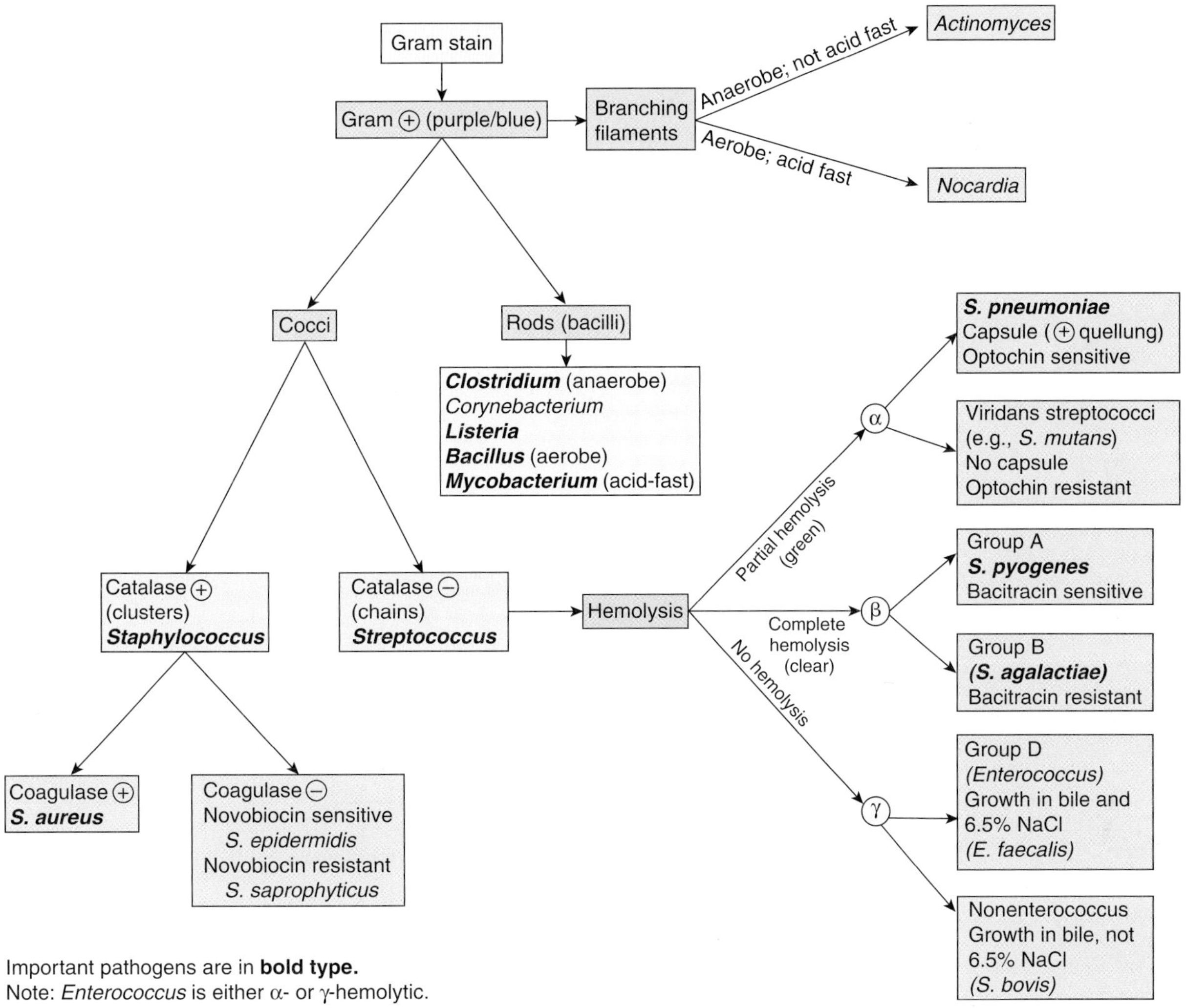

Important pathogens are in **bold type.**
Note: *Enterococcus* is either α- or γ-hemolytic.

Identification of gram-positive cocci

Staphylococci	NOvobiocin—*Saprophyticus* is Resistant; *Epidermidis* is Sensitive.	On the office's **staph** retreat, there was NO StRESs.
Streptococci	Optochin—*Viridans* is Resistant; *Pneumoniae* is Sensitive.	OVRPS (overpass).
	Bacitracin—group B strep are Resistant; group A strep are Sensitive.	B-BRAS.

α-hemolytic bacteria

Form green ring around colonies on blood agar. Include the following organisms:
- *Streptococcus pneumoniae* (catalase negative and optochin sensitive)
- Viridans streptococci (catalase negative and optochin resistant)

β-hemolytic bacteria

Form clear area of hemolysis on blood agar. Include the following organisms:
- *Staphylococcus aureus* (catalase and coagulase positive)
- *Streptococcus pyogenes*—group A strep (catalase negative and bacitracin sensitive)
- *Streptococcus agalactiae*—group B strep (catalase negative and bacitracin resistant)
- *Listeria monocytogenes* (tumbling motility, meningitis in newborns, unpasteurized milk)

Staphylococcus aureus

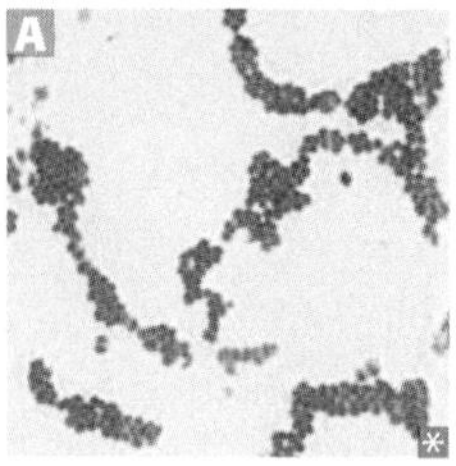

Gram-positive cocci in clusters A. Protein A (virulence factor) binds Fc-IgG, inhibiting complement fixation and phagocytosis.

Causes:
- Inflammatory disease—skin infections, organ abscesses, pneumonia
- Toxin-mediated disease—toxic shock syndrome (TSST-1), scalded skin syndrome (exfoliative toxin), rapid-onset food poisoning (enterotoxins)
- MRSA (methicillin-resistant S. *aureus*) infection—important cause of serious nosocomial and community-acquired infections; resistant to β-lactams because of altered penicillin-binding protein

TSST is a superantigen that binds to MHC II and T-cell receptor, resulting in polyclonal T-cell activation. Presents as fever, vomiting, rash, desquamation, shock, end-organ failure.

S. *aureus* food poisoning is due to ingestion of preformed toxin.

Causes acute bacterial endocarditis, osteomyelitis.

Staph make catalase because they have more "**staff**." Bad staph (*aureus*) make coagulase and toxins. Forms fibrin clot around self; can lead to abscess.

Staphylococcus epidermidis

Infects prosthetic devices and intravenous catheters by producing adherent biofilms. Component of normal skin flora; contaminates blood cultures.

Streptococcus pneumoniae

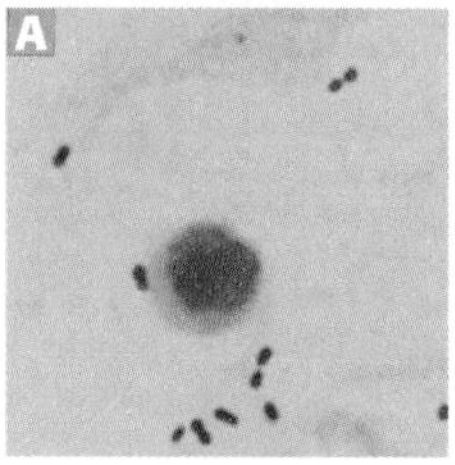

Most common cause of:
- **M**eningitis
- **O**titis media (in children)
- **P**neumonia
- **S**inusitis

Lancet-shaped, gram-positive diplococci A. Encapsulated. IgA protease.

S. *pneumoniae* **MOPS** are **M**ost **OP**tochin **S**ensitive.

Pneumococcus is associated with "rusty" sputum, sepsis in sickle cell anemia and splenectomy.

No virulence without capsule.

Viridans group streptococci

Viridans streptococci are α-hemolytic. They are normal flora of the oropharynx and cause dental caries (*Streptococcus mutans*) and subacute bacterial endocarditis at damaged valves (S. *sanguis*). Resistant to optochin, differentiating them from S. *pneumoniae*, which is α-hemolytic but is optochin sensitive.

Sanguis = blood. There is lots of blood in the heart (endocarditis). S. *sanguis* sticks to damaged valves by making glycocalyx.

Viridans group strep live in the mouth because they are not afraid **of-the-chin** (**op-to-chin** resistant).

***Streptococcus pyogenes* (group A streptococci)**	Causes: ▪ Pyogenic—pharyngitis, cellulitis, impetigo ▪ Toxigenic—scarlet fever, toxic shock–like syndrome, necrotizing fasciitis ▪ Immunologic—rheumatic fever, acute glomerulonephritis Bacitracin sensitive. Antibodies to M protein enhance host defenses against *S. pyogenes* but can give rise to rheumatic fever. ASO titer detects recent *S. pyogenes* infection.	**J♥NES** criteria to diagnose rheumatic fever: **J**oints—polyarthritis ♥—carditis **N**odules (subcutaneous) **E**rythema marginatum **S**ydenham's chorea **Ph**aryngitis can result in rheumatic "**ph**ever" and glomerulone**ph**ritis. Impetigo more commonly precedes glomerulonephritis than pharyngitis. Scarlet fever: scarlet rash sparing face, strawberry (scarlet) tongue, scarlet throat
***Streptococcus agalactiae* (group B streptococci)**	Bacitracin resistant, β-hemolytic, colonizes vagina; causes pneumonia, meningitis, and sepsis, mainly in **babies**. Produces CAMP factor, which enlarges the area of hemolysis formed by *S. aureus*. (Note: CAMP stands for the authors of the test, not cyclic AMP.) Hippurate test positive. Screen pregnant women at 35–37 weeks. Patients with positive culture receive intrapartum penicillin prophylaxis.	Group **B** for **B**abies!
Enterococci (group D streptococci) 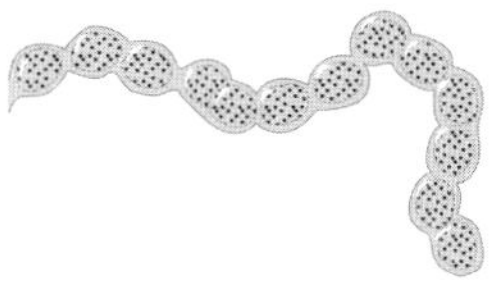	Enterococci (*Enterococcus faecalis* and *E. faecium*) are normal colonic flora that are penicillin G resistant and cause UTI, biliary tract infections, and subacute endocarditis. Lancefield group D includes the enterococci and the nonenterococcal group D streptococci. Lancefield grouping is based on differences in the C carbohydrate on the bacterial cell wall. Variable hemolysis. VRE (vancomycin-resistant enterococci) are an important cause of nosocomial infection.	Enterococci, hardier than nonenterococcal group D, can grow in 6.5% NaCl and bile (lab test). *Entero* = intestine, *faecalis* = feces, *strepto* = twisted (chains), *coccus* = berry.
***Streptococcus bovis* (group D streptococci)**	Colonizes the gut. Can cause bacteremia and subacute endocarditis in colon cancer patients.	Bovis in the blood = cancer in the colon.

Corynebacterium diphtheriae	Causes diphtheria via exotoxin encoded by β-prophage. Potent exotoxin inhibits protein synthesis via ADP-ribosylation of EF-2. Symptoms include pseudomembranous pharyngitis (grayish-white membrane) with lymphadenopathy, myocarditis, and arrhythmias. Lab diagnosis based on gram-positive rods with metachromatic (blue and red) granules and Elek's test for toxin. Toxoid vaccine prevents diphtheria.	*Coryne* = club shaped. Black colonies on cystine-tellurite agar. **ABCDEFG**: **A**DP-ribosylation **B**eta-prophage ***C**orynebacterium* ***D**iphtheria* **E**longation **F**actor 2 **G**ranules
Spores: bacterial	Some bacteria can form spores at the end of the stationary phase when nutrients are limited. Spores are highly resistant to heat and chemicals. Have dipicolinic acid in their core. Have no metabolic activity. Must autoclave to kill spores (as is done to surgical equipment) by steaming at 121°C for 15 minutes.	Spore-forming gram-positive bacteria found in soil: *Bacillus anthracis*, *Clostridium perfringens*, *C. tetani*. Other spore formers include *B. cereus*, *C. botulinum*, *Coxiella burnetii*.
Clostridia (with exotoxins)	Gram-positive, spore-forming, obligate anaerobic bacilli.	
C. tetani	Produces tetanospasmin, an exotoxin causing tetanus. Tetanus toxin (and botulinum toxin) are proteases that cleave releasing proteins for neurotransmitters.	**Tet**anus is **tet**anic paralysis (blocks glycine and GABA release [inhibitory neurotransmitters]) from Renshaw cells in spinal cord. Causes spastic paralysis, trismus (lockjaw), and risus sardonicus.
C. botulinum	Produces a preformed, heat-labile toxin that inhibits ACh release at the neuromuscular junction, causing botulism. In adults, disease is caused by ingestion of preformed toxin. In babies, ingestion of spores in honey causes disease (floppy baby syndrome).	***Bot**ulinum* is from bad **bot**tles of food and honey (causes a flaccid paralysis).
C. perfringens	Produces α toxin ("lecithinase," a phospholipase) that can cause myonecrosis (gas gangrene) and hemolysis.	***Perf**ringens* **perf**orates a gangrenous leg.
C. difficile	Produces 2 toxins. Toxin A, enterotoxin, binds to the brush border of the gut. Toxin B, cytotoxin, destroys the cytoskeletal structure of enterocytes, causing pseudomembranous colitis. Often 2° to antibiotic use, especially clindamycin or ampicillin. Diagnosed by detection of one or both toxins in stool.	***Di**fficile* causes **di**arrhea. Treatment: metronidazole or oral vancomycin.

Anthrax	Caused by *Bacillus anthracis*, a gram-positive, spore-forming rod that produces anthrax toxin. The only bacterium with a polypeptide capsule (contains D-glutamate).	
Cutaneous anthrax	Contact → black eschar (painless ulcer); can progress to bacteremia and death.	Black skin lesions—black eschar (necrosis) surrounded by edematous ring. Caused by lethal factor and edema factor.
Pulmonary anthrax	Inhalation of spores → flu-like symptoms that rapidly progress to fever, pulmonary hemorrhage, mediastinitis, and shock.	Woolsorters' disease—inhalation of spores from contaminated wool.

Bacillus cereus	Causes food poisoning. Spores survive cooking rice. Keeping rice warm results in germination of spores and enterotoxin formation. Emetic type usually seen with rice and pasta. Nausea and vomiting within 1–5 hours. Caused by cereulide, a preformed toxin. Diarrheal type causes watery, nonbloody diarrhea and GI pain in 8–18 hours.	Reheated rice syndrome.

Listeria monocytogenes

Facultative intracellular microbe; acquired by ingestion of unpasteurized milk/cheese and deli meats or by vaginal transmission during birth. Form "actin rockets" by which they move from cell to cell. Characteristic tumbling motility.

Can cause amnionitis, septicemia, and spontaneous abortion in pregnant women; granulomatosis infantiseptica; neonatal meningitis; meningitis in immunocompromised patients; mild gastroenteritis in healthy individuals. Treatment: gastroenteritis usually self-limited; ampicillin in infants, immunocompromised patients, and the elderly in empirical treatment of meningitis.

Actinomyces* vs. *Nocardia

Both form long, branching filaments resembling fungi.

Actinomyces	*Nocardia*
Gram-positive anaerobe	Gram-positive aerobe
Not acid fast	Acid fast
Normal oral flora	Found in soil
Causes oral/facial abscesses that drain through sinus tracts, forms yellow "sulfur granules"	Causes pulmonary infections in immunocompromised and cutaneous infections after trauma in immunocompetent
Treat with penicillin	Treat with sulfonamides

1° and 2° tuberculosis

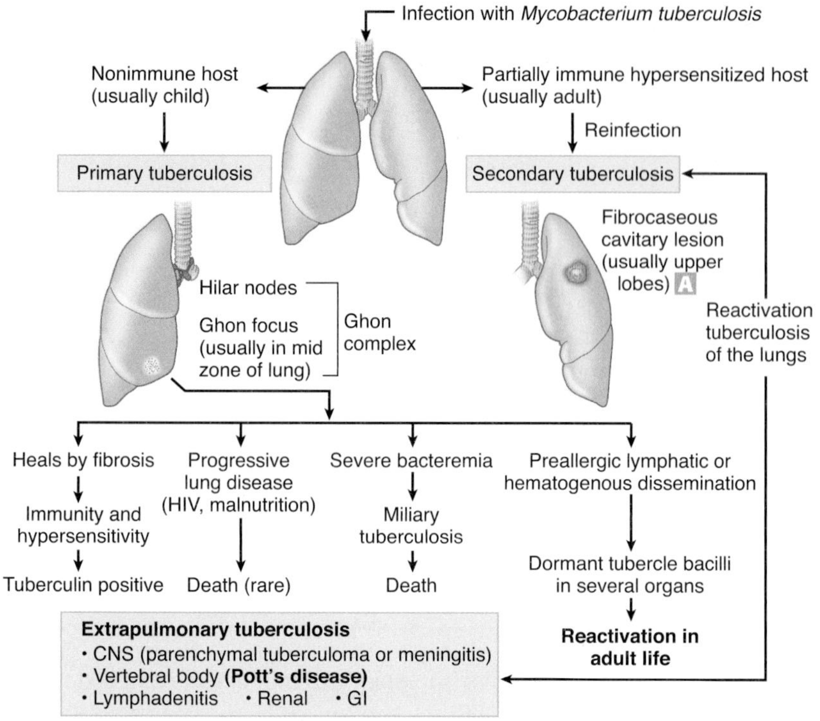
Infection with *Mycobacterium tuberculosis*
Nonimmune host (usually child)
Partially immune hypersensitized host (usually adult)
Reinfection
Primary tuberculosis
Secondary tuberculosis
Fibrocaseous cavitary lesion (usually upper lobes) A
Hilar nodes
Ghon focus (usually in mid zone of lung)
Ghon complex
Reactivation tuberculosis of the lungs
Heals by fibrosis
Immunity and hypersensitivity
Tuberculin positive
Progressive lung disease (HIV, malnutrition)
Death (rare)
Severe bacteremia
Miliary tuberculosis
Death
Preallergic lymphatic or hematogenous dissemination
Dormant tubercle bacilli in several organs
Reactivation in adult life
Extrapulmonary tuberculosis
• CNS (parenchymal tuberculoma or meningitis)
• Vertebral body **(Pott's disease)**
• Lymphadenitis • Renal • GI

PPD+ if current infection, past exposure, or BCG vaccinated.

PPD– if no infection or anergic (steroids, malnutrition, immunocompromise) and in sarcoidosis.

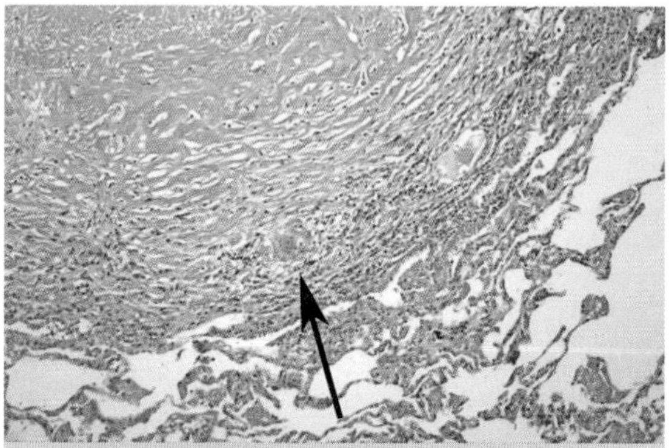

A **Caseating granuloma.** With multinucleated Langhan's giant cell (arrow).

Mycobacteria

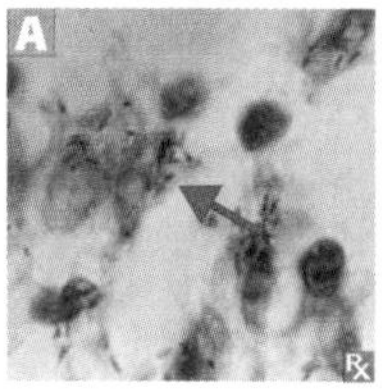
A

Mycobacterium tuberculosis (TB, often resistant to multiple drugs).

M. kansasii (pulmonary TB-like symptoms).

M. avium–intracellulare (causes disseminated, non-TB disease in AIDS; often resistant to multiple drugs). Prophylactic treatment with azithromycin.

All mycobacteria are acid-fast organisms A.

TB symptoms include fever, night sweats, weight loss, and hemoptysis.

Cord factor in virulent strains inhibits macrophage maturation and induces release of TNF-α. Sulfatides (surface glycolipids) inhibit phagolysosomal fusion.

Leprosy (Hansen's disease)

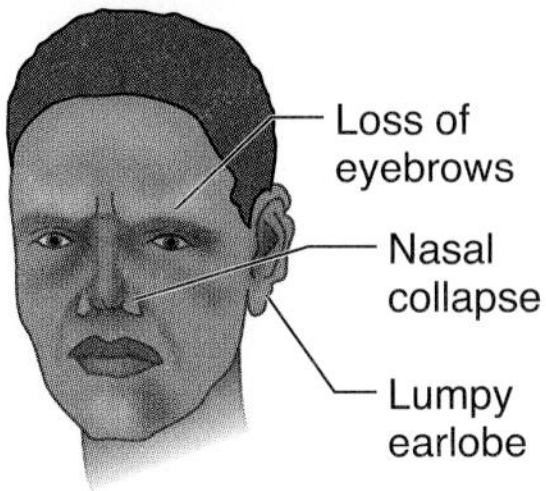
Loss of eyebrows
Nasal collapse
Lumpy earlobe

"Leonine facies" of lepromatous leprosy

Caused by *Mycobacterium leprae*, an acid-fast bacillus that likes cool temperatures (infects skin and superficial nerves—"glove and stocking" loss of sensation) and cannot be grown in vitro. Reservoir in United States: armadillos.

Hansen's disease has 2 forms:

- **Lepromatous**—presents diffusely over skin A and is communicable; characterized by low cell-mediated immunity with a humoral Th_2 response.
- **Tuberculoid**—limited to a few hypoesthetic, hairless skin plaques; characterized by high cell-mediated immunity with a largely Th_1-type immune response.

Multidrug therapy consisting of dapsone and rifampin for 6 months for tuberculoid form and dapsone, rifampin, and clofazimine for 2–5 years for lepromatous form.

Lepromatous can be lethal.

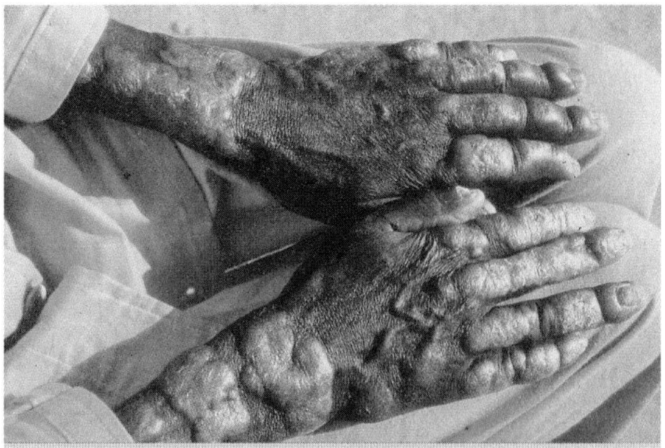

A **Leprosy.**

Gram-negative lab algorithm

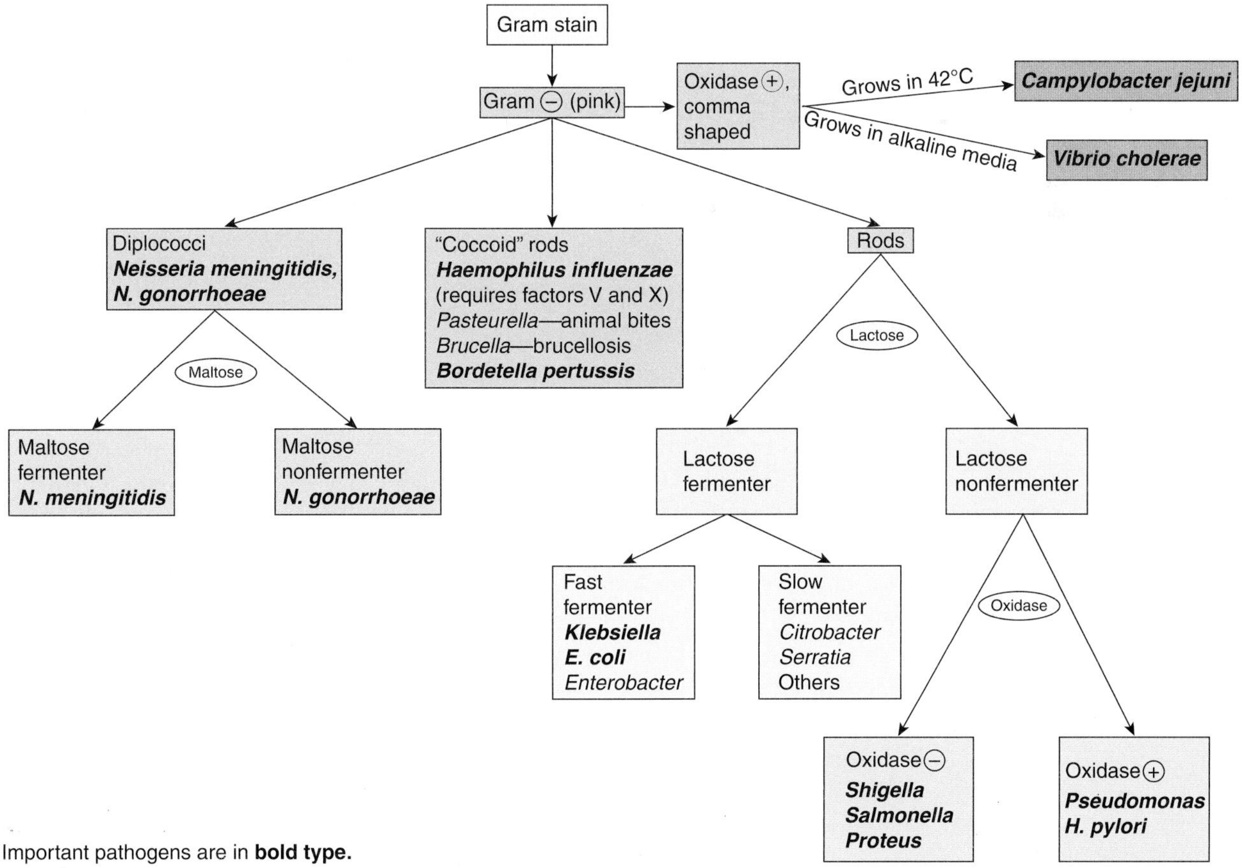
Gram stain
Gram ⊖ (pink)
Oxidase ⊕, comma shaped
Grows in 42°C
Campylobacter jejuni
Grows in alkaline media
Vibrio cholerae
Diplococci
Neisseria meningitidis, N. gonorrhoeae
Maltose
Maltose fermenter N. meningitidis
Maltose nonfermenter N. gonorrhoeae
"Coccoid" rods
Haemophilus influenzae (requires factors V and X)
Pasteurella—animal bites
Brucella—brucellosis
Bordetella pertussis
Rods
Lactose
Lactose fermenter
Lactose nonfermenter
Fast fermenter Klebsiella E. coli Enterobacter
Slow fermenter Citrobacter Serratia Others
Oxidase
Oxidase ⊖ Shigella Salmonella Proteus
Oxidase ⊕ Pseudomonas H. pylori

Important pathogens are in **bold type.**

Lactose-fermenting enteric bacteria

Grow pink colonies on MacConkey's agar. Examples include *Citrobacter, Klebsiella, E. coli, Enterobacter,* and *Serratia. E. coli* produces β-galactosidase, which breaks down lactose into glucose and galactose.

Lactose is **KEE**.
Test with MacCon**KEE'S** agar.
EMB agar—lactose fermenters grow as purple/black colonies. *E. coli* grows purple colonies with a green sheen.

Penicillin and gram-negative bugs

Gram-negative bacilli are resistant to penicillin G but may be susceptible to penicillin derivatives such as ampicillin and amoxicillin. The gram-negative outer membrane layer inhibits entry of penicillin G and vancomycin.

Neisseria

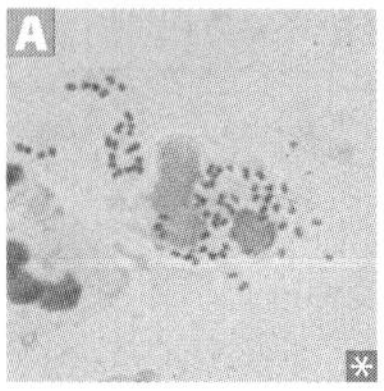

Gram-negative diplococci. Both ferment glucose and produce IgA proteases. *N. gonorrhoeae* within polymorphonuclear leukocytes A.

Menin**G**ococci ferment **M**altose and **G**lucose. **G**onococci ferment **G**lucose.

Gonococci	Meningococci
No polysaccharide capsule	Polysaccharide capsule
No maltose fermentation	Maltose fermentation
No vaccine (due to rapid antigenic variation of pilus proteins)	Vaccine (none for type B)
Sexually transmitted	Respiratory and oral secretions
Causes gonorrhea, septic arthritis, neonatal conjunctivitis, PID, and Fitz-Hugh–Curtis syndrome	Causes meningococcemia and meningitis, Waterhouse-Friderichsen syndrome
	Rifampin, ciprofloxacin, or ceftriaxone prophylaxis in close contacts
Treatment: ceftriaxone + (azithromycin or doxycycline) for possible chlamydia coinfection	Treatment: ceftriaxone or penicillin G

Haemophilus influenzae

HaEMOPhilus causes **E**piglottitis ("cherry red" in children), **M**eningitis, **O**titis media, and **P**neumonia. Small gram-negative (coccobacillary) rod. Aerosol transmission. Most invasive disease caused by capsular type B. Nontypeable strains cause mucosal infections (otitis media, conjunctivitis, bronchitis). Produces IgA protease. Culture on **chocolate** agar requires factors **V** (NAD^+) and **X** (hematin) for growth; can also be grown with *S. aureus*, which provides factor V.
Treat meningitis with ceftriaxone. Rifampin prophylaxis in close contacts.

When a child has "flu," mom goes to five (**V**) and dime (**X**) store to buy some **chocolate**.
Vaccine contains type B capsular polysaccharide (polyribosylribitol phosphate) conjugated to diphtheria toxoid or other protein. Given between 2 and 18 months of age.
Does not cause the flu (influenza virus does).

Legionella pneumophila	Legionnaires' disease = severe pneumonia, fever, GI and CNS symptoms. Pontiac fever = mild flu-like syndrome. Gram-negative rod. Gram stains poorly—use **silver** stain. Grow on **charcoal** yeast extract culture with **iron** and **cysteine**. Detected clinically by presence of antigen in urine. Aerosol transmission from environmental water source habitat. No person-to-person transmission. Treatment: macrolide or quinolone.	Think of a French **legionnaire** (soldier) with his **silver** helmet, sitting around a campfire (**charcoal**) with his **iron** dagger—he is no **sissy** (cysteine). Labs show hyponatremia.
Pseudomonas aeruginosa	*PSEUDOmonas* is associated with wound and burn infections, Pneumonia (especially in cystic fibrosis), Sepsis (black lesions on skin), External otitis (swimmer's ear), UTI, Drug use and Diabetic Osteomyelitis, and hot tub folliculitis. Malignant otitis externa in diabetics. Aerobic gram-negative rod. Non–lactose fermenting, oxidase positive. Produces pyocyanin (blue-green) pigment; has a grape-like odor. Water source. Produces endotoxin (fever, shock) and exotoxin A (inactivates EF-2). Treatment: aminoglycoside plus extended-spectrum penicillin (e.g., piperacillin, ticarcillin).	**Aer**uginosa—**aer**obic. Think water connection and blue-green pigment. Think *Pseudomonas* in burn victims. Chronic pneumonia in CF patients is associated with biofilm.
E. coli	*E. coli* virulence factors: fimbriae—cystitis and pyelonephritis; K capsule—pneumonia, neonatal meningitis; LPS endotoxin—septic shock.	

STRAIN	TOXIN AND MECHANISM	PRESENTATION
EIEC	Microbe invades intestinal mucosa and causes necrosis and inflammation. No toxins produced. Clinical manifestations similar to *Shigella*.	Invasive; dysentery.
ETEC	Labile toxin/stable toxin. No inflammation or invasion.	Traveler's diarrhea (watery).
EPEC	No toxin produced. Adheres to apical surface, flattens villi, prevents absorption.	Diarrhea usually in children (Pediatrics).
EHEC	O157:H7 is the most common serotype. Produces Shiga-like toxin and Hemolytic-uremic syndrome (triad of anemia, thrombocytopenia, and acute renal failure). Endothelium swells and narrows lumen, leading to mechanical hemolysis and reduced renal blood flow; damaged endothelium consumes platelets.	Dysentery (toxin alone causes necrosis and inflammation). Does not ferment sorbitol (distinguishes it from other *E. coli*).

Klebsiella	An intestinal flora that causes lobar pneumonia in alcoholics and diabetics when aspirated. Very mucoid colonies caused by abundant polysaccharide capsule. Red "currant jelly" sputum. Also cause of nosocomial UTIs.	4 A's: Aspiration pneumonia Abscess in lungs and liver Alcoholics di-**A**-betics

Salmonella* vs. *Shigella	***Salmonella***	***Shigella***
	Have flagella (**salmon** swim)	No flagella
	Can disseminate hematogenously	Cell to cell transmission; no hematogenous spread
	Have many animal reservoirs	Only reservoirs are humans and primates
	Produce hydrogen sulfide	Does not produce hydrogen sulfide
	Antibiotics may prolong symptoms	Antibiotics prolong excretion of organism in feces
	Invades intestinal mucosa and causes a monocytic response	Invades intestinal mucosa and causes PMN infiltration
	Can cause bloody diarrhea	Often causes bloody diarrhea
	Does not ferment lactose	Does not ferment lactose
Salmonella typhi	Causes typhoid fever. Found only in humans. Characterized by rose spots on the abdomen, fever, headache, and diarrhea. Can remain in gallbladder and cause a carrier state.	

Campylobacter jejuni	Major cause of bloody diarrhea, especially in children. Fecal-oral transmission through foods such as poultry, meat, unpasteurized milk. Comma or S-shaped, oxidase positive, grows at 42°C ("*Campylobacter* likes the hot **camp**fire"). Common antecedent to Guillain-Barré syndrome and reactive arthritis.
Vibrio cholerae	Produces profuse rice-water diarrhea via toxin that permanently activates G_s, ↑ cAMP. Comma shaped, oxidase positive, grows in alkaline media. Endemic to developing countries. Prompt oral rehydration is necessary.
Yersinia enterocolitica	Usually transmitted from pet feces (e.g., puppies), contaminated milk, or pork. Causes mesenteric adenitis that can mimic Crohn's or appendicitis.

Helicobacter pylori

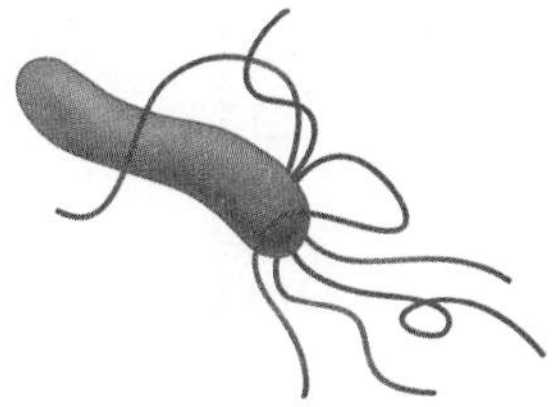

Causes gastritis and up to 90% of duodenal ulcers. Risk factor for peptic ulcer, gastric adenocarcinoma, and lymphoma. Curved gram-negative rod. Urease positive (can use urea breath test for diagnosis). Creates alkaline environment. Most common initial treatment is triple therapy: proton pump inhibitor; clarithromycin; amoxicillin or metronidazole.

Spirochetes

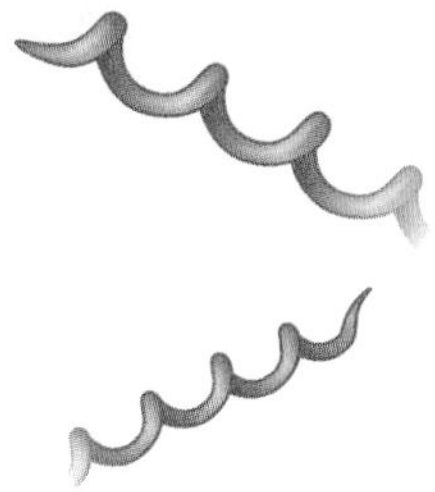

The spirochetes are spiral-shaped bacteria with axial filaments and include ***B**orrelia* (big size), *Leptospira*, and *Treponema*. Only *Borrelia* can be visualized using aniline dyes (Wright's or Giemsa stain) in light microscopy. *Treponema* is visualized by dark-field microscopy.

BLT.
B is **B**ig.

Leptospira interrogans

Found in water contaminated with animal urine, causes leptospirosis: flu-like symptoms, jaundice, photophobia with conjunctivitis. Prevalent among surfers and in tropics (i.e., Hawaii).

Weil's disease (icterohemorrhagic leptospirosis)—severe form with jaundice and azotemia from liver and kidney dysfunction; fever, hemorrhage, and anemia.

Lyme disease

Caused by *Borrelia burgdorferi*, which is transmitted by the tick *Ixodes* (also vector for *Babesia*). Natural reservoir is the mouse. Mice are important to tick life cycle.
Common in northeastern United States.
Treatment: doxycycline, ceftriaxone.
3 stages of **Lyme** disease:
- Stage 1—erythema chronicum migrans (expanding "bull's eye" red rash with central clearing), flu-like symptoms.
- Stage 2—neurologic (facial nerve palsy) and cardiac (AV nodal block) manifestations.
- Stage 3—musculoskeletal (chronic monoarthritis and migratory polyarthritis), neurological (encephalopathy and polyneuropathy), and cutaneous manifestations.

FAKE a Key **Lyme** pie:
Facial nerve palsy (typically bilateral)
Arthritis
Kardiac block
Erythema migrans

Syphilis — Caused by spirochete *Treponema pallidum*. Treatment: penicillin G.

1° syphilis

Localized disease presenting with *painless* chancre A. Screen with VDRL and confirm diagnosis with FTA-ABS.

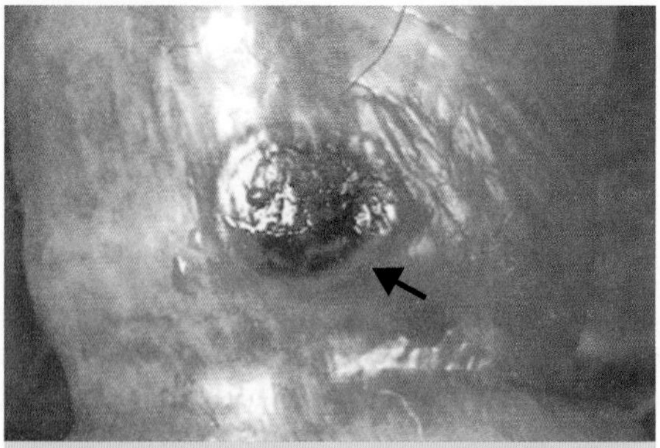

A Painless chancre.

2° syphilis

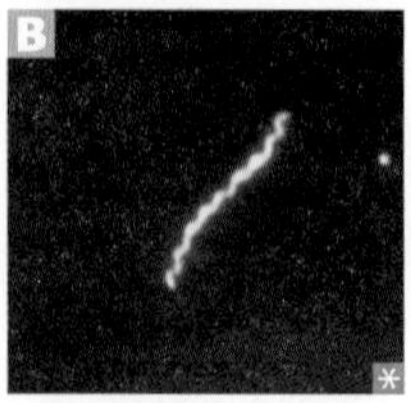

Disseminated disease with constitutional symptoms, maculopapular rash (palms and soles), condylomata lata. Treponemes are present in chancres of 1° and condylomata lata of 2° syphilis and may be directly visualized through dark-field microscopy B.

Screen with VDRL and confirm diagnosis with FTA-ABS.

Secondary syphilis = Systemic.

3° syphilis

Gummas (chronic granulomas), aortitis (vasa vasorum destruction), neurosyphilis (tabes dorsalis), Argyll Robertson pupil.

Signs: broad-based ataxia, positive Romberg, Charcot joint, stroke without hypertension.

Test spinal fluid with VDRL.

Congenital syphilis

Saber shins, saddle nose, CN VIII deafness, Hutchinson's teeth, mulberry molars.

Early prevention is key, as placental transmission typically occurs after first trimester.

Argyll Robertson pupil

Argyll Robertson pupil constricts with accommodation but is not reactive to light. Associated with 3° syphilis.

"Prostitute's pupil"—accommodates but does not react.

VDRL false positives

VDRL detects nonspecific antibody that reacts with beef cardiolipin. Used for diagnosis of syphilis, but many false positives, including viral infection (mononucleosis, hepatitis), some drugs, rheumatic fever, SLE, and leprosy.

VDRL:
- **V**iruses (mono, hepatitis)
- **D**rugs
- **R**heumatic fever
- **L**upus and leprosy

Jarisch-Herxheimer reaction

Flu-like syndrome immediately after antibiotics are started—due to killed bacteria releasing pyrogens.

Zoonotic bacteria Zoonosis: Infectious disease transmitted between animals and humans.

SPECIES	DISEASE	TRANSMISSION AND SOURCE
***Bartonella* spp.**	Cat scratch disease	Cat scratch
Borrelia burgdorferi	Lyme disease	*Ixodes* ticks (live on deer and mice)
Borrelia recurrentis	Recurrent fever	Louse (recurrent because of variable surface antigens)
***Brucella* spp.**	Brucellosis/undulant fever	Unpasteurized dairy
Campylobacter	Bloody diarrhea	Puppies, livestock (fecal-oral, ingestion of undercooked meat)
Chlamydophila psittaci	Psittacosis	Parrots, other birds
Coxiella burnetii	Q fever	Aerosols of cattle/sheep amniotic fluid
Ehrlichia chaffeensis	Ehrlichiosis	Lone Star tick
Francisella tularensis	Tularemia	Ticks, rabbits, deer fly
***Leptospira* spp.**	Leptospirosis	Animal urine
Mycobacterium leprae	Leprosy	Armadillos and humans with lepromatous leprosy
Pasteurella multocida	Cellulitis, osteomyelitis	Animal bite, cats, dogs
Rickettsia prowazekii	Epidemic typhus	Louse
Rickettsia rickettsii	Rocky Mountain spotted fever	*Dermacentor* tick bite
Rickettsia typhi	Endemic typhus	Fleas
Yersinia pestis	Plague	Fleas (rats and prairie dogs are reservoirs)

Gardnerella vaginalis

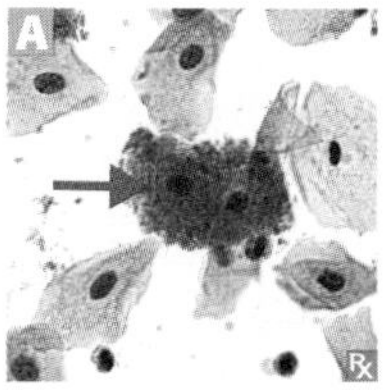

A pleomorphic, gram-variable rod that causes vaginosis presenting as a gray vaginal discharge with a **fishy** smell; nonpainful. Associated with sexual activity, but not an STD. Bacterial vaginosis is characterized by overgrowth of certain bacteria in vagina. **Clue** cells, or vaginal epithelial cells covered with bacteria, are visible under the microscope (arrow) A.

Treatment: metronidazole.

I don't have a **clue** why I smell **fish** in the **vagina garden**!

Rickettsial diseases and vector-borne illness	Treatment for all: doxycycline.	
Rash	Rocky Mountain spotted fever (tick)—*Rickettsia rickettsii.* Broadly distributed in US (in spite of name). Rash typically starts at wrists and ankles and then spreads to trunk, palms, and soles. Rickettsiae are obligate intracellular organisms that need CoA and NAD^+. Typhus: ▪ Endemic (fleas)—*R. typhi.* ▪ Epidemic (human body louse)—*R. prowazekii.* Rash starts centrally and spreads out, sparing palms and soles.	Classic triad—headache, fever, rash (vasculitis). "**R**ickettsii on the w**R**ists, **T**yphus on the **T**runk." **Palm** and **sole** rash is seen in **C**oxsackievirus **A** infection (hand, foot, and mouth disease), **R**ocky Mountain spotted fever, and secondary **S**yphilis (you drive **CARS** using your **palms** and **soles**).
No rash	Ehrlichiosis (tick)—*Ehrlichia.* Monocytes with morula (berry-like inclusions) in cytoplasm. Anaplasmosis (tick)—*Anaplasma.* Granulocytes with morula in cytoplasm.	
	Q fever (tick feces and cattle placenta release spores that are inhaled as aerosols)—*Coxiella burnetii.* No arthropod vector. Presents as pneumonia.	Q fever is Queer because it has no rash or vector and its causative organism can survive outside in its endospore form. Not in the *Rickettsia* genus, but closely related.

Chlamydiae	Chlamydiae cannot make their own ATP. They are obligate intracellular organisms that cause mucosal infections. 2 forms: ▪ **E**lementary body (small, dense) is "**E**nfectious" and **E**nters cell via **E**ndocytosis. ▪ **R**eticulate body **R**eplicates in cell by fission; form seen on tissue culture. *Chlamydia trachomatis* causes reactive arthritis, conjunctivitis, nongonococcal urethritis, and PID. *C. pneumoniae* and *C. psittaci* cause atypical pneumonia; transmitted by aerosol. Treatment: azithromycin (favored because one-time treatment) or doxycycline.	*Chlamys* = cloak (intracellular). *Chlamydophila psittaci*—notable for an avian reservoir. Lab diagnosis: cytoplasmic inclusions seen on Giemsa or fluorescent antibody–stained smear. The chlamydial cell wall is unusual in that it lacks muramic acid.

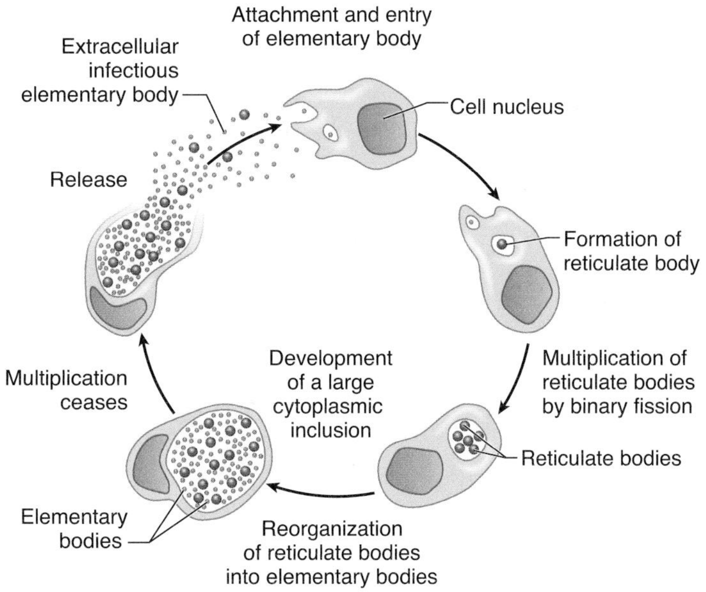

Chlamydia trachomatis serotypes

Types A, B, and C	Chronic infection, cause blindness due to follicular conjunctivitis in Africa.	ABC = Africa/Blindness/Chronic infection.
Types D–K	Urethritis/PID, ectopic pregnancy, neonatal pneumonia (staccato cough), or neonatal conjunctivitis.	D–K = everything else. Neonatal disease can be acquired during passage through infected birth canal.
Types L1, L2, and L3	Lymphogranuloma venereum.	

Mycoplasma pneumoniae 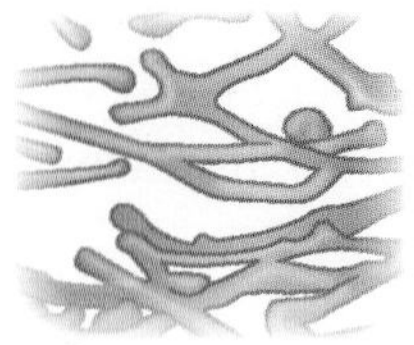	Classic cause of atypical "walking" pneumonia (insidious onset, headache, nonproductive cough, diffuse interstitial infiltrate). X-ray looks worse than patient. High titer of cold agglutinins (IgM), which can agglutinate or lyse RBCs. Grown on Eaton's agar. Treatment: macrolide or fluoroquinolone (penicillin ineffective since *Mycoplasma* have no cell wall).	No cell wall. Not seen on Gram stain. Bacterial membrane contains sterols for stability. Mycoplasmal pneumonia is more common in patients < 30 years of age. Frequent outbreaks in military recruits and prisons.

▸ MICROBIOLOGY—MYCOLOGY

Systemic mycoses

All of the following can cause pneumonia and can disseminate. All are caused by dimorphic fungi: cold (20°C) = mold; heat (37°C) = yeast. The only exception is coccidioidomycosis, which is a spherule (not yeast) in tissue. Treatment: fluconazole or itraconazole for **local** infection; amphotericin B for **systemic** infection. Systemic mycoses can mimic TB (granuloma formation), except, unlike TB, have no person-person transmission.

DISEASE	ENDEMIC LOCATION AND PATHOLOGIC FEATURES	NOTES
Histoplasmosis 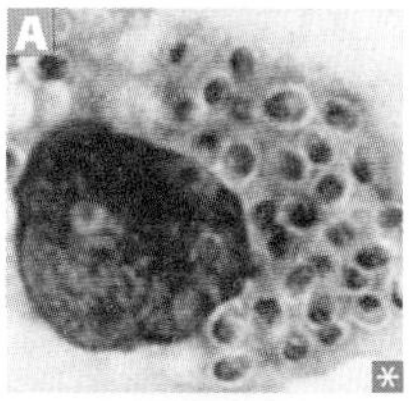	Mississippi and Ohio River valleys. Causes pneumonia. Macrophage filled with *Histoplasma* (smaller than RBC) A.	**H**isto **h**ides (within macrophages). Bird or bat droppings.
Blastomycosis 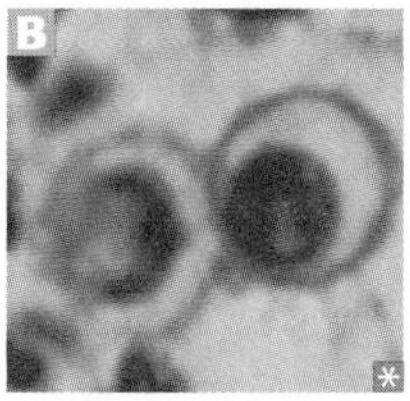	States east of Mississippi River and Central America. Causes inflammatory lung disease and can disseminate to skin and bone. Forms granulomatous nodules. Broad-base budding (same size as RBC) B.	**B**lasto **b**uds (**b**roadly).
Coccidioidomycosis 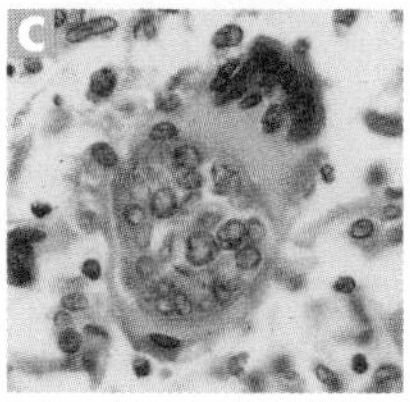	Southwestern United States, California. Causes pneumonia and meningitis; can disseminate to bone and skin. Case rate ↑ after earthquakes (spores in dust are thrown up in the air and become spherules in lungs). Spherule filled with endospores (much larger than RBC) C.	**C**occidio **c**rowds. San Joaquin Valley or desert (desert bumps) "valley fever."
Paracoccidioidomycosis 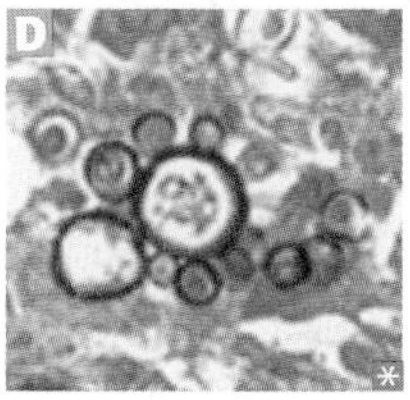	**Latin America.** Budding yeast with "**captain's wheel**" formation (much larger than RBC) D.	"Captain's wheel" appearance. Paracoccidio parasails with the **captain's wheel** all the way to **Latin America**.

Cutaneous mycoses

Tinea versicolor 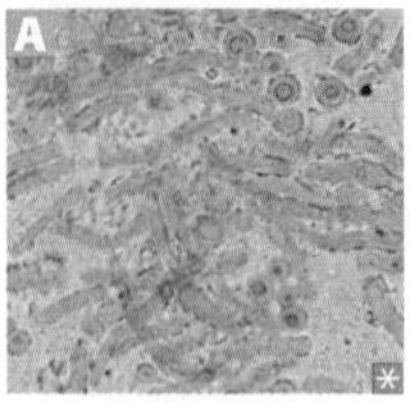	Caused by *Malassezia furfur*. Degradation of lipids produces acids that damage melanocytes and cause hypopigmented and/or hyperpigmented patches. Occurs in hot, humid weather. Treatment: topical miconazole, selenium sulfide (Selsun). "Spaghetti and meatball" appearance on KOH prep A.
Other tineae	Includes tinea pedis (foot), tinea cruris (groin), tinea corporis (ringworm, on body), tinea capitis (head, scalp), tinea unguium (onychomycosis, on fingernails). Pruritic lesions with central clearing resembling a ring, caused by dermatophytes (*Microsporum*, *Trichophyton*, and *Epidermophyton*). See mold hyphae in KOH prep, not dimorphic.

Opportunistic fungal infections

Candida albicans A

alba = white.

Systemic or superficial fungal infection.

Oral and esophageal thrush in immunocompromised (neonates, steroids, diabetes, AIDS), vulvovaginitis (diabetes, use of antibiotics), diaper rash, endocarditis in IV drug users, disseminated candidiasis (to any organ), chronic mucocutaneous candidiasis.

Treatment: topical azole for vaginal; fluconazole or caspofungin for oral/esophageal; fluconazole, amphotericin B, or caspofungin for systemic.

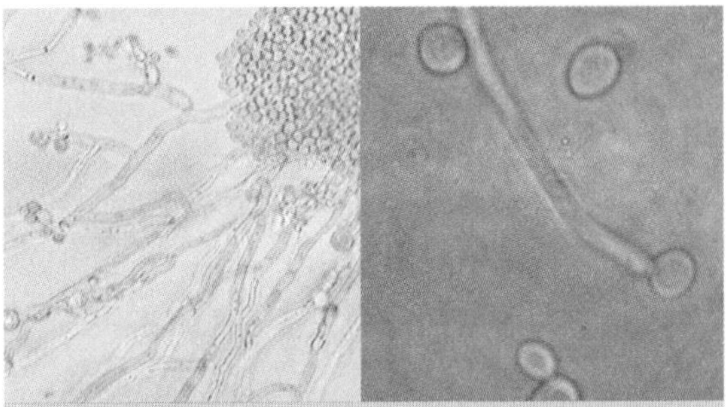

A **_Candida albicans._** Dimorphic yeast. Pseudohyphae and budding yeasts at 20°C (left). Germ tubes at 37°C (right).

Aspergillus fumigatus B

Invasive aspergillosis, especially in immunocompromised and those with chronic granulomatous disease.

Allergic bronchopulmonary aspergillosis (ABPA): with asthma or CF.

Aspergillomas in lung cavities, especially after TB infection.

Some species of *Aspergillus* produce aflatoxins, which are associated with HCC.

Think "**A**" for **A**cute **A**ngles in **A**spergillus. Not dimorphic.

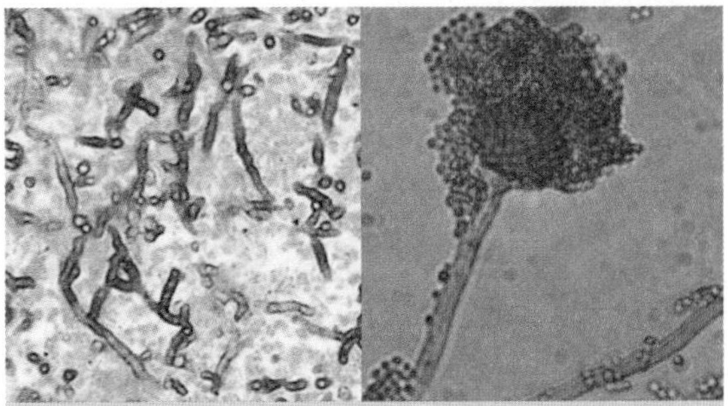

B **_Aspergillus fumigatus._** Septate hyphae that branch at 45° angle (left). Conidiophore with radiating chains of spores (right).

Cryptococcus neoformans C

Cryptococcal meningitis, cryptococcosis. Heavily encapsulated yeast. Not dimorphic. Found in soil, pigeon droppings. Acquired through inhalation with hematogenous dissemination to meninges. Culture on Sabouraud's agar. Stains with India ink. Latex agglutination test detects polysaccharide capsular antigen and is more specific. "Soap bubble" lesions in brain.

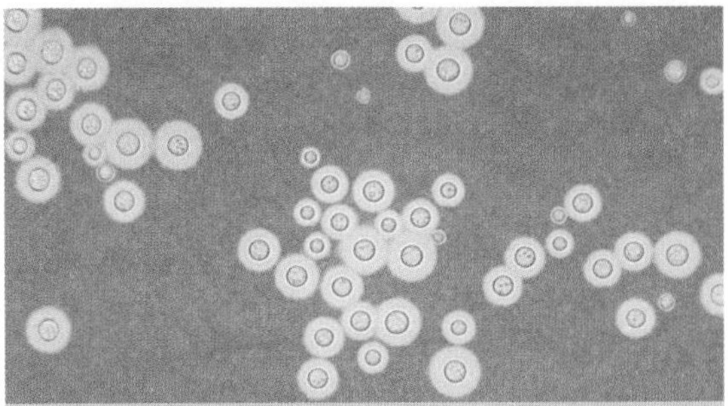

C **_Cryptococcus neoformans._** 5-10 μm yeasts with wide capsular halos and unequal budding in India ink stain.

Mucor D and _Rhizopus_ spp.

Mucormycosis. Disease mostly in ketoacidotic diabetic and leukemic patients. Fungi proliferate in blood vessel walls when there is excess ketone and glucose, penetrate cribriform plate, and enter brain. Rhinocerebral, frontal lobe abscesses. Headache, facial pain, black necrotic eschar on face; may have cranial nerve involvement.

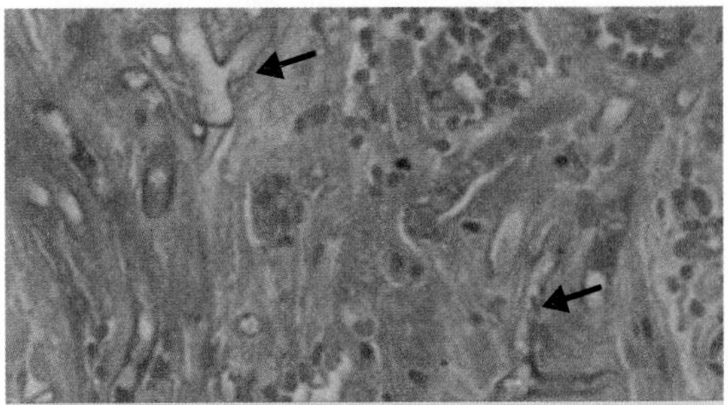

D **_Mucor._** Irregular, broad, nonseptate hyphae branching at wide angles (arrows).

Pneumocystis jirovecii

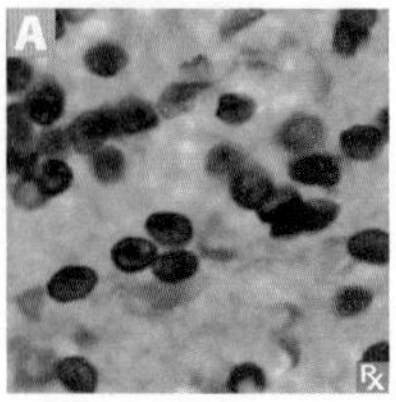

Causes *Pneumocystis* pneumonia (PCP), a diffuse interstitial pneumonia. Yeast (originally classified as protozoan). Inhaled. Most infections are asymptomatic. Immunosuppression (e.g., AIDS) predisposes to disease. Diffuse, bilateral CXR appearance. Diagnosed by lung biopsy or lavage. Disc-shaped yeast forms on methenamine silver stain of lung tissue A.

Treatment: TMP-SMX, pentamidine, dapsone. Start prophylaxis when CD4 drops < 200 cells/mm^3 in HIV patients.

Sporothrix schenckii

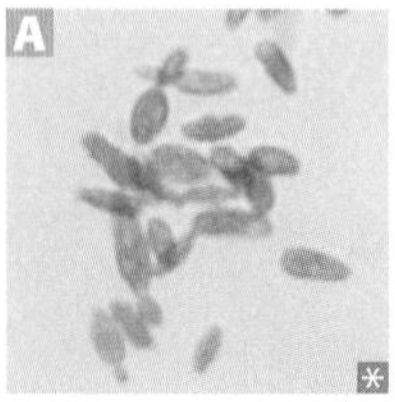

Sporotrichosis. Dimorphic, cigar-shaped budding yeast that lives on vegetation A. When spores are traumatically introduced into the skin, typically by a thorn ("**rose** gardener's" disease), causes local pustule or ulcer with nodules along draining lymphatics (ascending lymphangitis). Little systemic illness.

Treatment: itraconazole or **pot**assium iodide.

"Plant a **rose** in the **pot**."

▸ MICROBIOLOGY–PARASITOLOGY

Protozoa—GI infections

ORGANISM	DISEASE	TRANSMISSION	DIAGNOSIS	TREATMENT
Giardia lamblia 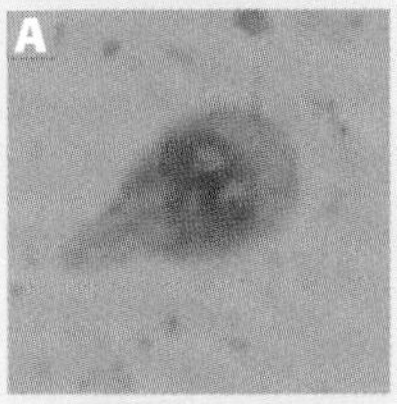	Giardiasis: bloating, flatulence, foul-smelling, fatty diarrhea (often seen in campers/hikers)—think **fat**-rich **Ghirardelli** chocolates for **fatty** stools of *Giardia*	Cysts in water	Trophozoites A or cysts (arrow) B in stool 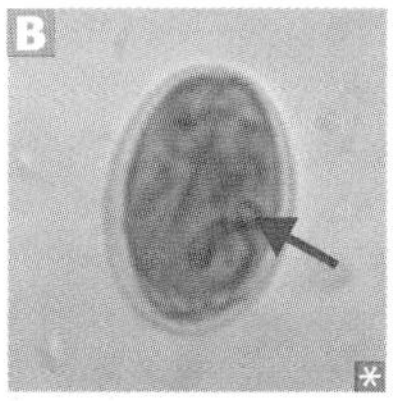	Metronidazole
Entamoeba histolytica 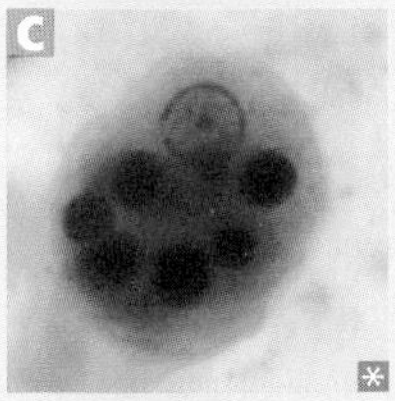	Amebiasis: bloody diarrhea (dysentery), liver abscess ("anchovy paste" exudate), RUQ pain (histology shows flask-shaped ulcer if submucosal abscess of colon ruptures)	Cysts in water	Serology and/or trophozoites (with RBCs in the cytoplasm) C or cysts (with multiple nuclei) D in stool 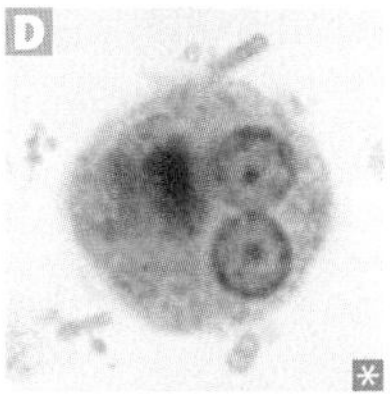	Metronidazole; iodoquinol for asymptomatic cyst passers
Cryptosporidium 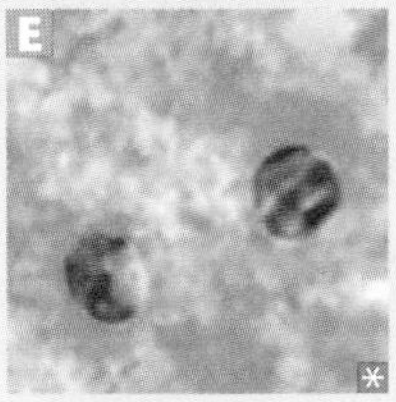	Severe diarrhea in AIDS Mild disease (watery diarrhea) in nonimmunocompromised	Cysts in water	Cysts on acid-fast stain E	Prevention (by filtering city water supplies); nitazoxanide in immunocompetent hosts

Protozoa—CNS infections

ORGANISM	DISEASE	TRANSMISSION	DIAGNOSIS	TREATMENT
Toxoplasma gondii 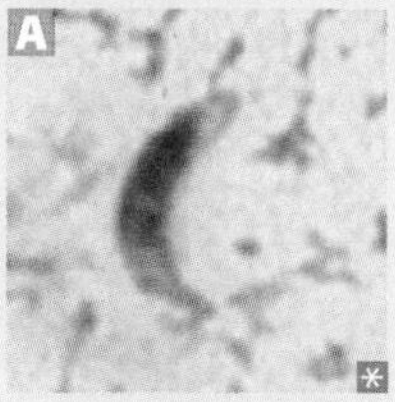	Brain abscess in HIV (seen as ring-enhancing brain lesions on CT/MRI); congenital toxoplasmosis = "classic triad" of chorioretinitis, hydrocephalus, and intracranial calcifications	Cysts in meat or cat feces; crosses placenta (pregnant women should avoid cats)	Serology, biopsy A	Sulfadiazine + pyrimethamine
Naegleria fowleri 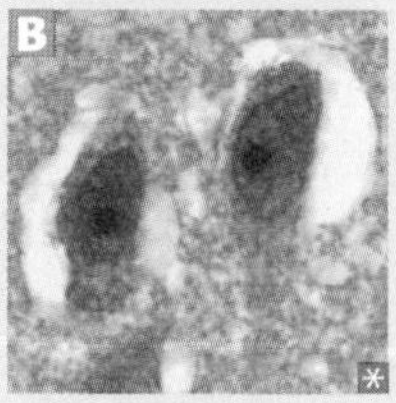	Rapidly fatal meningoencephalitis	Swimming in **freshwater** lakes (think **Nalgene** bottle filled with **freshwater** containing *Naegleria*); enters via cribriform plate	Amoebas in spinal fluid B	Amphotericin has been effective for a few survivors
Trypanosoma brucei ***T. gambiense*** ***T. rhodesiense*** 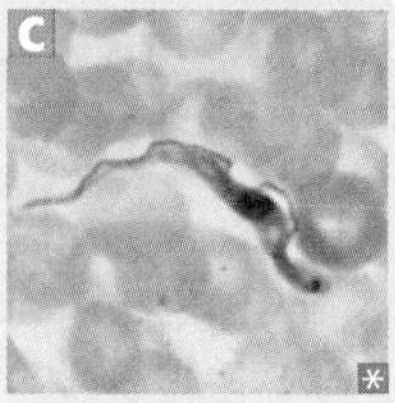	African sleeping sickness: enlarged lymph nodes, recurring fever (due to antigenic variation), somnolence, coma	Tsetse fly, a painful bite	Blood smear C	**Sur**amin for blood-borne disease or **mel**arsoprol for CNS penetration ("it **sure** is nice to go to sleep"; **mel**atonin helps with sleep)

Protozoa–Hematologic infections

ORGANISM	DISEASE	TRANSMISSION	DIAGNOSIS	TREATMENT
Plasmodium ***P. vivax/ovale*** ***P. falciparum*** ***P. malariae*** 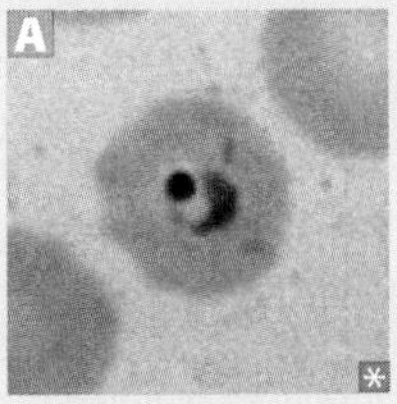	Malaria: fever, headache, anemia, splenomegaly *P. vivax/ovale*—48-hr cycle (tertian; includes fever on first day and third day, thus fevers are actually 48 hr apart); dormant form (hypnozoite) in liver *P. falciparum*—severe; irregular fever patterns; parasitized RBCs occlude capillaries in brain (cerebral malaria), kidneys, lungs *P. malariae*—72-hr cycle (quartan)	Mosquito (*Anopheles*)	Blood smear, trophozoite ring form A, RBC schizont with merozoites B 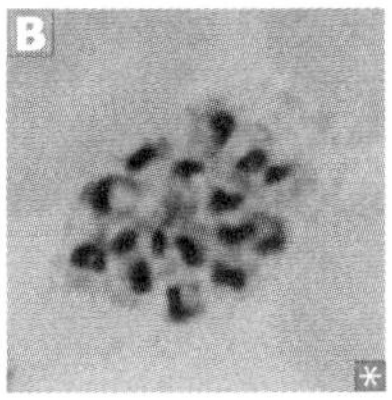	Begin with chloroquine, which blocks *Plasmodium* heme polymerase; if resistant, use mefloquine If life-threatening, use intravenous quinidine (test for G6PD deficiency) *Vivax/ovale*—add primaquine for hypnozoite (test for G6PD deficiency)
Babesia 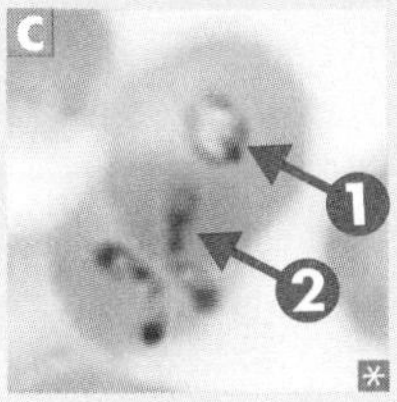	Babesiosis: fever and hemolytic anemia; predominantly in northeastern United States; asplenia ↑ risk of severe disease	*Ixodes* tick (same as *Borrelia burgdorferi* of Lyme disease; may often coinfect humans)	Blood smear, ring form C1, "Maltese cross" C2; PCR	Atovaquone + azithromycin

Protozoa—Others

ORGANISM	DISEASE	TRANSMISSION	DIAGNOSIS	TREATMENT
Visceral infections				
Trypanosoma cruzi 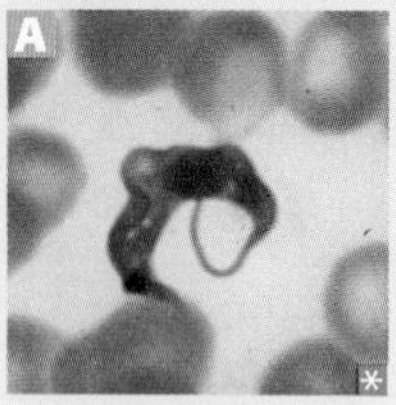	Chagas' disease: dilated cardiomyopathy, megacolon, megaesophagus; predominantly in South America	Reduviid bug ("kissing bug"), a painless bite (much like a kiss)	Blood smear A	Nifurtimox
Leishmania donovani 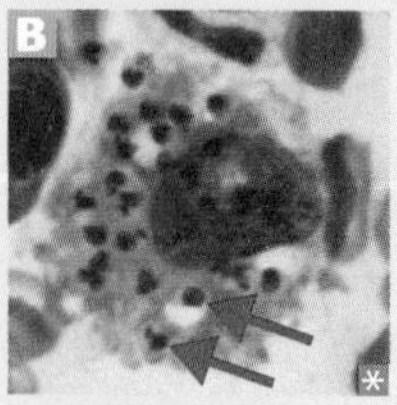	Visceral leishmaniasis (kala-azar): spiking fevers, hepatosplenomegaly, pancytopenia	Sandfly	Macrophages containing amastigotes B	Sodium stibogluconate
STDs				
Trichomonas vaginalis	Vaginitis: foul-smelling, greenish discharge; itching and burning; do not confuse with *Gardnerella vaginalis*, a gram-variable bacterium that causes vaginosis	Sexual (cannot exist outside human because it cannot form cysts)	Trophozoites (motile) on wet mount	Metronidazole for patient and partner (prophylaxis)

Nematodes (roundworms)

ORGANISM	TRANSMISSION	DISEASE	TREATMENT
Intestinal			
***Enterobius vermicularis* (pinworm)**	Food contaminated with eggs	Intestinal infection causing anal pruritus (diagnosed via the Scotch Tape test)	Bendazoles or pyrantel pamoate (worms are **bend**y; treat with me**bend**azole)
***Ascaris lumbricoides* (giant roundworm)**	Fecal-oral; eggs visible in feces under microscope	Intestinal infection	Bendazoles or pyrantel pamoate
Strongyloides stercoralis	Larvae in soil penetrate the skin	Intestinal infection causing vomiting, diarrhea, anemia	Ivermectin or albendazole
***Ancylostoma duodenale, Necator americanus* (hookworms)**	Larvae penetrate skin	Intestinal infection causing anemia by sucking blood from intestinal walls	Bendazoles or pyrantel pamoate
Tissue			
Dracunculus medinensis	In drinking water	Skin inflammation and ulceration	Slow extraction of worm
Onchocerca volvulus	Female blackfly bite	Hyperpigmented skin and river blindness (**black** flies, **black** skin nodules, "**black** sight"; allergic reaction to microfilaria possible	Ivermectin (**iver**mectin for **river** blindness)
Loa loa	Deer fly, horse fly, mango fly	Swelling in skin, worm in conjunctiva	Diethylcarbamazine
Wuchereria bancrofti	Female mosquito	Blocks lymphatic vessels: elephantiasis; takes 9 mo–1 yr after bite to become symptomatic	Diethylcarbamazine
Toxocara canis	Food contaminated with eggs	Visceral larva migrans	Albendazole or mebendazole

Nematode routes of infection

Ingested—*Enterobius, Ascaris, Trichinella.*
Cutaneous—*Strongyloides, Ancylostoma, Necator*

You'll get sick if you **EAT** these!
These get into your feet from the **SAN**d.

Cestodes (tapeworms)

ORGANISM	TRANSMISSION	DISEASE	TREATMENT
Taenia solium	Ingestion of larvae encysted in undercooked pork Ingestion of eggs	Intestinal infection Cysticercosis, neurocysticercosis	Praziquantel Praziquantel; -bendazoles for neurocysticercosis
Diphyllobothrium latum	Ingestion of larvae from raw freshwater fish	Vitamin B_{12} deficiency (tapeworm competes for B_{12} in intestine) → anemia	Praziquantel
Echinococcus granulosus	Ingestion of eggs from dog feces	Cysts in liver, causing anaphylaxis if antigens released (surgeons preinject with ethanol to kill cysts before removal)	-bendazoles

Trematodes (flukes)

ORGANISM	TRANSMISSION	DISEASE	TREATMENT
Schistosoma	Snails are host; cercariae penetrate skin of humans	Liver and spleen granulomas, fibrosis, and inflammation Chronic infection with *S. haematobium* can lead to squamous cell carcinoma of the bladder	Praziquantel
Clonorchis sinensis	Undercooked fish	Biliary tract inflammation → pigmented gallstones Associated with cholangiocarcinoma	Praziquantel
Paragonimus westermani	Undercooked crab meat	Lung inflammation and 2° bacterial infection, with hemoptysis	Praziquantel

Parasite hints

FINDINGS	ORGANISM
Brain cysts, seizures	*Taenia solium* (cysticercosis)
Liver cysts	*Echinococcus granulosus*
Vitamin B_{12} deficiency	*Diphyllobothrium latum*
Biliary tract disease, cholangiocarcinoma	*Clonorchis sinensis*
Hemoptysis	*Paragonimus westermani*
Portal hypertension	*Schistosoma mansoni*
Hematuria, bladder cancer	*Schistosoma haematobium*
Microcytic anemia	*Ancylostoma*, *Necator*
Perianal pruritus	*Enterobius*

▶ MICROBIOLOGY—VIROLOGY

Viral structure—general features

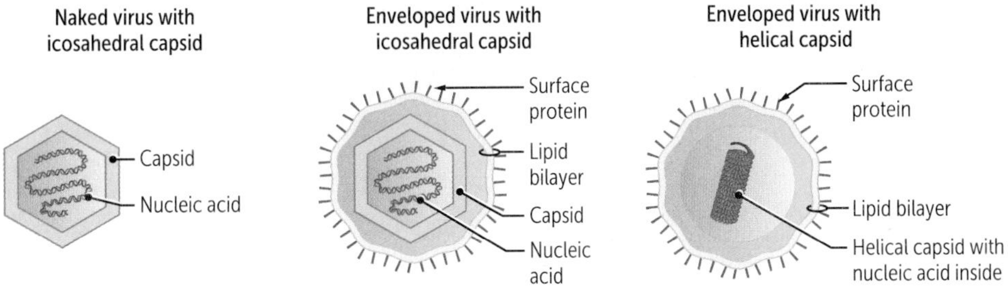
Naked virus with icosahedral capsid
Capsid
Nucleic acid
Enveloped virus with icosahedral capsid
Surface protein
Lipid bilayer
Capsid
Nucleic acid
Enveloped virus with helical capsid
Surface protein
Lipid bilayer
Helical capsid with nucleic acid inside

Viral genetics

Recombination	Exchange of genes between 2 chromosomes by crossing over within regions of significant base sequence homology.
Reassortment	When viruses with segmented genomes (e.g., influenza virus) exchange segments. High-frequency recombination. Cause of worldwide influenza pandemics.
Complementation	When 1 of 2 viruses that infect the cell has a mutation that results in a nonfunctional protein. The nonmutated virus "complements" the mutated one by making a functional protein that serves both viruses.
Phenotypic mixing	Occurs with simultaneous infection of a cell with 2 viruses. Genome of virus A can be partially or completely coated (forming pseudovirion) with the surface proteins of virus B. Type B protein coat determines the tropism (infectivity) of the hybrid virus. However, the progeny from this infection have a type A coat that is encoded by its type A genetic material.

Viral vaccines

Live attenuated vaccines	Induce humoral and cell-mediated immunity but have reverted to virulence on rare occasions. Killed/inactivated vaccines induce only humoral immunity but are stable. Live attenuated—**small**pox, **yellow** fever, **chicken**pox (VZV), **Sabin's** polio virus, **MMR**, Influenza (intranasal).	No booster needed for live attenuated vaccines. Dangerous to give live vaccines to immunocompromised patients or their close contacts. "**Live**! One night only! See **small yellow chickens** get vaccinated with **Sabin**'s and **MMR**! It's incredible!" MMR = measles, mumps, rubella (live attenuated vaccine that can be given to HIV-positive patients who do not show signs of immunodeficiency).
Killed	Rabies, Influenza (injected), Salk Polio, and HAV vaccines.	Sal**K** = **K**illed. **RIP A**lways.
Recombinant	HBV (antigen = recombinant HBsAg), HPV (types 6, 11, 16, and 18).	

DNA viral genomes	All DNA viruses except the Parvoviridae are dsDNA. All are linear except papilloma-, polyoma-, and hepadnaviruses (circular).	All are dsDNA (like our cells), except "**part-of-a-virus**" (**parvovirus**) is ssDNA. *Parvus* = small.

RNA viral genomes	All RNA viruses except Reoviridae are ssRNA. Positive-stranded RNA viruses: I went to a **retro** (**retro**virus) **toga** (**toga**virus) party, where I drank **flavored** (**flavi**virus) **Corona** (**corona**virus) and ate **hippy** (**hepe**virus) **Cali**fornia (**cali**civirus) **pic**kles (**pic**ornavirus).	All are ssRNA (like our mRNA), except "**repeato-virus**" (**reo**virus) is dsRNA.
Naked viral genome infectivity	Purified nucleic acids of most dsDNA (except poxviruses and HBV) and (+) strand ssRNA (≈ mRNA) viruses are infectious. Naked nucleic acids of (−) strand ssRNA and dsRNA viruses are not infectious. They require polymerases contained in the complete virion.	
Virus ploidy	All viruses are haploid (with 1 copy of DNA or RNA) except retroviruses, which have 2 identical ssRNA molecules (≈ diploid).	

Viral replication

DNA viruses	All replicate in the nucleus (except poxvirus).
RNA viruses	All replicate in the cytoplasm (except influenza virus and retroviruses).

Viral envelopes	**Naked** (nonenveloped) viruses include **P**apillomavirus, **A**denovirus, **P**icornavirus, **P**olyomavirus, **C**alcivirus, **P**arvovirus, **R**eovirus, and **He**pevirus. Generally, enveloped viruses acquire their envelopes from plasma membrane when they exit from cell. Exceptions include herpesviruses, which acquire envelopes from nuclear membrane.	Give **PAPP** smears and **CPR** to a **naked Heppy** (hippy). DNA = PAPP; RNA = CPR and hepevirus.

DNA virus characteristics

Some general rules—all DNA viruses:

GENERAL RULE	COMMENTS
Are **HHAPPPPy** viruses	**H**epadna, **H**erpes, **A**deno, **P**ox, **P**arvo, **P**apilloma, **P**olyoma.
Are double stranded	Except parvo (single stranded).
Are linear	Except papilloma and polyoma (circular, supercoiled) and hepadna (circular, incomplete).
Are icosahedral	Except pox (complex).
Replicate in the nucleus	Except pox (carries own DNA-dependent RNA polymerase).

DNA viruses

VIRAL FAMILY	ENVELOPE	DNA STRUCTURE	MEDICAL IMPORTANCE
Herpesviruses	Yes	DS and linear	HSV-1—oral (and some genital) lesions, spontaneous temporal lobe encephalitis, keratoconjunctivitis HSV-2—genital (and some oral) lesions VZV (HHV-3)—chickenpox, zoster (shingles); vaccine available EBV (HHV-4)—mononucleosis, Burkitt's lymphoma, Hodgkin's lymphoma CMV (HHV-5)—infection in immunosuppressed patients (AIDS retinitis), especially transplant recipients; congenital defects ("**sight**omegalovirus") HHV-6—roseola (exanthem subitum) HHV-7—less common cause of roseola HHV-8—Kaposi's sarcoma–associated herpesvirus (KSHV)
Hepadnavirus	Yes	DS and partial circular	HBV: ▪ Acute or chronic hepatitis ▪ Vaccine available—contains HBV surface antigen ▪ Not a retrovirus but has reverse transcriptase
Adenovirus	No	DS and linear	Febrile pharyngitis—sore throat; acute hemorrhagic cystitis Pneumonia Conjunctivitis—"pink eye"
Parvovirus	No	SS and linear (–) (smallest DNA virus)	B19 virus—aplastic crises in sickle cell disease, "slapped cheeks" rash in children—erythema infectiosum (fifth disease), RBC destruction in fetus leads to hydrops fetalis and death, pure RBC aplasia and rheumatoid arthritis–like symptoms in adults
Papillomavirus	No	DS and circular	HPV—warts (1, 2, 6, 11), CIN, cervical cancer (16, 18) vaccine available
Polyomavirus	No	DS and circular	JC virus—progressive multifocal leukoencephalopathy (PML) in HIV BK virus—transplant patients, commonly targets kidney (**J**C: **J**unky **C**erebrum; **BK**: **B**ad **K**idney)
Poxvirus	Yes	DS and linear (largest DNA virus)	Smallpox, although eradicated, could be used in germ warfare Vaccinia—cowpox ("milkmaid's blisters") Molluscum contagiosum—flesh-colored dome lesions with central dimple

DS, double-stranded; SS, single-stranded

Herpesviruses

VIRUS	DISEASES	ROUTE OF TRANSMISSION
HSV-1	Gingivostomatitis, keratoconjunctivitis, temporal lobe encephalitis (most common cause of sporadic encephalitis in the United States), herpes labialis A. Latent in trigeminal ganglia.	Respiratory secretions, saliva
HSV-2	Herpes genitalis B, neonatal herpes. Latent in sacral ganglia.	Sexual contact, perinatal
VZV	Varicella-zoster (chickenpox, shingles) C, encephalitis, pneumonia. Latent in dorsal root or trigeminal ganglia.	Respiratory secretions
EBV	Infectious mononucleosis, Burkitt's/Hodgkin's lymphoma, nasopharyngeal carcinoma. Latent in B cells.	Respiratory secretions, saliva
CMV	Congenital infection, mononucleosis (negative Monospot), pneumonia, retinitis. Infected cells have characteristic "owl's eye" inclusions D. Latent in mononuclear cells.	Congenital, transfusion, sexual contact, saliva, urine, transplant
HHV-6	Roseola: high fevers for several days that can cause seizures, followed by a diffuse macular rash.	Not determined
HHV-8	Kaposi's sarcoma (HIV patients).	Sexual contact

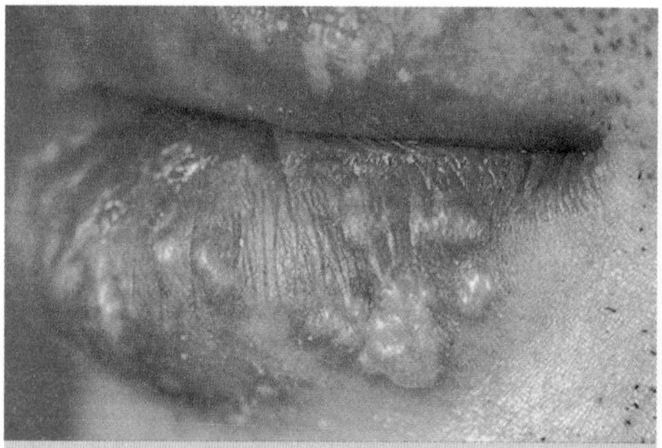

A **Herpes labialis.** Grouped and confluent vesicles with an erythematous rim.

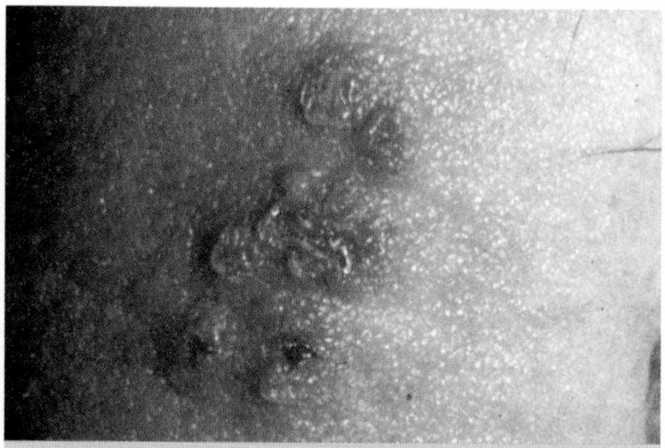

B **Herpes genitalis.** Ulcerating vesicles associated with HSV-2 and less frequently HSV-1.

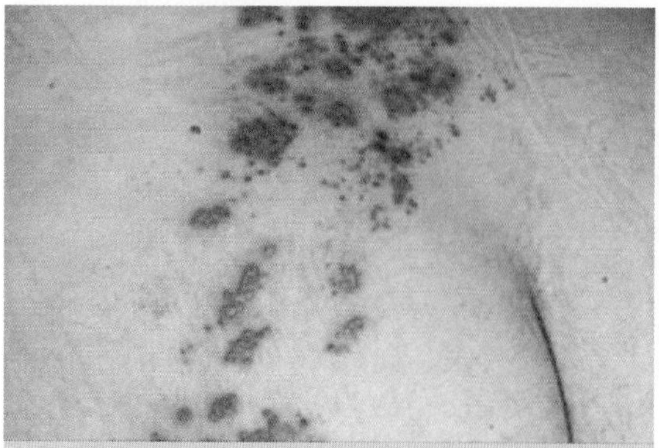

C **Zoster.** Hemorrhagic vesicles and pustules in dermatomal distribution.

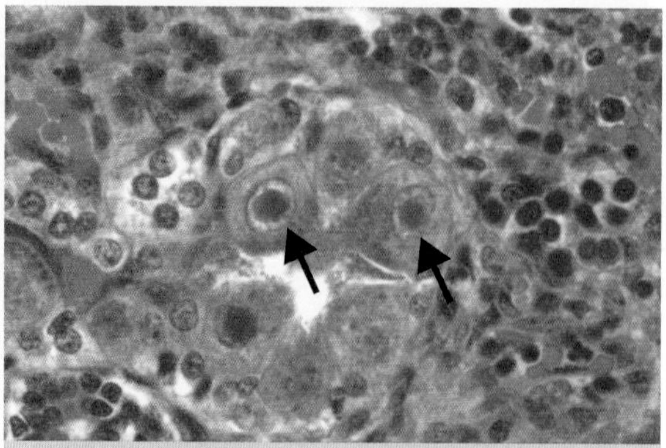

D **CMV.** Renal tubular cells in a neonate with congenital CMV infection. Note the "owl's eye" inclusions (arrows).

HSV identification	PCR is test of choice. Tzanck test—a smear of an opened skin vesicle to detect multinucleated giant cells commonly seen in HSV-1, HSV-2, and VZV. Infected cells also have intranuclear Cowdry A inclusions.	**Tzanck** heavens I do not have herpes.
EBV	A herpesvirus. Can cause mononucleosis. Infects B cells. Characterized by fever, hepatosplenomegaly, pharyngitis, and lymphadenopathy (especially posterior cervical nodes). Peak incidence 15–20 years of age. Atypical lymphocytes seen on peripheral blood smear A are not infected B cells but rather reactive cytotoxic T cells. Positive Monospot test—heterophile antibodies detected by agglutination of sheep or horse RBCs. Also associated with development of Hodgkin's and endemic Burkitt's lymphomas as well as nasopharyngeal carcinoma.	Most common during peak kissing years ("kissing disease"). 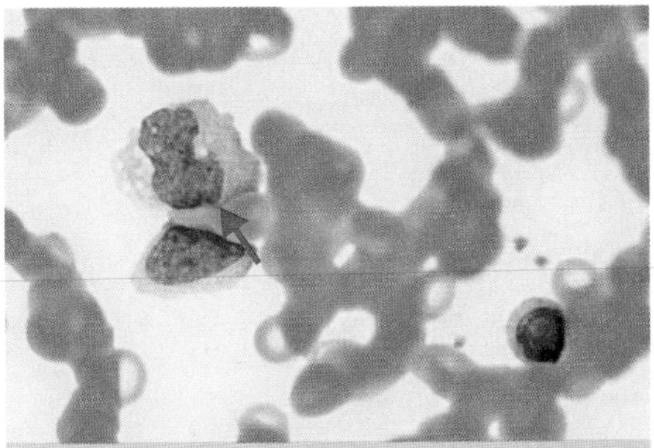 A **Atypical lymphocytes.** Seen with EBV infection. Note "hugging" of RBCs (arrow).

RNA viruses

VIRAL FAMILY	ENVELOPE	RNA STRUCTURE	CAPSID SYMMETRY	MEDICAL IMPORTANCE
Reoviruses	No	DS linear 10–12 segments	Icosahedral (double)	Coltivirus[a]—Colorado tick fever Rotavirus—#1 cause of fatal diarrhea in children
Picornaviruses	No	SS ⊕ linear	Icosahedral	**P**oliovirus—polio-Salk/Sabin vaccines—IPV/OPV **E**chovirus—aseptic meningitis **R**hinovirus—"common cold" **C**oxsackievirus—aseptic meningitis; herpangina (mouth blisters, fever); hand, foot, and mouth disease; myocarditis **H**AV—acute viral hepatitis **PERCH**
Hepevirus	No	SS ⊕ linear	Icosahedral	HEV
Caliciviruses	No	SS ⊕ linear	Icosahedral	Norovirus—viral gastroenteritis
Flaviviruses	Yes	SS ⊕ linear	Icosahedral	HCV Yellow fever[a] Dengue[a] St. Louis encephalitis[a] West Nile virus[a]
Togaviruses	Yes	SS ⊕ linear	Icosahedral	Rubella Eastern equine encephalitis[a] Western equine encephalitis[a]
Retroviruses	Yes	SS ⊕ linear	Icosahedral (HTLV), complex and conical (HIV)	Have reverse transcriptase HTLV—T-cell leukemia HIV—AIDS
Coronaviruses	Yes	SS ⊕ linear	Helical	Coronavirus—"common cold" and SARS
Orthomyxoviruses	Yes	SS ⊖ linear 8 segments	Helical	Influenza virus
Paramyxoviruses	Yes	SS ⊖ linear Nonsegmented	Helical	**P**a**R**a**M**yxovirus: **P**arainfluenza—croup **R**SV—bronchiolitis in babies; **R**x—**r**ibavirin **M**easles, **M**umps
Rhabdoviruses	Yes	SS ⊖ linear	Helical	Rabies
Filoviruses	Yes	SS ⊖ linear	Helical	Ebola/Marburg hemorrhagic fever—often fatal!
Arenaviruses	Yes	SS ⊖ circular 2 segments	Helical	LCMV—lymphocytic choriomeningitis virus Lassa fever encephalitis—spread by mice
Bunyaviruses	Yes	SS ⊖ circular 3 segments	Helical	California encephalitis[a] Sandfly/Rift Valley fevers[a] Crimean-Congo hemorrhagic fever[a] Hantavirus—hemorrhagic fever, pneumonia
Delta virus	Yes	SS ⊖ circular	Uncertain	HDV is a "defective" virus that requires HBV co-infection

SS, single-stranded; DS, double-stranded; ⊕, positive sense; ⊖, negative sense; [a]= arbovirus, transmitted by arthropods (mosquitoes, ticks).

(Adapted, with permission, from Levinson W, Jawetz E. *Medical Microbiology and Immunology: Examination and Board Review,* 6th ed. New York: McGraw-Hill, 2000: 182.)

Negative-stranded viruses	Must transcribe negative strand to positive. Virion brings its own RNA-dependent RNA polymerase. They include **A**renaviruses, **B**unyaviruses, **P**aramyxoviruses, **O**rthomyxoviruses, **F**iloviruses, and **R**habdoviruses.	**A**lways **B**ring **P**olymerase **O**r **F**ail **R**eplication.
Segmented viruses	All are RNA viruses. They include **B**unyaviruses, **O**rthomyxoviruses (influenza viruses), **A**renaviruses, and **R**eoviruses.	BOAR.
Picornavirus	Includes **P**oliovirus, **E**chovirus, **R**hinovirus, **C**oxsackievirus, **H**AV. RNA is translated into 1 large polypeptide that is cleaved by proteases into functional viral proteins. Can cause aseptic (viral) meningitis (except rhinovirus and HAV). All are enteroviruses (fecal-oral spread) except rhinovirus.	Pico**RNA**virus = small **RNA** virus. **PERCH** on a "**peak**" (**pico**).
Rhinovirus	A picornavirus. Nonenveloped RNA virus. Cause of common cold; > 100 serologic types. Acid labile—destroyed by stomach acid; therefore, does not infect the GI tract (unlike the other picornaviruses).	**Rhino** has a runny **nose**.
Yellow fever virus	A flavivirus (also an arbovirus) transmitted by *Aedes* mosquitoes. Virus has a monkey or human reservoir. Symptoms: high fever, black vomitus, and jaundice.	*Flavi* = yellow, jaundice.
Rotavirus 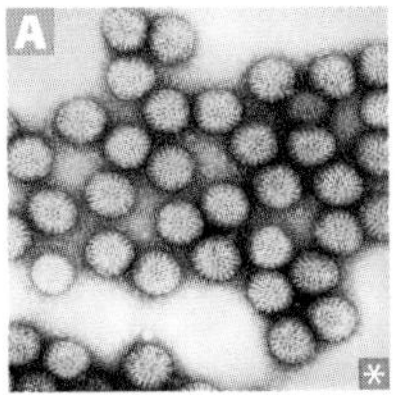	Rotavirus A, the most important global cause of infantile gastroenteritis, is a segmented dsRNA virus (a reovirus). Major cause of acute diarrhea in the United States during winter, especially in day-care centers, kindergartens. Villous destruction with atrophy leads to ↓ absorption of Na^+ and loss of K^+.	**ROTA**virus = **R**ight **O**ut **T**he **A**nus. CDC recommends routine vaccination of all infants.

Influenza viruses	Orthomyxoviruses. Enveloped, negative single-stranded RNA viruses with 8-segment genome. Contain hemagglutinin (promotes viral entry) and neuraminidase (promotes progeny virion release) antigens. Patients at risk for fatal bacterial superinfection. Rapid genetic changes.	Killed viral vaccine is major mode of protection; reformulated vaccine offered each fall. Vaccine containing live, temperature-sensitive mutant that replicates in the nose but not in the lung is also available. Used in children.
Genetic shift /antigenic shifts	Causes pandemics. Reassortment of viral genome; segments undergo high-frequency recombination, such as when human flu A virus recombines with swine flu A virus.	Sudden shift is more deadly than gradual drift.
Genetic drift	Causes epidemics. Minor (antigenic drift) changes based on random mutation.	

Rubella virus	A togavirus. Causes rubella, once known as German (3-day) measles. Fever, postauricular adenopathy, lymphadenopathy, arthralgias, fine truncal rash that starts at head and moves down. Causes mild disease in children but serious congenital disease (a ToRCHeS infection).
Paramyxoviruses	Paramyxoviruses cause disease in children. They include those that cause parainfluenza (croup: seal-like barking cough), mumps, and measles as well as RSV, which causes respiratory tract infection (bronchiolitis, pneumonia) in infants. All contain surface F (fusion) protein, which causes respiratory epithelial cells to fuse and form multinucleated cells. Palivizumab (monoclonal antibody against F protein) prevents pneumonia caused by RSV infection in premature infants.

Measles virus

A paramyxovirus that causes measles. Koplik spots A (red spots with blue-white center on buccal mucosa) and descending maculopapular rash B are characteristic. SSPE (subacute sclerosing panencephalitis, occurring years later), encephalitis (1:2000), and giant cell pneumonia (rarely, in immunosuppressed) are possible sequelae. Rash presents last and spreads from head to toe. Includes hands and feet (vs. truncal rash in rubella). Do not confuse with roseola (caused by HHV-6).

3 C's of measles:
Cough
Coryza
Conjunctivitis

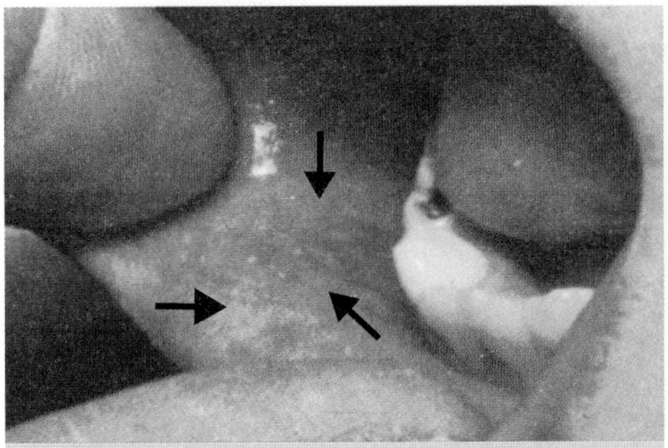

A **Koplik spots.** Note small white lesions with an erythematous halo that precede the measles rash by 1-2 days.

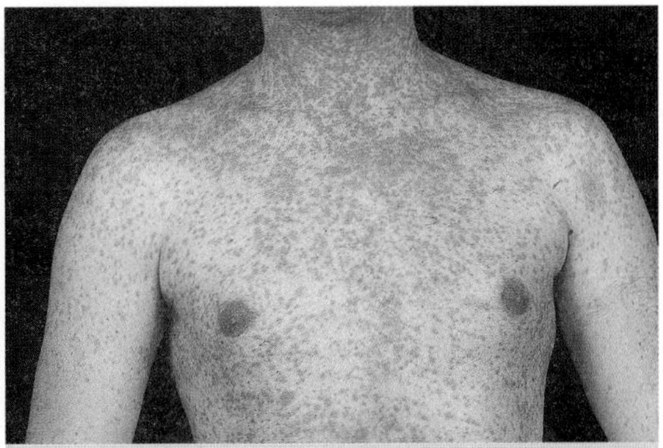

B **Rash of measles.** Discrete erythematous rash becomes confluent as it progresses downward.

Mumps virus

A paramyxovirus.
Symptoms: **P**arotitis A, **O**rchitis (inflammation of testes), and aseptic **M**eningitis. Can cause sterility (especially after puberty).

Mumps makes your parotid glands and testes as big as **POM-poms**.

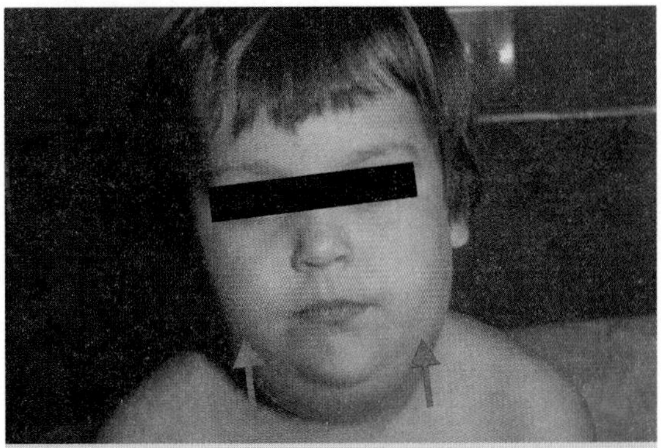

A **Mumps.** Swollen neck and parotid glands (arrows).

Rabies virus

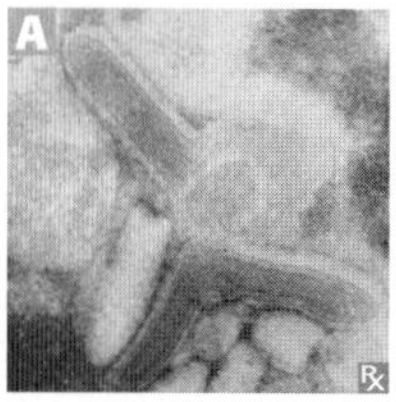

Bullet-shaped virus A. Negri bodies are characteristic cytoplasmic inclusions in neurons infected by rabies virus; commonly found in Purkinje cells of cerebellum B. Rabies has long incubation period (weeks to months) before symptom onset. Postexposure treatment is wound cleansing and vaccination ± rabies immune globulin.

Travels to the CNS by migrating in a retrograde fashion up nerve axons.

Progression of disease: fever, malaise → agitation, photophobia, hydrophobia → paralysis, coma → death.

More commonly from bat, raccoon, and skunk bites than from dog bites in the United States.

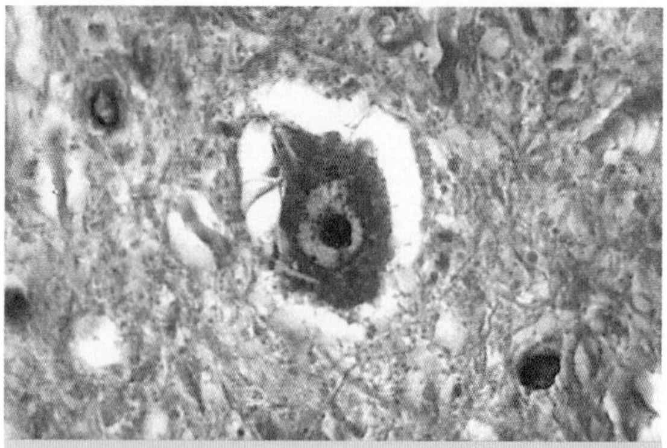

B Negri body.

Hepatitis viruses

	VIRUS	TRANSMISSION	CARRIER	INCUBATION	HCC RISK	NOTES
HAV[a]	RNA picornavirus	Fecal-oral	No	Short (weeks)	No	Asymptomatic (usually), Acute, Alone (no carriers)
HBV[b]	DNA hepadnavirus	Parenteral, sexual, maternal-fetal	Yes	Long (months)	Yes: integrates into host genome, acts as oncogene	
HCV	RNA flavivirus	Primarily blood, IVDU, post-transfusion	Yes	Long	Yes: from chronic inflammation	Chronic, Cirrhosis, Carcinoma, Carrier
HDV	RNA delta virus	Parenteral, sexual, maternal-fetal	Yes	Superinfection—short Co-infection—long	Yes	Defective virus Dependent on HBV; superinfection → ↓ prognosis
HEV[a]	RNA hepevirus	Fecal-oral, especially with waterborne epidemics	No	Short	No	High mortality in pregnant women; Enteric, Expectant mothers, Epidemic

Signs and symptoms of all hepatitis viruses: episodes of fever, jaundice, elevated ALT and AST.

[a]HAV and HEV are fecal-oral: The **vowels** hit your **bowels**. Naked viruses do not rely on an envelope so they are not destroyed by the gut.

[b]In HBV, the virus uses its own DNA-dependent DNA polymerase to make full double-stranded DNA. The host RNA polymerase transcribes mRNA from viral DNA and then makes viral proteins from the mRNAs.

Hepatitis serologic markers	
Anti-HAV (IgM)	IgM antibody to HAV; best test to detect active hepatitis A.
Anti-HAV (IgG)	IgG antibody indicates prior HAV infection and/or prior vaccination; protects against reinfection.
HBsAg	Antigen found on surface of HBV; indicates hepatitis B infection.
Anti-HBs	Antibody to HBsAg; indicates immunity to hepatitis B.
HBcAg	Antigen associated with core of HBV.
Anti-HBc	Antibody to HBcAg; IgM = acute/recent infection; IgG = prior exposure or chronic infection. Positive during window period.
HBeAg	A second, different antigenic determinant in the HBV core. HBeAg indicates active viral replication and therefore high transmissibility.
Anti-HBe	Antibody to e antigen; indicates low transmissibility.

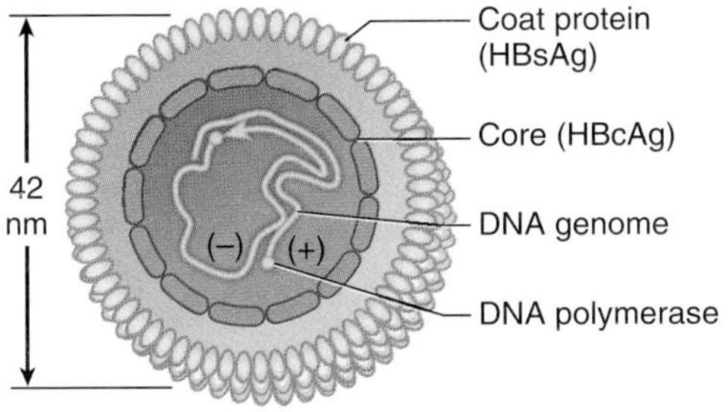

Virus particle

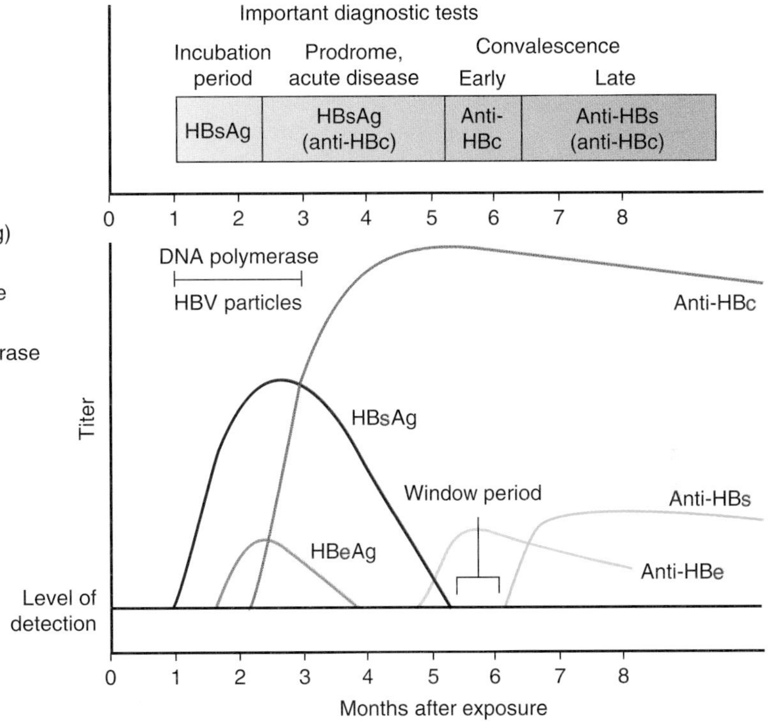

In viral hepatitis, ALT > AST.
In alcoholic hepatitis, AST > ALT.
SECES: SE are antigens, CES are antibodies; labeled on figure in order of appearance.

	HBsAg	Anti-HBs	HBeAg	Anti-HBe	Anti-HBc
Acute HBV	+		+		IgM
Window				+	IgM
Chronic HBV (high infectivity)	+		+		IgG
Chronic HBV (low infectivity)	+			+	IgG
Recovery		+		+	IgG
Immunized		+			

HIV

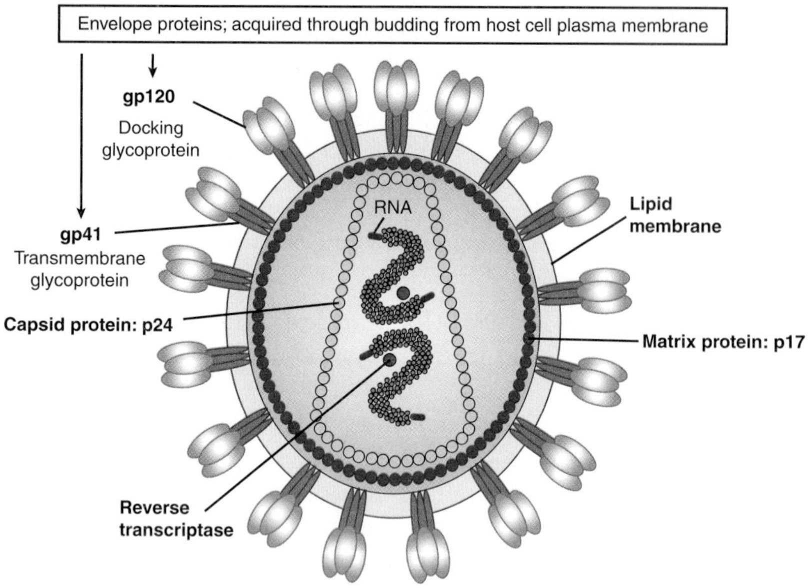

Envelope proteins; acquired through budding from host cell plasma membrane
gp120
Docking glycoprotein
gp41
Transmembrane glycoprotein
Capsid protein: p24
RNA
Lipid membrane
Matrix protein: p17
Reverse transcriptase

Diploid genome (2 molecules of RNA).

The 3 structural genes (protein coded for):

- *env* (gp120 and gp41):
  - Formed from cleavage of gp160 to form envelope proteins.
  - gp120—attachment to host CD4+ T cell.
  - gp41—fusion and entry.
- *gag* (p24)—capsid protein.
- *pol*—reverse transcriptase, aspartate protease, integrase.

Reverse transcriptase synthesizes dsDNA from RNA; dsDNA integrates into host genome.

Virus binds CCR5 (early) or CXCR4 (late) co-receptor and CD4 on T cells; binds CCR5 and CD4 on macrophages.

Homozygous CCR5 mutation = immunity.

Heterozygous CCR5 mutation = slower course.

HIV diagnosis

Presumptive diagnosis made with ELISA (sensitive, high false-positive rate and low threshold, **rule out** test); positive results are then confirmed with Western blot assay (specific, high false-negative rate and high threshold, **rule in** test).

HIV PCR/viral load tests determine the amount of viral RNA in the plasma. High viral load associated with poor prognosis. Also use viral load to monitor effect of drug therapy.

AIDS diagnosis ≤ 200 CD4+ cells/mm^3 (normal: 500–1500 cells/mm^3). HIV positive with AIDS-defining condition (e.g., *Pneumocystis* pneumonia, or PCP) or CD4/CD8 ratio < 1.5.

ELISA/Western blot tests look for antibodies to viral proteins; these tests often are falsely negative in the first 1–2 months of HIV infection and falsely positive initially in babies born to infected mothers (anti-gp120 crosses placenta).

Time course of HIV infection

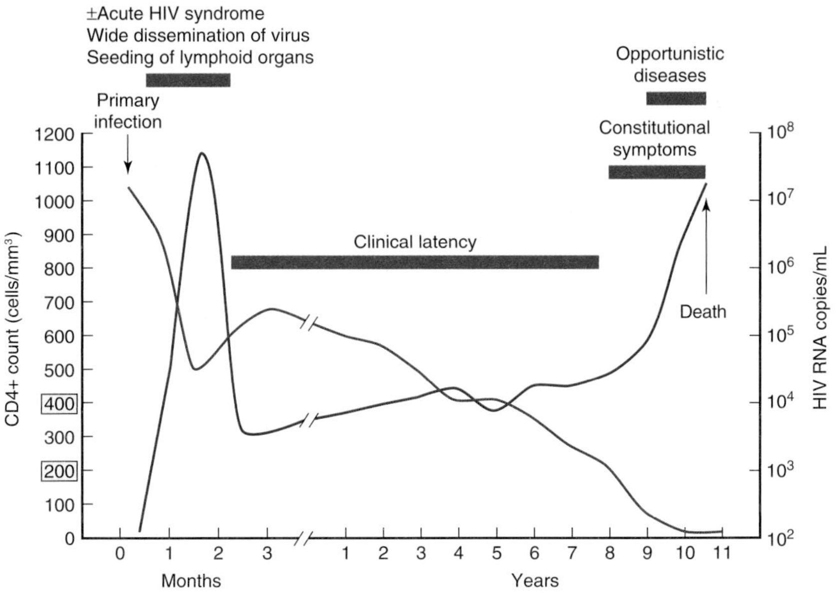

±Acute HIV syndrome
Wide dissemination of virus
Seeding of lymphoid organs
Primary infection
Opportunistic diseases
Constitutional symptoms
Clinical latency
Death
CD4+ count (cells/mm³)
1200
1100
1000
900
800
700
600
500
400
300
200
100
0
HIV RNA copies/mL
10⁸
10⁷
10⁶
10⁵
10⁴
10³
10²
0 1 2 3
Months
1 2 3 4 5 6 7 8 9 10 11
Years

Red line = CD4+ T-lymphocyte count (cells/mm^3); blue line = HIV RNA copies/mL plasma.

Blue boxes indicate immunocompromise (< 400 CD4+ cell/mm^3) and when AIDS-defining illnesses emerge (< 200 CD4+ cells/mm^3).

Four stages of infection:

1. Flu-like (acute)
2. Feeling fine (latent)
3. Falling count
4. Final crisis

During latent phase, virus replicates in lymph nodes.

Common diseases of HIV-positive adults

As CD4 count ↓, risk of reactivation of past infections (e.g., TB, HSV, shingles), dissemination of bacterial infections and fungal infections (e.g., coccidioidomycosis), and non-Hodgkin's lymphomas ↑.

CLINICAL PRESENTATION	FINDINGS/LABS	PATHOGEN
Systemic		
Low-grade fevers, cough, hepatosplenomegaly, tongue ulcer	Oval yeast cells within macrophages, CD4 < 100 cells/mm^3	*Histoplasma capsulatum* (causes only pulmonary symptoms in immunocompetent hosts)
Dermatologic		
Fluffy white cottage-cheese lesions	Pseudohyphae, commonly oral if CD4 < 400 cells/mm^3, esophageal if CD4 < 100 cells/mm^3	*C. albicans* (causes thrush)
Superficial vascular proliferation	Biopsy reveals neutrophilic inflammation	*Bartonella henselae* (causes bacillary angiomatosis)
Gastrointestinal		
Chronic, watery diarrhea	Acid-fast cysts seen in stool especially when CD4 < 200 cells/mm^3	*Cryptosporidium* spp.
Neurologic		
Encephalopathy	Due to reactivation of a latent virus; results in demyelination, CD4 < 200 cells/mm^3	JC virus reactivation (cause of PML)
Abscesses	Many ring-enhancing lesions on imaging, CD4 < 100 cells/mm^3	*Toxoplasma gondii*
Meningitis	India ink stain reveals yeast with narrow-based budding and large capsule, CD4 < 50 cells/mm^3	*Cryptococcus neoformans*
Retinitis	Cotton-wool spots on funduscopic exam and may also occur with esophagitis, CD4 < 50 cells/mm^3	CMV
Dementia	Must differentiate from other causes	Directly associated with HIV
Oncologic		
Superficial neoplastic proliferation of vasculature	Biopsy reveals lymphocytic inflammation	HHV-8 (causes Kaposi's sarcoma), do not confuse with bacillary angiomatosis caused by *B. henselae*
Hairy leukoplakia	Often on lateral tongue	EBV
Non-Hodgkin's lymphoma (large cell type)	Often on oropharynx (Waldeyer's ring)	May be associated with EBV
Squamous cell carcinoma	Often in anus (men who have sex with men) or cervix (females)	HPV
Primary CNS lymphoma	Focal or multiple, differentiate from toxoplasmosis	Often associated with EBV
Respiratory		
Interstitial pneumonia	Biopsy reveals cells with intranuclear (owl's eye) inclusion bodies	CMV
Invasive aspergillosis	Pleuritic pain, hemoptysis, infiltrates on imaging	*Aspergillus fumigatus*
Pneumonia	Especially with CD4 < 200 cells/mm^3	*Pneumocystis jirovecii*
Tuberculosis-like disease	Especially with CD4 < 50 cells/mm^3	*Mycobacterium avium–intracellulare*

Prions

Prion diseases are caused by the conversion of a normal cellular protein termed prion protein (PrP^c) to a β-pleated form (PrP^{sc}), which is transmissible. PrP^{sc} resists degradation and facilitates the conversion of still more PrP^c to PrP^{sc}. Accumulation of PrP^{sc} results in spongiform encephalopathy and dementia, ataxia, and death. It can be sporadic (Creutzfeldt-Jakob disease—rapidly progressive dementia), inherited (Gerstmann-Sträussler-Scheinker syndrome), or acquired (kuru).

▶ MICROBIOLOGY—SYSTEMS

Normal flora: dominant

LOCATION	MICROORGANISM
Skin	*Staphylococcus epidermidis*
Nose	*S. epidermidis*; colonized by *S. aureus*
Oropharynx	Viridans group streptococci
Dental plaque	*Streptococcus mutans*
Colon	*Bacteroides fragilis* > *E. coli*
Vagina	*Lactobacillus*, colonized by *E. coli* and group B strep

Neonates delivered by cesarean section have no flora but are rapidly colonized after birth.

Bugs causing food poisoning

S. aureus and *B. cereus* food poisoning starts quickly and ends quickly.

MICROORGANISM	SOURCE OF INFECTION
Vibrio parahaemolyticus and *V. vulnificus*[a]	Contaminated seafood
Bacillus cereus	Reheated rice. "Food poisoning from reheated rice? **Be serious!**" (***B. cereus***)
S. aureus	Meats, mayonnaise, custard; preformed toxin
Clostridium perfringens	Reheated meat dishes
C. botulinum	Improperly canned foods (sign is bulging cans)
E. coli O157:H7	Undercooked meat
Salmonella	Poultry, meat, and eggs

[a]*V. vulnificus* can also cause wound infections from contact with contaminated water or shellfish.

Bugs that can mimic appendicitis

Yersinia enterocolitica is most common cause of mesenteric adenitis, a disease that mimics appendicitis. Nontyphoidal *Salmonella* can also be a cause. *Camplyobacter jejuni* may also mimic appendicitis.

Bugs causing diarrhea

Bloody diarrhea	
Campylobacter	Comma- or S-shaped organisms; growth at 42°C
Salmonella	Lactose negative; flagellar motility; has animal reservoir, especially poultry and eggs
Shigella	Lactose negative; very low ID_{50}; produces Shiga toxin (human reservoir only)
Enterohemorrhagic *E. coli*	O157:H7; can cause HUS; makes Shiga-like toxin
Enteroinvasive *E. coli*	Invades colonic mucosa
Yersinia enterocolitica	Day-care outbreaks, pseudoappendicitis
Entamoeba histolytica	Protozoan
Watery diarrhea	
Enterotoxigenic *E. coli*	Traveler's diarrhea; produces ST and LT toxins
Vibrio cholerae	Comma-shaped organisms; rice-water diarrhea
C. difficile	Can also cause bloody diarrhea. Pseudomembranous colitis
C. perfringens	Also causes gas gangrene
Protozoa	*Giardia*, *Cryptosporidium* (in immunocompromised)
Viruses	Rotavirus, norovirus

Common causes of pneumonia

NEONATES (< 4 WK)	CHILDREN (4 WK–18 YR)	ADULTS (18–40 YR)	ADULTS (40–65 YR)	ELDERLY
Group B streptococci *E. coli*	Viruses (**R**SV) ***M**ycoplasma* ***C**hlamydia trachomatis* (infants–3 yr) ***C**. pneumoniae* (school-age children) ***S**treptococcus pneumoniae* **R**unts **M**ay **C**ough **C**hunky **S**putum	*Mycoplasma* *C. pneumoniae* *S. pneumoniae*	*S. pneumoniae* *H. influenzae* Anaerobes Viruses *Mycoplasma*	*S. pneumoniae* Influenza virus Anaerobes *H. influenzae* Gram-negative rods

Special groups	
Nosocomial (hospital acquired)	*Staphylococcus*, enteric gram-negative rods
Immunocompromised	*Staphylococcus*, enteric gram-negative rods, fungi, viruses, *Pneumocystis jirovecii*—with HIV
Aspiration	Anaerobes
Alcoholic/IV drug user	*S. pneumoniae*, *Klebsiella*, *Staphylococcus*
Cystic fibrosis	*Pseudomonas*, *S. aureus*, *S. pneumoniae*
Postviral	*Staphylococcus*, *H. influenzae*, *S. pneumoniae*
Atypical	*Mycoplasma*, *Legionella*, *Chlamydia*

Common causes of meningitis

NEWBORN (0–6 MO)	CHILDREN (6 MO–6 YR)	6–60 YR	60 YR +
Group B streptococci *E. coli* *Listeria*	*Streptococcus pneumoniae* *Neisseria meningitidis* *Haemophilus influenzae* type B Enteroviruses	*S. pneumoniae* *N. meningitidis* (#1 in teens) Enteroviruses HSV	*S. pneumoniae* Gram-negative rods *Listeria*

Give ceftriaxone and vancomycin empirically (add ampicillin if *Listeria* is suspected).
Viral causes of meningitis—enteroviruses (esp. coxsackievirus), HSV-2 (HSV-1 = encephalitis), HIV, West Nile virus, VZV.
In HIV—*Cryptococcus*, CMV, toxoplasmosis (brain abscess), JC virus (PML).
Note: Incidence of *H. influenzae* meningitis has ↓ greatly with introduction of the conjugate *H. influenzae* vaccine in last 10–15 years. Today, cases are usually seen in unimmunized children.

CSF findings in meningitis

	OPENING PRESSURE	CELL TYPE	PROTEIN	SUGAR
Bacterial	↑	↑ PMNs	↑	↓
Fungal/TB	↑	↑ lymphocytes	↑	↓
Viral	Normal/↑	↑ lymphocytes	Normal/↑	Normal

Osteomyelitis

CONDITION	CAUSE
Assume if no other information is available	*S. aureus*
Sexually active	*Neisseria gonorrhoeae* (rare), septic arthritis more common
Diabetics and IV drug users	*Pseudomonas aeruginosa*, *Serratia*
Sickle cell	*Salmonella*
Prosthetic replacement	*S. aureus* and *S. epidermidis*
Vertebral disease	*Mycobacterium tuberculosis* (Pott's disease)
Cat and dog bites or scratches	*Pasteurella multocida*

Most osteomyelitis occurs in children.
Elevated CRP and ESR classic but nonspecific.

Urinary tract infections

Cystitis presents with dysuria, frequency, urgency, suprapubic pain, and WBCs (but not WBC casts) in urine. Primarily caused by ascension of microbes from urethra to bladder. Males—infants with congenital defects, vesicoureteral reflux. Elderly—enlarged prostate. Ascension to kidney results in pyelonephritis, which presents with fever, chills, flank pain, CVA tenderness, hematuria, and WBC casts.

Ten times more common in women (shorter urethras colonized by fecal flora). Other predisposing factors include obstruction, kidney surgery, catheterization, GU malformation, diabetes, and pregnancy.

Diagnostic markers: positive leukocyte esterase test = bacterial UTI; positive nitrite test = gram-negative bacterial UTI.

UTI bugs

SPECIES	FEATURES	COMMENTS
Escherichia coli	Leading cause of UTI. Colonies show green metallic sheen on EMB agar.	Diagnostic markers: ⊕ Leukocyte esterase = bacterial. ⊕ Nitrite test = gram negative. ⊕ Urease test = urease-producing bugs (e.g., *Proteus*, *Klebsiella*). ⊖ Urease test = *E. coli*, *Enterococcus*.
Staphylococcus saprophyticus	2nd leading cause of community-acquired UTI in sexually active women.	
Klebsiella pneumoniae	3rd leading cause of UTI. Large mucoid capsule and viscous colonies.	
Serratia marcescens	Some strains produce a red pigment; often nosocomial and drug resistant.	
Enterobacter cloacae	Often nosocomial and drug resistant.	
Proteus mirabilis	Motility causes "swarming" on agar; produces urease; associated with struvite stones.	
Pseudomonas aeruginosa	Blue-green pigment and fruity odor; usually nosocomial and drug resistant.	

ToRCHeS infections

Microbes that may pass from mother to fetus. Transmission is transplacental in most cases, or via delivery (especially HSV-2). Nonspecific signs common to many **ToRCHeS** infections include hepatosplenomegaly, jaundice, thrombocytopenia, and growth retardation.

Other important infectious agents include *Streptococcus agalactiae* (group B streptococci), *E. coli*, and *Listeria monocytogenes*—all causes of meningitis in neonates. Parvovirus B19 causes hydrops fetalis.

AGENT	MODE OF TRANSMISSION	MATERNAL MANIFESTATIONS	NEONATAL MANIFESTIONS
Toxoplasma gondii	Cat feces or ingestion of undercooked meat	Usually asymptomatic; lymphadenopathy (rarely)	Classic triad: chorioretinitis, hydrocephalus, and intracranial calcifications
Rubella	Respiratory droplets	Rash, lymphadenopathy, arthritis	Classic triad: PDA (or pulmonary artery hypoplasia), cataracts, and deafness ± "blueberry muffin" rash
CMV	Sexual contact, organ transplants	Usually asymptomatic; mononucleosis-like illness	Hearing loss, seizures, petechial rash, "blueberry muffin" rash
HIV	Sexual contact, needlestick	Variable presentation depending on CD4+ count	Recurrent infections, chronic diarrhea
Herpes simplex virus-2	Skin or mucous membrane contact	Usually asymptomatic; herpetic (vesicular) lesions	Encephalitis, herpetic (vesicular) lesions
Syphilis	Sexual contact	Chancre (1°) and disseminated rash (2°) are the two stages likely to result in fetal infection	Often results in stillbirth, hydrops fetalis; if child survives, presents with facial abnormalities A B (notched teeth, saddle nose, short maxilla), saber shins, CN VIII deafness

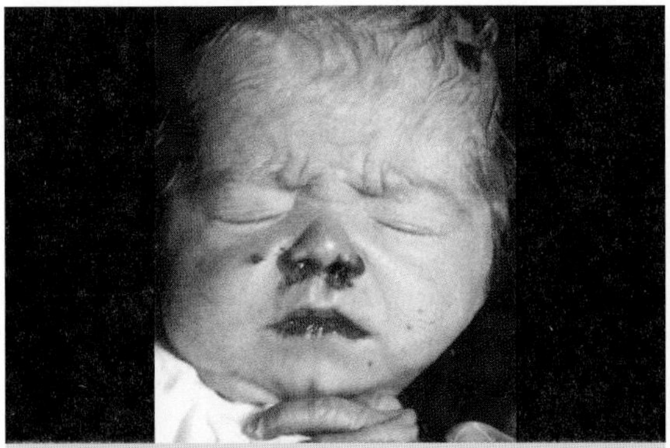

A **Congenital syphilis facies.** Skin is dry, wrinkled with yellow-brown hue. Note the hemorrhagic rhinitis.

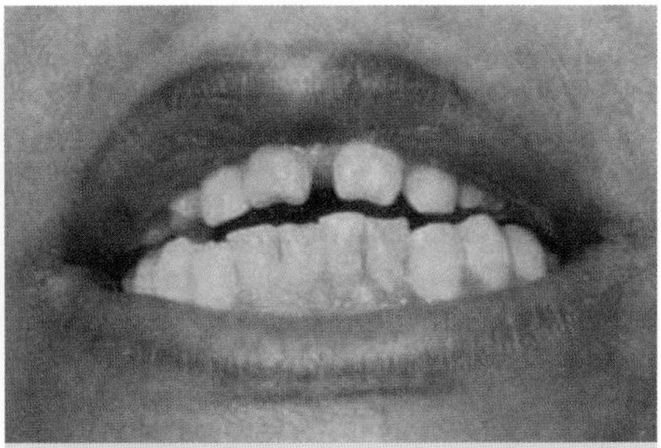

B **Hutchinson's teeth.** Note the centrally notched, widely spaced central incisors.

Red rashes of childhood

AGENT	ASSOCIATED SYNDROME/DISEASE	CLINICAL PRESENTATION
Rubella virus	Rubella	Rash begins at head and moves down; → fine truncal rash; postauricular lymphadenopathy
Measles virus	Measles	A paramyxovirus; beginning at head and moving down; rash is preceded by cough, coryza, conjunctivitis, and blue-white (Koplik) spots on buccal mucosa
VZV	Chickenpox	Vesicular rash begins on trunk; spreads to face and extremities with lesions of different age
HHV-6	Roseola	A macular rash over body appears after several days of high fever; can present with febrile seizures; usually affects infants
Parvovirus B19	Erythema infectiosum	"Slapped cheek" rash on face A (can cause hydrops fetalis in pregnant women)
Streptococcus pyogenes	Scarlet fever	Erythematous, sandpaper-like rash with fever and sore throat
Coxsackievirus type A	Hand-foot-mouth disease	Vesicular rash on palms and soles B; ulcers in oral mucosa

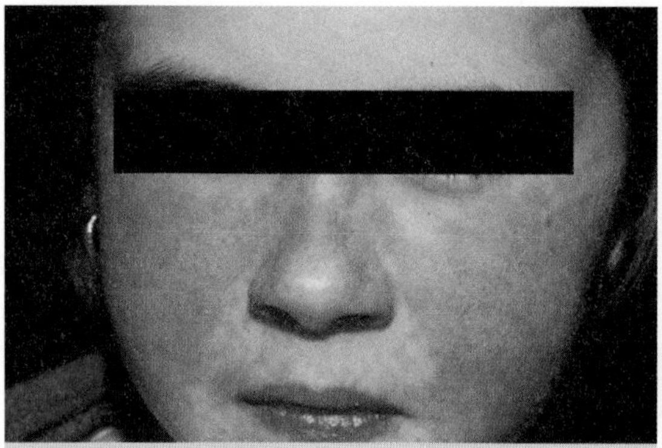

A **Erythema infectiosum.**

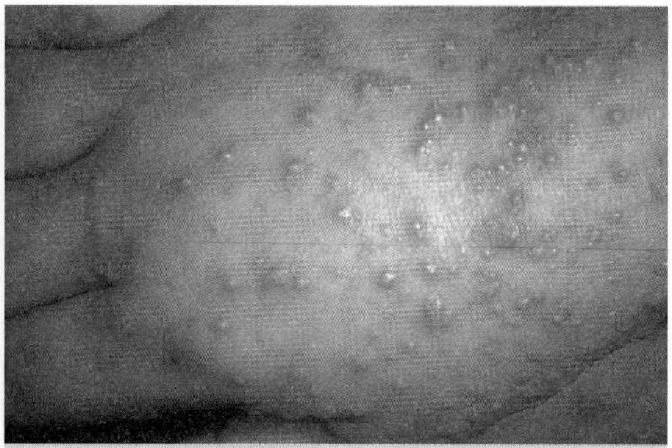

B **Hand-foot-mouth disease.**

Sexually transmitted diseases

DISEASE	CLINICAL FEATURES	ORGANISM
Gonorrhea	Urethritis, cervicitis, PID, prostatitis, epididymitis, arthritis, creamy purulent discharge	*Neisseria gonorrhoeae*
1° syphilis	Painless chancre	*Treponema pallidum*
2° syphilis	Fever, lymphadenopathy, skin rashes, condylomata lata	
3° syphilis	Gummas, tabes dorsalis, general paresis, aortitis, Argyll Robertson pupil	
Chancroid	Painful genital ulcer, inguinal adenopathy	*Haemophilus* ***ducreyi*** (it's so painful, you "**do cry**")
Genital herpes	Painful penile, vulvar, or cervical vesicles and ulcers; can cause systemic symptoms such as fever, headache, myalgia	HSV-2, less commonly HSV-1
Chlamydia	Urethritis, cervicitis, conjunctivitis, Reiter's syndrome, PID	*Chlamydia trachomatis* (D–K)
Lymphogranuloma venereum	Infection of lymphatics; genital ulcers, lymphadenopathy, rectal strictures	*C. trachomatis* (L1–L3)
Trichomoniasis	Vaginitis, strawberry-colored mucosa, motile in wet prep	*Trichomonas vaginalis*
AIDS	Opportunistic infections, Kaposi's sarcoma, lymphoma	HIV
Condylomata acuminata	Genital warts, koilocytes	HPV-6 and -11
Hepatitis B	Jaundice	HBV
Bacterial vaginosis	Noninflammatory, malodorous discharge (fishy smell); positive whiff test, clue cells, not exclusively an STD	*Gardnerella vaginalis*

Pelvic inflammatory disease

Top bugs—*Chlamydia trachomatis* (subacute, often undiagnosed), *Neisseria gonorrhoeae* (acute). *C. trachomatis*—the most common bacterial STD in the United States. Cervical motion tenderness (chandelier sign), purulent cervical discharge. PID may include salpingitis, endometritis, hydrosalpinx, and tubo-ovarian abscess. Can lead to Fitz-Hugh–Curtis syndrome—infection of the liver capsule and "violin string" adhesions of parietal peritoneum to liver.

Salpingitis is a risk factor for ectopic pregnancy, infertility, chronic pelvic pain, and adhesions.

Nosocomial infections

PATHOGEN	RISK FACTOR	NOTES
CMV, RSV	Newborn nursery	
E. coli, Proteus mirabilis	Urinary catheterization	The 2 most common causes of nosocomial infections are *E. coli* (UTI) and *S. aureus* (wound infection).
Pseudomonas aeruginosa	Respiratory therapy equipment	Presume *Pseudomonas* "***air**uginosa*" when **air** or burns are involved.
HBV	Work in renal dialysis unit	
Candida albicans	Hyperalimentation	
Legionella	Water aerosols	*Legionella* when water source is involved.

Bugs affecting unimmunized children

CLINICAL PRESENTATION	FINDINGS/LABS	PATHOGEN
Dermatologic		
Rash	Beginning at head and moving down with postauricular lymphadenopathy	Rubella virus
	Beginning at head and moving down; rash preceded by cough, coryza, conjunctivitis, and blue-white (Koplik) spots on buccal mucosa	Measles virus
Neurologic		
Meningitis	Microbe colonizes nasopharynx Can also lead to myalgia and paralysis	*H. influenzae* type B Poliovirus
Respiratory		
Pharyngitis	Grayish oropharyngeal exudate ("pseudomembranes" may obstruct airway); painful throat	*Corynebacterium diphtheriae* (elaborates toxin that causes necrosis in pharynx, cardiac, and CNS tissue)
Epiglottitis	Fever with dysphagia, drooling, and difficulty breathing due to edematous "cherry red" epiglottis	*H. influenzae* type B (also capable of causing epiglottitis in fully immunized children)

Bug hints (if all else fails)

CHARACTERISTIC	ORGANISM
Pus, empyema, abscess	*S. aureus*
Pediatric infection	*Haemophilus influenzae* (including epiglottitis)
Pneumonia in cystic fibrosis, burn infection	*Pseudomonas aeruginosa*
Branching rods in oral infection, sulfur granules	*Actinomyces israelii*
Traumatic open wound	*Clostridium perfringens*
Surgical wound	*S. aureus*
Dog or cat bite	*Pasteurella multocida*
"Currant jelly" sputum	*Klebsiella*
Positive PAS stain	*Tropheryma whipplei* (Whipple's disease)
Sepsis/meningitis in newborn	Group B strep
Health care provider	HBV (from needle stick)
Fungal infection in diabetic or immunocompromised patient	*Mucor* or *Rhizopus* spp.
Asplenic patient	Encapsulated microbes, especially **SHiN** (***S****. pneumoniae*, ***H****. **i**nfluenzae* type B, ***N****. meningitidis*)
Chronic granulomatous disease	Catalase-positive microbes, especially *S. aureus*
Neutropenic patients	*Candida albicans* (systemic), *Aspergillus*
Facial nerve palsy	*Borrelia burgdorferi* (Lyme disease)

▸ MICROBIOLOGY—ANTIMICROBIALS

Antimicrobial therapy

MECHANISM OF ACTION	DRUGS
❶ Block cell wall synthesis by inhibition of peptidoglycan cross-linking	Penicillin, methicillin, ampicillin, piperacillin, cephalosporins, aztreonam, imipenem
❷ Block peptidoglycan synthesis	Bacitracin, vancomycin
❸ Block nucleotide synthesis by inhibiting folic acid synthesis (involved in methylation)	Sulfonamides, trimethoprim
❹ Block DNA topoisomerases	Fluoroquinolones
❺ Block mRNA synthesis	Rifampin
❻ Damage DNA	Metronidazole
❼ Block protein synthesis at 50S ribosomal subunit	Chloramphenicol, macrolides, clindamycin, streptogramins (quinupristin, dalfopristin), linezolid
❽ Block protein synthesis at 30S ribosomal subunit	Aminoglycosides, tetracyclines

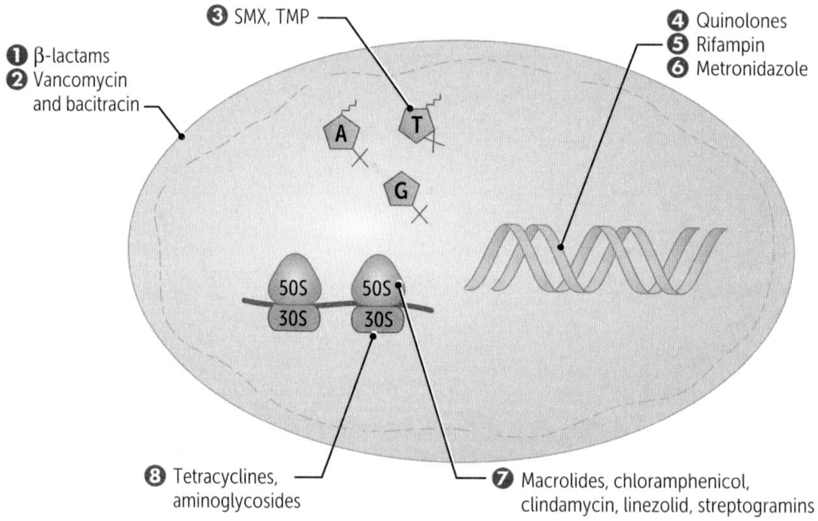

Penicillin

Penicillin	Penicillin G (IV and IM form), penicillin V (oral). Prototype β-lactam antibiotics.
MECHANISM	Bind penicillin-binding proteins (transpeptidases) Block transpeptidase cross-linking of peptidoglycan Activate autolytic enzymes
CLINICAL USE	Mostly used for gram-positive organisms (*S. pneumoniae, S. pyogenes, Actinomyces*). Also used for *Neisseria meningitidis, Treponema pallidum*, and syphilis. Bactericidal for gram-positive cocci, gram-positive rods, gram-negative cocci, and spirochetes. Not penicillinase resistant.
TOXICITY	Hypersensitivity reactions, hemolytic anemia.
RESISTANCE	β-lactamases cleave β-lactam ring.

Oxacillin, nafcillin, dicloxacillin (penicillinase-resistant penicillins)

MECHANISM	Same as penicillin. Narrow spectrum; penicillinase resistant because bulky R group blocks access of β-lactamase to β-lactam ring.	"Use **naf** (nafcillin) for **staph**."
CLINICAL USE	*S. aureus* (except MRSA; resistant because of altered penicillin-binding protein target site).	
TOXICITY	Hypersensitivity reactions, interstitial nephritis.	

Ampicillin, amoxicillin (aminopenicillins)

MECHANISM	Same as penicillin. Wider spectrum; penicillinase sensitive. Also combine with clavulanic acid to protect against β-lactamase. AmOxicillin has greater Oral bioavailability than ampicillin.	**AM**ino**P**enicillins are **AMP**ed-up penicillin.
CLINICAL USE	Extended-spectrum penicillin—*Haemophilus influenzae, E. coli, Listeria monocytogenes, Proteus mirabilis, Salmonella, Shigella,* enterococci.	Coverage: ampicillin/amoxicillin **HELPSS** kill enterococci.
TOXICITY	Hypersensitivity reactions; ampicillin rash; pseudomembranous colitis.	
RESISTANCE	β-lactamases cleave β-lactam ring.	

Ticarcillin, piperacillin (antipseudomonals)

MECHANISM	Same as penicillin. Extended spectrum.
CLINICAL USE	*Pseudomonas* spp. and gram-negative rods; susceptible to penicillinase; use with clavulanic acid.
TOXICITY	Hypersensitivity reactions.

β-lactamase inhibitors	Include Clavulanic Acid, Sulbactam, Tazobactam. Often added to penicillin antibiotics to protect the antibiotic from destruction by β-lactamase (penicillinase).	CAST.

Cephalosporins

MECHANISM	β-lactam drugs that inhibit cell wall synthesis but are less susceptible to penicillinases. Bactericidal.	Organisms typically not covered by cephalosporins are **LAME**: *Listeria*, **A**typicals (*Chlamydia*, *Mycoplasma*), **M**RSA, and **E**nterococci. Exception: ceftaroline covers MRSA.
CLINICAL USE	1st generation (cefazolin, cephalexin)—gram-positive cocci, *Proteus mirabilis*, *E. coli*, *Klebsiella pneumoniae*. Cefazolin used prior to surgery to prevent *S. aureus* wound infections.	1st generation—**PEcK**.
	2nd generation (cefoxitin, cefaclor, cefuroxime)—gram-positive cocci, *Haemophilus influenzae*, *Enterobacter aerogenes*, *Neisseria* spp., *Proteus mirabilis*, *E. coli*, *Klebsiella pneumoniae*, *Serratia marcescens*.	2nd generation—**HEN PEcKS**.
	3rd generation (ceftriaxone, cefotaxime, ceftazidime)—serious gram-negative infections resistant to other β-lactams.	Ceftriaxone—meningitis and gonorrhea. Ceftazidime—*Pseudomonas*.
	4th generation (cefepime)—↑ activity against *Pseudomonas* and gram-positive organisms.	
TOXICITY	Hypersensitivity reactions, vitamin K deficiency. Low cross-reactivity with penicillins. ↑ nephrotoxicity of aminoglycosides.	

Aztreonam

MECHANISM	A monobactam resistant to β-lactamases. Prevents peptidoglycan cross-linking by binding to PBP3. Synergistic with aminoglycosides. No cross-allergenicity with penicillins.
CLINICAL USE	Gram-negative rods only—No activity against gram-positives or anaerobes. For penicillin-allergic patients and those with renal insufficiency who cannot tolerate aminoglycosides.
TOXICITY	Usually nontoxic; occasional GI upset.

Imipenem/cilastatin, meropenem

MECHANISM	Imipenem is a broad-spectrum, β-lactamase-resistant carbapenem. Always administered with cilastatin (inhibitor of renal dehydropeptidase I) to ↓ inactivation of drug in renal tubules.	With imipenem, "the kill is **lastin'** with ci**lastatin**." Newer carbapenems include ertapenem and doripenem.
CLINICAL USE	Gram-positive cocci, gram-negative rods, and anaerobes. Wide spectrum, but the significant side effects limit use to life-threatening infections, or after other drugs have failed. Meropenem, however, has a reduced risk of seizures and is stable to dehydropeptidase I.	
TOXICITY	GI distress, skin rash, and CNS toxicity (seizures) at high plasma levels.	

Vancomycin

MECHANISM	Inhibits cell wall peptidoglycan formation by binding D-ala D-ala portion of cell wall precursors. Bactericidal.
CLINICAL USE	Gram positive only—serious, amultidrug-resistant organisms, including MRSA, enterococci, and *Clostridium difficile* (oral dose for pseudomembranous colitis).
TOXICITY	**N**ephrotoxicity, **O**totoxicity, **T**hrombophlebitis, diffuse flushing—**red man syndrome** (can largely prevent by pretreatment with antihistamines and slow infusion rate). Well tolerated in general—does **NOT** have many problems.
RESISTANCE	Occurs with amino acid change of **D-ala D-ala** to D-ala D-lac. "Pay back **2 D-ala**s (dollars) for **van**dalizing (**van**comycin)."

Protein synthesis inhibitors

Specifically target smaller bacterial ribosome (70S, made of 30S and 50S subunits), leaving human ribosome (80S) unaffected.

"Buy **AT 30**, **CCEL** (sell) at **50**."

30S inhibitors

A = Aminoglycosides [bactericidal]
T = Tetracyclines [bacteriostatic]

50S inhibitors

C = Chloramphenicol, Clindamycin [bacteriostatic]
E = Erythromycin (macrolides) [bacteriostatic]
L = Linezolid [variable]

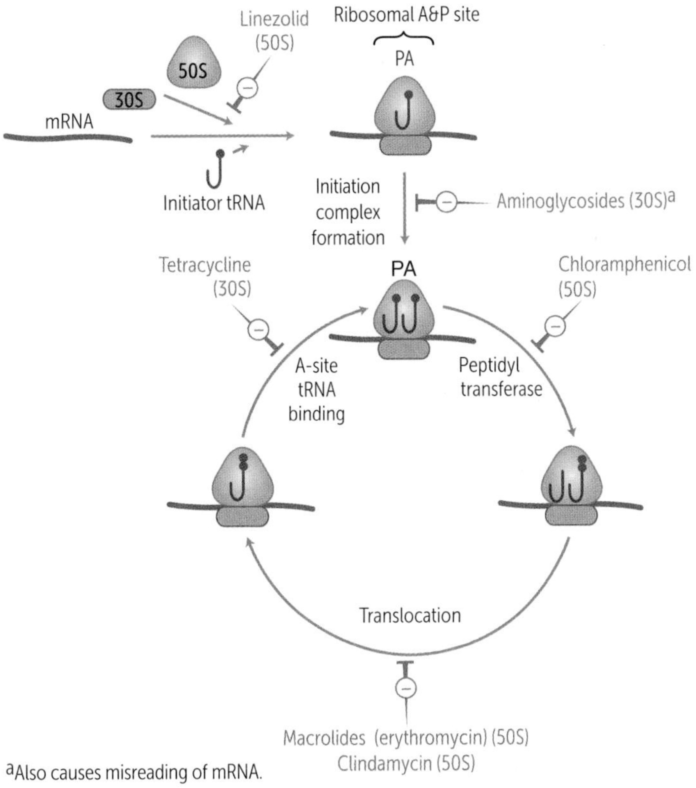

[a]Also causes misreading of mRNA.

Aminoglycosides	Gentamicin, Neomycin, Amikacin, Tobramycin, Streptomycin.	"**Mean**" (aminoglycoside) **GNATS caNNOT** kill anaerobes.
MECHANISM	Bactericidal; inhibit formation of initiation complex and cause misreading of mRNA. Also block translocation. Require O_2 for uptake; therefore ineffective against anaerobes.	**A** "initiates" the **A**lphabet.
CLINICAL USE	Severe gram-negative rod infections. Synergistic with β-lactam antibiotics. Neomycin for bowel surgery.	
TOXICITY	**N**ephrotoxicity (especially when used with cephalosporins), **N**euromuscular blockade, **O**totoxicity (especially when used with loop diuretics). **T**eratogen.	
RESISTANCE	Transferase enzymes that inactivate the drug by acetylation, phosphorylation, or adenylation.	

Tetracyclines	Tetracycline, doxycycline, demeclocycline, minocycline.	**D**emeclocycline—ADH antagonist; acts as a **D**iuretic in SIADH. Rarely used as antibiotic.
MECHANISM	Bacteriostatic; bind to 30S and prevent attachment of aminoacyl-tRNA; limited CNS penetration. Doxycycline is fecally eliminated and can be used in patients with renal failure. Do not take with milk, antacids, or iron-containing preparations because divalent cations inhibit its absorption in the gut.	
CLINICAL USE	*Borrelia burgdorferi*, *M. pneumoniae*. Drug's ability to accumulate intracellularly makes it very effective against *Rickettsia* and *Chlamydia*.	
TOXICITY	GI distress, discoloration of teeth and inhibition of bone growth in children, photosensitivity. Contraindicated in pregnancy.	
RESISTANCE	↓ uptake into cells or ↑ efflux out of cell by plasmid-encoded transport pumps.	

Macrolides	Azithromycin, clarithromycin, erythromycin.
MECHANISM	Inhibit protein synthesis by blocking translocation ("macro**slides**"); bind to the 23S rRNA of the 50S ribosomal subunit. Bacteriostatic.
CLINICAL USE	Atypical pneumonias (*Mycoplasma*, *Chlamydia*, *Legionella*), STDs (for *Chlamydia*), and gram-positive cocci (streptococcal infections in patients allergic to penicillin).
TOXICITY	**MACRO**: **M**otility issues, **A**rrhythmia caused by prolonged QT, acute **C**holestatic hepatitis, **R**ash, e**O**sinophilia. Increases serum concentration of theophyllines, oral anticoagulants.
RESISTANCE	Methylation of 23S rRNA binding site.

Chloramphenicol

MECHANISM	Blocks peptidyltransferase at 50S ribosomal subunit. Bacteriostatic.
CLINICAL USE	Meningitis (*Haemophilus influenzae, Neisseria meningitidis, Streptococcus pneumoniae*). Conservative use owing to toxicities but often still used in developing countries because of low cost.
TOXICITY	Anemia (dose dependent), aplastic anemia (dose independent), gray baby syndrome (in premature infants because they lack liver UDP-glucuronyl transferase).
RESISTANCE	Plasmid-encoded acetyltransferase that inactivates drug.

Clindamycin

MECHANISM	Blocks peptide transfer (transpeptidation) at 50S ribosomal subunit. Bacteriostatic.	
CLINICAL USE	Anaerobic infections (e.g., *Bacteroides fragilis, Clostridium perfringens*) in aspiration pneumonia or lung abscesses. Also oral infections with mouth anaerobes.	Treats anaerobes **above** the diaphragm vs. metronidazole (anaerobic infections **below** diaphragm).
TOXICITY	Pseudomembranous colitis (*C. difficile* overgrowth), fever, diarrhea.	

Sulfonamides

Sulfamethoxazole (SMX), sulfisoxazole, sulfadiazine.

MECHANISM	PABA antimetabolites inhibit dihydropteroate synthase. Bacteriostatic.
CLINICAL USE	Gram-positive, gram-negative, *Nocardia, Chlamydia*. Triple sulfas or SMX for simple UTI.
TOXICITY	Hypersensitivity reactions, hemolysis if G6PD deficient, nephrotoxicity (tubulointerstitial nephritis), photosensitivity, kernicterus in infants, displace other drugs from albumin (e.g., warfarin).
RESISTANCE	Altered enzyme (bacterial dihydropteroate synthase), ↓ uptake, or ↑ PABA synthesis.

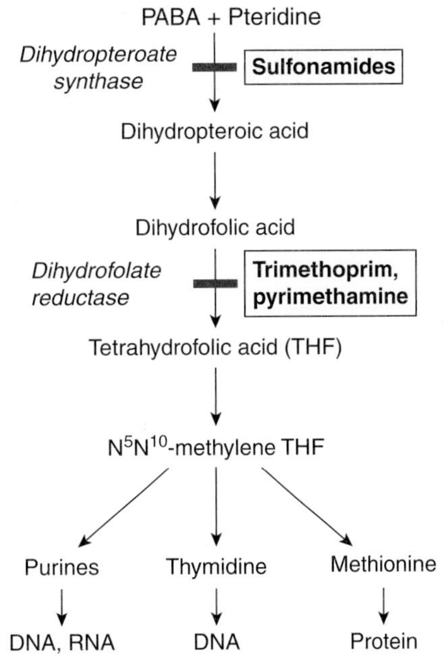
PABA + Pteridine
Dihydropteroate synthase
Sulfonamides
Dihydropteroic acid
Dihydrofolic acid
Dihydrofolate reductase
Trimethoprim, pyrimethamine
Tetrahydrofolic acid (THF)
N5N10-methylene THF
Purines
Thymidine
Methionine
DNA, RNA
DNA
Protein

(Adapted, with permission, from Katzung BG. *Basic and Clinical Pharmacology,* 7th ed. Stamford, CT: Appleton & Lange, 1997: 762.)

Trimethoprim

MECHANISM	Inhibits bacterial dihydrofolate reductase. Bacteriostatic.	
CLINICAL USE	Used in combination with sulfonamides (trimethoprim-sulfamethoxazole [TMP-SMX]), causing sequential block of folate synthesis. Combination used for UTIs, *Shigella, Salmonella, Pneumocystis jirovecii* pneumonia (treatment and prophylaxis).	
TOXICITY	Megaloblastic anemia, leukopenia, granulocytopenia. (May alleviate with supplemental folinic acid [leucovorin rescue].)	Abbreviated TMP. **TMP**: Treats **M**arrow **P**oorly.

Fluoroquinolones

Ciprofloxacin, norfloxacin, levofloxacin, ofloxacin, sparfloxacin, moxifloxacin, gatifloxacin, enoxacin (fluoroquinolones), nalidixic acid (a quinolone).

MECHANISM	Inhibit DNA gyrase (topoisomerase II) and topoisomerase IV. Bactericidal. Must not be taken with antacids.	
CLINICAL USE	Gram-negative rods of urinary and GI tracts (including *Pseudomonas*), *Neisseria*, some gram-positive organisms.	
TOXICITY	GI upset, superinfections, skin rashes, headache, dizziness. Less commonly, can cause tendonitis, tendon rupture, leg cramps, and myalgias. Contraindicated in pregnant women and in children because animal studies show damage to cartilage. Some may cause prolonged QT interval. May cause tendon rupture in people > 60 years old and in patients taking prednisone.	Fluoroquino**lones** hurt attachments to your **bones**.
RESISTANCE	Chromosome-encoded mutation in DNA gyrase, plasmid-mediated resistance, efflux pumps.	

Metronidazole

MECHANISM	Forms free radical toxic metabolites in the bacterial cell that damage DNA. Bactericidal, antiprotozoal.	
CLINICAL USE	Treats *Giardia, Entamoeba, Trichomonas, Gardnerella vaginalis*, Anaerobes (*Bacteroides, C. difficile*). Used with a proton pump inhibitor and clarithromycin for "triple therapy" against *H. Pylori.*	**GET GAP** on the **Metro** with **metro**nidazole! Treats anaerobic infection **below** the diaphragm vs. clindamycin (anaerobic infections **above** diaphragm).
TOXICITY	Disulfiram-like reaction with alcohol; headache, metallic taste.	

Antimycobacterial drugs

BACTERIUM	PROPHYLAXIS	TREATMENT
M. tuberculosis	Isoniazid	**R**ifampin, **I**soniazid, **P**yrazinamide, **E**thambutol (**RIPE** for treatment)
M. avium–intracellulare	Azithromycin	Azithromycin, rifampin, ethambutol, streptomycin
M. leprae	N/A	Long-term treatment with dapsone and rifampin for tuberculoid form. Add clofazimine for lepromatous form.

Isoniazid (INH)

MECHANISM	↓ synthesis of mycolic acids. Bacterial catalase-peroxidase (KatG) needed to convert INH to active metabolite.	**INH I**njures **N**eurons and **H**epatocytes.
CLINICAL USE	*Mycobacterium tuberculosis.* The only agent used as solo prophylaxis against TB.	Different INH half-lives in fast vs. slow acetylators.
TOXICITY	Neurotoxicity, hepatotoxicity. Pyridoxine (vitamin B_6) can prevent neurotoxicity, lupus.	

Rifampin

MECHANISM	Inhibits DNA-dependent RNA polymerase.	**R**ifampin's 4 **R**'s: **R**NA polymerase inhibitor **R**evs up microsomal P-450 **R**ed/orange body fluids **R**apid resistance if used alone
CLINICAL USE	*Mycobacterium tuberculosis*; delays resistance to dapsone when used for leprosy. Used for meningococcal prophylaxis and chemoprophylaxis in contacts of children with *Haemophilus influenzae* type B.	
TOXICITY	Minor hepatotoxicity and drug interactions (↑ P-450); orange body fluids (nonhazardous side effect).	

Pyrazinamide

MECHANISM	Mechanism uncertain. Thought to acidify intracellular environment via conversion to pyrazinoic acid. Effective in acidic pH of phagolysosomes, where TB engulfed by macrophages is found.
CLINICAL USE	*Mycobacterium tuberculosis.*
TOXICITY	Hyperuricemia, hepatotoxicity.

Ethambutol

MECHANISM	↓ carbohydrate polymerization of mycobacterium cell wall by blocking arabinosyltransferase.
CLINICAL USE	*Mycobacterium tuberculosis.*
TOXICITY	Optic neuropathy (red-green color blindness).

Antimicrobial prophylaxis

CONDITION	MEDICATION
Meningococcal infection	Ciprofloxacin (drug of choice), rifampin for children
Gonorrhea	Ceftriaxone
Syphilis	Benzathine penicillin G
History of recurrent UTIs	TMP-SMX
Endocarditis with surgical or dental procedures	Penicillins
Pregnant woman carrying group B strep	Ampicillin
Prophylaxis of strep pharyngitis in child with prior rheumatic fever	Oral penicillin
Prevention of postsurgical infection due to *S. aureus*	Cefazolin
Prevention of gonococcal or chlamydial conjunctivitis in newborn	Erythromycin ointment

HIV prophylaxis

CELL COUNT	PROPHYLAXIS	INFECTION
CD4 < 200 cells/mm^3	TMP-SMX[a]	*Pneumocystis* pneumonia
CD4 < 100 cells/mm^3	TMP-SMX[a]	*Pneumocystis* pneumonia and toxoplasmosis
CD4 < 50 cells/mm^3	Azithromycin	*Mycobacterium avium* complex

[a]Aerosolized pentamidine may be used if patient is unable to tolerate TMP-SMX, but this may not prevent toxoplasmosis infection concurrently.

Treatment of highly resistant bacteria

MRSA—vancomycin.
VRE—linezolid and streptogramins (quinupristin/dalfopristin).

Antifungal therapy

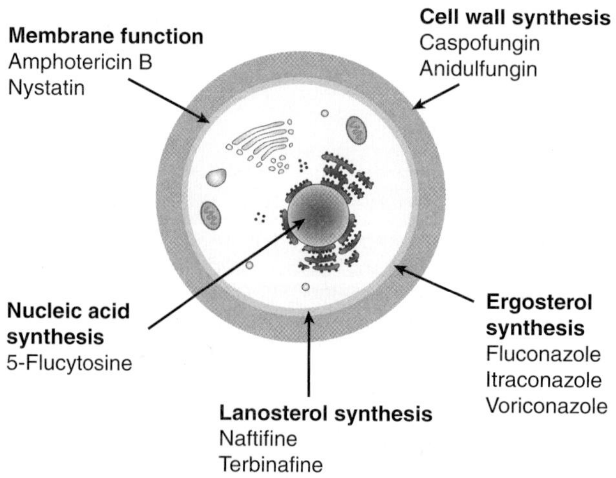
Membrane function
Amphotericin B
Nystatin
Cell wall synthesis
Caspofungin
Anidulfungin
Nucleic acid synthesis
5-Flucytosine
Ergosterol synthesis
Fluconazole
Itraconazole
Voriconazole
Lanosterol synthesis
Naftifine
Terbinafine

(Adapted, with permission, from Katzung BG, Trevor AJ. *USMLE Road Map: Pharmacology,* 1st ed. New York: McGraw-Hill, 2003: 120.)

Amphotericin B

MECHANISM	Binds ergosterol (unique to fungi); forms membrane pores that allow leakage of electrolytes.	Amphotericin "**tears**" holes in the fungal membrane by forming pores.
CLINICAL USE	Serious, systemic mycoses. *Cryptococcus* (amphotericin B with/without flucytosine for cryptococcal meningitis), *Blastomyces*, *Coccidioides*, *Histoplasma*, *Candida*, *Mucor*. Intrathecally for fungal meningitis. Supplement K and Mg because of altered renal tubule permeability.	
TOXICITY	Fever/chills ("shake and bake"), hypotension, nephrotoxicity, arrhythmias, anemia, IV phlebitis ("**amphoterrible**"). Hydration reduces nephrotoxicity. Liposomal amphotericin reduces toxicity.	

Nystatin

MECHANISM	Same as amphotericin B. Topical form because too toxic for systemic use.
CLINICAL USE	"Swish and swallow" for oral candidiasis (thrush); topical for diaper rash or vaginal candidiasis.

Azoles

Fluconazole, ketoconazole, clotrimazole, miconazole, itraconazole, voriconazole.

MECHANISM	Inhibit fungal sterol (ergosterol) synthesis, by inhibiting the P-450 enzyme that converts lanosterol to ergosterol.
CLINICAL USE	Local and less serious systemic mycoses. Fluconazole for chronic suppression of cryptococcal meningitis in AIDS patients and candidal infections of all types. Itraconazole for *Blastomyces*, *Coccidioides*, *Histoplasma*. Clotrimazole and miconazole for topical fungal infections.
TOXICITY	Testosterone synthesis inhibition (gynecomastia, esp. with ketoconazole), liver dysfunction (inhibits cytochrome P-450).

Flucytosine

MECHANISM	Inhibits DNA and RNA biosynthesis by conversion to 5-fluorouracil by cytosine deaminase.
CLINICAL USE	Used in systemic fungal infections (esp. meningitis caused by *Cryptococcus*) in combination with amphotericin B.
TOXICITY	Bone marrow suppression.

Caspofungin, micafungin

MECHANISM	Inhibits cell wall synthesis by inhibiting synthesis of β-glucan.
CLINICAL USE	Invasive aspergillosis, *Candida*.
TOXICITY	GI upset, flushing (by histamine release).

Terbinafine

MECHANISM	Inhibits the fungal enzyme squalene epoxidase.
CLINICAL USE	Used to treat dermatophytoses (especially onychomycosis—fungal infection of finger or toe nails).
TOXICITY	Abnormal LFTs, visual disturbances.

Griseofulvin

MECHANISM	Interferes with microtubule function; disrupts mitosis. Deposits in keratin-containing tissues (e.g., nails).
CLINICAL USE	Oral treatment of superficial infections; inhibits growth of dermatophytes (tinea, ringworm).
TOXICITY	Teratogenic, carcinogenic, confusion, headaches, ↑ P-450 and warfarin metabolism.

Antiprotozoan therapy Pyrimethamine (toxoplasmosis), suramin and melarsoprol (*Trypanosoma brucei*), nifurtimox (*T. cruzi*), sodium stibogluconate (leishmaniasis).

Chloroquine

MECHANISM	Blocks detoxification of heme into hemozoin. Heme accumulates and is toxic to plasmodia.
CLINICAL USE	Treatment of plasmodial species other than *P. falciparum* (frequency of resistance in *P. falciparum* is too high). Resistance due to membrane pump that ↓ intracellular concentration of drug. Treat *P. falciparum* with artemether/lumifantrine or atovaquone/proguanil. For life-threatening malaria, use quinidine in U.S. (quinine elsewhere) or artisunate.
TOXICITY	Retinopathy.

Antihelminthic therapy Mebendazole, pyrantel pamoate, ivermectin, diethylcarbamazine, praziquantel; immobilize helminths. Use praziquantel against flukes (trematodes) such as *Schistosoma*.

Antiviral therapy

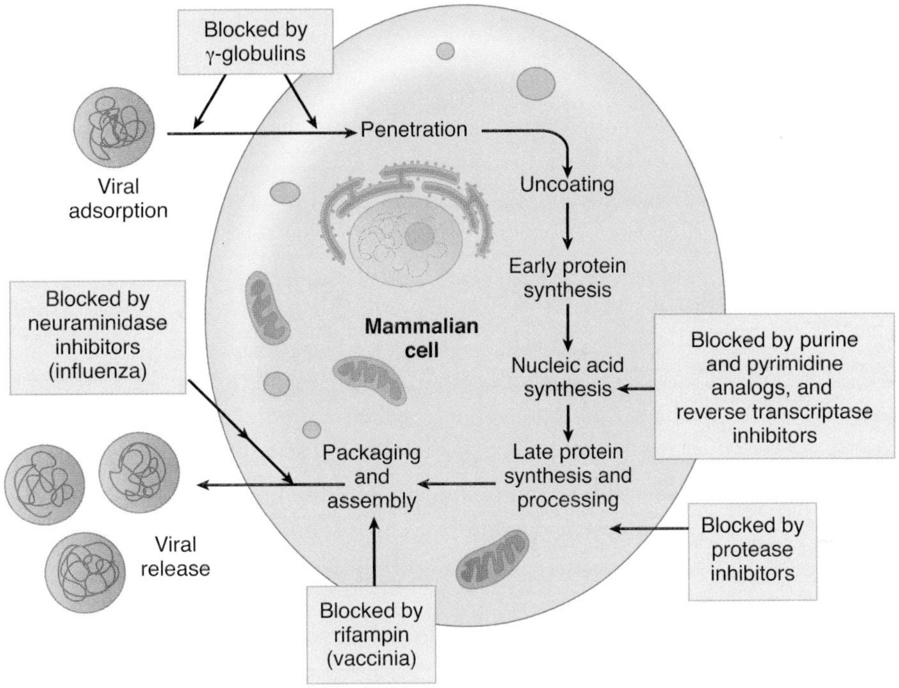

(Adapted, with permission, from Katzung BG, Trevor AJ. *USMLE Road Map: Pharmacology,* 1st ed. New York: McGraw-Hill, 2003: 120.)

Zanamivir, oseltamivir

MECHANISM	Inhibit influenza neuraminidase, decreasing the release of progeny virus.
CLINICAL USE	Treatment and prevention of both influenza A and B.

Ribavirin

MECHANISM	Inhibits synthesis of guanine nucleotides by competitively inhibiting IMP dehydrogenase.
CLINICAL USE	RSV, chronic hepatitis C.
TOXICITY	Hemolytic anemia. Severe teratogen.

Acyclovir

MECHANISM	Monophosphorylated by HSV/VZV thymidine kinase. Guanosine analog. Triphosphate formed by cellular enzymes. Preferentially inhibits viral DNA polymerase by chain termination.
CLINICAL USE	HSV and VZV. Weak activity against EBV. No activity against CMV. Used for HSV-induced mucocutaneous and genital lesions as well as for encephalitis. Prophylaxis in immunocompromised patients. No effect on latent forms of HSV and VZV. Valacyclovir, a prodrug of acyclovir, has better oral bioavailability. For herpes zoster, use a related agent, famciclovir.
TOXICITY	Few serious adverse effects.
MECHANISM OF RESISTANCE	Mutated viral thymidine kinase.

Ganciclovir

MECHANISM	5′-monophosphate formed by a CMV viral kinase. Guanosine analog. Triphosphate formed by cellular kinases. Preferentially inhibits viral DNA polymerase.
CLINICAL USE	CMV, especially in immunocompromised patients. Valganciclovir, a prodrug of ganciclovir, has better oral bioavailability.
TOXICITY	Leukopenia, neutropenia, thrombocytopenia, renal toxicity. More toxic to host enzymes than acyclovir.
MECHANISM OF RESISTANCE	Mutated CMV DNA polymerase or lack of viral kinase.

Foscarnet

MECHANISM	Viral DNA polymerase inhibitor that binds to the pyrophosphate-binding site of the enzyme. Does not require activation by viral kinase.	**Fos**carnet = pyro**fos**phate analog.
CLINICAL USE	CMV retinitis in immunocompromised patients when ganciclovir fails; acyclovir-resistant HSV.	
TOXICITY	Nephrotoxicity.	
MECHANISM OF RESISTANCE	Mutated DNA polymerase.	

Cidofovir

MECHANISM	Preferentially inhibits viral DNA polymerase. Does not require phosphorylation by viral kinase.
CLINICAL USE	CMV retinitis in immunocompromised patients; acyclovir-resistant HSV. Long half-life.
TOXICITY	Nephrotoxicity (coadminister with probenecid and IV saline to reduce toxicity).

HIV therapy

Highly active antiretroviral therapy (HAART): initiated when patients present with AIDS-defining illness, low CD4 cell counts (< 500 cells/mm^3), or high viral load. Regimen consists of 3 drugs to prevent resistance:

[2 nucleoside reverse transcriptase inhibitors (NRTIs)] +
[1 non-nucleoside reverse transcriptase inhibitor (NNRTI) OR 1 protease inhibitor OR 1 integrase inhibitor]

DRUG	MECHANISM	TOXICITY
Protease inhibitors		
Lopinavir Atazanavir Darunavir Fosamprenavir Saquinavir Ritonavir Indinavir	Assembly of virions depends on HIV-1 protease (*pol* gene), which cleaves the polypeptide products of HIV mRNA into their functional parts. Thus, protease inhibitors prevent maturation of new viruses. Ritonavir can "boost" other drug concentrations by inhibiting cytochrome P-450. All protease inhibitors end in *-navir.* **Navir** (never) **tease** a **protease**.	Hyperglycemia, GI intolerance (nausea, diarrhea), lipodystrophy. Nephropathy, hematuria (indinavir).
NRTIs		
Tenofovir (TDF) Emtricitabine (FTC) Abacavir (ABC) Lamivudine (3TC) Zidovudine (ZDV, formerly AZT) Didanosine (ddI) Stavudine (d4T)	Competitively inhibit nucleotide binding to reverse transcriptase and terminate the DNA chain (lack a 3′ OH group). Tenofovir is a nucleotide analog and does not have to be activated; the others are nucleoside analogs and do need to be phosphorylated to be active. ZDV is used for general prophylaxis and during pregnancy to reduce risk of fetal transmission. Have **you dined (vudine)** with my **nuclear** (**nucleo**sides) family?	Bone marrow suppression (can be reversed with G-CSF and erythropoietin), peripheral neuropathy, lactic acidosis (nucleosides), rash (non-nucleosides), anemia (ZDV).
NNRTIs		
Nevirapine Efavirenz Delavirdine	Bind to reverse transcriptase at site different from NRTIs. Do not require phosphorylation to be active or compete with nucleotides.	Same as NRTIs.
Integrase inhibitors		
Raltegravir	Inhibits HIV genome integration into host cell chromosome by reversibly inhibiting HIV integrase.	Hypercholesterolemia.

Interferons

MECHANISM	Glycoproteins synthesized by virus-infected cells; block replication of both RNA and DNA viruses.
CLINICAL USE	IFN-α—chronic hepatitis B and C, Kaposi's sarcoma. IFN-β—MS. IFN-γ—NADPH oxidase deficiency.
TOXICITY	Neutropenia, myopathy.

Antibiotics to avoid in pregnancy

ANTIBIOTIC	ADVERSE EFFECT
Sulfonamides	Kernicterus
Aminoglycosides	Ototoxicity
Fluoroquinolones	Cartilage damage
Clarithromycin	Embryotoxic
Tetracyclines	Discolored teeth, inhibition of bone growth
Ribavirin (antiviral)	Teratogenic
Griseofulvin (antifungal)	Teratogenic
Chloramphenicol	"Gray baby"

SAFe Children Take Really Good Care.

HIGH-YIELD PRINCIPLES IN

Immunology

"I hate to disappoint you, but my rubber lips are immune to your charms."
—Batman & Robin

"No State shall abridge the privileges or immunities of its citizens."
—The United States Constitution

The immunology content on USMLE exams has been expanded and reclassified into a new category called the immune system. Mastery of the basic principles and facts in this area will be useful. Cell surface markers are important to know because they are clinically useful (e.g., in identifying specific types of immune deficiency or cancer) and are functionally critical to the jobs immune cells carry out. By spending a little extra effort here, it is possible to turn a traditionally difficult subject into one that is high yield.

▸ IMMUNOLOGY–LYMPHOID STRUCTURES

Lymph node

A 2° lymphoid organ that has many afferents, 1 or more efferents. Encapsulated, with trabeculae. Functions are nonspecific filtration by macrophages, storage and activation of B and T cells, antibody production.

Follicle

Site of B-cell localization and proliferation. In outer cortex. 1° follicles are dense and dormant. 2° follicles have pale central germinal centers and are active.

Medulla

Consists of medullary cords (closely packed lymphocytes and plasma cells) and medullary sinuses. Medullary sinuses communicate with efferent lymphatics and contain reticular cells and macrophages.

Paracortex

Houses T cells. Region of cortex between follicles and medulla. Contains high endothelial venules through which T and B cells enter from blood. In an extreme cellular immune response, paracortex becomes greatly enlarged. Not well developed in patients with DiGeorge syndrome.

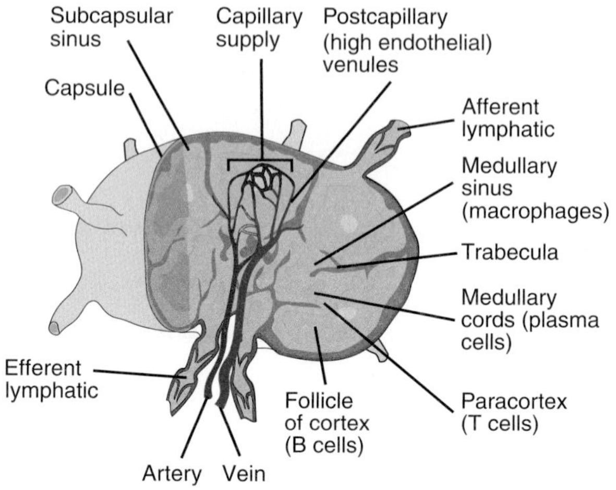

Paracortex enlarges in an extreme cellular immune response (i.e., viral).

Lymph drainage

AREA OF BODY	1° LYMPH NODE DRAINAGE SITE
Upper limb, lateral breast	Axillary
Stomach	Celiac
Duodenum, jejunum	Superior mesenteric
Sigmoid colon	Colic → inferior mesenteric
Rectum (lower portion) of anal canal (above pectinate line)	Internal iliac
Anal canal (below pectinate line)	Superficial inguinal
Testes	Superficial and deep plexuses → para-aortic
Scrotum	Superficial inguinal
Thigh (superficial)	Superficial inguinal
Lateral side of dorsum of foot	Popliteal

Right lymphatic duct—drains right arm, right chest, and right half of head.
Thoracic duct—drains everything else.

Sinusoids of spleen

Long, vascular channels in red pulp with fenestrated "barrel hoop" basement membrane. Macrophages found nearby.

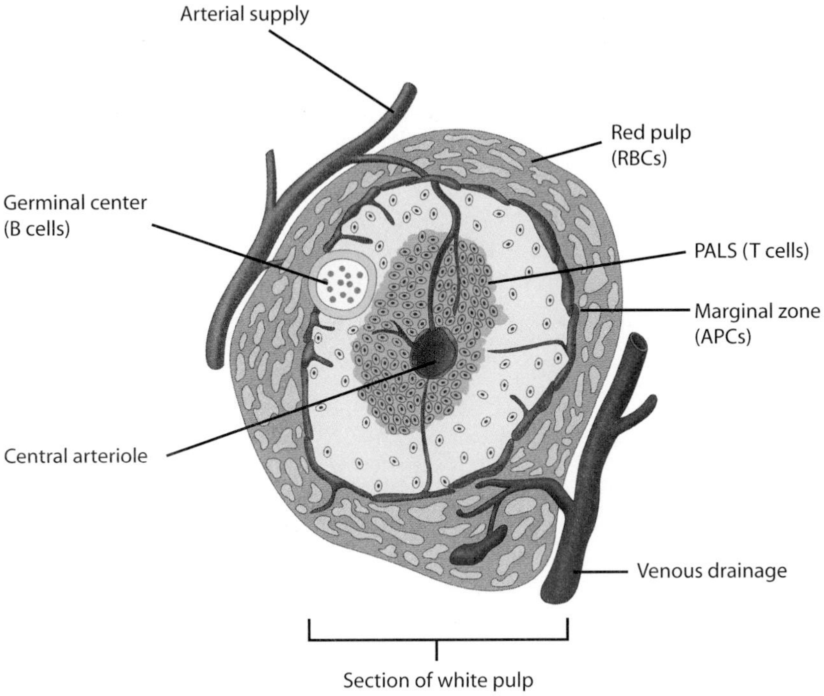
Arterial supply
Red pulp (RBCs)
Germinal center (B cells)
PALS (T cells)
Marginal zone (APCs)
Central arteriole
Venous drainage
Section of white pulp

(Reproduced, with permission, from Junqueira LC, Carneiro J: *Basic Histology: Text and Atlas,* 11th ed. New York: McGraw-Hill, 2005.)

T cells are found in the periarterial lymphatic sheath (PALS) within the white pulp of the spleen. B cells are found in follicles within the white pulp of the spleen.

Macrophages in the spleen remove encapsulated bacteria.

Splenic dysfunction: ↓ IgM → ↓ complement activation → ↓ C3b opsonization → ↑ susceptibility to encapsulated organisms:

- ***S**treptococcus pneumoniae*
- ***H**aemophilus **i**nfluenzae* type B
- ***N**eisseria meningitidis*
- ***S**almonella*
- ***K**lebsiella pneumoniae*
- Group B **S**treptococci (**SHiN SKiS**)

Postsplenectomy:

- Howell-Jolly bodies (nuclear remnants)
- Target cells
- Thrombocytosis

Thymus

Site of T-cell differentiation and maturation. Encapsulated. From epithelium of 3rd branchial pouches. Lymphocytes of mesenchymal origin. Cortex is dense with immature T cells; medulla is pale with mature T cells and epithelial reticular cells containing Hassall's corpuscles. Positive selection (MHC restriction) occurs in the cortex and negative selection (nonreactive to self) occurs in the medulla.

T cells = **T**hymus.
B cells = **B**one marrow.

▶ IMMUNOLOGY—LYMPHOCYTES

Innate vs. adaptive immunity

Innate	Receptors that recognize pathogens are germline encoded. Response to pathogens is fast and nonspecific. No memory. Consists of neutrophils, macrophages, dendritic cells, natural killer cells (lymphoid origin), and complement.
Adaptive	Receptors that recognize pathogens undergo V(D)J recombination during lymphocyte development. Response is slow on first exposure, but memory response is faster and more robust. Consists of T cells, B cells, and circulating antibody.

MHC I and II	MHC = major histocompatibility complex, encoded by human leukocyte antigen (HLA) genes; present antigen fragments to T cells and bind TCR.
MHC I	HLA-A, HLA-B, HLA-C. Binds TCR and CD8. Expressed on all nucleated cells. Not expressed on RBC. Antigen is loaded in RER with mostly intracellular peptides. Mediates viral immunity. Pairs with β_2-microglobulin (aids in transport to cell surface).
MHC II	HLA-DR, HLA-DP, HLA-DQ. Binds TCR and CD4. Expressed only on antigen-presenting cells (APCs). Antigen is loaded following release of invariant chain in an acidified endosome.

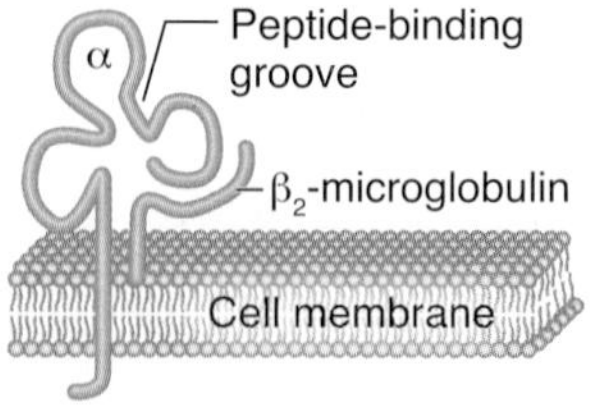
α
Peptide-binding
groove
β2-microglobulin
Cell membrane

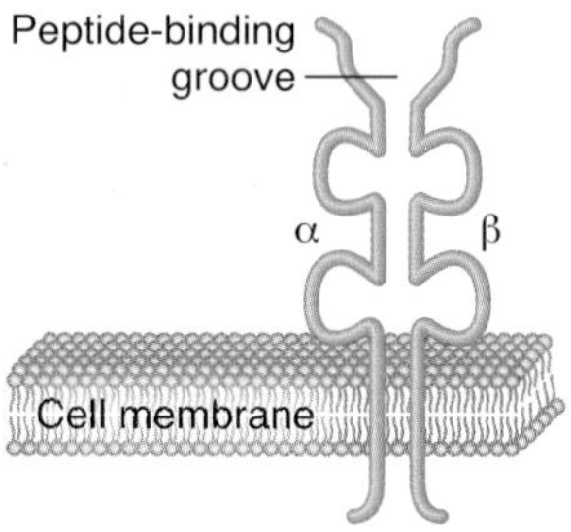
Peptide-binding
groove
α
β
Cell membrane

HLA subtypes associated with diseases

A3	Hemochromatosis.
B27	**P**soriasis, **A**nkylosing spondylitis, **I**nflammatory bowel disease, **R**eiter's syndrome. **PAIR.**
DQ2/DQ8	Celiac disease.
DR2	Multiple sclerosis, hay fever, SLE, Goodpasture's.
DR3	Diabetes mellitus type 1, Graves' disease.
DR4	Rheumatoid arthritis, diabetes mellitus type 1.
DR5	Pernicious anemia → B_{12} deficiency, Hashimoto's thyroiditis.

Natural killer cells	Use perforin and granzymes to induce apoptosis of virally infected cells and tumor cells. Only lymphocyte member of innate immune system. Activity enhanced by IL-2, IL-12, IFN-β, and IFN-α. Induced to kill when exposed to a nonspecific activation signal on target cell and/or to an absence of class I MHC on target cell surface.

Major functions of B and T cells

B cell functions	Make antibody—opsonize bacteria, neutralize viruses (IgG); activate complement (IgM, IgG); sensitize mast cells (IgE). Allergy (type I hypersensitivity): IgE. Cytotoxic (type II) and immune complex (type III) hypersensitivity: IgG. Hyperacute and humorally mediated acute and chronic organ rejection.
T cell functions	CD4+ T cells help B cells make antibody and produce cytokines to activate other cells of immune system. CD8+ T cells kill virus-infected cells directly. Delayed cell-mediated hypersensitivity (type IV). Acute and chronic cellular organ rejection.

Differentiation of T cells

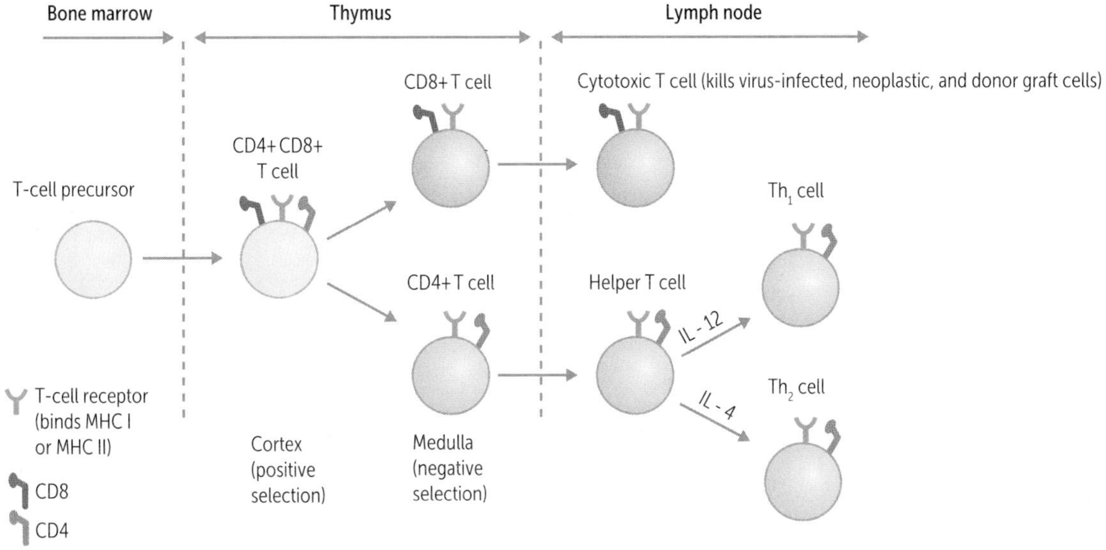

Positive selection	Thymic cortex. T cells expressing TCRs capable of binding surface self MHC molecules survive.
Negative selection	Medulla. T cells expressing TCRs with high affinity for self antigens undergo apoptosis.

T and B cell activation

Antigen-presenting cells (APCs):
- Dendritic cell (only APC that can activate naive T-cell)
- Macrophage
- B cell

Two signals are required for T cell activation and B cell activation and class switching.

Naive T cell activation

1. Foreign body is phagocytosed by dendritic cell.
2. Foreign antigen is presented on MHC II and recognized by TCR on Th (helper) cell. Antigen is presented on MHC I to Tc (cytotoxic) cells (signal 1).
3. "Costimulatory signal" is given by interaction of B7 and CD28 (signal 2).
4. Th cell activates and produces cytokines. Tc cell activates and is able to recognize and kill virus-infected cell.

B cell activation and class switching

1. Helper T cell activation as above.
2. B cell receptor-mediated endocytosis; foreign antigen is presented on MHC II and recognized by TCR on Th cell (signal 1).
3. CD40 receptor on B cell binds CD40 ligand on Th cell (signal 2).
4. Th cell secretes cytokines that determine Ig class switching of B cell. B cell activates and undergoes class switching, affinity maturation, and antibody production.

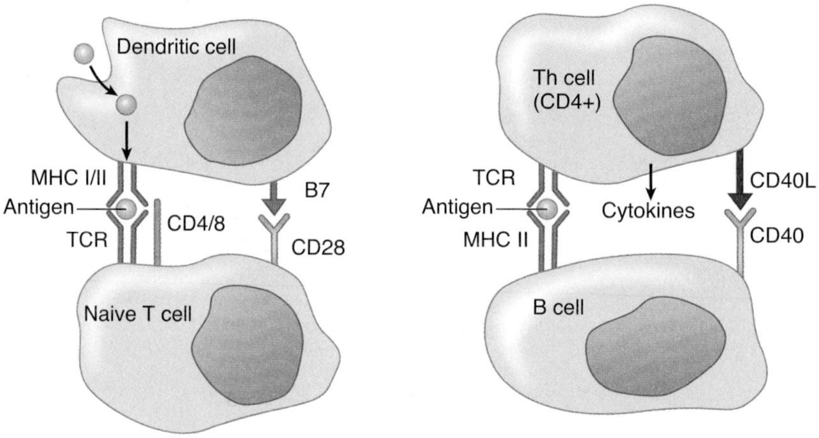

Helper T cells

Th_1 cell	Th_2 cell
Secretes IFN-γ	Secretes IL-4, IL-5, IL-10, IL-13
Activates macrophages	Recruits eosinophils for parasite defense and promotes IgE production by B cells
Inhibited by IL-4 and IL-10 (from Th_2 cell)	Inhibited by IFN-γ (from Th_1 cell)

Macrophage-lymphocyte interaction—activated lymphocytes (release IFN-γ) and macrophages (release IL-1, TNF-α) stimulate one another.

Helper T cells have CD4, which binds to MHC II on APCs.

Cytotoxic T cells

Kill virus-infected, neoplastic, and donor graft cells by inducing apoptosis.
Release cytotoxic granules containing preformed proteins (perforin—helps to deliver the content of granules into target cell; granzyme—a serine protease, activates apoptosis inside target cell; granulysin—antimicrobial, induces apoptosis).
Cytotoxic T cells have CD8, which binds to MHC I on virus-infected cells.

Regulatory T cells

Help maintain specific immune tolerance by suppressing CD4 and CD8 T-cell effector functions.
Express CD3, CD4, CD25 (α chain of IL-2 receptor) cell surface markers.
Activated regulatory T cells produce anti-inflammatory cytokines like IL-10 and TGF-β.

Antibody structure and function

Variable part of L and H chains recognizes antigens. Fc portion of IgM and IgG fixes complement. Heavy chain contributes to Fc and Fab fractions. Light chain contributes only to Fab fraction.

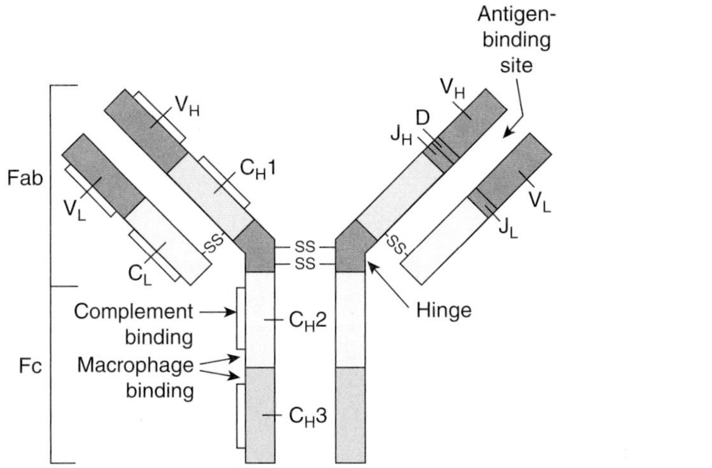
Antigen-binding site
V_H
D
J_H
C_H1
Fab
V_L
J_L
C_L
SS
SS
SS
SS
Hinge
Complement binding
C_H2
Fc
Macrophage binding
C_H3

(Adapted, with permission, from Ganong WF. *Review of Medical Physiology*, 22nd ed. New York: McGraw-Hill, 2005: 528.)

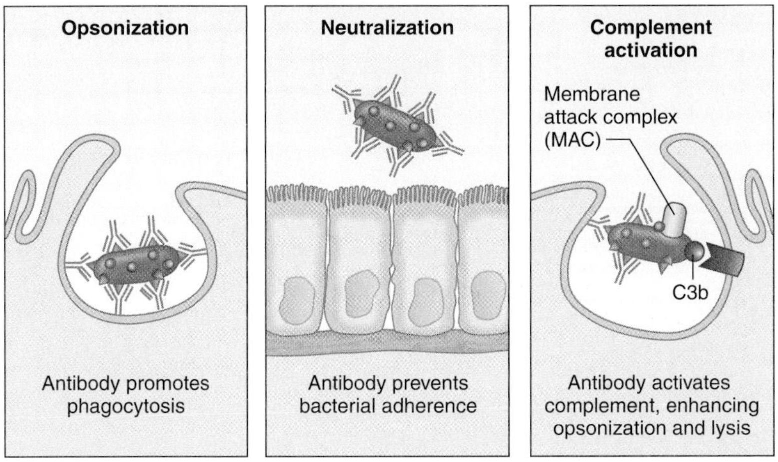
Opsonization
Antibody promotes phagocytosis
Neutralization
Antibody prevents bacterial adherence
Complement activation
Membrane attack complex (MAC)
C3b
Antibody activates complement, enhancing opsonization and lysis

Fab:
- Antigen-binding fragment
- Determines idiotype: unique antigen-binding pocket; only 1 antigenic specificity expressed per B cell

Fc:
- Constant
- Carboxy terminal
- Complement binding at C_H2 (IgG + IgM only)
- Carbohydrate side chains
- Determines isotype (IgM, IgD, etc.)

Antibody diversity is generated by:
- Random "recombination" of VJ (light-chain) or V(D)J (heavy-chain) genes
- Random combination of heavy chains with light chains
- Somatic hypermutation (following antigen stimulation)
- Addition of nucleotides to DNA during recombination (see 1st entry in this list) by terminal deoxynucleotidyl transferase

Immunoglobulin isotypes	Mature B lymphocytes express IgM and IgD on their surfaces. They may differentiate by isotype switching (gene rearrangement; mediated by cytokines and CD40 ligand) into plasma cells that secrete IgA, IgE, or IgG.
IgG	Main antibody in 2° (**delayed**) response to an antigen. Most abundant isotype. Fixes complement, crosses the placenta (provides infants with passive immunity), opsonizes bacteria, neutralizes bacterial toxins and viruses.
IgA	Prevents attachment of bacteria and viruses to mucous membranes; does not fix complement. Monomer (in circulation) or dimer (when secreted). Crosses epithelial cells by transcytosis. Found in secretions (tears, saliva, mucus) and early breast milk (known as colostrum). Picks up secretory component from epithelial cells before secretion.
IgM	Produced in the 1° (**immediate**) response to an antigen. Fixes complement but does not cross the placenta. Antigen receptor on the surface of B cells. Monomer on B cell or pentamer. Shape of pentamer allows it to efficiently trap free antigens out of tissue while humoral response evolves.
IgD	Unclear function. Found on the surface of many B cells and in serum.
IgE	Binds mast cells and basophils; cross-links when exposed to allergen, mediating immediate (type I) hypersensitivity through release of inflammatory mediators such as histamine. Mediates immunity to worms by activating eosinophils. Lowest concentration in serum.

Antigen type and memory

Thymus-independent antigens	Antigens lacking a peptide component; cannot be presented by MHC to T cells (e.g., lipopolysaccharide from cell envelope of gram-negative bacteria and polysaccharide capsular antigen). Stimulate release of antibodies and do not result in immunologic memory.
Thymus-dependent antigens	Antigens containing a protein component (e.g., diphtheria vaccine). Class switching and immunologic memory occur as a result of direct contact of B cells with Th cells (CD40–CD40 ligand interaction).

▶ IMMUNOLOGY—IMMUNE RESPONSES

Complement

Overview	System of interacting proteins that play a role in innate immunity and inflammation. Membrane attack complex (MAC) of complement defends against gram-negative bacteria.	
Activation	**Classic** pathway—**IgG** or **IgM** mediated. Alternative pathway—microbe surface molecules. Lectin pathway—mannose or other sugars on microbe surface.	**GM** makes **classic** cars.
Functions	C3b—opsonization. C3**a**, C5**a**—**a**naphylaxis. C5a—neutrophil chemotaxis. C5b-9—cytolysis by MAC.	C3**b b**inds **b**acteria.
Opsonins	C3b and IgG are the two 1° opsonins in bacterial defense; C3b also helps clear immune complexes.	
Inhibitors	Decay-accelerating factor (DAF) and C1 esterase inhibitor help prevent complement activation on self cells (e.g., RBC).	

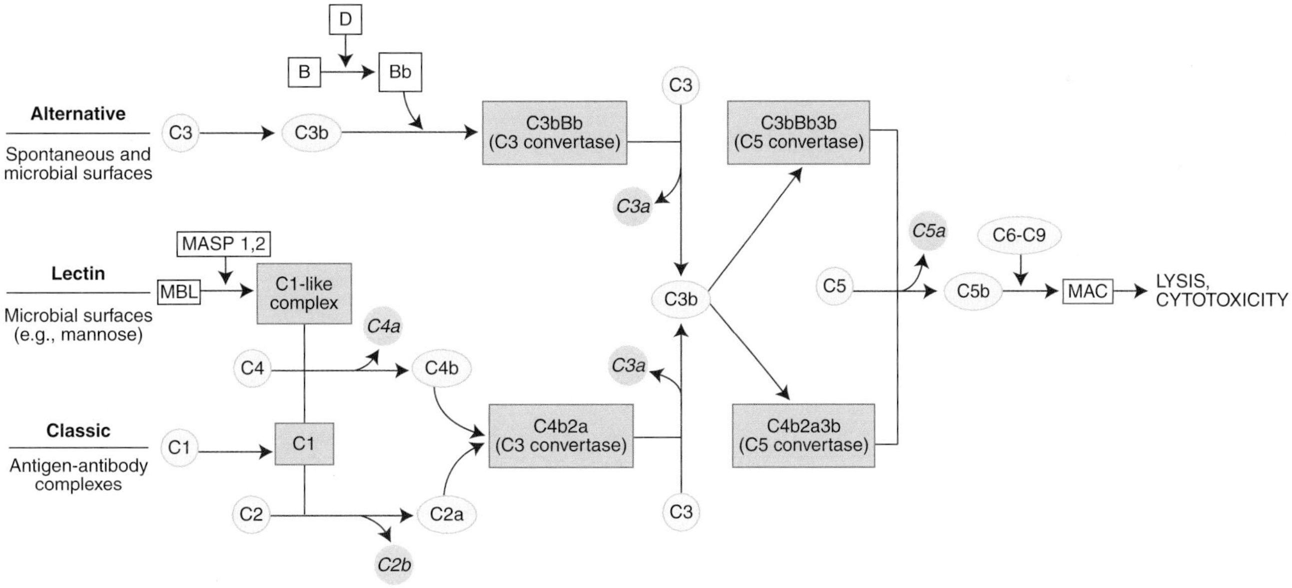

Complement disorders

C1 esterase inhibitor deficiency	→ hereditary angioedema. ACE inhibitors are contraindicated.
C3 deficiency	→ severe, recurrent pyogenic sinus and respiratory tract infections; ↑ susceptibility to type III hypersensitivity reactions.
C5–C9 deficiencies	→ recurrent *Neisseria* bacteremia.
DAF (GPI anchored enzyme) deficiency	→ complement-mediated lysis of RBCs and paroxysmal nocturnal hemoglobinuria (PNH).

Important cytokines

SECRETED BY MACROPHAGES		
IL-1	An endogenous pyrogen. Causes fever, acute inflammation. Activates endothelium to express adhesion molecules; induces chemokine secretion to recruit leukocytes.	"**Hot T-Bone** st**EA**k": IL-1: fever (**hot**). IL-2: stimulates **T** cells. IL-3: stimulates **Bone** marrow. IL-4: stimulates Ig**E** production. IL-5: stimulates Ig**A** production.
IL-6	An endogenous pyrogen. Also secreted by Th_2 cells. Causes fever and stimulates production of acute-phase proteins.	
IL-8	Major chemotactic factor for neutrophils.	"**Clean up** on **aisle** 8." Neutrophils are recruited by **IL-8** to **clear** infections.
IL-12	Induces differentiation of T cells into Th_1 cells. Activates NK cells. Also secreted by B cells.	
TNF-α	Mediates septic shock. Activates endothelium. Causes leukocyte recruitment, vascular leak.	
SECRETED BY ALL T CELLS		
IL-2	Stimulates growth of helper, cytotoxic, and regulatory T cells.	
IL-3	Supports the growth and differentiation of bone marrow stem cells. Functions like GM-CSF.	
FROM Th_1 CELLS		
Interferon-γ	Activates macrophages and Th_1 cells. Suppresses Th_2 cells. Has antiviral and antitumor properties.	
FROM Th_2 CELLS		
IL-4	Induces differentiation into Th_2 cells. Promotes growth of B cells. Enhances class switching to IgE and IgG.	
IL-5	Promotes differentiation of B cells. Enhances class switching to IgA. Stimulates the growth and differentiation of eosinophils.	
IL-10	Modulates inflammatory response. Inhibits actions of activated T cells and Th_1. Also secreted by regulatory T cells.	TGF-β has similar actions to IL-10, because it is involved in inhibiting inflammation.

Interferon mechanism	Interferons (α, β, γ) are proteins that place uninfected cells in an antiviral state. Interferons induce the production of a ribonuclease that inhibits viral protein synthesis by degrading viral mRNA (but not host mRNA).	**Interfer**es with viruses: ▪ α- and β-interferons inhibit viral protein synthesis. ▪ γ-interferons ↑ MHC I and II expression and antigen presentation in all cells. ▪ Activates NK cells to kill virus-infected cells.
Cell surface proteins	All cells except mature RBCs have MHC I.	
T cells	TCR (binds antigen-MHC complex) CD3 (associated with TCR for signal transduction) CD28 (binds B7 on APC)	
Helper T cells	CD4, CD40 ligand	
Cytotoxic T cells	CD8	
B cells	Ig (binds antigen) CD19, CD20, CD21 (receptor for EBV), CD40 MHC II, B7	You can drink **B**eer at the **B**ar when you're **21**: **B** cells, Epstein-**B**arr virus; CD-**21**.
Macrophages	CD14, CD40 MHC II, B7 Fc and C3b receptors (enhanced phagocytosis)	
NK cells	CD16 (binds Fc of IgG), CD56 (unique marker for NK)	
Anergy	Self-reactive T cells become nonreactive without costimulatory molecule. B cells also become anergic, but tolerance is less complete than in T cells.	
Effects of bacterial toxins	Superantigens (*S. pyogenes* and *S. aureus*)—cross-link the β region of the T-cell receptor to the MHC class II on APCs. Can activate any T cell, leading to massive release of cytokines. Endotoxins/lipopolysaccharide (gram-negative bacteria)—directly stimulate macrophages by binding to endotoxin receptor CD14; Th cells are not involved.	
Antigen variation	Classic examples: ▪ Bacteria—*Salmonella* (2 flagellar variants), *Borrelia* (relapsing fever), *Neisseria gonorrhoeae* (pilus protein). ▪ Virus—influenza (major = shift, minor = drift). ▪ Parasites—trypanosomes (programmed rearrangement).	Some mechanisms for variation include DNA rearrangement and RNA segment reassortment (e.g., influenza major shift).

Passive vs. active immunity

	Passive	Active
MEANS OF ACQUISITION	Receiving preformed antibodies	Exposure to foreign antigens
ONSET	Rapid	Slow
DURATION	Short span of antibodies (half-life = 3 weeks)	Long-lasting protection (memory)
EXAMPLES	IgA in breast milk, antitoxin, humanized monoclonal antibody	Natural infection, vaccines, toxoid
NOTES	After exposure to **T**etanus toxin, **B**otulinum toxin, **H**BV, or **R**abies virus, patients are given preformed antibodies (passive)—"**T**o **B**e **H**ealed **R**apidly"	Combined passive and active immunizations can be given in case of hepatitis B or rabies exposure.

Vaccination

Vaccines are used to induce an active immune response (humoral and/or cellular) to specific pathogens.

VACCINE TYPE	DESCRIPTION	PROS/CONS	EXAMPLES
Live attenuated vaccine	Microorganism loses its pathogenicity but retains capacity for transient growth within inoculated host. Mainly induces a **cellular response.**	Pro: induces strong, often life-long immunity. Con: may revert to virulent form.	Measles, mumps, polio (Sabin), rubella, varicella, yellow fever.
Inactivated or killed vaccine	Pathogen is inactivated by heat or chemicals; maintaining epitope structure on surface antigens is important for immune response. **Humoral immunity** induced.	Pro: stable and safer than live vaccines. Con: weaker immune response; booster shots usually required.	Cholera, hepatitis A, polio (Salk), rabies.

Hypersensitivity types

Type I

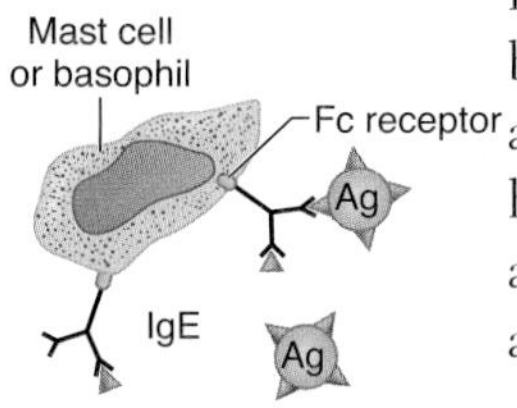
Mast cell
or basophil
Fc receptor
Ag
IgE
Ag

Anaphylactic and atopic—free antigen cross-links IgE on presensitized mast cells and basophils, triggering release of vasoactive amines that act at postcapillary venules (i.e., histamine). Reaction develops rapidly after antigen exposure because of preformed antibody.

First (type) and Fast (anaphylaxis). Types I, II, and III are all antibody mediated.
Test: skin test for specific IgE.

Type II

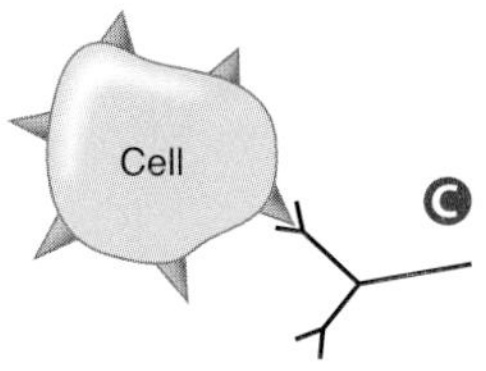
Cell
C

C = complement

Cytotoxic (antibody mediated)—IgM, IgG bind to fixed antigen on "enemy" cell, leading to cellular destruction.
3 mechanisms:
- Opsonization leading to phagocytosis or complement activation
- Complement-mediated lysis
- Antibody-dependent cell-mediated cytotoxicity (ADCC), usually due to NK cells

Type **II** is cy-2-toxic.
Antibody and complement lead to membrane attack complex (MAC).
Test: direct and indirect Coombs'.

Type III

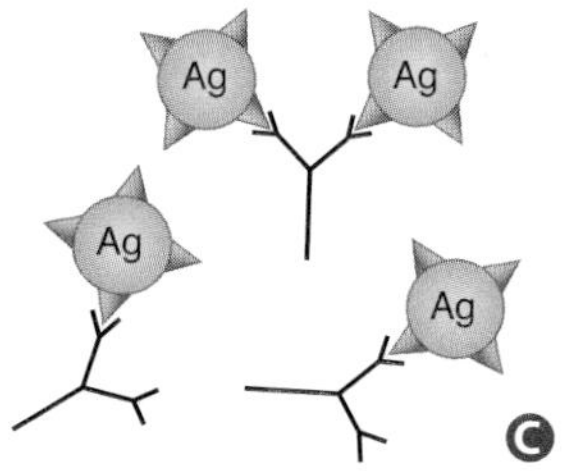
Ag
Ag
Ag
Ag
C

Immune complex—antigen-antibody (IgG) complexes activate complement, which attracts neutrophils; neutrophils release lysosomal enzymes.

In type **III** reaction, imagine an immune complex as **3** things stuck together: antigen-antibody-complement.

Serum sickness—an immune complex disease (type III) in which antibodies to the foreign proteins are produced (takes 5 days). Immune complexes form and are deposited in membranes, where they fix complement (leads to tissue damage). More common than Arthus reaction.

Most serum sickness is now caused by drugs (not serum) acting as haptens. Fever, urticaria, arthralgias, proteinuria, lymphadenopathy 5–10 days after antigen exposure.

Arthus reaction—a local subacute antibody-mediated hypersensitivity (type III) reaction. Intradermal injection of antigen induces antibodies, which form antigen-antibody complexes in the skin. Characterized by edema, necrosis, and activation of complement.

Antigen-antibody complexes cause the Arthus reaction.
Test: immunofluorescent staining.

Type IV

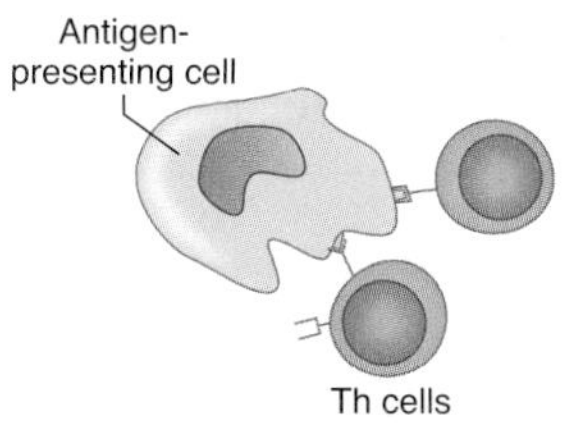
Antigen-
presenting cell
Th cells

Delayed (T-cell-mediated) type—sensitized T lymphocytes encounter antigen and then release lymphokines (leads to macrophage activation; no antibody involved).

4th and **last**—delayed. Cell mediated; therefore, it is not transferable by serum.
4 T's = **T** lymphocytes, **T**ransplant rejections, **T**B skin tests, **T**ouching (contact dermatitis).
Test: patch test, PPD.

ACID:
- **A**naphylactic and **A**topic (type I)
- **C**ytotoxic (antibody mediated) (type II)
- **I**mmune complex (type III)
- **D**elayed (cell mediated) (type IV)

Hypersensitivity disorders

REACTION	EXAMPLES	PRESENTATION
Type I	Anaphylaxis (e.g., bee sting, some food/drug allergies) Allergic and atopic disorders (e.g., rhinitis, hay fever, eczema, hives, asthma)	Immediate, anaphylactic, atopic
Type II	Autoimmune hemolytic anemia (AIHA) Pernicious anemia Idiopathic thrombocytopenic purpura Erythroblastosis fetalis Acute hemolytic transfusion reactions Rheumatic fever Goodpasture's syndrome Bullous pemphigoid Pemphigus vulgaris	Disease tends to be specific to tissue or site where antigen is found
Type III	SLE Polyarteritis nodosa Poststreptococcal glomerulonephritis Serum sickness Arthus reaction (e.g., swelling and inflammation following tetanus vaccine)	Can be associated with vasculitis and systemic manifestations
Type IV	Multiple sclerosis Guillain-Barré syndrome Graft-versus-host disease PPD (test for *M. tuberculosis*) Contact dermatitis (e.g., poison ivy, nickel allergy)	Response is delayed and does **not** involve antibodies (vs. types I, II, and III)

Blood transfusion reactions

TYPE	PATHOGENESIS	CLINICAL PRESENTATION
Allergic reaction	Type I hypersensitivity reaction against plasma proteins in transfused blood.	Urticaria, pruritus, wheezing, fever. Treat with antihistamines.
Anaphylactic reaction	Severe reaction. IgA-deficient individuals must receive blood products that lack IgA.	Dyspnea, bronchospasm, hypotension, respiratory arrest, shock.
Febrile nonhemolytic transfusion reaction (FNHTR)	Type II hypersensitivity reaction. Host antibodies against donor HLA antigens and leukocytes.	Fever, headaches, chills, flushing.
Acute hemolytic transfusion reaction (HTR)	Type II hypersensitivity reaction. Intravascular hemolysis (ABO blood group incompatibility) or extravascular hemolysis (host antibody reaction against foreign antigen on donor RBCs).	Fever, hypotension, tachypnea, tachycardia, flank pain, hemoglobinemia (intravascular), jaundice (extravascular hemolysis).

Autoantibodies

AUTOANTIBODY	ASSOCIATED DISORDER
Antinuclear antibodies (ANA)	SLE, nonspecific
Anti-dsDNA, anti-Smith	SLE
Antihistone	Drug-induced lupus
Rheumatoid factor, anti-CCP	Rheumatoid arthritis
Anticentromere	Scleroderma (CREST syndrome)
Anti-Scl-70 (anti-DNA topoisomerase I)	Scleroderma (diffuse)
Antimitochondrial	1° biliary cirrhosis
IgA antiendomysial, IgA anti-tissue transglutaminase	Celiac disease
Anti–basement membrane	Goodpasture's syndrome
Anti-desmoglein	Pemphigus vulgaris
Antimicrosomal, antithyroglobulin	Hashimoto's thyroiditis
Anti-Jo-1, anti-SRP, anti-Mi-2	Polymyositis, dermatomyositis
Anti-SSA (anti-Ro)	Sjögren's syndrome
Anti-SSB (anti-La)	Sjögren's syndrome
Anti-U1 RNP (ribonucleoprotein)	Mixed connective tissue disease
Anti–smooth muscle	Autoimmune hepatitis
Anti–glutamate decarboxylase	Type 1 diabetes mellitus
c-ANCA (PR3-ANCA)	Granulomatosis with polyangiitis (Wegener's)
p-ANCA (MPO-ANCA)	Microscopic polyangiitis, Churg-Strauss syndrome

Infections in immunodeficiency

PATHOGEN	NO T CELLS	NO B CELLS	NO GRANULOCYTE	NO COMPLEMENT
Bacteria	Sepsis	Encapsulated: *Streptococcus pneumoniae*, *Haemophilus influenzae* type B, *Neisseria meningitidis*, *Salmonella*, *Klebsiella pneumoniae*, group B Strep (SHiN SKiS)	*Staphylococcus*, *Burkholderia cepacia*, *Serratia*, *Nocardia*	*Neisseria* (no membrane attack complex)
Virus	CMV, EBV, VZV, chronic infection with respiratory/GI viruses	Enteroviral encephalitis, poliovirus (live vaccine contraindicated)	N/A	N/A
Fungi/parasites	*Candida*, PCP	GI giardiasis (no IgA)	*Candida*, *Aspergillus*	N/A

Note: B-cell deficiencies tend to produce recurrent bacterial infections, whereas T-cell deficiencies produce more fungal and viral infections.

Immune deficiencies

DISEASE	DEFECT	PRESENTATION	FINDINGS
B-cell disorders			
X-linked (Bruton's) agammaglobulinemia	X-linked recessive (↑ in **B**oys). Defect in *BTK*, a tyrosine kinase gene → no **B** cell maturation.	Recurrent bacterial infections after 6 months (↓ maternal IgG) as a result of opsonization defect.	Normal pro-B, ↓ maturation, ↓ number of B cells, ↓ immunoglobulins of all classes.
Selective IgA deficiency	Unknown. Most common primary immunodeficiency.	Majority asymptomatic. Can see sinopulmonary infections, GI infections, autoimmune disease, **A**naphylaxis to Ig**A**-containing blood products.	IgA < 7 mg/dL with normal IgG, IgM, and IgG vaccine titers. False-positive β-HCG tests due to presence of heterophile antibody.
Common variable immunodeficiency (CVID)	Defect in B-cell maturation; many causes.	Can be acquired in 20s–30s; ↑ risk of autoimmune disease, lymphoma, sinopulmonary infections.	Normal number of B cells; ↓ plasma cells, immunoglobulin.
T-cell disorders			
Thymic aplasia (DiGeorge syndrome)	22q11 deletion; failure to develop 3rd and 4th pharyngeal pouches.	Tetany (hypocalcemia), recurrent viral/fungal infections (T-cell deficiency), congenital heart and great vessel defects.	Thymus and parathyroids fail to develop → ↓ T cells, ↓ PTH, ↓ Ca^{2+}. Absent thymic shadow on CXR.
IL-12 receptor deficiency	↓ Th_1 response.	Disseminated mycobacterial infections.	↓ IFN-γ.
Hyper-IgE syndrome (Job's syndrome)	Th_1 cells fail to produce IFN-γ → inability of neutrophils to respond to chemotactic stimuli.	**FATED**: coarse **F**acies, cold (noninflamed) staphylococcal **A**bscesses, retained primary **T**eeth, ↑ Ig**E**, **D**ermatologic problems (eczema).	↑ IgE.
Chronic mucocutaneous candidiasis	T-cell dysfunction.	*Candida albicans* infections of skin and mucous membranes.	

Immune deficiencies *(continued)*

DISEASE	DEFECT	PRESENTATION	FINDINGS
B- and T-cell disorders			
Severe combined immunodeficiency (SCID)	Several types: defective IL-2 receptor (most common, X-linked), adenosine deaminase deficiency.	Failure to thrive, chronic diarrhea, thrush. Recurrent viral, bacterial, fungal, and protozoal infections. Absence of thymic shadow, germinal centers (lymph node biopsy), and B cells (peripheral blood smear). Treatment: bone marrow transplant (no allograft rejection).	↓ T-cell recombinant excision circles (TRECs). Absence of thymic shadow, germinal centers (lymph node biopsy), and T cells (flow cytometry).
Ataxia-telangiectasia	Defects in the *ATM* gene, which codes for DNA repair enzymes.	Triad: cerebellar defects (ataxia), spider angiomas (telangiectasia), IgA deficiency.	↑ AFP.
Hyper-IgM syndrome	Most commonly defective CD40L on helper T cells = inability to class switch.	Severe pyogenic infections early in life.	↑ IgM; ↓↓ IgG, IgA, IgE.
Wiskott-Aldrich syndrome	X-linked; in *WAS* gene on X chromosome → T cells unable to reorganize actin cytoskeleton.	Triad (**TIE**): **T**hrombocytopenic purpura, **I**nfections, **E**czema.	↑ IgE, IgA; ↓ IgM. Thrombocytopenia.
Phagocyte dysfunction			
Leukocyte adhesion deficiency (type 1)	Defect in LFA-1 integrin (CD18) protein on phagocytes.	Recurrent bacterial infections, absent pus formation, delayed separation of umbilical cord.	Neutrophilia.
Chédiak-Higashi syndrome	Autosomal recessive; defect in lysosomal trafficking regulator gene (*LYST*). Microtubule dysfunction in phagosome-lysosome fusion.	Recurrent pyogenic infections by staphylococci and streptococci; partial albinism, peripheral neuropathy.	Giant granules in neutrophils.
Chronic granulomatous disease	Lack of NADPH oxidase → ↓ reactive oxygen species (e.g., superoxide) and absent respiratory burst in neutrophils.	↑ susceptibility to catalase-positive organisms (e.g., *S. aureus*, *E. coli*, *Aspergillus*).	Abnormal dihydrorhodamine (DHR) flow cytometry test. Nitroblue tetrazolium dye reduction test no longer preferred.

Grafts

Autograft	From self.
Syngeneic graft	From identical twin or clone.
Allograft	From nonidentical individual of same species.
Xenograft	From different species.

Transplant rejection

TYPE OF REJECTION	ONSET AFTER TRANSPLANTATION	PATHOGENESIS	FEATURES
Hyperacute	Within minutes	Antibody mediated (type II) because of the presence of preformed anti-donor antibodies in the transplant recipient.	Occludes graft vessels, causing ischemia and necrosis.
Acute	Weeks later	Cell-mediated due to CTLs reacting against foreign MHCs. Reversible with immunosuppressants (e.g., cyclosporine, muromonab-CD3).	Vasculitis of graft vessels with dense interstitial lymphocytic infiltrate.
Chronic	Months to years	Class I-$MHC_{non\text{-}self}$ is perceived by CTLs as class I-MHC_{self} presenting a non-self antigen.	Irreversible. T-cell and antibody-mediated vascular damage (obliterative vascular fibrosis); fibrosis of graft tissue and blood vessels.
Graft-versus-host	Varies	Grafted immunocompetent T cells proliferate in the irradiated immunocompromised disease host and reject cells with "foreign" proteins, resulting in severe organ dysfunction.	Maculopapular rash, jaundice, hepatosplenomegaly, and diarrhea. Usually in bone marrow and liver transplant (organs rich in lymphocytes). Potentially beneficial in bone marrow transplant.

▶ IMMUNOLOGY–IMMUNOSUPPRESSANTS

Cyclosporine

MECHANISM	Binds to cyclophilins. Complex blocks the differentiation and activation of T cells by inhibiting calcineurin, thus preventing the production of IL-2 and its receptor.
CLINICAL USE	Suppresses organ rejection after transplantation; selected autoimmune disorders.
TOXICITY	Nephrotoxicity, hypertension, hyperlipidemia, hyperglycemia, tremor, gingival hyperplasia, hirsutism.

Tacrolimus (FK-506)

MECHANISM	Similar to cyclosporine; binds to FK-binding protein, inhibiting calcineurin and secretion of IL-2 and other cytokines.
CLINICAL USE	Potent immunosuppressive used in organ transplant recipients.
TOXICITY	Similar to cyclosporine except no gingival hyperplasia and hirsutism.

Sirolimus (rapamycin)

MECHANISM	Inhibits mTOR. Inhibits T-cell proliferation in response to IL-2.
CLINICAL USE	Immunosuppression after kidney transplantation in combination with cyclosporine and corticosteroids. Also used with drug-eluting stents.
TOXICITY	Hyperlipidemia, thrombocytopenia, leukopenia.

Azathioprine

MECHANISM	Antimetabolite precursor of 6-mercaptopurine that interferes with the metabolism and synthesis of nucleic acids. Toxic to proliferating lymphocytes.
CLINICAL USE	Kidney transplantation, autoimmune disorders (including glomerulonephritis and hemolytic anemia).
TOXICITY	Bone marrow suppression. Active metabolite mercaptopurine is metabolized by xanthine oxidase; thus, toxic effects may be increased by allopurinol.

Muromonab-CD3 (OKT3)

MECHANISM	Monoclonal antibody that binds to CD3 (epsilon chain) on the surface of T cells. Blocks cellular interaction with CD3 protein responsible for T-cell signal transduction.
CLINICAL USE	Immunosuppression after kidney transplantation.
TOXICITY	Cytokine release syndrome, hypersensitivity reaction.

Recombinant cytokines and clinical uses

AGENT	CLINICAL USES
Aldesleukin (interleukin-2)	Renal cell carcinoma, metastatic melanoma
Epoetin alfa (erythropoietin)	Anemias (especially in renal failure)
Filgrastim (granulocyte colony-stimulating factor)	Recovery of bone marrow
Sargramostim (granulocyte-macrophage colony-stimulating factor)	Recovery of bone marrow
α-interferon	Hepatitis B and C, Kaposi's sarcoma, leukemias, malignant melanoma
β-interferon	Multiple sclerosis
γ-interferon	Chronic granulomatous disease
Oprelvekin (interleukin-11)	Thrombocytopenia
Thrombopoietin	Thrombocytopenia

Therapeutic antibodies

AGENT	TARGET	CLINICAL USE
Muromonab-CD3 (OKT3)	CD3	Prevent acute transplant rejection
Digoxin Immune Fab	Digoxin	Antidote for digoxin intoxication
Infliximab	TNF-α	Crohn's disease, rheumatoid arthritis, psoriatic arthritis, ankylosing spondylitis
Adalimumab	TNF-α	Crohn's disease, rheumatoid arthritis, psoriatic arthritis
Abciximab	Glycoprotein IIb/IIIa	Prevent cardiac ischemia in unstable angina and in patients treated with percutaneous coronary intervention
Trastuzumab (Herceptin)	HER2	HER2–overexpressing breast cancer
Rituximab	CD20	B-cell non-Hodgkin's lymphoma
Omalizumab	IgE	Additional line of treatment for severe asthma

HIGH-YIELD PRINCIPLES IN

Pathology

"Digressions, objections, delight in mockery, carefree mistrust are signs of health; everything unconditional belongs in pathology."

—Friedrich Nietzsche

The fundamental principles of pathology are key to understanding diseases in all organ systems. Major topics such as inflammation and neoplasia appear frequently in questions across different organ systems, and such topics are definitely high yield. For example, the concepts of cell injury and inflammation are key to understanding the inflammatory response that follows myocardial infarction, a very common subject of board questions. Similarly, a familiarity with the early cellular changes that culminate in the development of neoplasias—for example, esophageal or colon cancer—is critical. Finally, make sure you recognize the major tumor-associated genes and are comfortable with key cancer concepts such as tumor staging and metastasis.

▸ PATHOLOGY–INFLAMMATION

Apoptosis

Programmed cell death; ATP required. Intrinsic or extrinsic pathway; both pathways → activation of cytosolic caspases that mediate cellular breakdown. No significant inflammation.

Characterized by cell shrinkage, nuclear shrinkage (pyknosis) and basophilia, membrane blebbing, nuclear fragmentation (karyorrhexis), and formation of apoptotic bodies, which are then phagocytosed.

Intrinsic pathway

Involved in tissue remodeling in embryogenesis. Occurs when a growth factor is withdrawn from a proliferating cell population (e.g., ↓ IL-2 after a completed immune reaction → apoptosis of proliferating effector cells). Also occurs after exposure to injurious stimuli (e.g., radiation, toxins, hypoxia).

Changes in proportions of anti- and pro-apoptotic factors lead to increased mitochondria permeability and cytochrome c release.

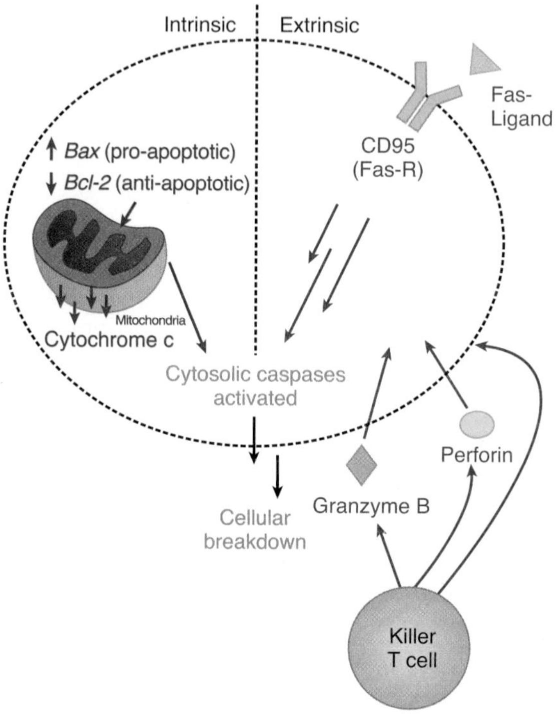
Intrinsic
Extrinsic
Fas-
Ligand
CD95
(Fas-R)
↑ *Bax* (pro-apoptotic)
↓ *Bcl-2* (anti-apoptotic)
Mitochondria
Cytochrome c
Cytosolic caspases
activated
Cellular
breakdown
Granzyme B
Perforin
Killer
T cell

Extrinsic pathway

2 pathways:

- Ligand receptor interactions (Fas ligand binding to Fas [CD95]).
- Immune cell (cytotoxic T-cell release of perforin and granzyme B).

Necrosis

Enzymatic degradation and protein denaturation of a cell resulting from exogenous injury. Intracellular components extravasate. Inflammatory process (unlike apoptosis).

Types of necrosis:

- Coagulative—heart, liver, kidney
- Liquefactive—brain, bacterial abscess, pleural effusion
- Caseous—TB, systemic fungi
- Fatty—peripancreatic fat (saponification via lipase)
- Fibrinoid—blood vessels
- Gangrenous—dry (ischemic coagulative) or wet (with bacteria); common in limbs and in GI tract

Cell injury

REVERSIBLE WITH O_2	IRREVERSIBLE
↓ ATP synthesis Cellular swelling (no ATP → impaired Na^+/K^+ pump) Nuclear chromatin clumping ↓ glycogen Fatty change Ribosomal detachment (↓ protein synthesis)	Nuclear pyknosis, karyolysis, karyorrhexis Ca^{2+} influx → caspase activation Plasma membrane damage Lysosomal rupture Mitochondrial permeability

Ischemia: susceptible areas

Areas susceptible to hypoxia and ischemia/infarction:

ORGAN	LOCATION
Brain	ACA/MCA/PCA boundary areas[a,b]
Heart	Subendocardium (LV)
Kidney	Straight segment of proximal tubule (medulla) Thick ascending limb (medulla)
Liver	Area around central vein (zone III)
Colon	Splenic flexure,[a] rectum[a]

[a]Watershed areas receive dual blood supply from most distal branches of 2 arteries, which protects these areas from single-vessel focal blockage. However, these areas are susceptible to ischemia from systemic hypoperfusion.

[b]Hypoxic ischemic encephalopathy (HIE) affects pyramidal cells of hippocampus and Purkinje cells.

Infarcts: red vs. pale

Red (hemorrhagic) infarcts occur in loose tissues with collaterals, such as liver, lungs, or intestine, or following reperfusion.

Pale infarcts occur in solid tissues with a single blood supply, such as heart, kidney, and spleen.

Red = reperfusion.

Reperfusion injury is due to damage by free radicals.

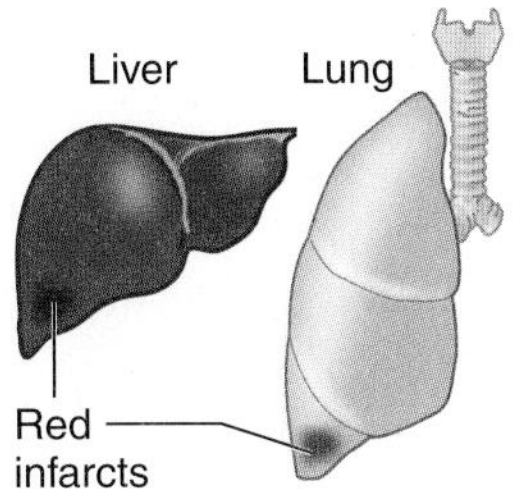
Liver
Lung
Red infarcts

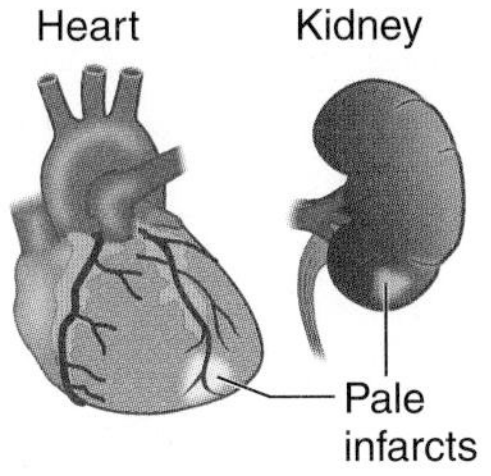
Heart
Kidney
Pale infarcts

Shock

Hypovolemic/cardiogenic	Septic
Low-output failure	High-output failure
↑ TPR	↓ TPR
Low cardiac output	Dilated arterioles, high venous return
Cold, clammy patient (vasoconstriction)	Hot patient (vasodilation)

Atrophy

Reduction in the size or number of cells. Causes include:

- ↓ hormones (uterus/vagina)
- ↓ innervation (motor neuron damage)
- ↓ blood flow
- ↓ nutrients
- ↑ pressure (nephrolithiasis)
- Occlusion of secretory ducts (cystic fibrosis)

Inflammation

Characterized by *rubor* (redness), *dolor* (pain), *calor* (heat), *tumor* (swelling), and *functio laesa* (loss of function).

Vascular component

↑ vascular permeability, vasodilation, endothelial injury.

Cellular component

Neutrophils extravasate from circulation to injured tissue to participate in inflammation through phagocytosis, degranulation, and inflammatory mediator release.

Acute

Neutrophil, eosinophil, and antibody mediated. Acute inflammation is rapid onset (seconds to minutes), lasts minutes to days. Outcomes include complete resolution, abscess formation, and progression to chronic inflammation.

Chronic

Mononuclear cell mediated: characterized by persistent destruction and repair. Associated with blood vessel proliferation, fibrosis. Granuloma: nodular collections of epithelioid macrophages and giant cells. Outcomes include scarring and amyloidosis.

Leukocyte extravasation

Neutrophils exit from blood vessels at sites of tissue injury and inflammation in 4 steps:

STEP	VASCULATURE/STROMA	LEUKOCYTE
❶ Rolling	E-selectin P-selectin	Sialyl-Lewis^X
❷ Tight binding	ICAM-1	LFA-1 ("integrin")
❸ Diapedesis—leukocyte travels between endothelial cells and exits blood vessel	PECAM-1	PECAM-1
❹ Migration—leukocyte travels through interstitium to site of injury or infection guided by chemotactic signals	Bacterial products: C5a, IL-8, LTB_4, and Kallikrein (CILK)	Various

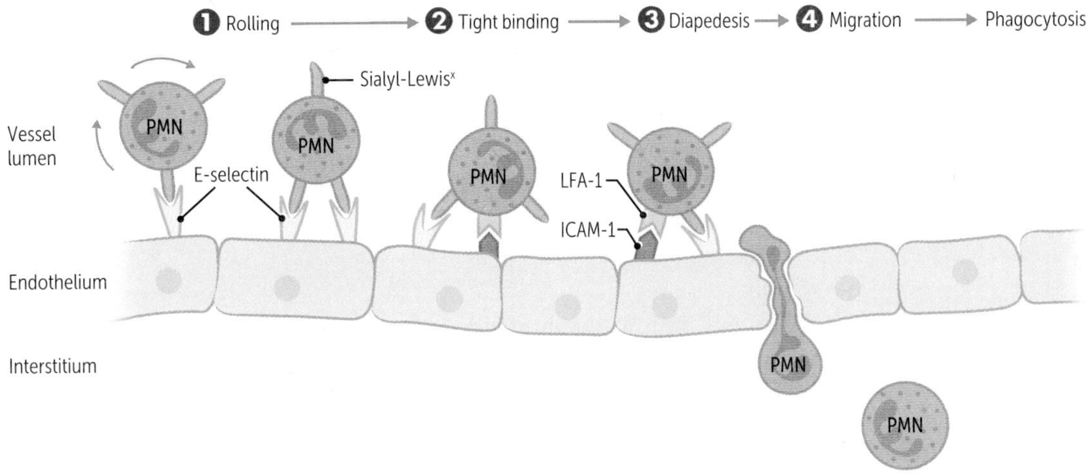

Free radical injury

Free radicals damage cells via membrane lipid peroxidation, protein modification, and DNA breakage.

Initiated via radiation exposure, metabolism of drugs (phase I), redox reaction, nitric oxide, transition metals, leukocyte oxidative burst.

Free radicals can be eliminated by enzymes (catalase, superoxide dismutase, glutathione peroxidase), spontaneous decay, antioxidants (vitamins A, C, E).

Pathologies include:

- Retinopathy of prematurity
- Bronchopulmonary dysplasia
- Carbon tetrachloride, leading to liver necrosis (fatty change)
- Acetaminophen overdose (fulminant hepatitis)
- Iron overload (hemochromatosis)
- Reperfusion after anoxia (e.g., superoxide), especially after thrombolytic therapy

Wound healing

PHASE	MEDIATORS	CHARACTERISTICS
Inflammatory (immediate)	Platelets, neutrophils, macrophages	Clot formation, ↑ vessel permeability and neutrophil migration into tissue; macrophages clear debris 2 days later
Proliferative (2–3 days after wound)	Fibroblasts, myofibroblasts, endothelial cells, keratinocytes, macrophages	Deposition of granulation tissue and collagen, angiogenesis, epithelial cell proliferation, dissolution of clot, and wound contraction (mediated by myofibroblasts)
Remodeling (1 week after wound)	Fibroblasts	Type III collagen replaced by type I collagen, ↑ tensile strength of tissue

Granulomatous diseases

Mycobacterium tuberculosis
Fungal infections (e.g., histoplasmosis), coccidioidomycosis)
Treponema pallidum (syphilis)
M. leprae (leprosy)
Bartonella henselae (cat scratch disease)
Sarcoidosis
Crohn's disease
Granulomatosis with polyangiitis (Wegener's)
Churg-Strauss syndrome
Berylliosis, silicosis

Th_1 cells secrete γ-interferon, activating macrophages. TNF-α from macrophages induce and maintain granuloma formation. Anti-TNF drugs can, as a side effect, cause sequestering granulomas to breakdown, leading to disseminated disease.

Transudate vs. exudate

Transudate	Exudate
Hypocellular	Cellular
Protein poor	Protein rich
Specific gravity < 1.012	Specific gravity > 1.020
Due to: ▪ ↑ hydrostatic pressure ▪ ↓ oncotic pressure ▪ Na^+ retention	Due to: ▪ Lymphatic obstruction ▪ Inflammation

Erythrocyte sedimentation rate

Products of inflammation (e.g., fibrinogen) coat RBCs and cause aggregation. When aggregated, RBCs fall at a faster rate within the test tube.

↑ ESR	↓ ESR
Infections Inflammation (e.g., temporal arteritis) Cancer Pregnancy SLE	Sickle cell (altered shape) Polycythemia (too many) CHF (unknown)

Iron poisoning

One of the leading causes of fatality from toxicologic agents in children.

MECHANISM	Cell death due to peroxidation of membrane lipids.
SYMPTOMS	Acute—gastric bleeding. Chronic—metabolic acidosis, scarring leading to GI obstruction.

Amyloidosis

Abnormal aggregation of proteins or their fragments into β-pleated sheet structures, leading to cell damage and apoptosis A. Affected tissue has waxy appearance.

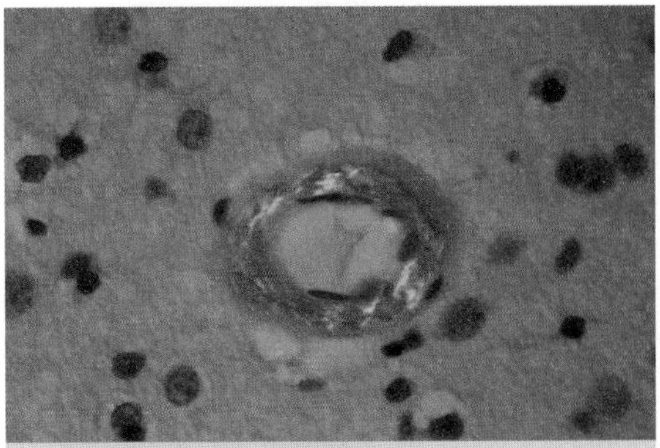

A **Amyloidosis.** Note the apple-green birefringence (Congo red stain) of the amyloid deposits in the artery wall.

COMMON TYPES	DESCRIPTION
AL (primary)	Due to deposition of proteins from Ig **L**ight chains. Can occur as a plasma cell disorder or associated with multiple myeloma. Often multiple organ sytem impact, including renal (nephrotic syndrome), cardiac (heart failure, arrhythmia), hematologic (easy bruising), hepatomegaly, and neuropathy.
AA (secondary)	Seen with chronic diseases like RA, IBD, spondyloarthropathy, chronic infections. Fibrils composed of serum **A**myloid **A**. Often multisystem like AL amyloidosis.
Dialysis-related	Fibrils composed of β_2-microglobulin in patients with ESRD and long-term dialysis. Often presents as carpal tunnel syndrome and other joint issues.
Heritable	Heterogeneous group of disorders. Example is ATTR neurologic/cardiac amyloidosis due to transthyretin (TTR or prealbumin) gene mutation.
Age-related (senile) systemic	Due to deposition of normal (wild-type) TTR in myocardium and other sites. Slower progression of cardiac dysfunction vs. AL amyloidosis.
Organ-specific	Amyloid deposition localized to a single organ. Most important form is amyloidosis in Alzheimer's disease due to deposition of amyloid-β protein cleaved from amyloid precursor protein (APP).

▶ PATHOLOGY—NEOPLASIA

Neoplastic progression Hallmarks of cancer—evasion of apoptosis, self-sufficiency in growth signals, insensitivity to anti-growth signals, sustained angiogenesis, limitless replicative potential, tissue invasion, and metastasis.

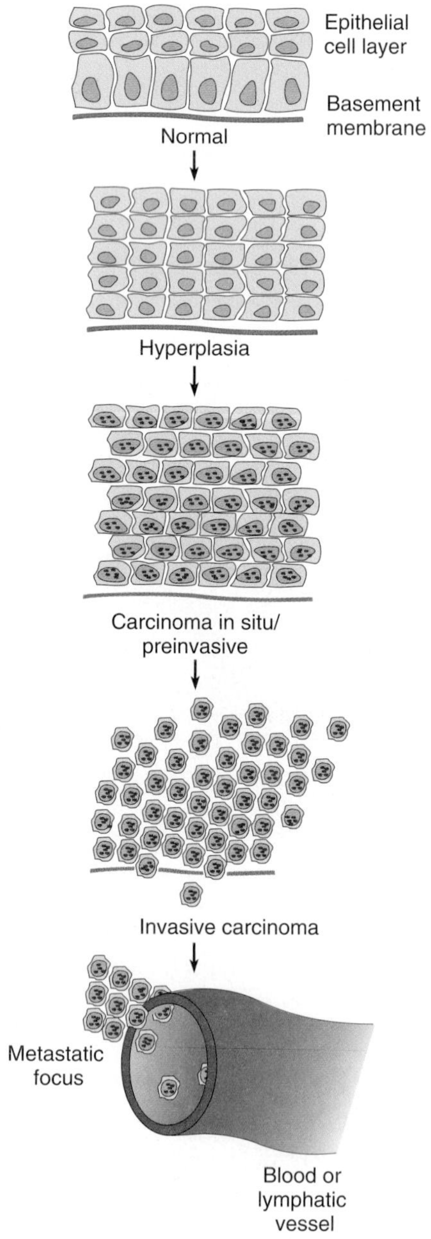

- Normal cells with basal → apical differentiation

- Cells have increased in number—**hyperplasia**
- Abnormal proliferation of cells with loss of size, shape, and orientation—**dysplasia**

Carcinoma in situ
- Neoplastic cells have not invaded basement membrane
- High nuclear/cytoplasmic ratio and clumped chromatin
- Neoplastic cells encompass entire thickness

- Cells have invaded basement membrane using **collagenases** and **hydrolases** (metalloproteinases)
- Can metastasize if they reach a blood or lymphatic vessel

Metastasis—spread to distant organ
- Must survive immune attack
- "Seed and soil" theory of metastasis
  - Seed = tumor embolus
  - Soil = target organ—liver, lungs, bone, brain, etc.

-plasia definitions

REVERSIBLE	
Hyperplasia	↑ in number of cells.
Metaplasia	One adult cell type is replaced by another. Often 2° to irritation and/or environmental exposure (e.g., squamous metaplasia in trachea and bronchi of smokers).
Dysplasia	Abnormal growth with loss of cellular orientation, shape, and size in comparison to normal tissue maturation; commonly preneoplastic.
IRREVERSIBLE	
Anaplasia	Abnormal cells lacking differentiation; resemble primitive cells of same tissue, often equated with undifferentiated malignant neoplasms. Little or no resemblance to tissue of origin.
Neoplasia	A clonal proliferation of cells that is uncontrolled and excessive. Neoplasia may be benign or malignant.
Desmoplasia	Fibrous tissue formation in response to neoplasm.

Tumor grade vs. stage

Grade	Degree of cellular differentiation based on histologic appearance of individual tumor. Usually graded 1–4; 1 = low grade, well differentiated to 4 = high grade, poorly differentiated, anaplastic.	Stage usually has more prognostic value than grade.
Stage	Degree of localization/spread based on site and size of 1° lesion, spread to regional lymph nodes, presence of metastases; spread of tumor in a specific patient. Based on clinical (c) or pathology (p) findings. Example: cT3N1M0	TNM staging system (Stage = Spread): **T** = **T**umor size **N** = **N**ode involvement **M** = **M**etastases (important prognostic factor)

Tumor nomenclature

CELL TYPE	BENIGN	MALIGNANT[a]
Epithelium	Adenoma, papilloma	Adenocarcinoma, papillary carcinoma
Mesenchyme		
Blood cells		Leukemia, lymphoma
Blood vessels	Hemangioma	Angiosarcoma
Smooth muscle	Leiomyoma	Leiomyosarcoma
Striated muscle	Rhabdomyoma	Rhabdomyosarcoma
Connective tissue	Fibroma	Fibrosarcoma
Bone	Osteoma	Osteosarcoma
Fat	Lipoma	Liposarcoma

[a]The term **carcinoma** implies epithelial origin, whereas **sarcoma** denotes mesenchymal origin. Both terms imply malignancy.

Tumor differences

Benign	Usually well differentiated, slow growing, well demarcated, no metastasis.
Malignant	May be poorly differentiated, erratic growth, locally invasive/diffuse, may metastasize.

Cachexia

Weight loss, muscle atrophy, and fatigue that occur in chronic disease (e.g., cancer, AIDS, heart failure, tuberculosis). Mediated by TNF-α (nicknamed cachectin), IFN-γ, and IL-6.

Disease conditions associated with neoplasms

CONDITION	NEOPLASM
Down syndrome	**ALL** ("we **ALL** fall **Down**"), AML
Xeroderma pigmentosum, albinism	Melanoma, basal cell carcinoma, and especially squamous cell carcinomas of skin
Chronic atrophic gastritis, pernicious anemia, postsurgical gastric remnants	Gastric adenocarcinoma
Tuberous sclerosis (facial angiofibroma, seizures, mental retardation)	Giant cell astrocytoma, renal angiomyolipoma, and cardiac rhabdomyoma
Actinic keratosis	Squamous cell carcinoma of skin
Barrett's esophagus (chronic GI reflux)	Esophageal adenocarcinoma
Plummer-Vinson syndrome (↓ iron)	Squamous cell carcinoma of esophagus
Cirrhosis (alcoholic, hepatitis B or C)	Hepatocellular carcinoma
Ulcerative colitis	Colonic adenocarcinoma
Paget's disease of bone	2° osteosarcoma and fibrosarcoma
Immunodeficiency states	Malignant lymphomas
AIDS	Aggressive malignant lymphomas (non-Hodgkin's) and Kaposi's sarcoma
Autoimmune diseases (e.g., Hashimoto's thyroiditis, myasthenia gravis)	Lymphoma
Acanthosis nigricans (hyperpigmentation and epidermal thickening)	Visceral malignancy (stomach, lung, uterus)
Dysplastic nevus	Malignant melanoma
Radiation exposure	Leukemia, sarcoma, papillary thyroid cancer, and breast cancer.

Oncogenes Gain of function → ↑ cancer risk. Need damage to only 1 allele.

GENE	ASSOCIATED TUMOR	GENE PRODUCT
abl	CML	Tyrosine kinase
c-myc	Burkitt's lymphoma	Transcription factor
bcl-2	Follicular and undifferentiated lymphomas (inhibits apoptosis)	Anti-apoptotic molecule
HER2/neu (c-erbB2)	Breast, ovarian, and gastric carcinomas	Tyrosine kinase
ras	Colon carcinoma	GTPase
L-*myc*	**L**ung tumor	Transcription factor
N-*myc*	**N**euroblastoma	Transcription factor
ret	Multiple endocrine neoplasia (MEN) types 2A and 2B	Tyrosine kinase
c-kit	Gastrointestinal stromal tumor (GIST)	Cytokine receptor

Tumor suppressor genes Loss of function → ↑ cancer risk; both alleles must be lost for expression of disease.

GENE	ASSOCIATED TUMOR	GENE PRODUCT
Rb	**R**etino**b**lastoma, osteosarcoma	Inhibits E2F; blocks G1 → S phase
p53	Most human cancers, Li-Fraumeni syndrome	Transcription factor for p21, blocks G1 → S phase
BRCA1	**Br**east and ovarian **ca**ncer	DNA repair protein
BRCA2	**Br**east and ovarian **ca**ncer	DNA repair protein
p16	Melanoma	
BRAF	Melanoma	B-raf
APC	Colorectal cancer (associated with FAP)	
WT1	**W**ilms' **T**umor (nephroblastoma)	
NF1	**N**euro**F**ibromatosis type **1**	RAS GTPase activating protein (RAS-GAP)
NF2	**N**euro**F**ibromatosis type **2**	Merlin (schwannomin) protein
DPC4	Pancreatic cancer	**DPC**—**D**eleted in **P**ancreatic **C**ancer
DCC	Colon cancer	**DCC**—**D**eleted in **C**olon **C**ancer

Tumor markers

PSA	Prostate-specific antigen. Used to follow prostate carcinoma. Can also be elevated in BPH and prostatitis. Questionable risk/benefit for screening.	Tumor markers should not be used as the 1° tool for cancer diagnosis. They may be used to confirm diagnosis, to monitor for tumor recurrence, and to monitor response to therapy.
Prostatic acid phosphatase	Prostate carcinoma.	
CEA	**C**arcino**E**mbryonic **A**ntigen. Very nonspecific but produced by ~ 70% of colorectal and pancreatic cancers; also produced by gastric, breast, and medullary thyroid carcinomas.	
α-fetoprotein	Normally made by fetus. Hepatocellular carcinomas. Nonseminomatous germ cell tumors (e.g., testis, ovary).	
β-hCG	**H**ydatidiform moles and **C**horiocarcinomas (**G**estational trophoblastic disease).	hCG is commonly associated with pregnancy.
CA-125	Ovarian cancer.	
S-100	Melanoma, neural tumors, schwannomas.	
Alkaline phosphatase	Metastases to bone, liver, Paget's disease of bone.	
Bombesin	Neuroblastoma, lung and gastric cancer.	
TRAP	**T**artrate-**R**esistant **A**cid **P**hosphatase (**TRAP**). **Hairy** cell leukemia—a B-cell neoplasm.	**TRAP** the **hairy** animal.
CA-19-9	Pancreatic adenocarcinoma.	
Calcitonin	Medullary thyroid carcinoma.	

Oncogenic microbes

Microbe	Associated cancer
HTLV-1	Adult T-cell leukemia/lymphoma
HBV, HCV	Hepatocellular carcinoma
EBV	Burkitt's lymphoma, Hodgkin's lymphoma, nasopharyngeal carcinoma, CNS lymphoma (in immunocompromised patients)
HPV	Cervical carcinoma (16, 18), penile/anal carcinoma, upper respiratory SCC
HHV-8 (Kaposi's sarcoma–associated herpesvirus)	Kaposi's sarcoma, body cavity fluid B-cell lymphoma
H. pylori	Gastric adenocarcinoma and lymphoma
Schistosoma haematobium	Bladder cancer (squamous cell)
Liver fluke *(Clonorchis sinensis)*	Cholangiocarcinoma

Chemical carcinogens

TOXIN	ORGAN	IMPACT
Aflatoxins (*Aspergillus*)	Liver	Hepatocellular carcinoma
Vinyl chloride	Liver	Angiosarcoma
Carbon tetrachloride	Liver	Centrilobular necrosis, fatty change
Nitrosamines (smoked foods)	Stomach	Gastric cancer
Cigarette smoke	Larynx Lung Kidney Bladder Pancreas	Squamous cell carcinoma Squamous cell and small cell carcinoma Renal cell carcinoma Transitional cell carcinoma Pancreatic adenocarcinoma
Asbestos	Lung	Bronchogenic carcinoma > mesothelioma
Arsenic	Skin Liver	Squamous cell carcinoma Angiosarcoma
Naphthalene (aniline) dyes	Bladder	Transitional cell carcinoma
Alkylating agents	Blood	Leukemia

Paraneoplastic syndromes

HORMONE/AGENT	EFFECT	NEOPLASM(S)
ACTH or ACTH-like peptide	Cushing's syndrome	Small cell lung carcinoma
ADH	SIADH	Small cell lung carcinoma and intracranial neoplasms
PTHrP	Hypercalcemia	Squamous cell lung carcinoma, renal cell carcinoma, breast cancer
1,25-$(OH)_2$ D_3 (calcitriol)	Hypercalcemia	Hodgkin's lymphoma, some non-Hodgkin's lymphomas
Erythropoietin	Polycythemia	Renal cell carcinoma, hemangioblastoma, hepatocellular carcinoma, pheochromocytoma
Antibodies against presynaptic Ca^{2+} channels at NMJ	Lambert-Eaton syndrome (muscle weakness)	Small cell lung carcinoma

Psammoma bodies	Laminated, concentric, calcific spherules seen in: ▪ Papillary adenocarcinoma of thyroid ▪ Serous papillary cystadenocarcinoma of ovary ▪ Meningioma ▪ Malignant mesothelioma	**PS**a**MM**oma: **P**apillary (thyroid) **S**erous (ovary) **M**eningioma **M**esothelioma

Cancer epidemiology

	MALE	FEMALE	NOTES
Incidence	Prostate (32%) Lung (16%) Colon/rectum (12%)	Breast (32%) Lung (13%) Colon/rectum (13%)	Lung cancer incidence has dropped in men, but has not changed significantly in women
Mortality	Lung (33%) Prostate (13%)	Lung (23%) Breast (18%)	Cancer is the 2nd leading cause of death in the United States (heart disease is 1st)

Common metastases

SITE OF METASTASIS	1° TUMOR	NOTES
Brain	Lung > breast > genitourinary > osteosarcoma > melanoma > GI.	50% of brain tumors are from metastases. Typically multiple well-circumscribed tumors at gray/white matter junction.
Liver	Colon >> stomach > pancreas.	Liver and lung are the most common sites of metastasis after the regional lymph nodes.
Bone	Prostate, breast > lung > thyroid, testes.	Bone metastasis >> primary bone tumors. Whole-body bone scan shows tumor predilection for axial skeleton. Lung = lytic. Prostate = blastic. Breast = lytic and blastic.

HIGH-YIELD PRINCIPLES IN

Pharmacology

"Take me, I am the drug; take me, I am hallucinogenic."

—Salvador Dali

"I was under medication when I made the decision not to burn the tapes."

—Richard Nixon

"I wondher why ye can always read a doctor's bill an' ye niver can read his purscription."

—Finley Peter Dunne

"Once you get locked into a serious drug collection, the tendency is to push it as far as you can."

—Hunter S. Thompson

Preparation for questions on pharmacology is straightforward. Memorizing all the key drugs and their characteristics (e.g., mechanisms, clinical use, and important side effects) is high yield. Focus on understanding the prototype drugs in each class. Avoid memorizing obscure derivatives. Learn the "classic" and distinguishing toxicities of the major drugs. Specific drug dosages or trade names are generally not testable. Reviewing associated biochemistry, physiology, and microbiology can be useful while studying pharmacology. There is a strong emphasis on ANS, CNS, antimicrobial, and cardiovascular agents as well as on NSAIDs. Much of the material is clinically relevant. Newer drugs on the market are also fair game.

▸ PHARMACOLOGY–PHARMACOKINETICS & PHARMACODYNAMICS

Enzyme kinetics

Michaelis-Menten kinetics

[S] = concentration of substrate; V = velocity.

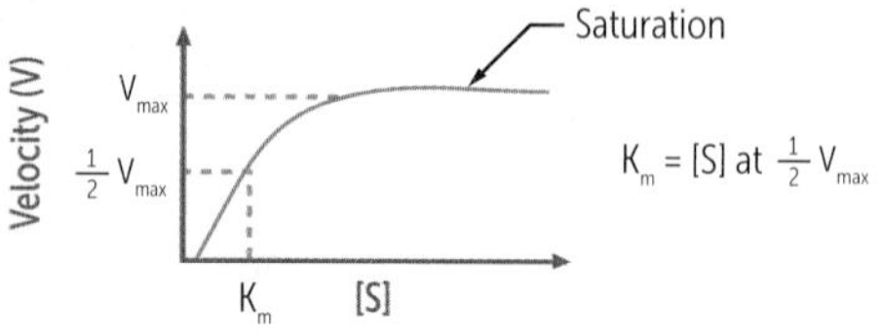

K_m is inversely related to the affinity of the enzyme for its substrate.

V_{max} is directly proportional to the enzyme concentration.

Most enzymatic reactions follow a hyperbolic curve (follow Michaelis-Menten kinetics); however, enzymatic reactions that follow cooperative kinetics (i.e., hemoglobin) have a sigmoid curve.

Lineweaver-Burk plot

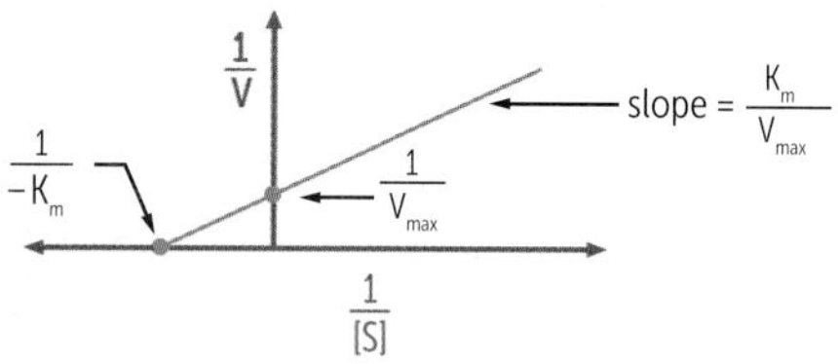

↑ y-intercept, ↓ V_{max}.

The further to the right the x-intercept, the greater the K_m and the lower the affinity.

Enzyme inhibition

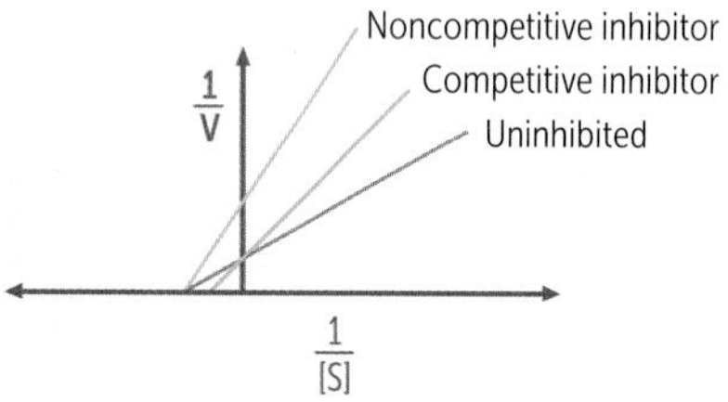

Competitive inhibitors cross each other competitively, whereas noncompetitive inhibitors do not.

	COMPETITIVE INHIBITORS	NONCOMPETITIVE INHIBITORS
Resemble substrate	Yes	No
Overcome by ↑ [S]	Yes	No
Bind active site	Yes	No
Effect on V_{max}	Unchanged	↓
Effect on K_m	↑	Unchanged
Pharmacodynamics	↓ potency	↓ efficacy

Pharmacokinetics

Bioavailability (F)

Fraction of administered drug that reaches systemic circulation unchanged. For an IV dose, F = 100%.

Orally: F typically <100% to incomplete absorption and first-pass metabolism.

Volume of distribution (V_d)

Theoretical fluid volume required to maintain the total absorbed drug amount at the plasma concentration. V_d of plasma protein–bound drugs can be altered by liver and kidney disease (↓ protein binding, ↑ V_d).

$$V_d = \frac{\text{amount of drug in the body}}{\text{plasma drug concentration}}$$

V_d	DISTRIBUTION	DRUG TYPES
Low (4–8 L)	Blood	Large/charged molecules; plasma protein bound
Medium	ECF	Small hydrophilic molecules
High	All tissues	Small lipophilic molecules, especially if bound to tissue protein

Half-life ($t_{1/2}$)

The time required to change the amount of drug in the body by ½ during elimination (or constant infusion). Property of first-order elimination. A drug infused at a constant rate takes 4–5 half-lives to reach steady state.

$$t_{1/2} = \frac{0.7 \times V_d}{CL}$$

# of half-lives	1	2	3	4
% remaining	50%	25%	12.5%	6.25%

Clearance (CL)

Relates the rate of elimination to the plasma concentration. Clearance may be impaired with defects in cardiac, hepatic, or renal function.

$$CL = \frac{\text{rate of elimination of drug}}{\text{plasma drug concentration}} = V_d \times K_e \text{ (elimination constant)}$$

Dosage calculations

Loading dose = $C_p \times V_d/F$.
Maintenance dose = $C_p \times CL/F$.
C_p = target plasma concentration.

In renal or liver disease, maintenance dose ↓ and loading dose is unchanged.
Time to steady state depends primarily on $t_{1/2}$ and is independent of dosing frequency or size.

Elimination of drugs

Zero-order elimination	Rate of elimination is constant regardless of C_p (i.e., constant **amount** of drug eliminated per unit time). C_p ↓ linearly with time. Examples of drugs—**P**henytoin, **E**thanol, and **A**spirin (at high or toxic concentrations).	Capacity-limited elimination. **PEA.** (A pea is round, shaped like the "0" in "**zero**-order.")
First-order elimination	Rate of elimination is directly proportional to the drug concentration (i.e., constant **fraction** of drug eliminated per unit time). C_p ↓ exponentially with time.	Flow-dependent elimination.

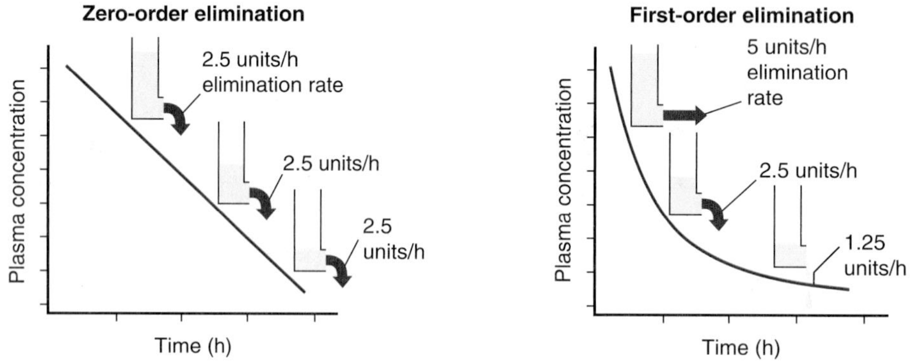
Zero-order elimination
2.5 units/h elimination rate
2.5 units/h
2.5 units/h
Plasma concentration
Time (h)
First-order elimination
5 units/h elimination rate
2.5 units/h
1.25 units/h
Plasma concentration
Time (h)

(Adapted, with permission, from Katzung BG, Trevor AJ. *Pharmacology: Examination & Board Review,* 5th ed. Stamford, CT: Appleton & Lange, 1998: 5.)

Urine pH and drug elimination

Ionized species are trapped in urine and cleared quickly. Neutral forms can be reabsorbed.

Weak acids

Examples: phenobarbital, methotrexate, aspirin. Trapped in basic environments. Treat overdose with bicarbonate.

$$\underset{\text{(lipid soluble)}}{RCOOH} \rightleftharpoons \underset{\text{(trapped)}}{RCOO^- + H^+}$$

Weak bases

Example: amphetamines. Trapped in acidic environments. Treat overdose with ammonium chloride.

$$\underset{\text{(trapped)}}{RNH_3^+} \rightleftharpoons \underset{\text{(lipid soluble)}}{RNH_2 + H^+}$$

Drug metabolism

Phase I	Reduction, oxidation, hydrolysis with cytochrome P-450 usually yield slightly polar, water-soluble metabolites (often still active).	Geriatric patients lose phase I first.
Phase II	Conjugation (**G**lucuronidation, **A**cetylation, **S**ulfation) usually yields very polar, inactive metabolites (renally excreted).	Geriatric patients have **GAS** (phase II). Patients who are slow acetylators have greater side effects from certain drugs because of ↓ rate of metabolism.

Efficacy vs. potency

Efficacy	Maximal effect a drug can produce. High-efficacy drug classes are analgesic (pain) medications, antibiotics, antihistamines, and decongestants. Partial agonists have less efficacy than full agonists.
Potency	Amount of drug needed for a given effect. ↑ potency, ↑ affinity for receptor. Highly potent drug classes include chemotherapeutic (cancer) drugs, antihypertensive (blood pressure) drugs, and antilipid (cholesterol) drugs.

Receptor binding

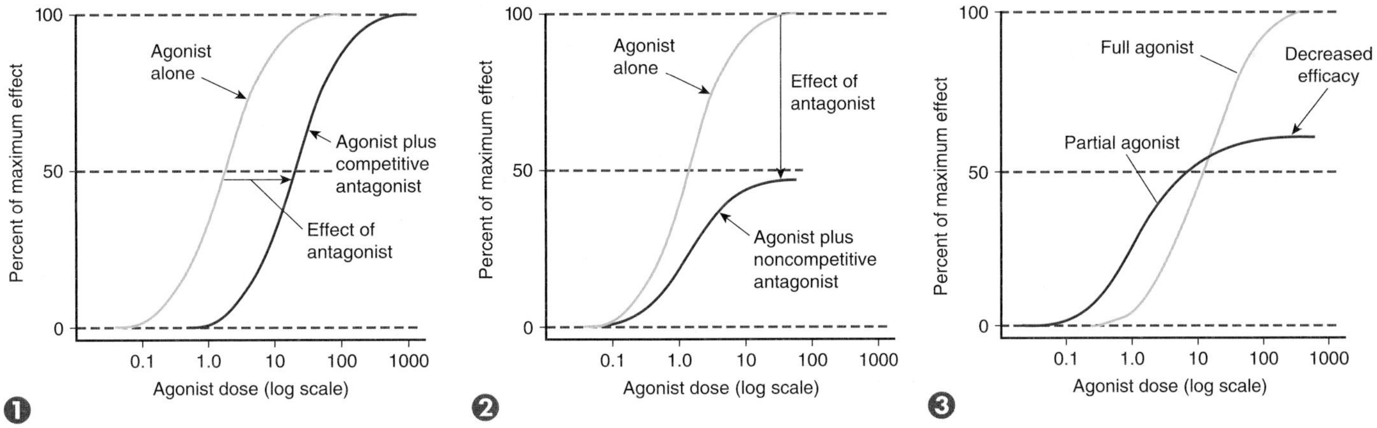

(Image A and B reproduced, with permission, from Trevor AJ et al. *Katzung & Trevor's Pharmacology: Examination & Board Review,* 8th ed. New York: McGraw-Hill, 2008: 14. Image C adapted, with permission, from Katzung BG. *Basic and Clinical Pharmacology,* 7th ed. Stamford, CT: Appleton & Lange, 1997: 13.)

FIGURE	EFFECT	EXAMPLE
❶ Competitive antagonist	Shifts curve to right → ↓ potency, no change in efficacy. Can be overcome by increasing the concentration of agonist substrate.	Diazepam + flumazenil on GABA receptor.
❷ Noncompetitive antagonist	Shifts curve down → ↓ efficacy. Cannot be overcome by increasing agonist substrate concentration.	NE + phenoxybenzamine on α-receptors.
❸ Partial agonist	Acts at same site as full agonist, but with reduced maximal effect → ↓ efficacy. Potency is a different variable and can be ↑ or ↓.	Morphine (full agonist) + buprenorphine (partial agonist) at opioid μ-receptor.

Therapeutic index	Measurement of drug safety. $\frac{LD_{50}}{ED_{50}} = \frac{\text{median lethal dose}}{\text{median effective dose}}$	TILE: Therapeutic Index = LD_{50} / ED_{50}. Safer drugs have higher TI values. Examples of drugs with low TI values include digoxin, lithium, theophylline, and warfarin.
Therapeutic window	Measure of clinical drug safety. Range of minimum effective dose to minimum toxic dose.	

▶ PHARMACOLOGY–AUTONOMIC DRUGS

Central and peripheral nervous system

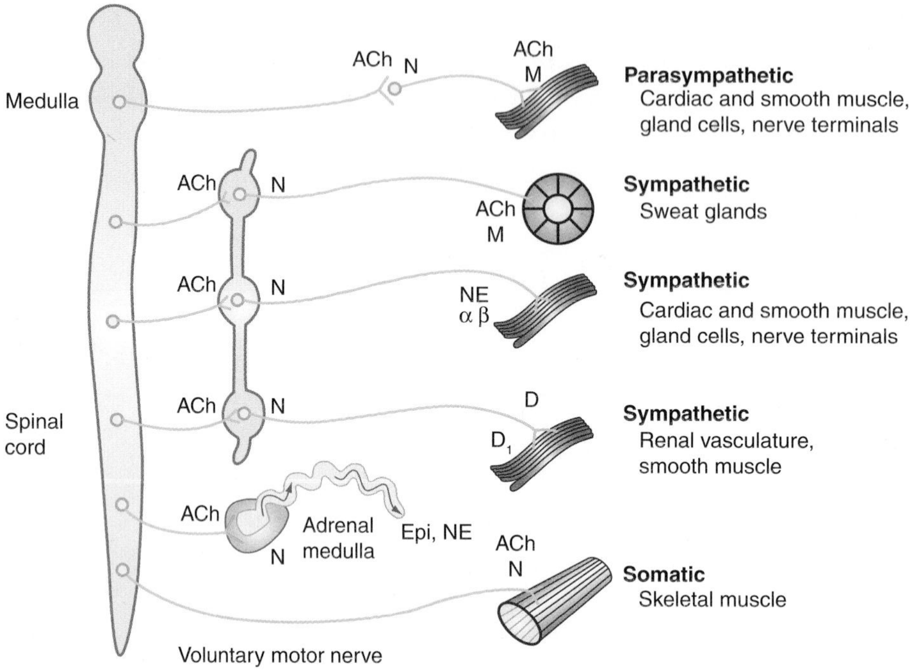

(Adapted, with permission, from Katzung BG. *Basic and Clinical Pharmacology,* 10th ed. New York: McGraw-Hill, 2007: 76.)

Note that the adrenal medulla and sweat glands are part of the sympathetic nervous system but are innervated by cholinergic fibers.

Botulinum toxin prevents release of neurotransmitter at all cholinergic terminals.

ACh receptors

Nicotinic ACh receptors are ligand-gated Na^+/K^+ channels; N_N (found in autonomic ganglia) and N_M (found in neuromuscular junction) subtypes.

Muscarinic ACh receptors are G-protein–coupled receptors that act through 2nd messengers; 5 subtypes: M_1, M_2, M_3, M_4, and M_5.

G-protein–linked 2nd messengers

RECEPTOR	G-PROTEIN CLASS	MAJOR FUNCTIONS
Sympathetic		
α_1	q	↑ vascular smooth muscle contraction, ↑ pupillary dilator muscle contraction (mydriasis), ↑ intestinal and bladder sphincter muscle contraction
α_2	i	↓ sympathetic outflow, ↓ insulin release ↓ lipolysis, ↑ platelet aggregation
β_1	s	↑ heart rate, ↑ contractility, ↑ renin release, ↑ lipolysis
β_2	s	Vasodilation, bronchodilation, ↑ heart rate, ↑ contractility, ↑ lipolysis, ↑ insulin release, ↓ uterine tone (tocolysis), ciliary muscle relaxation, ↑ aqueous humor production
Parasympathetic		
M_1	q	CNS, enteric nervous system
M_2	i	↓ heart rate and contractility of atria
M_3	q	↑ exocrine gland secretions (e.g., lacrimal, gastric acid), ↑ gut peristalsis, ↑ bladder contraction, bronchoconstriction, ↑ pupillary sphincter muscle contraction (miosis), ciliary muscle contraction (accommodation)
Dopamine		
D_1	s	Relaxes renal vascular smooth muscle
D_2	i	Modulates transmitter release, especially in brain
Histamine		
H_1	q	↑ nasal and bronchial mucus production, contraction of bronchioles, pruritus, and pain
H_2	s	↑ gastric acid secretion
Vasopressin		
V_1	q	↑ vascular smooth muscle contraction
V_2	s	↑ H_2O permeability and reabsorption in the collecting tubules of the kidney (V_2 is found in the 2 kidneys)

"**Qiss** (kiss) and **qiq** (kick) till you're **siq** (sick) of **sqs** (super qinky sex)."

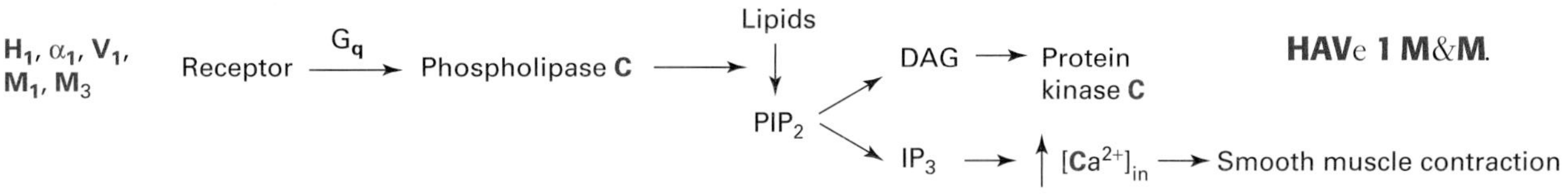
H1, α1, V1, M1, M3
Receptor
Gq
Phospholipase C
Lipids
PIP2
DAG
Protein kinase C
IP3
[Ca2+]in
Smooth muscle contraction

HAVe **1 M**&**M**.

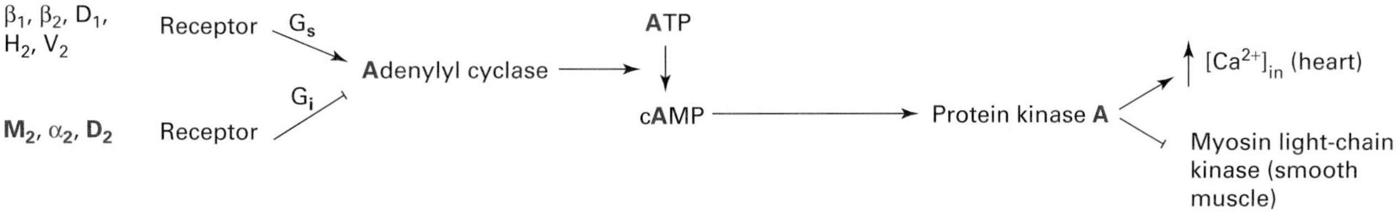
β1, β2, D1, H2, V2
Receptor
Gs
Adenylyl cyclase
Gi
M2, α2, D2
Receptor
ATP
cAMP
Protein kinase A
[Ca2+]in (heart)
Myosin light-chain kinase (smooth muscle)

MAD 2's.

Autonomic drugs

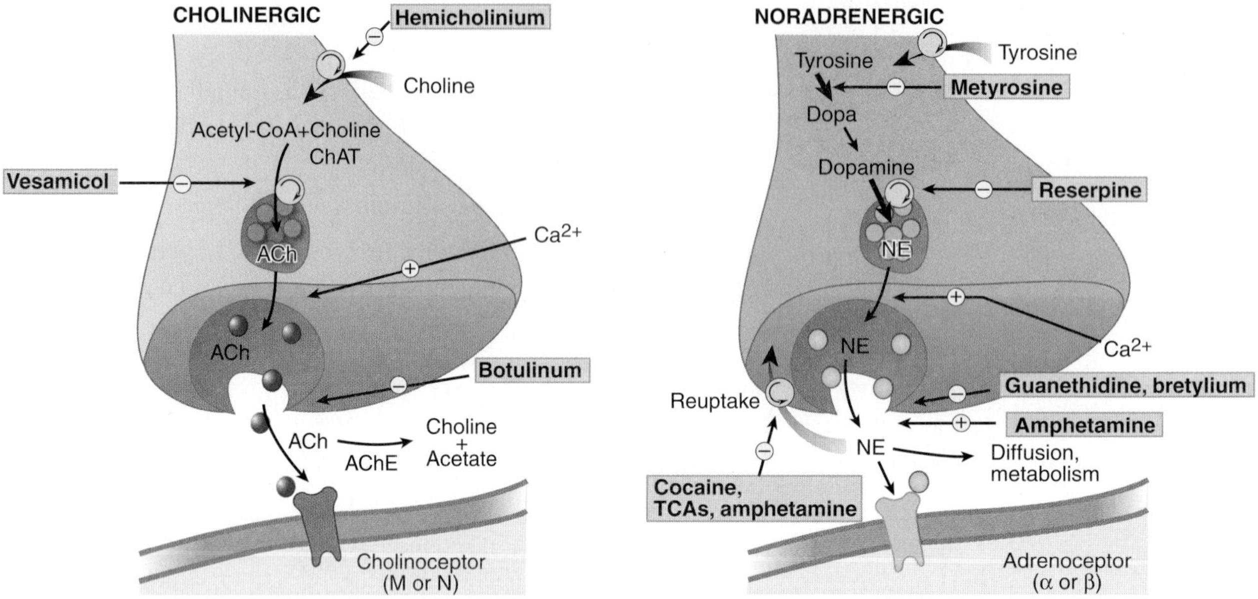

Circles with rotating arrows represent transporters. (Adapted, with permission, from Katzung BG, Trevor AJ. *Pharmacology: Examination & Board Review,* 5th ed. Stamford, CT: Appleton & Lange, 1998: 42.)

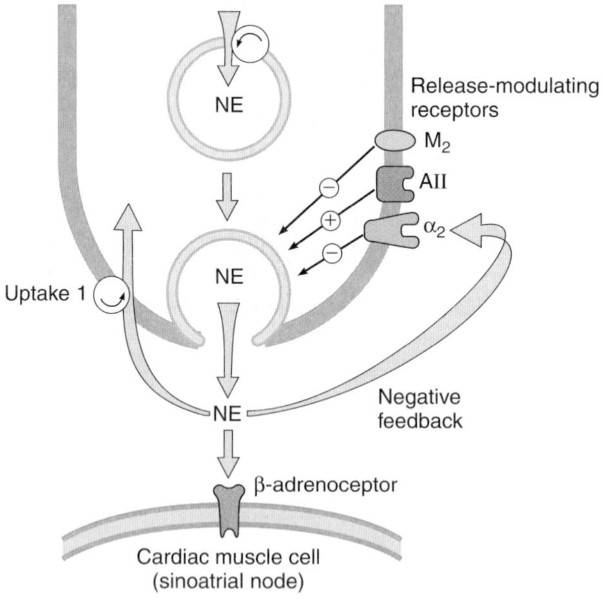

(Adapted, with permission, from Katzung BG, Trevor AJ. *Pharmacology: Examination & Board Review,* 5th ed. Stamford, CT: Appleton & Lange, 1998: 42.)

Release of NE from a sympathetic nerve ending is modulated by NE itself, acting on presynaptic α_2-autoreceptors, and by ACh, angiotensin II, and other substances.

Cholinomimetic agents

DRUG	CLINICAL APPLICATIONS	ACTION
Direct agonists		
Bethanechol	Postoperative ileus, neurogenic ileus, and urinary retention	Activates bowel and bladder smooth muscle; resistant to AChE. "**Bethany, call** (**bethanechol**) me, maybe, if you want to activate your bowels and bladder."
Carbachol	Glaucoma, pupillary contraction, and relief of intraocular pressure	**Carbon** copy of acetyl**chol**ine.
Pilocarpine	Potent stimulator of sweat, tears, and saliva Open-angle and closed-angle glaucoma	Contracts ciliary muscle of eye (open-angle glaucoma), pupillary sphincter (closed-angle glaucoma); resistant to AChE. "You cry, drool, and sweat on your '**pilo**w.'"
Methacholine	Challenge test for diagnosis of asthma	Stimulates muscarinic receptors in airway when inhaled.
Indirect agonists (anticholinesterases)		
Neostigmine	Postoperative and neurogenic ileus and urinary retention, myasthenia gravis, reversal of neuromuscular junction blockade (postoperative)	↑ endogenous ACh. **Neo** CNS = **No** CNS penetration.
Pyridostigmine	Myasthenia gravis (long acting); does not penetrate CNS	↑ endogenous ACh; ↑ strength. Py**rid**ostig**m**ine gets **rid** of **m**yasthenia **g**ravis.
Edrophonium	Diagnosis of myasthenia gravis (extremely short acting)	↑ endogenous ACh.
Physostigmine	Anticholinergic toxicity (crosses blood-brain barrier → CNS)	↑ endogenous ACh. **Phys**ostigmine "**phyx**es" atropine overdose.
Donepezil	Alzheimer's disease	↑ endogenous ACh.

Note: With all cholinomimetic agents, watch for exacerbation of COPD, asthma, and peptic ulcers when giving to susceptible patients.

Cholinesterase inhibitor poisoning	Often due to organophosphates, such as parathion, that **irreversibly** inhibit AChE. Causes **D**iarrhea, **U**rination, **M**iosis, **B**ronchospasm, **B**radycardia, **E**xcitation of skeletal muscle and CNS, **L**acrimation, **S**weating, and **S**alivation. Antidote—atropine + pralidoxime (regenerates active AChE).	DUMBBELSS. Organophosphates are components of insecticides; poisoning usually seen in farmers.

Muscarinic antagonists

DRUGS	ORGAN SYSTEMS	APPLICATIONS
Atropine, homatropine, tropicamide	Eye	Produce mydriasis and cycloplegia
Benztropine	CNS	**Park**inson's disease—"**Park** my **Benz**"
Scopolamine	CNS	Motion sickness
Ipratropium, tiotropium	Respiratory	COPD, asthma ("**I pray** I can breathe soon!")
Oxybutynin	Genitourinary	Reduce urgency in mild cystitis and reduce bladder spasms
Glycopyrrolate	Gastrointestinal, respiratory	Parenteral: preoperative use to reduce airway secretions Oral: drooling, peptic ulcer

Atropine

Muscarinic antagonist. Used to treat bradycardia and for ophthalmic applications.

ORGAN SYSTEM	ACTION	
Eye	↑ pupil dilation, cycloplegia	Blocks **DUMBBeLSS**. Skeletal muscle and CNS excitation mediated by nicotinic receptors. See previous page.
Airway	↓ secretions	
Stomach	↓ acid secretion	
Gut	↓ motility	
Bladder	↓ urgency in cystitis	
TOXICITY	↑ body **temperature** (due to ↓ sweating); rapid pulse; dry mouth; **dry, flushed skin**; **cycloplegia**; constipation; **disorientation** Can cause acute angle-closure glaucoma in elderly (due to mydriasis), urinary retention in men with prostatic hyperplasia, and hyperthermia in infants	Side effects: **Hot** as a hare **Dry** as a bone **Red** as a beet **Blind** as a bat **Mad** as a hatter Jimson weed (*Datura*) → gardener's pupil (mydriasis due to plant alkaloids)

Sympathomimetics

DRUG	α_1	α_2	β_1	β_2	D_1	APPLICATIONS
Direct sympathomimetics						
Epinephrine	+++	+++	++++	++++	0	Anaphylaxis, glaucoma (open angle), asthma, hypotension
Norepinephrine	++++	++++	++	0	0	Hypotension (but ↓ renal perfusion)
Isoproterenol	0	0	++++	++++	0	Torsade de pointes (tachycardia decreases ↓ QT interval), bradyarrhythmias (but can worsen ischemia)
Dopamine	+++ (high dose)	+++ (high dose)	+++ (medium dose)	++ (medium dose)	+++ (low dose)	Shock (renal perfusion), heart failure; inotropic and chronotropic
Dobutamine	+	+	++++	+	0	Heart failure, cardiac stress testing; inotropic and chronotropic
Phenylephrine	+++	++	0	0	0	Hypotension (vasoconstrictor), ocular procedures (mydriatic), rhinitis (decongestant)
Albuterol, salmeterol, terbutaline	0	0	++	++++	0	Metaproterenol and albuterol for acute asthma; salmeterol for long-term asthma or COPD control; terbutaline to reduce premature uterine contractions
Ritodrine	0	0	0	++++	0	Reduces premature uterine contractions
Indirect sympathomimetics						
Amphetamine	Indirect general agonist, releases stored catecholamines					Narcolepsy, obesity, attention deficit disorder
Ephedrine	Indirect general agonist, releases stored catecholamines					Nasal decongestion, urinary incontinence, hypotension
Cocaine	Indirect general agonist, reuptake inhibitor					Causes vasoconstriction and local anesthesia; never give β-blockers if cocaine intoxication is suspected (can lead to unopposed α_1 activation and extreme hypertension)

Norepinephrine vs. isoproterenol

Norepinephrine causes an increase in systolic and diastolic pressures as a result of α_1-mediated vasoconstriction → ↑ mean arterial pressure → bradycardia. However, isoproterenol has little α effect but causes β_2-mediated vasodilation, resulting in ↓ mean arterial pressure and ↑ heart rate through β_1 and reflex activity.

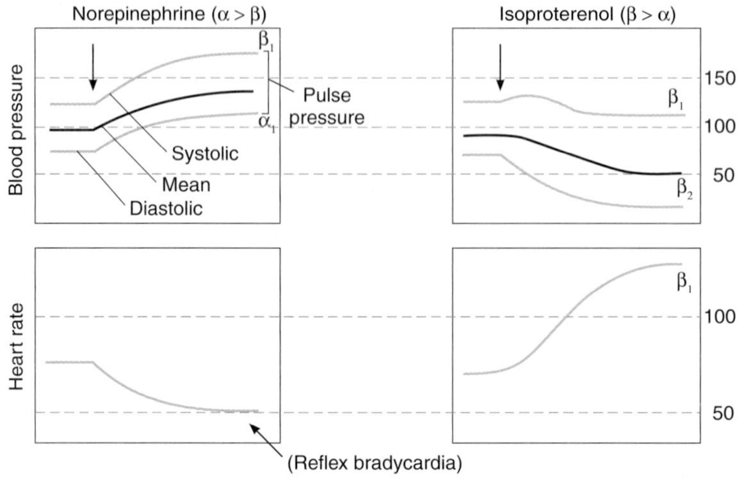

(Adapted, with permission, from Katzung BG, Trevor AJ. *Pharmacology: Examination & Board Review,* 5th ed. Stamford, CT: Appleton & Lange, 1998: 72.)

Sympathoplegics

Clonidine, α-methyldopa	Centrally acting α_2-agonists, ↓ central sympathetic outflow	Application: hypertension, especially with renal disease (no decrease in blood flow to kidney)

α-blockers

DRUG	APPLICATIONS	TOXICITY
Nonselective		
Phenoxybenzamine (irreversible)	Pheochromocytoma (use phenoxybenzamine before removing tumor, since high levels of released catecholamines will not be able to overcome blockage)	Orthostatic hypotension, reflex tachycardia
Phentolamine (reversible)	Give to patients on MAO inhibitors who eat tyramine-containing foods	
α_1 selective (-osin ending)		
Prazosin, terazosin, doxazosin, tamsulosin	Hypertension, urinary retention in BPH	1st-dose orthostatic hypotension, dizziness, headache
α_2 selective		
Mirtazapine	Depression	Sedation, ↑ serum cholesterol, ↑ appetite

α-blockade of epinephrine vs. phenylephrine

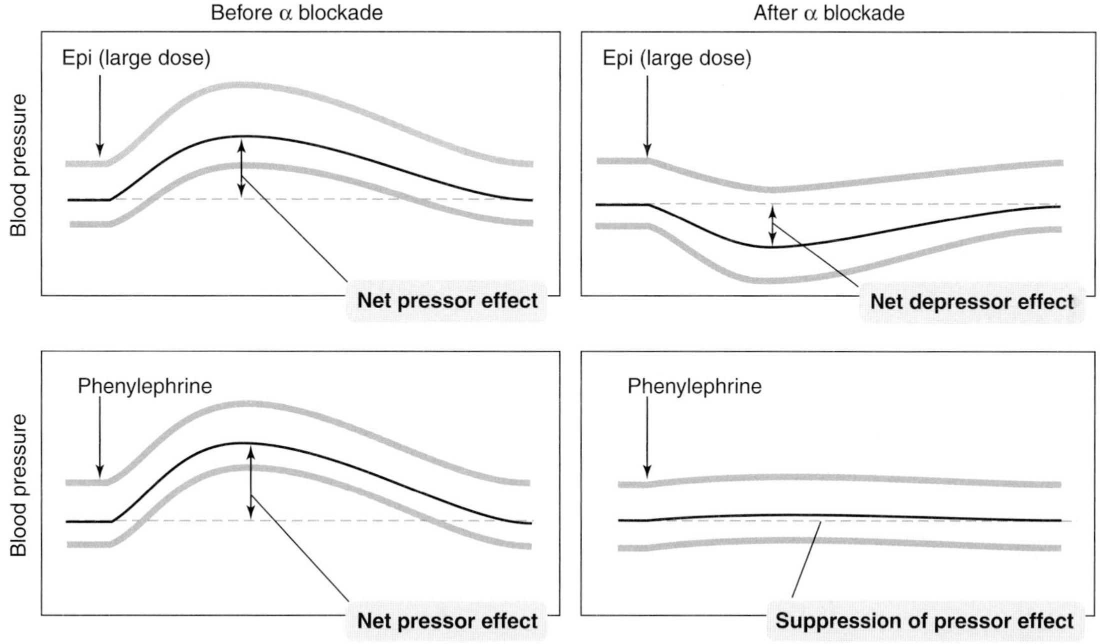

(Adapted, with permission, from Katzung BG, Trevor AJ. *Pharmacology: Examination & Board Review,* 5th ed. Stamford, CT: Appleton & Lange, 1998: 80.)

Shown above are the effects of an α-blocker (e.g., phentolamine) on blood pressure responses to epinephrine and phenylephrine. The epinephrine response exhibits reversal of the mean blood pressure change, from a net increase (the α response) to a net decrease (the β_2 response). The response to phenylephrine is suppressed but not reversed because phenylephrine is a "pure" α-agonist without β action.

β-blockers	Acebutolol, betaxolol, esmolol, atenolol, metoprolol, propranolol, timolol, pindolol, labetalol.	
APPLICATION	EFFECTS	
Angina pectoris	↓ heart rate and contractility, resulting in ↓ O_2 consumption	
MI	β-blockers ↓ mortality	
SVT (metoprolol, esmolol)	↓ AV conduction velocity (class II antiarrhythmic)	
Hypertension	↓ cardiac output, ↓ renin secretion (due to β_1-receptor blockade on JGA cells)	
CHF	Slows progression of chronic failure	
Glaucoma (timolol)	↓ secretion of aqueous humor	
TOXICITY	Impotence, exacerbation of asthma, cardiovascular adverse effects (bradycardia, AV block, CHF), CNS adverse effects (seizures, sedation, sleep alterations); use with caution in diabetics	
SELECTIVITY	β_1-selective antagonists ($\beta_1 > \beta_2$)—**A**cebutolol (partial agonist), **B**etaxolol, **E**smolol (short acting), **A**tenolol, **M**etoprolol	**A BEAM** of β_1-blockers. Advantageous in patients with comorbid pulmonary disease.
	Nonselective antagonists ($\beta_1 = \beta_2$)—**P**ropranolol, **T**imolol, **N**adolol, and **P**indolol	**P**lease **T**ry **N**ot **β**eing **P**icky.
	Nonselective (vasodilatory) α- and β-antagonists—carvedilol, labetalol	
	Partial β-**A**gonists—**P**indolol, **A**cebutolol	**PAPA.**

▶ PHARMACOLOGY—TOXICITIES AND SIDE EFFECTS

Specific antidotes

TOXIN	ANTIDOTE/TREATMENT
Acetaminophen	N-acetylcysteine (replenishes glutathione)
Salicylates	$NaHCO_3$ (alkalinize urine), dialysis
Amphetamines (basic)	NH_4Cl (acidify urine)
Acetylcholinesterase inhibitors, organophosphates	Atropine, pralidoxime
Antimuscarinic, anticholinergic agents	Physostigmine salicylate, control hyperthermia
β-blockers	Glucagon
Digitalis	Normalize **K**$^+$, **L**idocaine, **A**nti-dig Fab fragments, **M**g^{2+} (**KLAM**)
Iron	Deferoxamine, deferasirox
Lead	CaEDTA, dimercaprol, succimer, penicillamine
Mercury, arsenic, gold	Dimercaprol (BAL), succimer
Copper, arsenic, gold	Penicillamine
Cyanide	Nitrite + thiosulfate, hydroxocobalamin
Methemoglobin	**Meth**ylene blue, vitamin C
Carbon monoxide	100% O_2, hyperbaric O_2
Methanol, ethylene glycol (antifreeze)	Fomepizole > ethanol, dialysis
Opioids	Naloxone/naltrexone
Benzodiazepines	Flumazenil
TCAs	$NaHCO_3$ (plasma alkalinization)
Heparin	Protamine
Warfarin	Vitamin K, fresh frozen plasma
tPA, streptokinase, urokinase	Aminocaproic acid
Theophylline	β-blocker

Drug reactions

DRUG REACTION BY SYSTEM	CAUSAL AGENTS	
Cardiovascular		
Coronary vasospasm	Cocaine, sumatriptan, ergot alkaloids	
Cutaneous flushing	**V**ancomycin, **A**denosine, **N**iacin, **C**a^{2+} channel blockers	VANC
Dilated cardiomyopathy	Doxorubicin (Adriamycin), daunorubicin	
Torsades de pointes	Class III (sotalol) and class IA (quinidine) antiarrhythmics	
Hematologic		
Agranulocytosis	**C**lozapine, **C**arbamazepine, **C**olchicine, **P**ropylthiouracil, **M**ethimazole, **D**apsone	Agranulocytosis **C**ould **C**ertainly **C**ause **P**retty **M**ajor **D**amage
Aplastic anemia	Chloramphenicol, benzene, NSAIDs, propylthiouracil, methimazole	
Direct Coombs-positive hemolytic anemia	Methyldopa, penicillin	
Gray baby syndrome	Chloramphenicol	
Hemolysis in G6PD-deficient patients	**I**soniazid (INH), **S**ulfonamides, **P**rimaquine, **A**spirin, **I**buprofen, **N**itrofurantoin	Hemolysis **IS PAIN**
Megaloblastic anemia	**P**henytoin, **M**ethotrexate, **S**ulfa drugs	Having a **blast** with **PMS**
Thrombotic complications	OCPs (e.g., estrogens)	
Respiratory		
Cough	ACE inhibitors	Note: ARBs like losartan—no cough
Pulmonary fibrosis	**BL**eomycin, **A**miodarone, **B**usulfan	It's hard to **BLAB** when you have pulmonary fibrosis
GI		
Acute cholestatic hepatitis, jaundice	Erythromycin	
Focal to massive hepatic necrosis	**H**alothane, *Amanita phalloides*, **V**alproic acid, **Ac**etaminophen	Liver "**HAVAc**"
Hepatitis	INH	
Pseudomembranous colitis	Clindamycin, ampicillin	
Reproductive/endocrine		
Adrenocortical insufficiency	Glucocorticoid withdrawal (HPA suppression)	
Gynecomastia	**S**pironolactone, **D**igitalis, **C**imetidine, chronic **A**lcohol use, estrogens, **K**etoconazole	**S**ome **D**rugs **C**reate **A**wkward **K**nockers
Hot flashes	Tamoxifen, clomiphene	
Hyperglycemia	Niacin, tacrolimus, protease inhibitors, HCTZ, corticosteroids	
Hypothyroidism	Lithium, amiodarone, sulfonamides	

Drug reactions *(continued)*

DRUG REACTION BY SYSTEM	CAUSAL AGENTS	
Musculoskeletal/connective tissue		
Fat redistribution	Glucocorticoids, protease inhibitors	
Gingival hyperplasia	Phenytoin, verapamil	
Gout	Furosemide, thiazides, niacin, cyclosporine	
Myopathies	Fibrates, Niacin, Colchicine, Hydroxychloroquine, Interferon-α, Penicillamine, Statins, Glucocorticoids	Fish N CHIPS Give you myopathies
Osteoporosis	Corticosteroids, heparin	
Photosensitivity	Sulfonamides, Amiodarone, Tetracycline	SAT for a photo
Rash (Stevens-Johnson syndrome)	Penicillin, Ethosuximide, Carbamazepine, Sulfa drugs, Lamotrigine, Allopurinol, Phenytoin, Phenobarbital	Bad rash after a PEC SLAPP
SLE-like syndrome	Hydralazine, INH, Procainamide, Phenytoin	It's not HIPP to have lupus
Teeth (kids)	Tetracyclines	
Tendonitis, tendon rupture, and cartilage damage	Fluoroquinolones	
Renal/GU		
Diabetes insipidus	Lithium, demeclocycline	
Fanconi's syndrome	Expired tetracycline	
Hemorrhagic cystitis	Cyclophosphamide, ifosfamide (prevent by coadministering with mesna)	
Interstitial nephritis	Methicillin, NSAIDs, furosemide	
SIADH	Carbamazepine, cyclophosphamide	
Neurologic		
Cinchonism	Quinidine, quinine	
Parkinson-like syndrome	Antipsychotics, reserpine, metoclopramide	
Seizures	Isoniazid, Bupropion, Imipenem/cilastatin, Tramadol, Enflurane, Metoclopramide	With seizures, I BITE My tongue
Tardive dyskinesia	Antipsychotics	
Multiorgan		
Antimuscarinic	Atropine, TCAs, H_1-blockers, neuroleptics	
Disulfiram-like reaction	Metronidazole, certain cephalosporins, procarbazine, 1st-generation sulfonylureas	
Nephrotoxicity/ototoxicity	Aminoglycosides, vancomycin, loop diuretics, cisplatin	

P-450 interactions	**Inducers (+)**	**Inhibitors (–)**
	Modafinil Barbiturates St. John's wort Phenytoin Rifampin Griseofulvin Carbamazepine Chronic alcohol use Momma Barb Steals Phen-phen and Refuses Greasy Carbs Chronically.	Macrolides Amiodarone Grapefruit juice Isoniazid Cimetidine Ritonavir Acute alcohol abuse Ciprofloxacin Ketoconazole Sulfonamides Gemfibrozil Quinidine MAGIC RACKS in GQ.
Sulfa drugs	Probenecid, Furosemide, Acetazolamide, Celecoxib, Thiazides, Sulfonamide antibiotics, Sulfasalazine, Sulfonylureas Patients with sulfa allergies may develop fever, urinary tract infection, pruritic rash, Stevens-Johnson syndrome, hemolytic anemia, thrombocytopenia, agranulocytosis, and urticaria (hives). Symptoms range from mild to life-threatening.	Popular FACTSSS

▸ PHARMACOLOGY–MISCELLANEOUS

Drug name

ENDING	CATEGORY	EXAMPLE
Antimicrobial		
-azole	Antifungal	Ketoconazole
-cillin	Penicillin	Methicillin
-cycline	Antibiotic, protein synthesis inhibitor	Tetracycline
-navir	Protease inhibitor	Saquinavir
CNS		
-triptan	5-$HT_{1B/1D}$ agonists (migraine)	Sumatriptan
-ane	Inhalational general anesthetic	Halothane
-caine	Local anesthetic	Lidocaine
-operidol	Butyrophenone (neuroleptic)	Haloperidol
-azine	Phenothiazine (neuroleptic, antiemetic)	Chlorpromazine
-barbital	Barbiturate	Phenobarbital
-zolam	Benzodiazepine	Alprazolam
-azepam	Benzodiazepine	Diazepam
-etine	SSRI	Fluoxetine
-ipramine	TCA	Imipramine
-triptyline	TCA	Amitriptyline
Autonomic		
-olol	β-antagonist	Propranolol
-terol	β_2-agonist	Albuterol
-zosin	α_1-antagonist	Prazosin
Cardiovascular		
-oxin	Cardiac glycoside (inotropic agent)	Digoxin
-pril	ACE inhibitor	Captopril
-afil	Erectile dysfunction	Sildenafil
Other		
-tropin	Pituitary hormone	Somatotropin
-tidine	H_2 antagonist	Cimetidine

NOTES

SECTION III

High-Yield Organ Systems

"Symptoms, then, are in reality nothing but the cry from suffering organs."
—Jean-Martin Charcot

"Man is an intelligence in servitude to his organs."
—Aldous Huxley

▶ APPROACHING THE ORGAN SYSTEMS

In this section, we have divided the High-Yield Facts into the major **Organ Systems.** Within each Organ System are several subsections, including **Embryology, Anatomy, Physiology, Pathology,** and **Pharmacology.** As you progress through each Organ System, refer back to information in the previous subsections to organize these basic science subsections into a "vertical" framework for learning. Below is some general advice for studying the organ systems by these subsections.

Embryology

For 2013, we have shifted Embryology into the Organ Systems section. Relevant embryology is tied to each organ system subsection. Embryology tends to correspond well with the relevant Anatomy, especially with regard to congenital malformations.

Anatomy

Several topics fall under this heading, including gross anatomy, histology, and neuroanatomy. Do not memorize all the small details; however, do not ignore anatomy altogether. Review what you have already learned and what you wish you had learned. Many questions require two steps. The first step is to identify a structure on anatomic cross section, electron micrograph, or photomicrograph. The second step may require an understanding of the clinical significance of the structure.

When studying, stress clinically important material. For example, be familiar with gross anatomy related to specific diseases (e.g., Pancoast tumor, Horner's syndrome), traumatic injuries (e.g., fractures, sensory and motor nerve deficits), procedures (e.g., lumbar puncture), and common surgeries (e.g., cholecystectomy). There are also many questions on the exam involving x-rays, CT scans, and neuro MRI scans. Many students suggest browsing through a general radiology atlas, pathology atlas, and histology atlas. Focus on learning basic anatomy at key levels in the body (e.g., sagittal brain MRI; axial CT of the midthorax, abdomen, and pelvis). Basic neuroanatomy (especially pathways, blood supply, and functional anatomy) also has good yield. Use this as an opportunity to learn associated neuropathology and neurophysiology.

Physiology

The portion of the examination dealing with physiology is broad and concept oriented and thus does not lend itself as well to fact-based review. Diagrams are often the best study aids, especially given the increasing number of questions requiring the interpretation of diagrams. Learn to apply basic physiologic relationships in a variety of ways (e.g., the Fick equation, clearance equations). You are seldom asked to perform complex calculations. Hormones are the focus of many questions, so learn their sites of production and action as well as their regulatory mechanisms.

A large portion of the physiology tested on the USMLE Step 1 is now clinically relevant and involves understanding physiologic changes associated with pathologic processes (e.g., changes in pulmonary function with COPD). Thus, it is worthwhile to review the physiologic changes that are found with common pathologies of the major organ systems (e.g., heart, lungs, kidneys, GI tract) and endocrine glands.

Pathology

Questions dealing with this discipline are difficult to prepare for because of the sheer volume of material involved. Review the basic principles and hallmark characteristics of the key diseases. Given the increasingly clinical orientation of Step 1, it is no longer sufficient to know only the "buzz word" associations of certain diseases (e.g., café-au-lait macules and neurofibromatosis); you must also know the clinical descriptions of these findings.

Given the clinical slant of the USMLE Step 1, it is also important to review the classic presenting signs and symptoms of diseases as well as their associated laboratory findings. Delve into the signs, symptoms, and pathophysiology of major diseases that have a high prevalence in the United States (e.g., alcoholism, diabetes, hypertension, heart failure, ischemic heart disease, infectious disease). Be prepared to think one step beyond the simple diagnosis to treatment or complications.

The examination includes a number of color photomicrographs and photographs of gross specimens that are presented in the setting of a brief clinical history. However, read the question and the choices carefully before looking at the illustration, because the history will help you identify the pathologic process. Flip through an illustrated pathology textbook, color atlases, and appropriate Web sites in order to look at the pictures in the days before the exam. Pay attention to potential clues such as age, sex, ethnicity, occupation, recent activities and exposures, and specialized lab tests.

Pharmacology

Preparation for questions on pharmacology is straightforward. Memorizing all the key drugs and their characteristics (e.g., mechanisms, clinical use, and important side effects) is high yield. Focus on understanding the prototype drugs in each class. Avoid memorizing obscure derivatives. Learn the "classic" and distinguishing toxicities of the major drugs. Do not bother with drug dosages or trade names. Reviewing associated biochemistry, physiology, and microbiology can be useful while studying pharmacology. There is a strong emphasis on ANS, CNS, antimicrobial, and cardiovascular agents as well as on NSAIDs. Much of the material is clinically relevant. Newer drugs on the market are also fair game.

▶ NOTES

HIGH-YIELD SYSTEMS

Cardiovascular

"As for me, except for an occasional heart attack, I feel as young as I ever did."

—Robert Benchley

"Hearts will never be practical until they are made unbreakable."

—The Wizard of Oz

"As the arteries grow hard, the heart grows soft."

—H. L. Mencken

"Nobody has ever measured, not even poets, how much the heart can hold."

—Zelda Fitzgerald

"Only from the heart can you touch the sky."

—Rumi

▸ CARDIOVASCULAR—EMBRYOLOGY

Heart embryology

EMBRYONIC STRUCTURE	GIVES RISE TO
Truncus arteriosus (TA)	Ascending aorta and pulmonary trunk
Bulbus cordis	Smooth parts (outflow tract) of left and right ventricles
Primitive ventricle	Trabeculated left and right ventricles
Primitive atria	Trabeculated left and right atria
Left horn of sinus venosus (SV)	Coronary sinus
Right horn of SV	Smooth part of right atrium
Right common cardinal vein and right anterior cardinal vein	SVC

Truncus arteriosus

Neural crest migration → truncal and bulbar ridges that spiral and fuse to form the aorticopulmonary (AP) septum → ascending aorta and pulmonary trunk.

Pathology—transposition of great vessels (failure to spiral), tetralogy of Fallot (skewed AP septum development), persistent TA (partial AP septum development).

Interventricular septum development

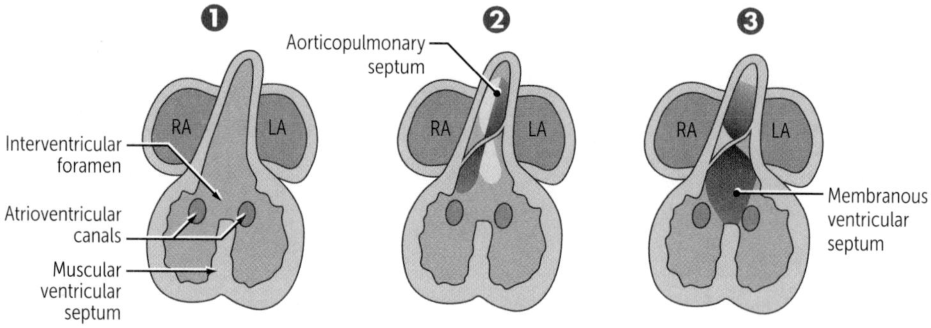

❶ Muscular ventricular septum forms. Opening is called interventricular foramen.

❷ AP septum rotates and fuses with muscular ventricular septum to form membranous interventricular septum, closing interventricular foramen.

❸ Growth of endocardial cushions separates atria from ventricles and contributes to both atrial separation and membranous portion of the interventricular septum.

Pathology—improper neural crest migration into the TA can result in transposition of the great arteries or a persistent TA. Membranous septal defect causes an initial left-to-right shunt, which later reverses to a right-to-left shunt due to the onset of pulmonary hypertension (Eisenmenger's syndrome).

Interatrial septum development

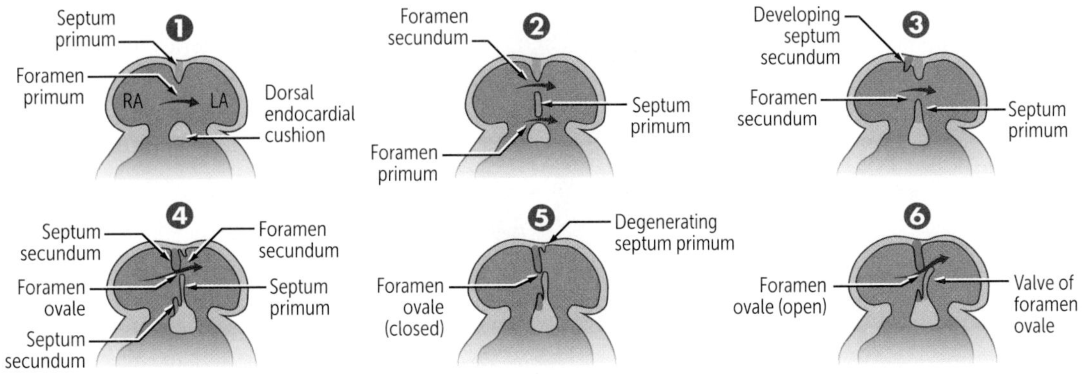

❶ Foramen primum narrows as septum primum grows toward endocardial cushions.
❷ Perforations in septum primum form foramen secundum (foramen primum disappears).
❸ Foramen secundum maintains right-to-left shunt as septum secundum begins to grow.
❹ Septum secundum contains a permanent opening (foramen ovale).
❺ Foramen secundum enlarges and upper part of septum primum degenerates.
❻ Remaining portion of septum primum forms valve of foramen ovale.
7. (Not shown) Septum secundum and septum primum fuse to form the atrial septum.
8. (Not shown) Foramen ovale usually closes soon after birth because of ↑ LA pressure.

Pathology—patent foramen ovale, caused by failure of the septum primum and septum secundum to fuse after birth.

Fetal erythropoiesis

Fetal erythropoiesis occurs in:
- Yolk sac (3–10 wk)
- Liver (6 wk–birth)
- Spleen (15–30 wk)
- Bone marrow (22 wk to adult)

Young Liver Synthesizes Blood.
Fetal hemoglobin = $\alpha_2\gamma_2$.
Adult hemoglobin = $\alpha_2\beta_2$.

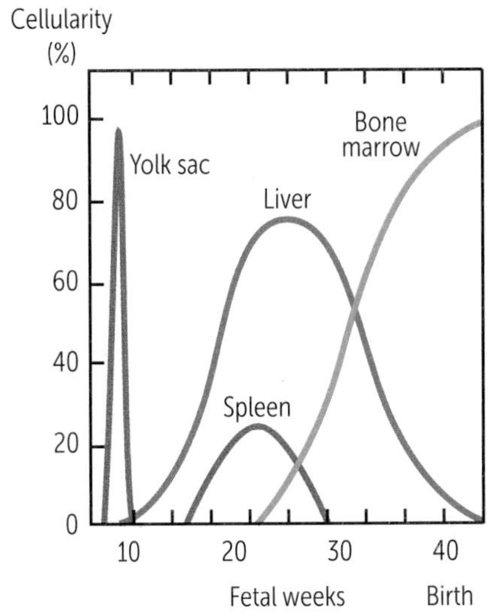

Fetal circulation

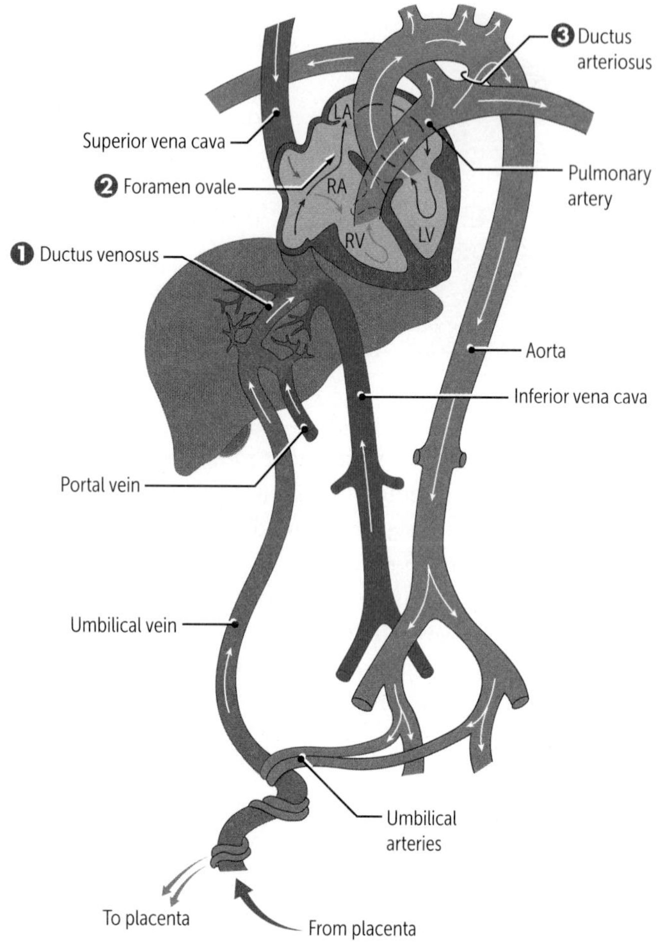

❸ Ductus arteriosus
LA
Superior vena cava
❷ Foramen ovale
RA
Pulmonary artery
RV
LV
❶ Ductus venosus
Aorta
Inferior vena cava
Portal vein
Umbilical vein
Umbilical arteries
To placenta
From placenta

Blood in umbilical vein has a PO_2 of ≈ 30 mmHg and is ≈ 80% saturated with O_2. Umbilical arteries have low O_2 saturation.

3 important shunts:

❶ Blood entering the fetus through the umbilical vein is conducted via the **ductus venosus** into the IVC to bypass the hepatic circulation

❷ Most oxygenated blood reaching the heart via the IVC is diverted through the **foramen ovale** and pumped out the aorta to the head and body

❸ Deoxygenated blood entering the RA from the SVC enters the RV, is expelled into the pulmonary artery, and then passes through the **ductus arteriosus** into the descending aorta.

At birth, infant takes a breath; ↓ resistance in pulmonary vasculature causes ↑ left atrial pressure vs. right atrial pressure; foramen ovale closes (now called fossa ovalis); ↑ in O_2 leads to ↓ in prostaglandins, causing closure of ductus arteriosus.

Indomethacin helps close PDA.

Prostaglandins E_1 and E_2 keep PDA open.

Fetal-postnatal derivatives

Umbilical vein	Ligamentum teres hepatis	Contained in falciform ligament.
UmbiLical arteries	MediaL umbilical ligaments	
Ductus arteriosus	Ligamentum arteriosum	
Ductus venosus	Ligamentum venosum	
Foramen ovale	Fossa ovalis	
AllaNtois	Urachus-mediaN umbilical ligament	The urachus is the part of the allantoic duct between the bladder and the umbilicus. Urachal cyst or sinus is a remnant.
Notochord	Nucleus pulposus of intervertebral disc	

▸ CARDIOVASCULAR–ANATOMY

Coronary artery anatomy

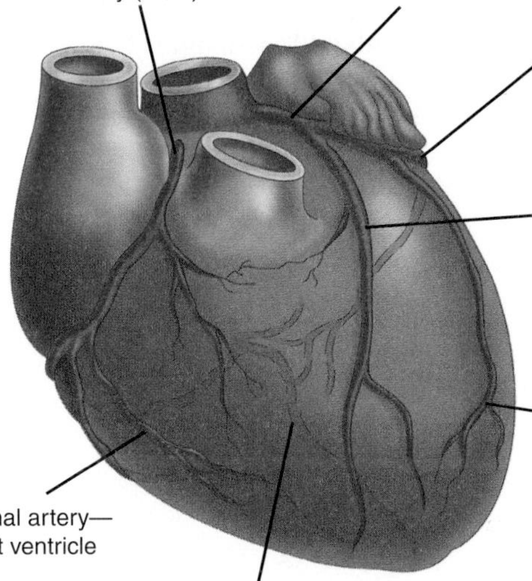
Right coronary artery (RCA)
Left main coronary artery (LCA)
Left circumflex coronary artery (LCX)—supplies lateral and posterior walls of left ventricle
Left anterior descending artery (LAD)—supplies anterior 2/3 of interventricular septum, anterior papillary muscle, and anterior surface of left ventricle
Left marginal artery
Acute marginal artery—supplies right ventricle
Posterior descending/interventricular artery (PD)—supplies posterior 1/3 of interventricular septum and posterior walls of ventricles

SA and AV nodes are usually supplied by RCA.

Right-dominant circulation = 85% = PD arises from RCA.

Left-dominant circulation = 8% = PD arises from LCX.

Codominant circulation = 7% = PD arises from both LCX and RCA.

Coronary artery occlusion most commonly occurs in the LAD.

Coronary arteries fill during **diastole**.

The most posterior part of the heart is the left atrium; enlargement can cause dysphagia (due to compression of the esophagus) or hoarseness (due to compression of the left recurrent laryngeal nerve, a branch of the vagus). Transesophageal echocardiography is useful for diagnosing left atrial enlargement, aortic dissection, and thoracic aortic aneurysm.

▸ CARDIOVASCULAR–PHYSIOLOGY

Cardiac output

CO = stroke volume (SV) × heart rate (HR).

Fick principle:

$$CO = \frac{\text{rate of } O_2 \text{ consumption}}{\text{arterial } O_2 \text{ content} - \text{venous } O_2 \text{ content}}$$

$$\text{Mean arterial pressure (MAP)} = \left(\text{cardiac output}\right) \times \left(\text{total peripheral resistance}\right)$$

MAP = ⅔ diastolic pressure + ⅓ systolic pressure.
Pulse pressure = systolic pressure – diastolic pressure.
Pulse pressure ∝ stroke volume.

$$SV = \frac{CO}{HR} = EDV - ESV$$

During the early stages of exercise, CO is maintained by ↑ HR and ↑ SV. During the late stages of exercise, CO is maintained by ↑ HR only (SV plateaus).
If HR is too high, diastolic filling is incomplete and CO ↓ (e.g., ventricular tachycardia).

Cardiac output variables

Stroke **V**olume affected by **C**ontractility, **A**fterload, and **P**reload. ↑ SV when ↑ preload, ↓ afterload, or ↑ contractility.

Contractility (and SV) ↑ with:
- Catecholamines (↑ activity of Ca^{2+} pump in sarcoplasmic reticulum)
- ↑ intracellular Ca^{2+}
- ↓ extracellular Na^+ (↓ activity of Na^+/Ca^{2+} exchanger)
- Digitalis (blocks Na^+/K^+ pump → ↑ intracellular Na^+ → ↓ Na^+/Ca^{2+} exchanger activity → ↑ intracellular Ca^{2+})

Contractility (and SV) ↓ with:
- β_1-blockade (↓ cAMP)
- Heart failure (systolic dysfunction)
- Acidosis
- Hypoxia/hypercapnea (↓ P_{O_2}/↑ P_{CO_2})
- Non-dihydropyridine Ca^{2+} channel blockers

SV CAP.

SV ↑ in anxiety, exercise, and pregnancy.

A failing heart has ↓ SV.

Myocardial O_2 demand is ↑ by:
- ↑ afterload (∝ arterial pressure)
- ↑ contractility
- ↑ heart rate
- ↑ heart size (↑ wall tension)

Preload and afterload

Preload = ventricular EDV.

Afterload = mean arterial pressure (proportional to peripheral resistance).

VEnodilators (e.g., nitroglycerin) ↓ pr**E**load.

VAsodilators (e.g., hydr**A**lazine) ↓ **A**fterload (**a**rterial).

Preload ↑ with:
- Exercise (slightly).
- ↑ blood volume (e.g., overtransfusion).
- Excitement (↑ sympathetic activity).

Starling curve

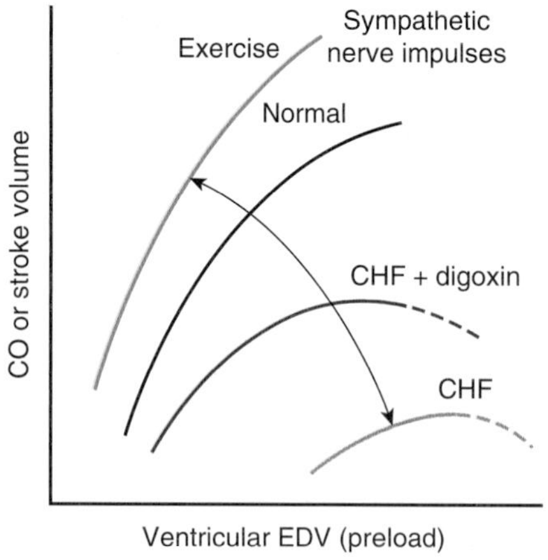

Force of contraction is proportional to end-diastolic length of cardiac muscle fiber (preload).

↑ contractility with sympathetic stimulation, catecholamines, digoxin.

↓ contractility with loss of myocardium (MI), β-blockers, calcium channel blockers.

Ejection fraction (EF)

$$EF = \frac{SV}{EDV} = \frac{EDV - ESV}{EDV}$$

EF is an index of ventricular contractility.

EF is normally ≥ 55%.

EF ↓ in systolic heart failure.

Resistance, pressure, flow

$\Delta P = \dot{Q} \times R$

Similar to Ohm's law: $\Delta V = IR$

Resistance

$$= \frac{\text{driving pressure } (\Delta P)}{\text{flow } (\dot{Q})} = \frac{8\eta \text{ (viscosity)} \times \text{length}}{\pi r^4}$$

Total resistance of vessels in series

$= R_1 + R_2 + R_3 \ldots$

1/Total resistance of vessels in parallel

$= 1/R_1 + 1/R_2 + 1/R_3 \ldots$

Viscosity depends mostly on hematocrit.

Viscosity ↑ in:

- Polycythemia
- Hyperproteinemic states (e.g., multiple myeloma)
- Hereditary spherocytosis

Viscosity ↓ in anemia.

Pressure gradient drives flow from high pressure to low pressure.

Resistance is directly proportional to viscosity and vessel length and inversely proportional to the radius to the 4th power.

Arterioles account for most of total peripheral resistance → regulate capillary flow.

Cardiac and vascular function curves

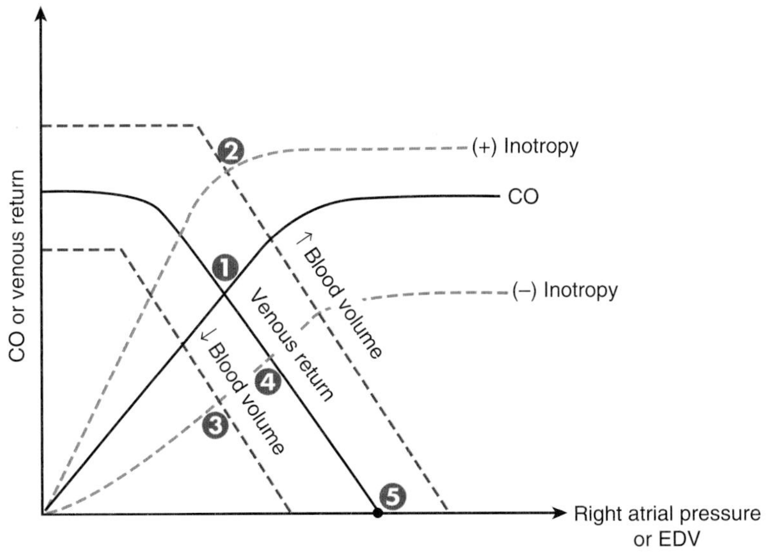

❶ Operating point of heart (cardiac output and venous return are equal)

❷ ↓ TPR, e.g., exercise, AV shunt

❸ ↑ TPR, e.g., hemorrhage before compensation can occur

❹ As in heart failure, narcotic overdose

❺ X-intercept of venous return curve = mean systemic filling pressure

Cardiac cycle

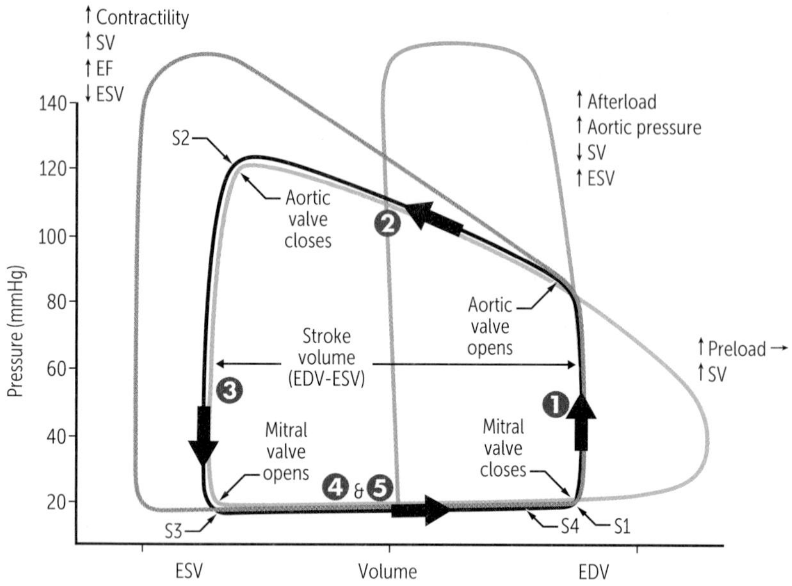

Phases—left ventricle:

1. Isovolumetric contraction—period between mitral valve closure and aortic valve opening; period of highest O_2 consumption
2. Systolic ejection—period between aortic valve opening and closing
3. Isovolumetric relaxation—period between aortic valve closing and mitral valve opening
4. Rapid filling—period just after mitral valve opening
5. Reduced filling—period just before mitral valve closure

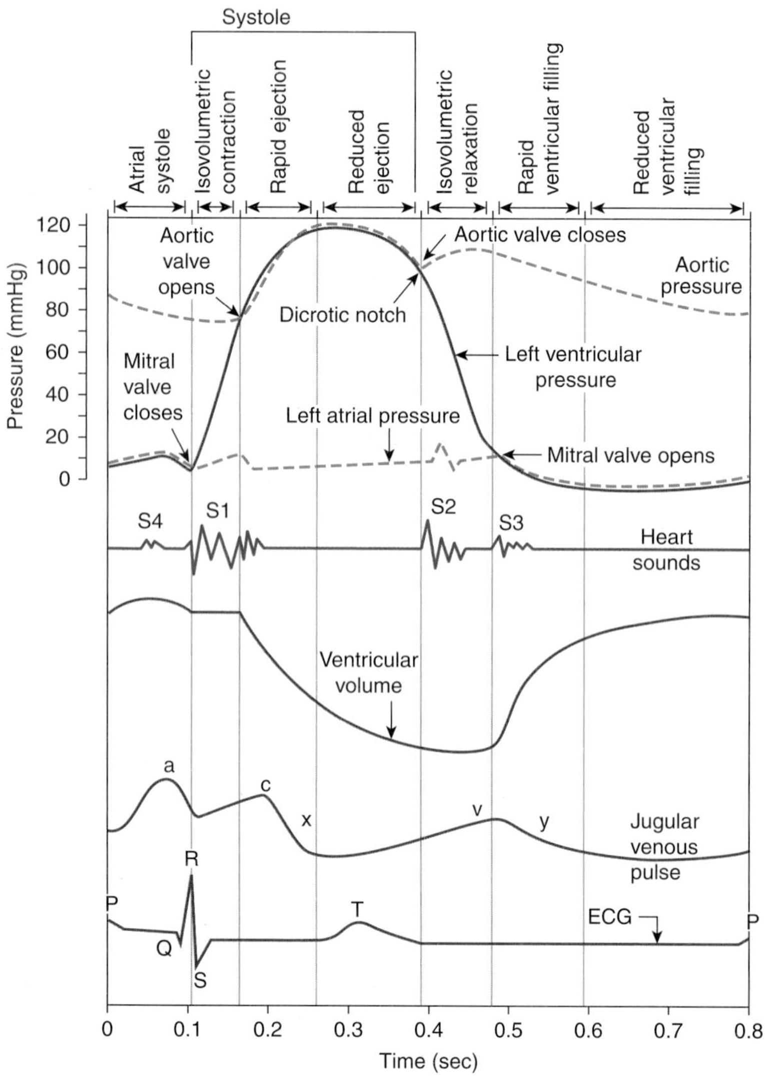

Sounds:

S1—mitral and tricuspid valve closure. Loudest at mitral area.

S2—aortic and pulmonary valve closure. Loudest at left sternal border.

S3—in early diastole during rapid ventricular filling phase. Associated with ↑ filling pressures (e.g., mitral regurgitation, CHF) and more common in dilated ventricles (but normal in children and pregnant women).

S4 ("atrial kick")—in late diastole. High atrial pressure. Associated with ventricular hypertrophy. Left atrium must push against stiff LV wall.

Jugular venous pulse (JVP):

a wave—**a**trial contraction.

c wave—RV **c**ontraction (closed tricuspid valve bulging into atrium).

x descent—atrial relaxation and downward displacement of closed tricuspid valve during ventricular contraction.

v wave—↑ right atrial pressure due to filling against closed tricuspid valve.

y descent—blood flow from RA to RV.

Splitting

Normal splitting	Inspiration → drop in intrathoracic pressure →↑ venous return to the RV → increased RV stroke volume →↑ RV ejection time → delayed closure of pulmonic valve. ↓ pulmonary impedance (↑ capacity of the pulmonary circulation) also occurs during inspiration, which contributes to delayed closure of pulmonic valve.	Expiration: S1 | A2 P2 || Inspiration: S1 | A2 | P2 |
Wide splitting	Seen in conditions that delay RV emptying (pulmonic stenosis, right bundle branch block). Delay in RV emptying causes delayed pulmonic sound (regardless of breath). An exaggeration of normal splitting.	Expiration: S1 | A2 | P2 | Inspiration: S1 | A2 | P2 |
Fixed splitting	Seen in ASD. ASD → left-to-right shunt →↑ RA and RV volumes →↑ flow through pulmonic valve such that, regardless of breath, pulmonic closure is greatly delayed.	Expiration: S1 | A2 | P2 | Inspiration: S1 | A2 | P2 |
Paradoxical splitting	Seen in conditions that delay LV emptying (aortic stenosis, left bundle branch block). Normal order of valve closure is reversed so that P2 sound occurs before delayed A2 sound. Therefore on inspiration, P2 closes later and moves closer to A2, thereby "paradoxically" eliminating the split.	Expiration: S1 | P2 | A2 | Inspiration: S1 | P2 A2 ||

Auscultation of the heart

Where to listen: APT M

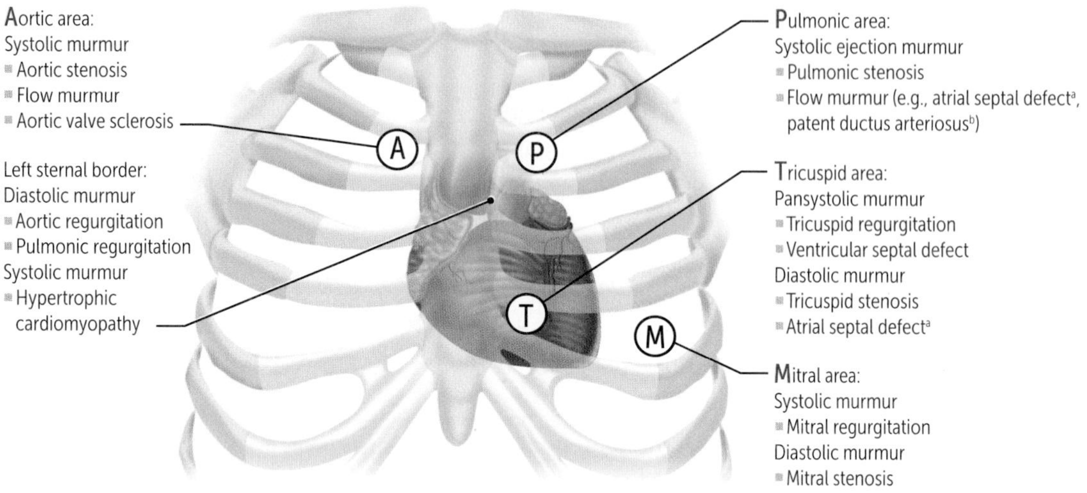
Aortic area:
Systolic murmur
Aortic stenosis
Flow murmur
Aortic valve sclerosis
Left sternal border:
Diastolic murmur
Aortic regurgitation
Pulmonic regurgitation
Systolic murmur
Hypertrophic cardiomyopathy
A
P
T
M
Pulmonic area:
Systolic ejection murmur
Pulmonic stenosis
Flow murmur (e.g., atrial septal defect[a], patent ductus arteriosus[b])
Tricuspid area:
Pansystolic murmur
Tricuspid regurgitation
Ventricular septal defect
Diastolic murmur
Tricuspid stenosis
Atrial septal defect[a]
Mitral area:
Systolic murmur
Mitral regurgitation
Diastolic murmur
Mitral stenosis

[a] ASD commonly presents with a pulmonary flow murmur (↑ flow through pulmonary valve) and a diastolic rumble (↑ flow across tricuspid); blood flow across the actual ASD does not cause a murmur because there is no pressure gradient. The murmur later progresses to a louder diastolic murmur of pulmonic regurgitation from dilatation of the pulmonary artery.

[b] The continuous, machine-like murmur of PDA is best appreciated in the left infraclavicular region.

BEDSIDE MANEUVER	EFFECT
Inspiration	↑ intensity of right heart sounds
Expiration	↑ intensity of left heart sounds
Hand grip (↑ systemic vascular resistance)	↑ intensity of MR, AR, VSD, MVP murmurs ↓ intensity of AS, hypertrophic cardiomyopathy murmurs
Valsalva (↓ venous return)	↓ intensity of most murmurs ↑ intensity of MVP, hypertrophic cardiomyopathy murmurs
Rapid squatting (↑ venous return, ↑ preload, ↑ afterload with prolonged squatting)	↓ intensity of MVP, hypertrophic cardiomyopathy murmurs

Systolic heart sounds include aortic/pulmonic stenosis, mitral/tricuspid regurgitation, ventricular septal defect.
Diastolic heart sounds include aortic/pulmonic regurgitation, mitral/tricuspid stenosis.

Heart murmurs

Systolic	
Mitral/tricuspid regurgitation (MR/TR) 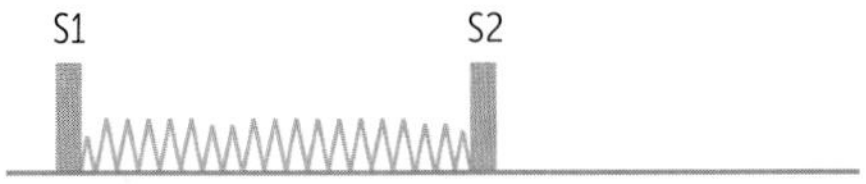S1 S2	Holosystolic, high-pitched "blowing murmur." Mitral—loudest at apex and radiates toward axilla. Enhanced by maneuvers that ↑ TPR (e.g., squatting, hand grip) or LA return (e.g., expiration). MR is often due to ischemic heart disease, mitral valve prolapse, or LV dilation. Tricuspid—loudest at tricuspid area and radiates to right sternal border. Enhanced by maneuvers that ↑ RA return (e.g., inspiration). TR can be caused by RV dilation. Rheumatic fever and infective endocarditis can cause either MR or TR.
Aortic stenosis (AS) 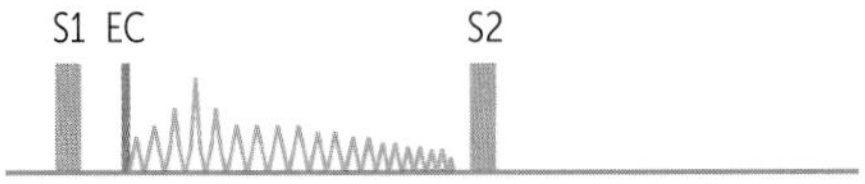S1 EC S2	Crescendo-decrescendo systolic ejection murmur following ejection click (EC; due to abrupt halting of valve leaflets). LV >> aortic pressure during systole. Radiates to carotids/heart base. "Pulsus parvus et tardus"—pulses are weak with a delayed peak. Can lead to **S**yncope, **A**ngina, and **D**yspnea on exertion (**SAD**). Often due to age-related calcific aortic stenosis or bicuspid aortic valve.
VSD 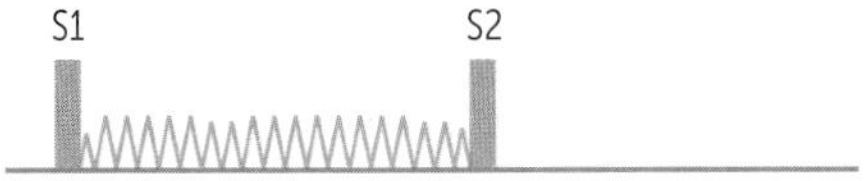S1 S2	Holosystolic, harsh-sounding murmur. Loudest at tricuspid area, accentuated with hand grip maneuver due to increased afterload.
Mitral valve prolapse (MVP) 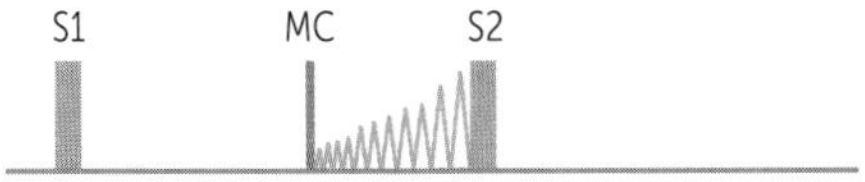S1 MC S2	Late systolic crescendo murmur with midsystolic click (MC; due to sudden tensing of chordae tendineae). Most frequent valvular lesion. Best heard over apex. Loudest at S2. Usually benign. Can predispose to infective endocarditis. Can be caused by myxomatous degeneration, rheumatic fever, or chordae rupture. Enhanced by maneuvers that ↓ venous return (e.g., standing or Valsalva).
Diastolic	
Aortic regurgitation (AR) 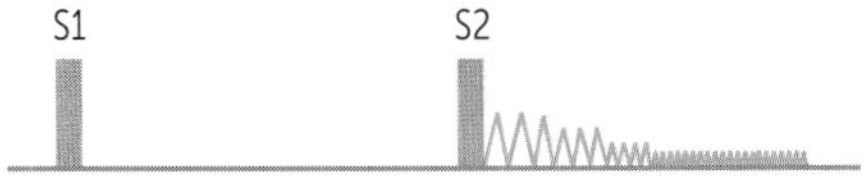S1 S2	Immediate high-pitched "blowing" diastolic decrescendo murmur. Wide pulse pressure when chronic; can present with bounding pulses and head bobbing. Often due to aortic root dilation, bicuspid aortic valve, endocarditis, or rheumatic fever. ↑ murmur during hand grip. Vasodilators ↓ intensity of murmur.
Mitral stenosis (MS) 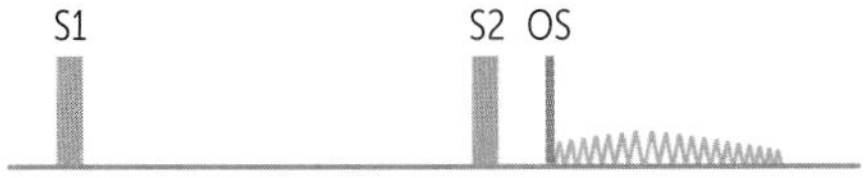S1 S2 OS	Follows opening snap (OS; due to abrupt halt in leaflet motion in diastole, after rapid opening due to fusion at leaflet tips). Delayed rumbling late diastolic murmur. LA >> LV pressure during diastole. Often occurs 2° to rheumatic fever. Chronic MS can result in LA dilation. Enhanced by maneuvers that ↑ LA return (e.g., expiration).
Continuous	
PDA 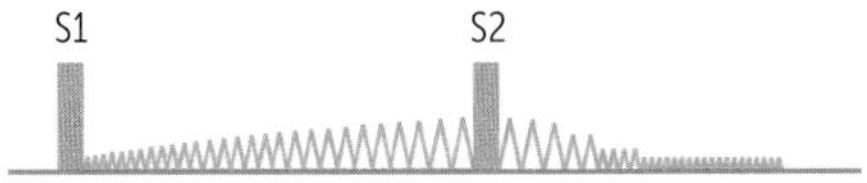S1 S2	Continuous machine-like murmur. Loudest at S2. Often due to congenital rubella or prematurity. Best heard at left infraclavicular area.

Ventricular action potential

Also occurs in bundle of His and Purkinje fibers.

Phase 0 = rapid upstroke—voltage-gated Na^+ channels open.

Phase 1 = initial repolarization—inactivation of voltage-gated Na^+ channels. Voltage-gated K^+ channels begin to open.

Phase 2 = plateau—Ca^{2+} influx through voltage-gated Ca^{2+} channels balances K^+ efflux. Ca^{2+} influx triggers Ca^{2+} release from sarcoplasmic reticulum and myocyte contraction.

Phase 3 = rapid repolarization—massive K^+ efflux due to opening of voltage-gated slow K^+ channels and closure of voltage-gated Ca^{2+} channels.

Phase 4 = resting potential—high K^+ permeability through K^+ channels.

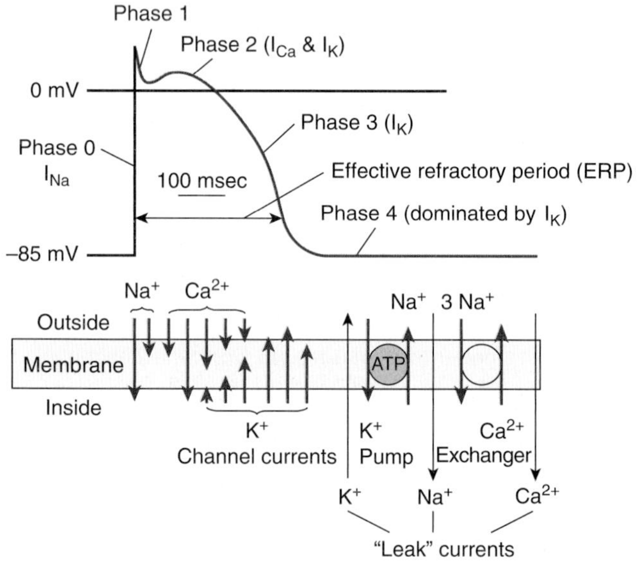

In contrast to skeletal muscle:

- Cardiac muscle AP has a plateau, which is due to Ca^{2+} influx and K^+ efflux; myocyte contraction occurs due to Ca^{2+}-induced Ca^{2+} release from the sarcoplasmic reticulum.
- Cardiac nodal cells spontaneously depolarize during diastole resulting in automaticity due to I_f channels ("funny current" channels responsible for a slow, mixed Na^+/K^+ inward current).
- Cardiac myocytes are electrically coupled to each other by gap junctions.

Pacemaker action potential

Occurs in the SA and AV nodes. Key differences from the ventricular action potential include:

Phase 0 = upstroke—opening of voltage-gated Ca^{2+} channels. Fast voltage-gated Na^+ channels are permanently inactivated because of the less negative resting voltage of these cells. Results in a slow conduction velocity that is used by the AV node to prolong transmission from the atria to ventricles.

Phase 2 = plateau is absent.

Phase 3 = inactivation of the Ca^{2+} channels and ↑ activation of K^+ channels → ↑ K^+ efflux.

Phase 4 = slow diastolic depolarization—membrane potential spontaneously depolarizes as Na^+ conductance ↑ (I_f different from I_{Na} in phase 0 of ventricular action potential). Accounts for automaticity of SA and AV nodes. The slope of phase 4 in the SA node determines heart rate. ACh/adenosine ↓ the rate of diastolic depolarization and ↓ heart rate, while catecholamines ↑ depolarization and ↑ heart rate. Sympathetic stimulation ↑ the chance that I_f channels are open and thus ↑ HR.

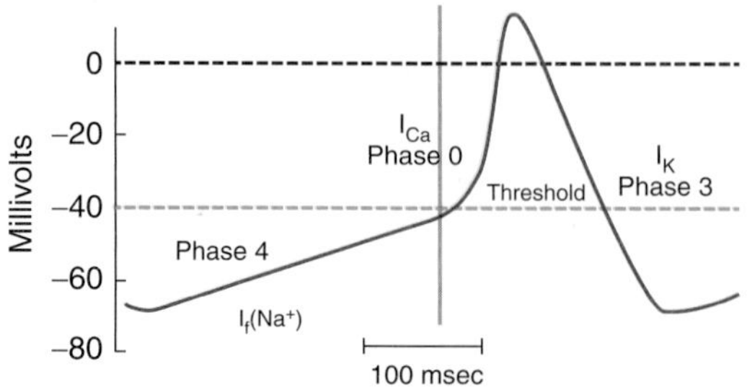

Electrocardiogram

P wave—atrial depolarization. Atrial repolarization is masked by QRS complex.

PR interval—conduction delay through AV node (normally < 200 msec).

QRS complex—ventricular depolarization (normally < 120 msec).

QT interval—mechanical contraction of the ventricles.

T wave—ventricular repolarization. T-wave inversion may indicate recent MI.

ST segment—isoelectric, ventricles depolarized.

U wave—caused by hypokalemia, bradycardia.

Speed of conduction—Purkinje > atria > ventricles > AV node.

Pacemakers—SA > AV > bundle of His/Purkinje/ventricles.

Conduction pathway—SA node → atria → AV node → common bundle → bundle branches → Purkinje fibers → ventricles.

SA node "pacemaker" inherent dominance with slow phase of upstroke.

AV node—100-msec delay—atrioventricular delay; allows time for ventricular filling.

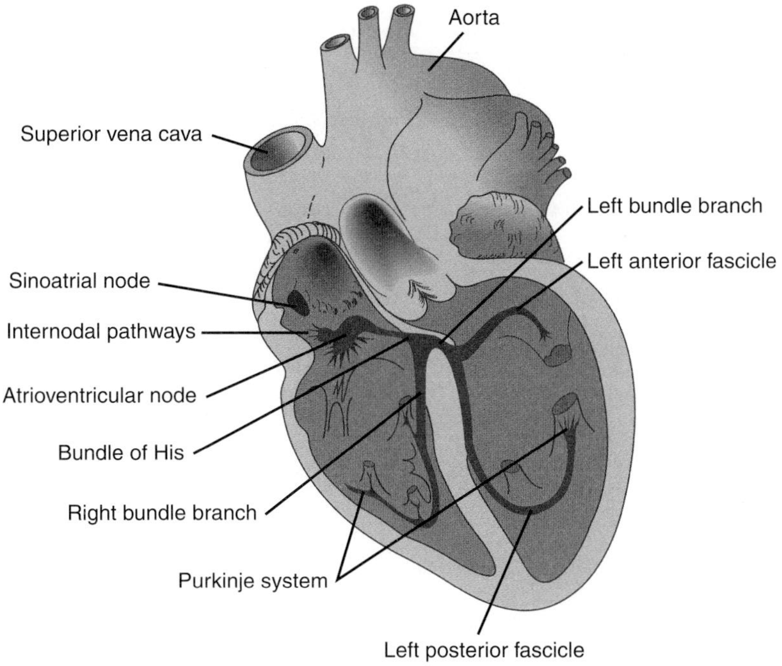

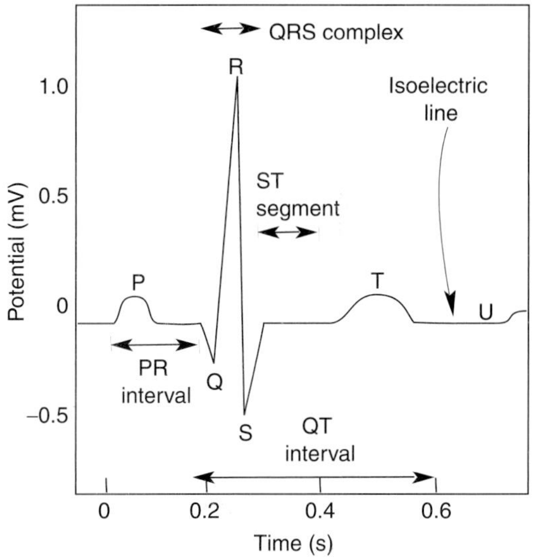

Torsades de pointes

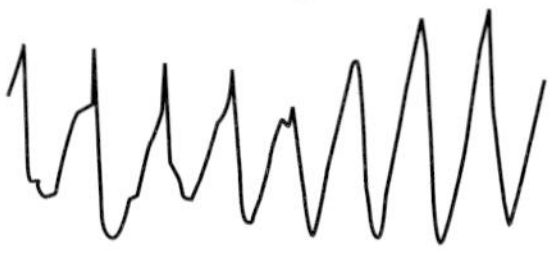

Ventricular tachycardia, characterized by shifting sinusoidal waveforms on ECG, can progress to ventricular fibrillation. Anything that prolongs the QT interval can predispose to torsades de pointes. Treatment includes magnesium sulfate.

Congenital long QT syndromes are most often due to defects in cardiac sodium or potassium channels. Can present with severe congenital sensorineural deafness (**Jervell and Lange-Nielsen syndrome**).

ECG tracings

Atrial fibrillation

Chaotic and erratic baseline (irregularly irregular) with no discrete P waves in between irregularly spaced QRS complexes. Can result in atrial stasis and lead to stroke. Treatment includes rate control, anticoagulation, and possible cardioversion.

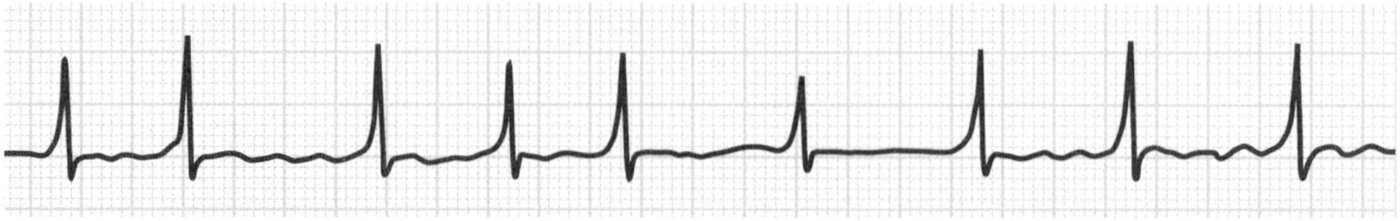

Atrial flutter

A rapid succession of identical, back-to-back atrial depolarization waves. The identical appearance accounts for the "sawtooth" appearance of the flutter waves. Pharmacologic conversion to sinus rhythm: class IA, IC, or III antiarrhythmics. Rate control: β-blocker or calcium channel blocker.

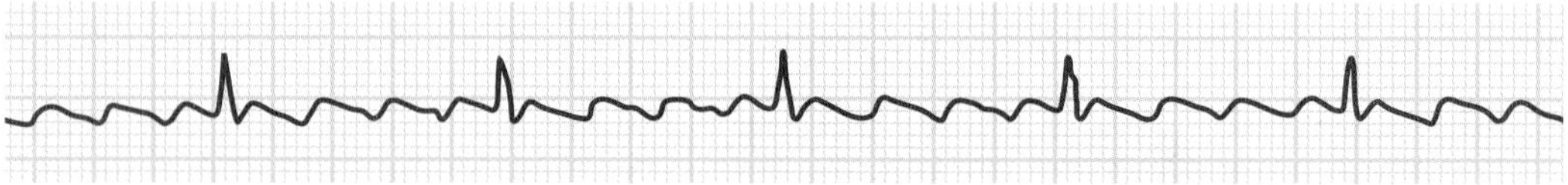

Ventricular fibrillation

A completely erratic rhythm with no identifiable waves. Fatal arrhythmia without immediate CPR and defibrillation.

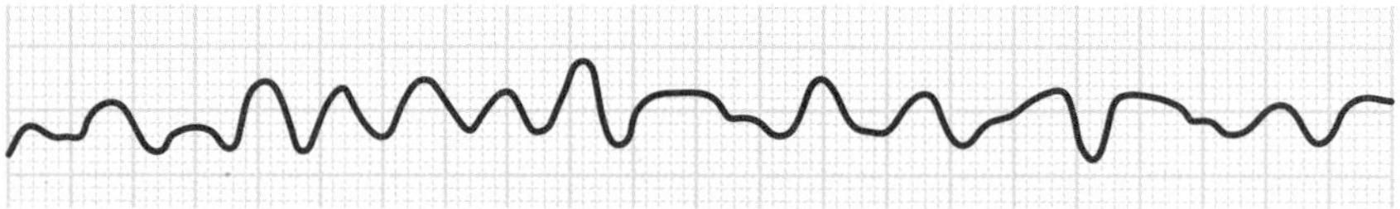

AV block

1st degree

The PR interval is prolonged (> 200 msec). Asymptomatic.

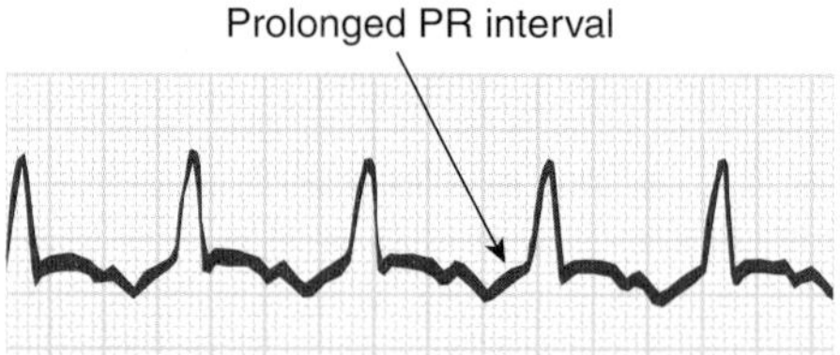
Prolonged PR interval

2nd degree

Mobitz type I (Wenckebach)

Progressive lengthening of the PR interval until a beat is "dropped" (a P wave not followed by a QRS complex). Usually asymptomatic.

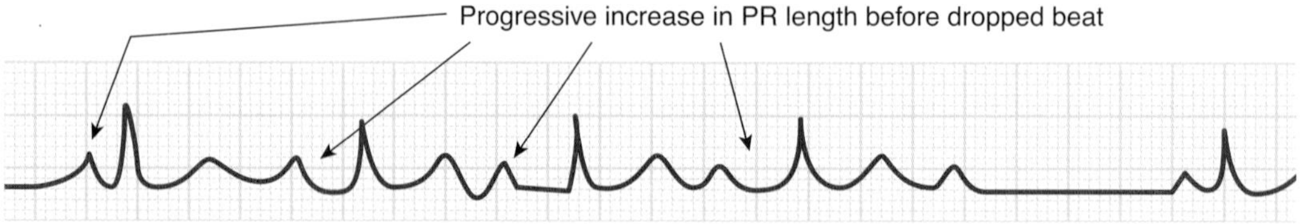
Progressive increase in PR length before dropped beat

ECG tracings *(continued)*

Mobitz type II

Dropped beats that are not preceded by a change in the length of the PR interval (as in type I). These abrupt, nonconducted P waves result in a pathologic condition. It is often found as 2:1 block, where there are 2 or more P waves to 1 QRS response. May progress to 3rd-degree block. Often treated with pacemaker.

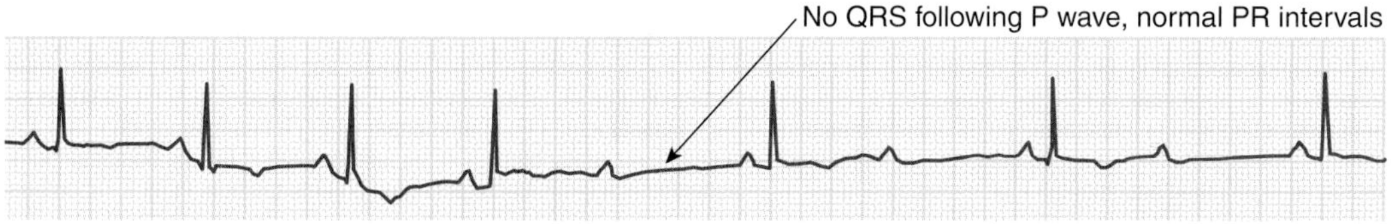
No QRS following P wave, normal PR intervals

3rd degree (complete)

The atria and ventricles beat independently of each other. Both P waves and QRS complexes are present, although the P waves bear no relation to the QRS complexes. The atrial rate is faster than the ventricular rate. Usually treated with pacemaker. Lyme disease can result in 3rd-degree heart block.

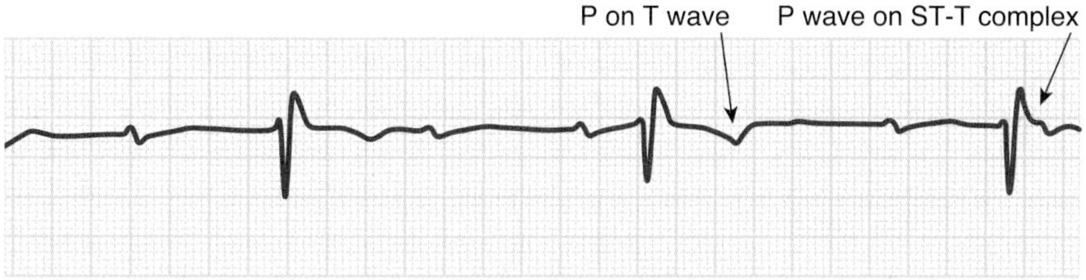
P on T wave
P wave on ST-T complex

Atrial natriuretic peptide

ANP is released from atrial myocytes in response to ↑ blood volume and atrial pressure. Causes generalized vascular relaxation and ↓ Na^+ reabsorption at the medullary collecting tubule. Constricts efferent renal arterioles and dilates afferent arterioles (cGMP mediated), promoting diuresis and contributing to the "escape from aldosterone" mechanism.

Baroreceptors and chemoreceptors

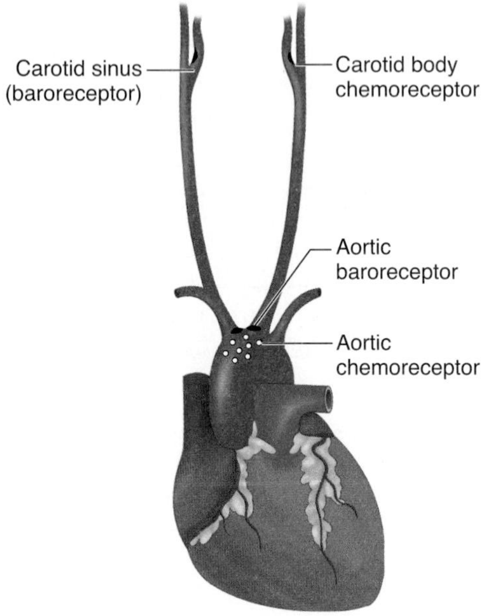

Carotid sinus (baroreceptor)
Carotid body chemoreceptor
Aortic baroreceptor
Aortic chemoreceptor

Receptors:

- Aortic arch transmits via vagus nerve to solitary nucleus of medulla (responds **only** to ↑ BP).
- Carotid sinus transmits via glossopharyngeal nerve to solitary nucleus of medulla (responds to ↓ and ↑ in BP).

Baroreceptors:

- Hypotension—↓ arterial pressure → ↓ stretch → ↓ afferent baroreceptor firing → ↑ efferent sympathetic firing and ↓ efferent parasympathetic stimulation → vasoconstriction, ↑ HR, ↑ contractility, ↑ BP. Important in the response to severe hemorrhage.
- Carotid massage—↑ pressure on carotid artery → ↑ stretch → ↑ afferent baroreceptor firing → ↓ HR.
- Contributes to Cushing reaction (triad of hypertension, bradycardia, and respiratory depression) ↑ intracranial pressure constricts arterioles → cerebral ischemia and reflex sympathetic increase in perfusion pressure (hypertension) → ↑ stretch → reflex baroreceptor induced–bradycardia.

Chemoreceptors:

- Peripheral—carotid and aortic bodies are stimulated by ↓ P_{O_2} (< 60 mmHg), ↑ P_{CO_2}, and ↓ pH of blood.
- Central—are stimulated by changes in pH and P_{CO_2} of brain interstitial fluid, which in turn are influenced by arterial CO_2. Do not directly respond to P_{O_2}.

Circulation through organs

Lung	Organ with largest blood flow (100% of cardiac output).
Liver	Largest share of systemic cardiac output.
Kidney	Highest blood flow per gram of tissue.
Heart	Largest arteriovenous O_2 difference because O_2 extraction is ~ 80%. Therefore ↑ O_2 demand is met by ↑ coronary blood flow, not by ↑ extraction of O_2.

Normal pressures

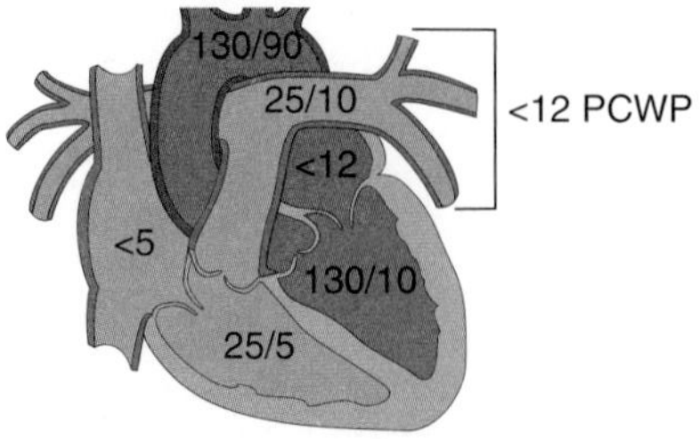

130/90
25/10
<12 PCWP
<12
<5
130/10
25/5

PCWP—pulmonary capillary wedge pressure (in mmHg) is a good approximation of left atrial pressure. In mitral stenosis, PCWP > LV diastolic pressure.

Measured with pulmonary artery catheter (Swan-Ganz catheter).

Autoregulation How blood flow to an organ remains constant over a wide range of perfusion pressures.

ORGAN	FACTORS DETERMINING AUTOREGULATION	
Heart	Local metabolites (vasodilatory)–CO_2, adenosine, NO	Note: the pulmonary vasculature is unique in that hypoxia causes vasoconstriction so that only well-ventilated areas are perfused. In other organs, hypoxia causes vasodilation.
Brain	Local metabolites (vasodilatory)–CO_2 (pH)	
Kidneys	Myogenic and tubuloglomerular feedback	
Lungs	Hypoxia causes vasoconstriction	
Skeletal muscle	Local metabolites—lactate, adenosine, K^+	
Skin	Sympathetic stimulation most important mechanism—temperature control	

Capillary fluid exchange

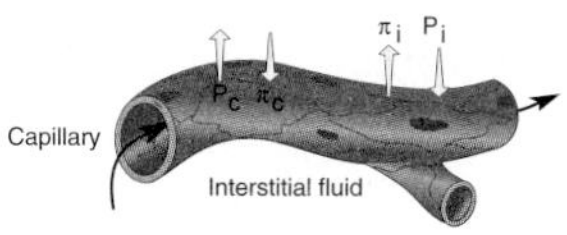

Starling forces determine fluid movement through capillary membranes:

- P_c = capillary pressure—pushes fluid out of capillary
- P_i = interstitial fluid pressure—pushes fluid into capillary
- π_c = plasma colloid osmotic pressure—pulls fluid into capillary
- π_i = interstitial fluid colloid osmotic pressure—pulls fluid out of capillary

Thus, net filtration pressure = $P_{net} = [(P_c - P_i) - (\pi_c - \pi_i)]$.

K_f = filtration constant (capillary permeability).

J_v = net fluid flow = $(K_f)(P_{net})$.

Edema—excess fluid outflow into interstitium commonly caused by:

- ↑ capillary pressure (↑ P_c; heart failure)
- ↓ plasma proteins (↓ π_c; nephrotic syndrome, liver failure)
- ↑ capillary permeability (↑ K_f; toxins, infections, burns)
- ↑ interstitial fluid colloid osmotic pressure (↑ π_i; lymphatic blockage)

▸ CARDIOVASCULAR–PATHOLOGY

Congenital heart disease

Right-to-left shunts (early cyanosis)—"blue babies"	Tetralogy of Fallot (most common cause of early cyanosis) Transposition of great vessels Persistent Truncus arteriosus—failure of truncus arteriosus to divide into pulmonary trunk and aorta; most patients have accompanying VSD Tricuspid atresia—characterized by absence of tricuspid valve and hypoplastic RV; requires both ASD and VSD for viability Total anomalous pulmonary venous return (TAPVR)—pulmonary veins drain into right heart circulation (SVC, coronary sinus, etc.); associated with ASD and sometimes PDA to allow for right-to-left shunting to maintain CO	The 5 T's: Tetralogy Transposition Truncus Tricuspid TAPVR
Left-to-right shunts (late cyanosis)—"blue kids"	VSD (most common congenital cardiac anomaly) ASD (loud S1; wide, fixed split S2) PDA (close with indomethacin)	Frequency: VSD > ASD > PDA

Eisenmenger's syndrome

Uncorrected VSD, ASD, or PDA causes compensatory pulmonary vascular hypertrophy, which results in progressive pulmonary hypertension. As pulmonary resistance ↑, the shunt reverses from left-to-right to right-to-left, which causes late cyanosis, clubbing, and polycythemia.

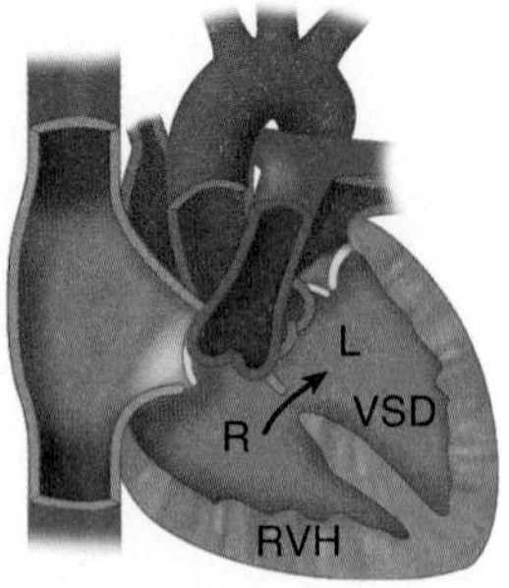

Tetralogy of Fallot

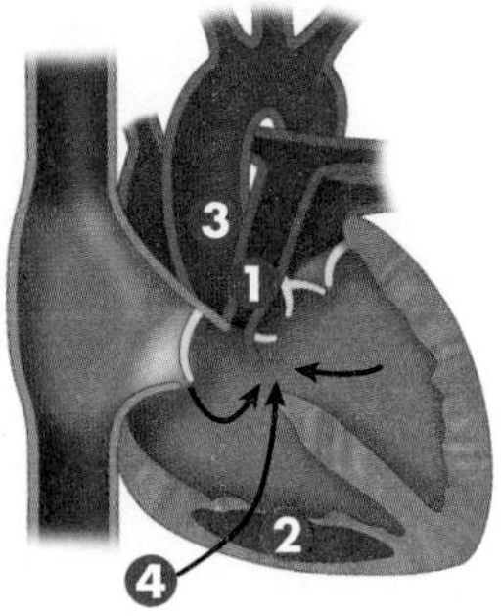

Tetralogy of Fallot is caused by anterosuperior displacement of the infundibular septum.

❶ Pulmonary infundibular stenosis (most important determinant for prognosis)
❷ RVH
❸ Overriding aorta (overrides the VSD)
❹ VSD

Early cyanosis ("tet spells") caused by a right-to-left shunt across the VSD. Isolated VSDs usually flow left to right (acyanotic). In tetralogy, pulmonary stenosis forces right-to-left (cyanotic) flow and causes RVH (on x-ray, boot-shaped heart).

PROVe.

Older patients historically learned to squat to relieve cyanotic symptoms. Squatting reduced blood flow to the legs, ↑ peripheral vascular resistance (PVR), and thus ↓ the cyanotic right-to-left shunt across the VSD.

Preferred treatment is early, primary surgical correction.

D-transposition of great vessels

Aorta leaves RV (anterior) and pulmonary trunk leaves LV (posterior) → separation of systemic and pulmonary circulations. Not compatible with life unless a shunt is present to allow adequate mixing of blood (e.g., VSD, PDA, or patent foramen ovale).

Due to failure of the aorticopulmonary septum to spiral.

Without surgical correction, most infants die within the first few months of life.

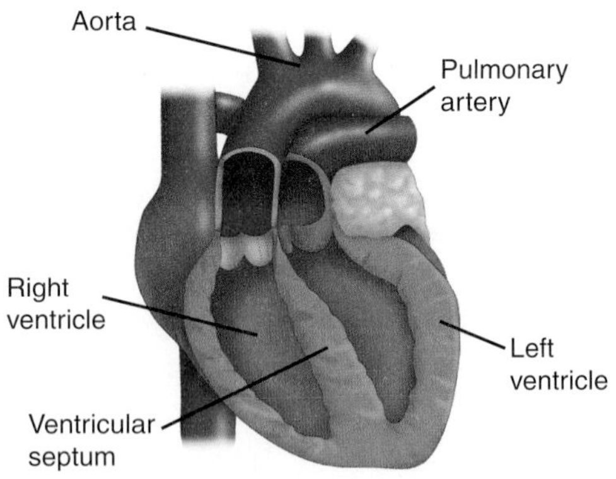

Coarctation of the aorta

Can result in aortic regurgitation.

Infantile type—aortic stenosis proximal to insertion of ductus arteriosus (preductal). Associated with Turner syndrome.

Infantile: **in** close to the heart. Check femoral pulses on physical exam.

Adult type—stenosis is distal to ligamentum arteriosum (postductal). Associated with notching of the ribs (due to collateral circulation), hypertension in upper extremities, weak pulses in lower extremities.

Adult: **d**istal to **d**uctus. Most commonly associated with bicuspid aortic valve.

Patent ductus arteriosus

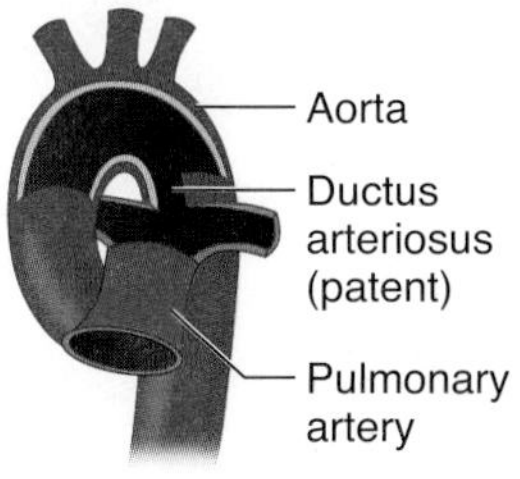
Aorta
Ductus arteriosus (patent)
Pulmonary artery

In fetal period, shunt is right to left (normal). In neonatal period, lung resistance ↓ and shunt becomes left to right with subsequent RVH and/or LVH and failure (abnormal). Associated with a continuous, "machine-like" murmur. Patency is maintained by PGE synthesis and low O_2 tension.

Uncorrected PDA can eventually result in late cyanosis in the lower extremities (differential cyanosis).

Endomethacin (indomethacin) **end**s patency of PDA; PGE k**EE**ps it open (may be necessary to sustain life in conditions such as transposition of the great vessels).

PDA is normal in utero and normally closes only after birth.

Congenital cardiac defect associations

DISORDER	DEFECT
22q11 syndromes	Truncus arteriosus, tetralogy of Fallot
Down syndrome	ASD, VSD, AV septal defect (endocardial cushion defect)
Congenital rubella	Septal defects, PDA, pulmonary artery stenosis
Turner syndrome	Coarctation of aorta (preductal)
Marfan's syndrome	Aortic insufficiency and dissection (late complication)
Infant of diabetic mother	Transposition of great vessels

Hypertension	Defined as BP ≥ 140/90 mmHg.
RISK FACTORS	↑ age, obesity, diabetes, smoking, genetics, black > white > Asian.
FEATURES	90% of hypertension is 1° (essential) and related to ↑ CO or ↑ TPR; remaining 10% mostly 2° to renal disease. Malignant hypertension is severe (> 180/120 mmHg) and rapidly progressing.
PREDISPOSES TO	Atherosclerosis, left ventricular hypertrophy, stroke, CHF, renal failure, retinopathy, and aortic dissection.

Hyperlipidemia signs

Atheromas	Plaques in blood vessel walls.
Xanthomas	Plaques or nodules composed of lipid-laden histiocytes in the skin, especially the eyelids (xanthelasma).
Tendinous xanthoma	Lipid deposit in tendon, especially Achilles.
Corneal arcus	Lipid deposit in cornea, nonspecific (arcus senilis).

Arteriosclerosis

Mönckeberg	Calcification in the media of the arteries, especially radial or ulnar. Usually benign; "pipestem" arteries. Does not obstruct blood flow; intima not involved.
Arteriolosclerosis	Two types: hyaline (thickening of small arteries in essential hypertension or diabetes mellitus) and hyperplastic ("onion skinning" in malignant hypertension).
Atherosclerosis	Fibrous plaques and atheromas form in intima of arteries.

Atherosclerosis

Disease of elastic arteries and large- and medium-sized muscular arteries.

RISK FACTORS	Modifiable: smoking, hypertension, hyperlipidemia, diabetes. Non-modifiable: age, gender (↑ in men and postmenopausal women), and positive family history.
PROGRESSION	Inflammation important in pathogenesis. Endothelial cell dysfunction → macrophage and LDL accumulation → foam cell formation → fatty streaks → smooth muscle cell migration (involves PDGF and FGF), proliferation, and extracellular matrix deposition → fibrous plaque → complex atheromas A.
COMPLICATIONS	Aneurysms, ischemia, infarcts, peripheral vascular disease, thrombus, emboli.
LOCATION	Abdominal aorta > coronary artery > popliteal artery > carotid artery.
SYMPTOMS	Angina, claudication, but can be asymptomatic.

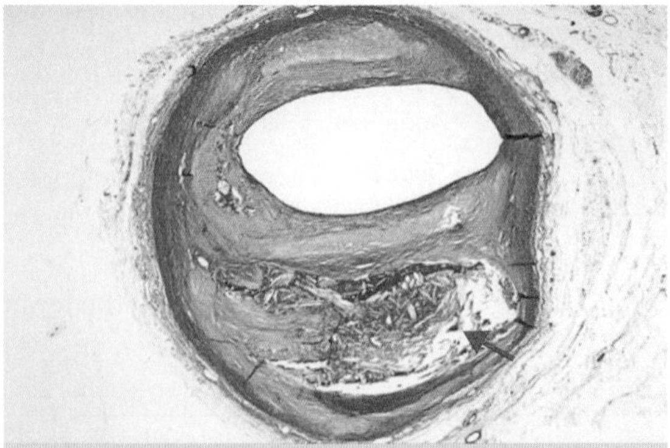

A **Atherosclerosis.** Atherosclerotic plaque in the LAD coronary artery. Note the cholesterol crystals (arrow).

Aortic aneurysms

Localized pathologic dilation of blood vessel.

Abdominal aortic aneurysm	Associated with atherosclerosis. Occurs more frequently in hypertensive male smokers > 50 years of age.
Thoracic aortic aneurysm	Associated with hypertension, cystic medial necrosis (Marfan's syndrome) and historically 3° syphilis.

Aortic dissection

Longitudinal intraluminal tear forming a false lumen A. Associated with hypertension, bicuspid aortic valve, cystic medial necrosis, and inherited connective tissue disorders (e.g., Marfan's syndrome). Presents with tearing chest pain radiating to the back. CXR shows mediastinal widening. The false lumen can be limited to the ascending aorta, propagate from the ascending aorta, or propagate from the descending aorta. Can result in pericardial tamponade, aortic rupture, and death.

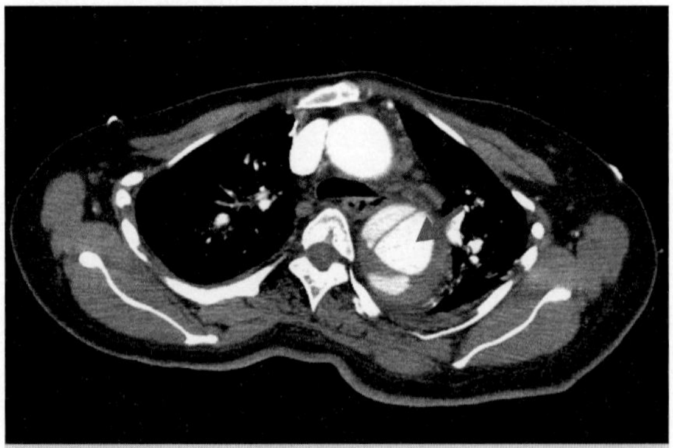

A **Aortic dissection (CT).** Note intraluminal tear forming a "flap" that separates the true and false lumina in the descending aorta (arrow).

Ischemic heart disease manifestations

Angina	CAD narrowing > 75%; no myocyte necrosis: ▪ Stable—mostly 2° to atherosclerosis; ST depression on ECG (retrosternal chest pain with exertion) ▪ Prinzmetal's variant—occurs at rest 2° to coronary artery spasm; ST elevation on ECG ▪ Unstable/crescendo—thrombosis with incomplete coronary artery occlusion; ST depression on ECG (worsening chest pain at rest or with minimal exertion)
Coronary steal syndrome	Vasodilator may aggravate ischemia by shunting blood from area of critical stenosis to an area of higher perfusion.
Myocardial infarction	Most often acute thrombosis due to coronary artery atherosclerosis with complete occlusion of coronary artery and myocyte necrosis; ECG initially shows ST depression progressing to ST elevation with continued ischemia and transmural necrosis.
Sudden cardiac death	Death from cardiac causes within 1 hour of onset of symptoms, most commonly due to a lethal arrhythmia (e.g., ventricular fibrillation). Associated with CAD (up to 70% of cases).
Chronic ischemic heart disease	Progressive onset of CHF over many years due to chronic ischemic myocardial damage.

Evolution of MI

Coronary artery occlusion: LAD > RCA > circumflex.

Symptoms: diaphoresis, nausea, vomiting, severe retrosternal pain, pain in left arm and/or jaw, shortness of breath, fatigue.

TIME	GROSS	LIGHT MICROSCOPE	RISK
0–4 hr	None	None	Arrhythmia, CHF exacerbation, cardiogenic shock
4–12 hr	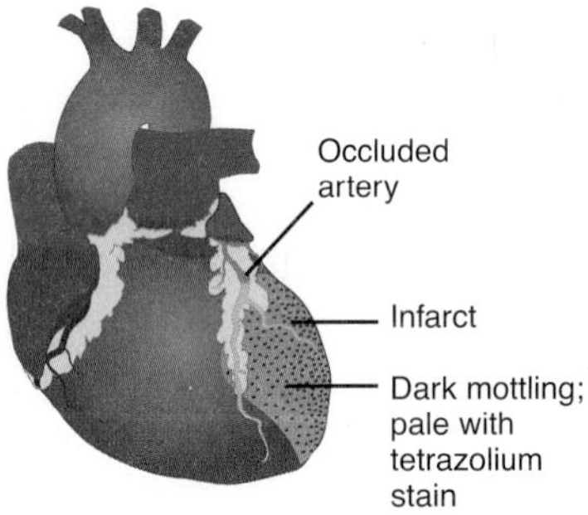Occluded artery Infarct Dark mottling; pale with tetrazolium stain	Early coagulative necrosis, edema, hemorrhage, wavy fibers. 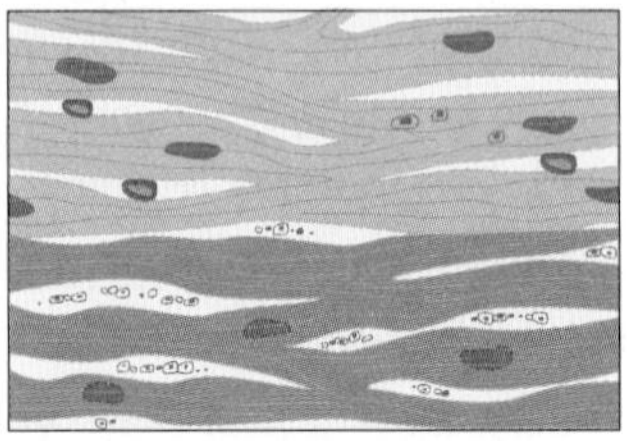	Arrhythmia
12–24 hr		Contraction bands from reperfusion injury. Release of necrotic cell content into blood. Beginning of neutrophil migration.	Arrhythmia
1–3 days	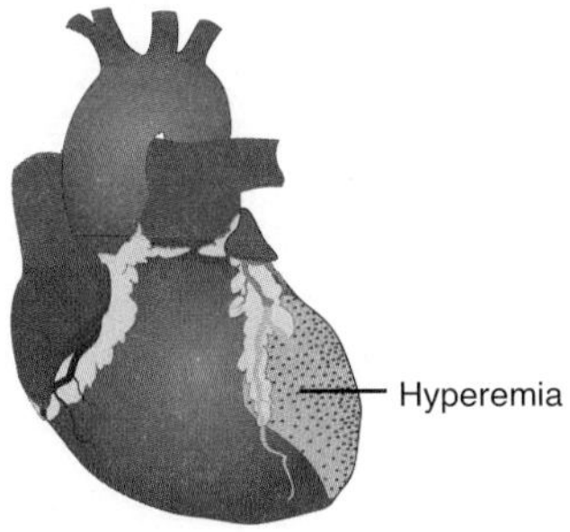Hyperemia	Extensive coagulative necrosis. Tissue surrounding infarct shows acute inflammation. Neutrophil migration. 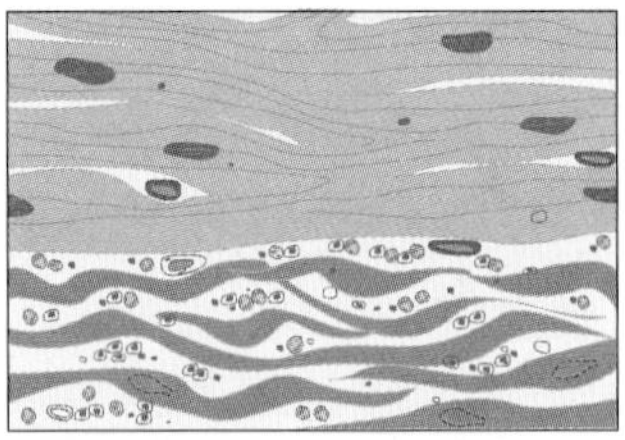	Fibrinous pericarditis
3–14 days	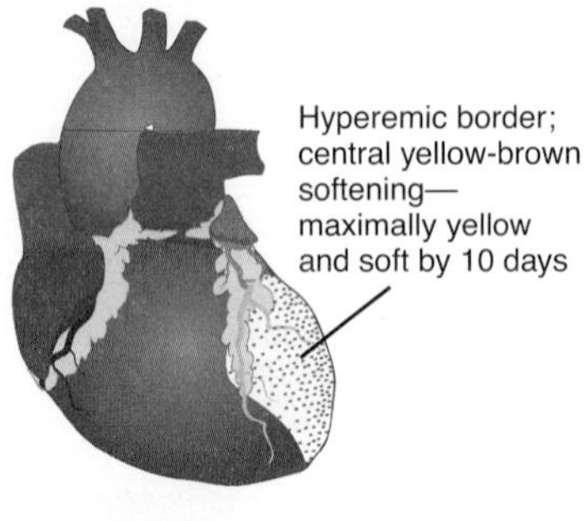Hyperemic border; central yellow-brown softening—maximally yellow and soft by 10 days	Macrophage infiltration followed by granulation tissue at the margins. 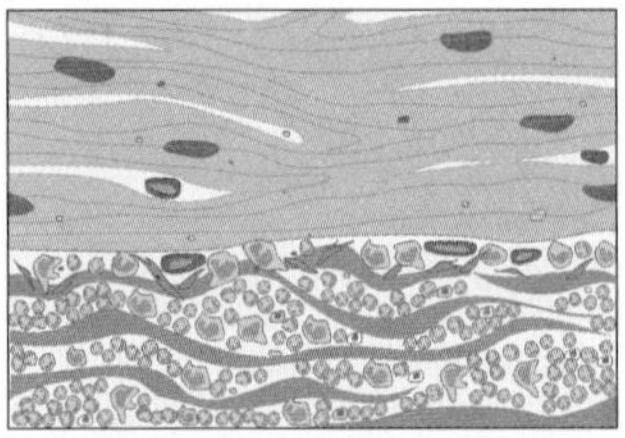	Free wall rupture leading to tamponade, papillary muscle rupture, ventricular aneurysm, interventricular septal rupture due to macrophages that have degraded important structural components
2 weeks to several months	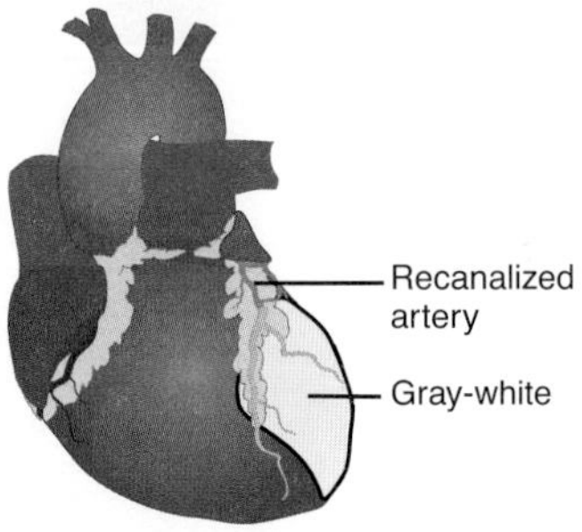Recanalized artery Gray-white	Contracted scar complete. 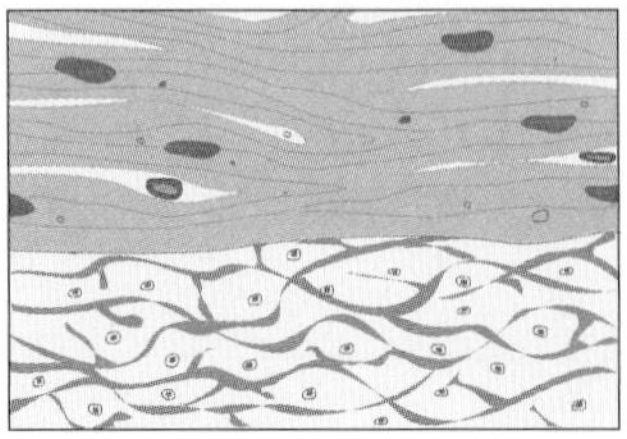	Dressler's syndrome

Diagnosis of MI

In the first 6 hours, ECG is the gold standard.
Cardiac troponin I rises after 4 hours and is elevated for 7–10 days; more specific than other protein markers.
CK-MB is predominantly found in myocardium but can also be released from skeletal muscle. Useful in diagnosing reinfarction following acute MI because levels return to normal after 48 hours.
ECG changes can include ST elevation (transmural infarct), ST depression (subendocardial infarct), and pathologic Q waves (transmural infarct).

Types of infarcts

Transmural infarcts	Subendocardial infarcts
↑ necrosis	Due to ischemic necrosis of < 50% of ventricle wall
Affects entire wall	Subendocardium especially vulnerable to ischemia
ST elevation on ECG, Q waves	ST depression on ECG

ECG diagnosis of MI

INFARCT LOCATION	LEADS WITH Q WAVES
Anterior wall (LAD)	V1–V4
Anteroseptal (LAD)	V1–V2
Anterolateral (LCX)	V4–V6
Lateral wall (LCX)	I, aVL
Inferior wall (RCA)	II, III, aVF

MI complications

Cardiac arrhythmia—important cause of death before reaching hospital; common in first few days
LV failure and pulmonary edema.
Cardiogenic shock (large infarct—high risk of mortality).
Ventricular free wall rupture → cardiac tamponade; papillary muscle rupture → severe mitral regurgitation; and interventricular septum rupture → VSD.
Ventricular aneurysm formation—↓ CO, risk of arrhythmia, embolus from mural thrombus; greatest risk approximately 1 week post-MI.
Postinfarction fibrinous pericarditis—friction rub (1–3 days post-MI).
Dressler's syndrome—autoimmune phenomenon resulting in fibrinous pericarditis (several weeks post-MI).

Cardiomyopathies

Dilated (congestive) cardiomyopathy	Most common cardiomyopathy (90% of cases). Often idiopathic (up to 50% of cases may be familial). Other etiologies include chronic **A**lcohol abuse, wet **B**eriberi, **C**oxsackie B virus myocarditis, chronic **C**ocaine use, **C**hagas' disease, **D**oxorubicin toxicity, hemochromatosis, and peripartum cardiomyopathy. Findings: S3, dilated heart on ultrasound, balloon appearance on chest x-ray. Treatment: Na^+ restriction, ACE inhibitors, diuretics, digoxin, heart transplant.	Systolic dysfunction ensues. Eccentric hypertrophy (sarcomeres added in series). **ABCCCD**.
Hypertrophic cardiomyopathy	Hypertrophied interventricular septum is "too close" to mitral valve leaflet, leading to outflow tract obstruction A. 60–70% of cases are familial, autosomal dominant (commonly a β-myosin heavy chain mutation). Associated with Friedreich's ataxia. Disoriented, tangled, hypertrophied myocardial fibers. Cause of sudden death in young athletes. Findings: normal-sized heart, S4, apical impulses, systolic murmur. Treatment: β-blocker or non-dihydropyridine calcium channel blocker (e.g., verapamil).	Diastolic dysfunction ensues. Asymmetric concentric hypertrophy (sarcomeres added in parallel). Proximity of hypertrophied interventricular septum to mitral leaflet obstructs outflow tract, resulting in systolic murmur and syncopal episodes. 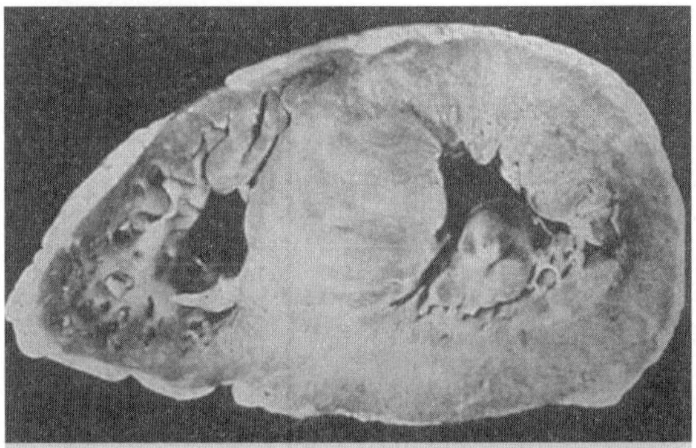 A **Hypertrophic cardiomyopathy.**
Restrictive/ obliterative cardiomyopathy	Major causes include sarcoidosis, amyloidosis, postradiation fibrosis, endocardial fibroelastosis (thick fibroelastic tissue in endocardium of young children), **Löffler's syndrome** (endomyocardial fibrosis with a prominent eosinophilic infiltrate), and hemochromatosis (dilated cardiomyopathy can also occur).	Diastolic dysfunction ensues.

CHF

A clinical syndrome that occurs in patients with an inherited or acquired abnormality of cardiac structure or function, which is characterized by a constellation of clinical symptoms (dyspnea, fatigue) and signs (edema, rales).

Right heart failure most often results from left heart failure. Isolated right heart failure is usually due to cor pulmonale.

ACE inhibitors, β-blockers (except in acute decompensated HF), angiotensin receptor antagonists, and spironolactone reduce mortality. Thiazide or loop diuretics are used mainly for symptomatic relief. Hydralazine with nitrate therapy improves both symptoms and mortality in select patients.

ABNORMALITY	CAUSE
Cardiac dilation	Greater ventricular end-diastolic volume.
Dyspnea on exertion	Failure of cardiac output to ↑ during exercise.
Left heart failure	
Pulmonary edema, paroxysmal nocturnal dyspnea	↑ pulmonary venous pressure → pulmonary venous distention and transudation of fluid. Presence of hemosiderin-laden macrophages ("heart failure" cells) in the lungs.
Orthopnea (shortness of breath when supine)	↑ venous return in supine position exacerbates pulmonary vascular congestion.
Right heart failure	
Hepatomegaly (nutmeg liver)	↑ central venous pressure → ↑ resistance to portal flow. Rarely, leads to "cardiac cirrhosis."
Peripheral edema	↑ venous pressure → fluid transudation.
Jugular venous distention	↑ venous pressure.

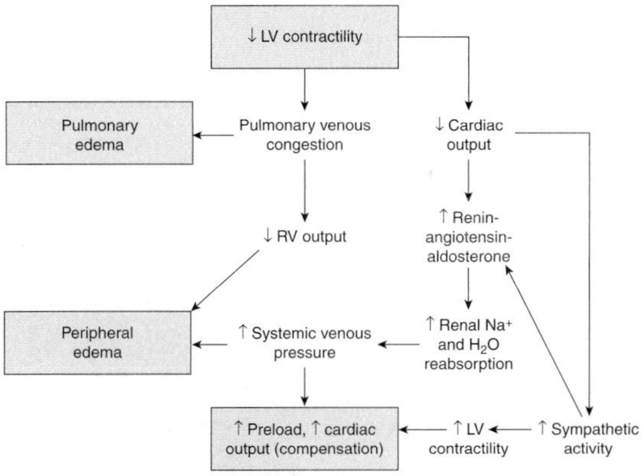

Bacterial endocarditis

Fever (most common symptom), Roth's spots (round white spots on retina surrounded by hemorrhage), Osler's nodes (tender raised lesions on finger or toe pads), new murmur, Janeway lesions (small, painless, erythematous lesions on palm or sole), anemia, splinter hemorrhages A on nail bed. Multiple blood cultures necessary for diagnosis.

- Acute—*S. aureus* (high virulence). Large vegetations on previously normal valves B. Rapid onset.
- Subacute—viridans streptococci (low virulence). Smaller vegetations on congenitally abnormal or diseased valves. Sequela of dental procedures. More insidious onset.

Endocarditis may also be nonbacterial 2° to malignancy, hypercoagulable state, or lupus (marantic/thrombotic endocarditis). *S. bovis* is present in colon cancer, *S. epidermidis* on prosthetic valves.

Mitral valve is most frequently involved.

Tricuspid valve endocarditis is associated with IV **drug** abuse (don't **tri drugs**). Associated with *S. aureus*, *Pseudomonas*, and *Candida*.

Complications: chordae rupture, glomerulonephritis, suppurative pericarditis, emboli.

Bacteria **FROM JANE**:
Fever
Roth's spots
Osler's nodes
Murmur
Janeway lesions
Anemia
Nail-bed hemorrhage
Emboli

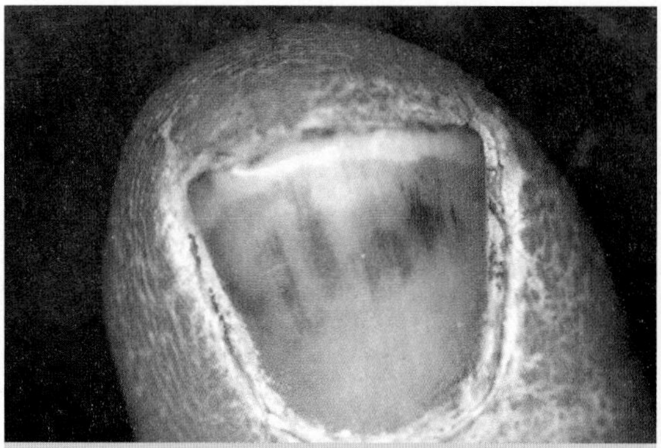

A Splinter hemorrhage.

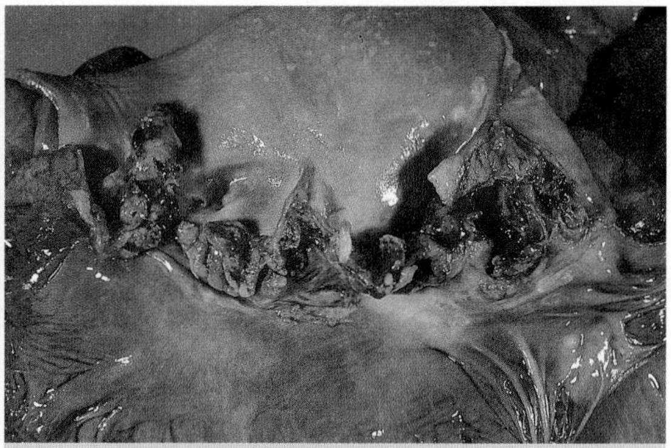

B Acute bacterial endocarditis.

Rheumatic fever

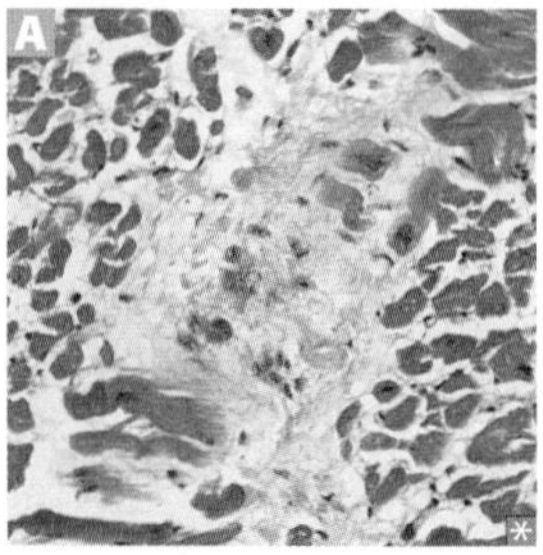

A consequence of pharyngeal infection with group A β-hemolytic streptococci. Early deaths due to myocarditis. Late sequelae include rheumatic heart disease, which affects heart valves—mitral > aortic >> tricuspid (high-pressure valves affected most). Early lesion is mitral valve regurgitation; late lesion is mitral stenosis. Associated with Aschoff bodies (granuloma with giant cells) A, Anitschkow's cells (activated histiocytes), elevated ASO titers.

Immune mediated (type II hypersensitivity); not a direct effect of bacteria. Antibodies to M protein.

FEVERSS:
Fever
Erythema marginatum
Valvular damage (vegetation and fibrosis)
ESR ↑
Red-hot joints (migratory polyarthritis)
Subcutaneous nodules
St. Vitus' dance (Sydenham's chorea)

Acute pericarditis

Commonly presents with sharp pain, aggravated by inspiration, and relieved by sitting up and leaning forward. Presents with friction rub. ECG changes include widespread ST-segment elevation and/or PR depression.

- **Fibrinous**—caused by Dressler's syndrome, uremia, radiation. Presents with loud friction rub.
- **Serous**—viral pericarditis (often resolves spontaneously); noninfectious inflammatory diseases (e.g., rheumatoid arthritis, SLE).
- **Suppurative/purulent**—usually caused by bacterial infections (e.g., *Pneumococcus*, *Streptococcus*). Rare now with antibiotics.

Cardiac tamponade

Compression of heart by fluid (e.g., blood, effusions) in pericardium, leading to ↓ CO. Equilibration of diastolic pressures in all 4 chambers.
Findings: hypotension, ↑ venous pressure (JVD), distant heart sounds, ↑ HR, pulsus paradoxus.

Pulsus paradoxus—↓ in amplitude of systolic blood pressure by ≥ 10 mmHg during inspiration. Seen in severe cardiac tamponade, asthma, obstructive sleep apnea, pericarditis, and croup.

Syphilitic heart disease

3° syphilis disrupts the vasa vasorum of the aorta with consequent atrophy of the vessel wall and dilation of the aorta and valve ring.
May see calcification of the aortic root and ascending aortic arch. Leads to "tree bark" appearance of the aorta.

Can result in aneurysm of the ascending aorta or aortic arch and aortic insufficiency.

Cardiac tumors

Myxomas—most common 1° cardiac tumor in adults A. 90% occur in the atria (mostly left atrium). Myxomas are usually described as a "ball valve" obstruction in the left atrium (associated with multiple syncopal episodes).

Rhabdomyomas—most frequent 1° cardiac tumor in children (associated with tuberous sclerosis).

Most common heart tumor is a metastasis (from melanoma, lymphoma).

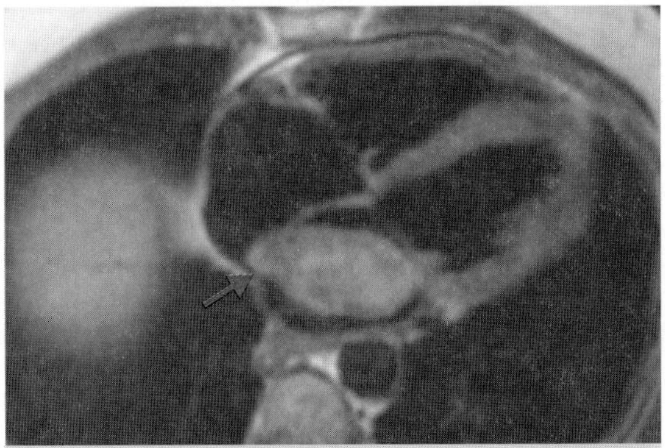

A **Left atrial myxoma (MRI).**

Kussmaul's sign

↑ in JVP on inspiration instead of a normal ↓.
Inspiration → negative intrathoracic pressure not transmitted to heart → impaired filling of right ventricle → blood backs up into venae cavae → JVD. May be seen with constrictive pericarditis, restrictive cardiomyopathies, right atrial or ventricular tumors, or cardiac tamponade.

Raynaud's phenomenon	↓ blood flow to the skin due to arteriolar vasospasm in response to cold temperature or emotional stress. Most often in the fingers and toes A. Called Raynaud's disease when primary (idiopathic), Raynaud's syndrome when secondary to a disease process such as mixed connective tissue disease, SLE, or CREST (limited form of systemic sclerosis) syndrome.	Affects small vessels.

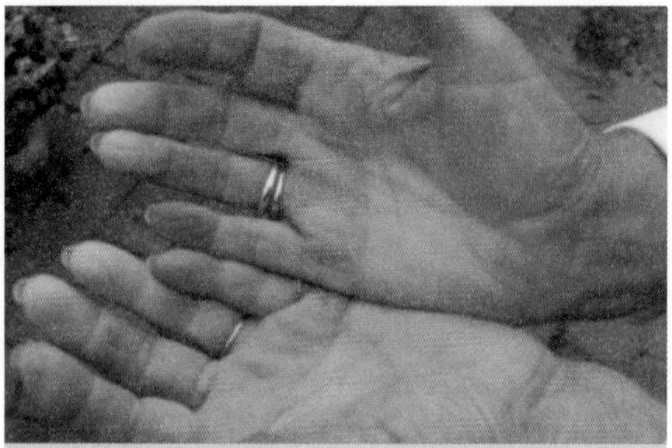

A **Raynaud's phenomenon.** Note the fingertip cyanosis (arrow).

Vasculitis

	EPIDEMIOLOGY/PRESENTATION	PATHOLOGY/LABS
Large-vessel vasculitis		
Temporal (giant cell) arteritis	Generally elderly females. Unilateral headache (temporal artery), jaw claudication. May lead to irreversible blindness due to ophthalmic artery occlusion. Associated with polymyalgia rheumatica.	Most commonly affects branches of carotid artery. Focal granulomatous inflammation. ↑ ESR. Treat with high-dose corticosteroids.
Takayasu's arteritis	Asian females < 40 years of age. "Pulseless disease" (weak upper extremity pulses), fever, night sweats, arthritis, myalgias, skin nodules, ocular disturbances.	Granulomatous thickening of aortic arch, proximal great vessels. ↑ ESR. Treat with corticosteroids.
Medium-vessel vasculitis		
Polyarteritis nodosa	Young adults. Hepatitis B seropositivity in 30% of patients. Fever, weight loss, malaise, headache. GI: abdominal pain, melena. Hypertension, neurologic dysfunction, cutaneous eruptions, renal damage.	Typically involves renal and visceral vessels, not pulmonary arteries. Immune-complex mediated. Transmural inflammation of the arterial wall with fibrinoid necrosis. Lesions are of different ages. Many aneurysms and constrictions on arteriogram. Treat with corticosteroids, cyclophosphamide.
Kawasaki disease	Asian children < 4 years of age. Fever, cervical lymphadenitis, conjunctival injection, changes in lips/oral mucosa ("strawberry tongue"), hand-foot erythema, and desquamating rash.	May develop coronary aneurysms → MI, rupture. Treat with IV immunoglobulin and aspirin.
Buerger's disease (thromboangiitis obliterans)	Heavy smokers, males < 40 years of age. Intermittent claudication may lead to gangrene, autoamputation of digits, superficial nodular phlebitis. Raynaud's phenomenon is often present.	Segmental thrombosing vasculitis. Treat with smoking cessation.

Vasculitis *(continued)*

	EPIDEMIOLOGY/PRESENTATION	PATHOLOGY/LABS
Small-vessel vasculitis		
Microscopic polyangiitis	Necrotizing vasculitis commonly involving lung, kidneys, and skin with pauci-immune glomerulonephritis and palpable purpura.	No granulomas. p-ANCA. Treat with cyclophosphamide and corticosteroids.
Wegener's granulomatosis (granulomatosis with polyangiitis)	Upper respiratory tract: perforation of nasal septum, chronic sinusitis, otitis media, mastoiditis. Lower respiratory tract: hemoptysis, cough, dyspnea. Renal: hematuria, red cell casts.	Triad: ▪ Focal necrotizing vasculitis ▪ Necrotizing granulomas in the lung and upper airway ▪ Necrotizing glomerulonephritis. c-ANCA. Chest x-ray: large nodular densities. Treat with cyclophosphamide, corticosteroids.
Churg-Strauss syndrome	Asthma, sinusitis, palpable purpura, peripheral neuropathy (e.g., wrist/foot drop). Can also involve heart, GI, kidneys (pauci-immune glomerulonephritis).	Granulomatous, necrotizing vasculitis with eosinophilia. p-ANCA, elevated IgE level.
Henoch-Schönlein purpura	Most common childhood systemic vasculitis. Often follows URI. Classic triad: ▪ Skin: palpable purpura on buttocks/legs ▪ Arthralgia ▪ GI: abdominal pain, melena, multiple lesions of same age	Vasculitis secondary to IgA complex deposition. Associated with IgA nephropathy.

Vascular tumors

Strawberry hemangioma	Benign capillary hemangioma of infancy. Appears in first few weeks of life (1/200 births); grows rapidly and regresses spontaneously at 5–8 years of age.
Cherry hemangioma	Benign capillary hemangioma of the elderly. Does not regress. Frequency ↑ with age.
Pyogenic granuloma	Polypoid capillary hemangioma that can ulcerate and bleed. Associated with trauma and pregnancy.
Cystic hygroma	Cavernous lymphangioma of the neck. Associated with Turner syndrome.
Glomus tumor	Benign, painful, red-blue tumor under fingernails. Arises from modified smooth muscle cells of glomus body.
Bacillary angiomatosis	Benign capillary skin papules found in AIDS patients. Caused by *Bartonella henselae* infections. Frequently mistaken for Kaposi's sarcoma.
Angiosarcoma	Rare blood vessel malignancy typically occurring in the head, neck, and breast areas. Associated with patients receiving radiation therapy, especially for breast cancer and Hodgkin's lymphoma. Very aggressive and difficult to resect due to delay in diagnosis.
Lymphangiosarcoma	Lymphatic malignancy associated with persistent lymphedema (e.g., post–radical mastectomy).
Kaposi's sarcoma	Endothelial malignancy most commonly of the skin, but also mouth, GI tract, and respiratory tract. Associated with HHV-8 and HIV. Frequently mistaken for bacillary angiomatosis.

Sturge-Weber disease	Congenital vascular disorder that affects capillary-sized blood vessels. Manifests with port-wine stain (nevus flammeus) on face, ipsilateral leptomeningeal angiomatosis (intracerebral AVM), seizures, and early-onset glaucoma.	Affects small vessels.

▸ CARDIOVASCULAR–PHARMACOLOGY

Antihypertensive therapy

Essential hypertension	Diuretics, ACE inhibitors, angiotensin II receptor blockers (ARBs), calcium channel blockers.	See the Renal chapter for more details about diuretics and ACE inhibitors/ARBs.
CHF	Diuretics, ACE inhibitors/ARBs, β-blockers (compensated CHF), K^+-sparing diuretics.	β-blockers must be used cautiously in decompensated CHF, and are contraindicated in cardiogenic shock.
Diabetes mellitus	ACE inhibitors/ARBs, calcium channel blockers, diuretics, β-blockers, α-blockers.	ACE inhibitors are protective against diabetic nephropathy. See the Pharmacology chapter for more details about α-blockers.

Calcium channel blockers

Nifedipine, verapamil, diltiazem, amlodipine.

MECHANISM	Block voltage-dependent L-type calcium channels of cardiac and smooth muscle and thereby reduce muscle contractility. Vascular smooth muscle—amlodipine = nifedipine > diltiazem > verapamil. Heart—verapamil > diltiazem > amlodipine = nifedipine (verapamil = ventricle).
CLINICAL USE	Hypertension, angina, arrhythmias (not nifedipine), Prinzmetal's angina, Raynaud's.
TOXICITY	Cardiac depression, AV block, peripheral edema, flushing, dizziness, and constipation.

Hydralazine

MECHANISM	↑ cGMP → smooth muscle relaxation. Vasodilates arterioles > veins; afterload reduction.
CLINICAL USE	Severe hypertension, CHF. First-line therapy for hypertension in pregnancy, with methyldopa. Frequently coadministered with a β-blocker to prevent reflex tachycardia.
TOXICITY	Compensatory tachycardia (contraindicated in angina/CAD), fluid retention, nausea, headache, angina. Lupus-like syndrome.

Malignant hypertension treatment

Commonly used drugs include nitroprusside, nicardipine, clevidipine, labetalol, and fenoldopam.

Nitroprusside	Short acting; ↑ cGMP via direct release of NO. Can cause cyanide toxicity (releases cyanide).
Fenoldopam	Dopamine D_1 receptor agonist—coronary, peripheral, renal, and splanchnic vasodilation. ↓ BP and ↑ natriuresis.

Nitroglycerin, isosorbide dinitrate

MECHANISM	Vasodilate by releasing nitric oxide in smooth muscle, causing ↑ in cGMP and smooth muscle relaxation. Dilate veins >> arteries. ↓ preload.
CLINICAL USE	Angina, pulmonary edema.
TOXICITY	Reflex tachycardia, hypotension, flushing, headache, "Monday disease" in industrial exposure: development of tolerance for the vasodilating action during the work week and loss of tolerance over the weekend results in tachycardia, dizziness, and headache upon reexposure.

Antianginal therapy

Goal—reduction of myocardial O_2 consumption (MVO_2) by decreasing 1 or more of the determinants of MVO_2: end-diastolic volume, blood pressure, heart rate, contractility, ejection time.

COMPONENT	NITRATES (AFFECT PRELOAD)	β-BLOCKERS (AFFECT AFTERLOAD)	NITRATES + β-BLOCKERS
End-diastolic volume	↓	↑	No effect or ↓
Blood pressure	↓	↓	↓
Contractility	↑ (reflex response)	↓	Little/no effect
Heart rate	↑ (reflex response)	↓	↓
Ejection time	↓	↑	Little/no effect
MVO_2	↓	↓	↓↓

Calcium channel blockers—**n**ifedipine is similar to **n**itrates in effect; verapamil is similar to β-blockers in effect.
Pindolol and acebutolol—partial β-agonists contraindicated in angina.

Lipid-lowering agents

DRUG	EFFECT ON LDL "BAD CHOLESTEROL"	EFFECT ON HDL "GOOD CHOLESTEROL"	EFFECT ON TRIGLYCERIDES	MECHANISMS OF ACTION	SIDE EFFECTS/PROBLEMS
HMG-CoA reductase inhibitors (lovastatin, pravastatin, simvastatin, atorvastatin, rosuvastatin)	↓↓↓	↑	↓	Inhibit conversion of HMG-CoA to mevalonate, a cholesterol precursor	Hepatotoxicity (↑ LFTs), rhabdomyolysis
Niacin (vitamin B_3)	↓↓	↑↑	↓	Inhibits lipolysis in adipose tissue; reduces hepatic VLDL secretion into circulation	Red, flushed face, which is ↓ by aspirin or long-term use Hyperglycemia (acanthosis nigricans) Hyperuricemia (exacerbates gout)
Bile acid resins (cholestyramine, colestipol, colesevelam)	↓↓	Slightly ↑	Slightly ↑	Prevent intestinal reabsorption of bile acids; liver must use cholesterol to make more	Patients hate it—tastes bad and causes GI discomfort, ↓ absorption of fat-soluble vitamins Cholesterol gallstones
Cholesterol absorption blockers (ezetimibe)	↓↓	—	—	Prevent cholesterol reabsorption at small intestine brush border	Rare ↑ LFTs, diarrhea
Fibrates (gemfibrozil, clofibrate, bezafibrate, fenofibrate)	↓	↑	↓↓↓	Upregulate LPL → ↑ TG clearance	Myositis, hepatotoxicity (↑ LFTs), cholesterol gallstones

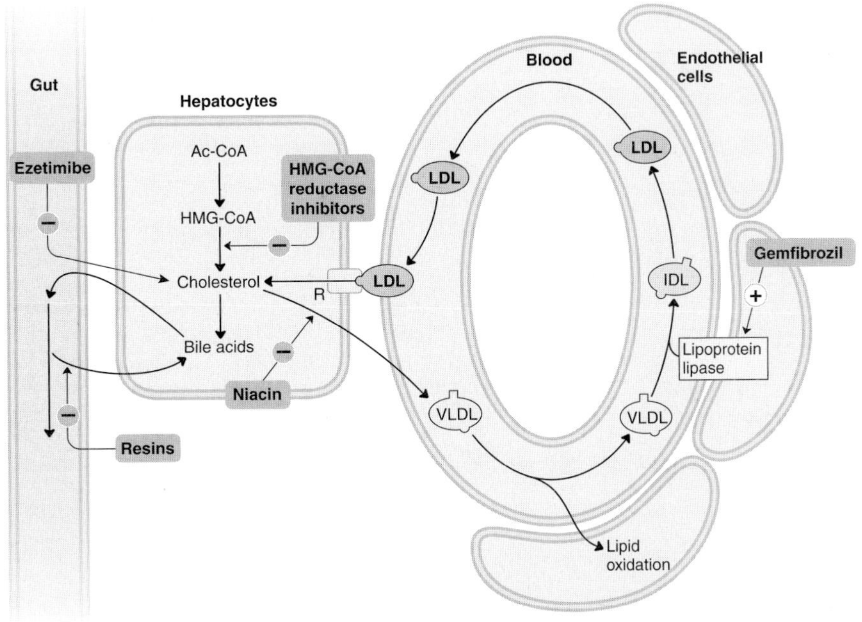

(Adapted, with permission, from Katzung BG, Trevor AJ. *USMLE Road Map: Pharmacology,* 1st ed. New York: McGraw-Hill, 2003: 56.)

Cardiac glycosides	Digoxin—75% bioavailability, 20–40% protein bound, $t_{1/2}$ = 40 hours, urinary excretion.
MECHANISM	Direct inhibition of Na^+/K^+ ATPase leads to indirect inhibition of Na^+/Ca^{2+} exchanger/antiport. ↑ $[Ca^{2+}]_i$ → positive inotropy. Stimulates vagus nerve → ↓ HR.
CLINICAL USE	CHF (↑ contractility); atrial fibrillation (↓ conduction at AV node and depression of SA node).
TOXICITY	Cholinergic—nausea, vomiting, diarrhea, blurry yellow vision (think Van Gogh). ECG—↑ PR, ↓ QT, ST scooping, T-wave inversion, arrhythmia, AV block. Can lead to hyperkalemia, a poor prognostic indicator. Factors predisposing to toxicity—renal failure (↓ excretion), hypokalemia (permissive for digoxin binding at K^+-binding site on Na^+/K^+ ATPase), quinidine (↓ digoxin clearance; displaces digoxin from tissue-binding sites).
ANTIDOTE	Slowly normalize K^+, lidocaine, cardiac pacer, anti-digoxin Fab fragments, Mg^{2+}.

Antiarrhythmics—Na⁺ channel blockers (class I)	Local anesthetics. Slow or block (↓) conduction (especially in depolarized cells). ↓ slope of phase 0 depolarization and ↑ threshold for firing in abnormal pacemaker cells. Are state dependent (selectively depress tissue that is frequently depolarized [e.g., tachycardia]). Hyperkalemia causes ↑ toxicity for all class I drugs.	
Class IA	**Q**uinidine, **P**rocainamide, **Disopyramide**. ↑ AP duration, ↑ effective refractory period (ERP), ↑ QT interval. Affect both atrial and ventricular arrhythmias, especially reentrant and ectopic supraventricular and ventricular tachycardia. Toxicity: quinidine (cinchonism—headache, tinnitus); procainamide (reversible SLE-like syndrome); disopyramide (heart failure); thrombocytopenia; torsades de pointes due to ↑ QT interval.	"The **Q**ueen **P**roclaims **Diso**'s **pyramid**."
Class IB	**Lid**ocaine, **Mex**iletine, Tocainide. ↓ AP duration. Preferentially affect ischemic or depolarized Purkinje and ventricular tissue. Useful in acute ventricular arrhythmias (especially post-MI) and in digitalis-induced arrhythmias. Toxicity: local anesthetic. CNS stimulation/depression, cardiovascular depression.	"I'd **B**uy **Lid**y's **Mex**ican Tacos." Phenytoin can also fall into the IB category. **IB** is **B**est post-MI.
Class IC	Flecainide, propafenone. No effect on AP duration. Useful in ventricular tachycardias that progress to VF and in intractable SVT. Usually used only as last resort in refractory tachyarrhythmias. For patients without structural abnormalities. Toxicity: proarrhythmic, especially post-MI (contraindicated). Significantly prolongs refractory period in AV node.	**IC** is **C**ontraindicated in structural heart disease and post-MI.

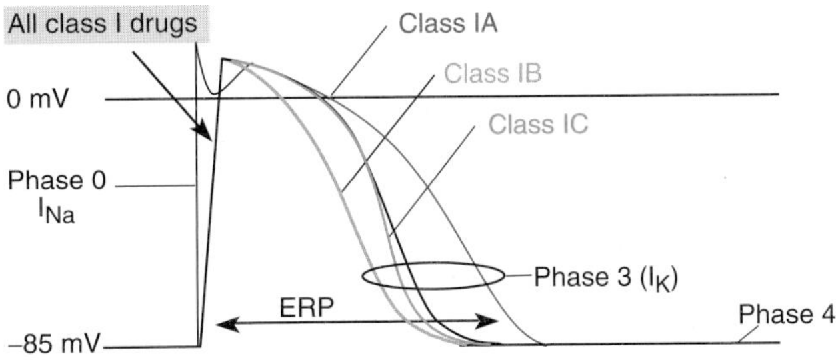

(Adapted, with permission, from Katzung BG, Trevor AJ. *Pharmacology: Examination & Board Review,* 5th ed. Stamford, CT: Appleton & Lange, 1998: 118.)

Antiarrhythmics—β-blockers (class II)	Metoprolol, propranolol, esmolol, atenolol, timolol.
MECHANISM	Decreases SA and AV nodal activity by ↓ cAMP, ↓ Ca^{2+} currents. Suppress abnormal pacemakers by ↓ slope of phase 4. AV node particularly sensitive—↑ PR interval. Esmolol very short acting.
CLINICAL USE	Ventricular tachycardia, SVT, slowing ventricular rate during atrial fibrillation and atrial flutter.
TOXICITY	Impotence, exacerbation of asthma, cardiovascular effects (bradycardia, AV block, CHF), CNS effects (sedation, sleep alterations). May mask the signs of hypoglycemia. Metoprolol can cause dyslipidemia. Treat overdose with glucagon. Propranolol can exacerbate vasospasm in Prinzmetal's angina.

Antiarrhythmics—K^+ channel blockers (class III)	Amiodarone, Ibutilide, Dofetilide, Sotalol.	"AIDS."
MECHANISM	↑ AP duration, ↑ ERP. Used when other antiarrhythmics fail. ↑ QT interval.	
TOXICITY	Sotalol—torsades de pointes, excessive β block; ibutilide—torsades; amiodarone—pulmonary fibrosis, hepatotoxicity, hypothyroidism/hyperthyroidism (amiodarone is 40% iodine by weight), corneal deposits, skin deposits (blue/gray) resulting in photodermatitis, neurologic effects, constipation, cardiovascular effects (bradycardia, heart block, CHF). Amiodarone has class I, II, III, and IV effects because it alters the lipid membrane.	Remember to check PFTs, LFTs, and TFTs when using amiodarone.

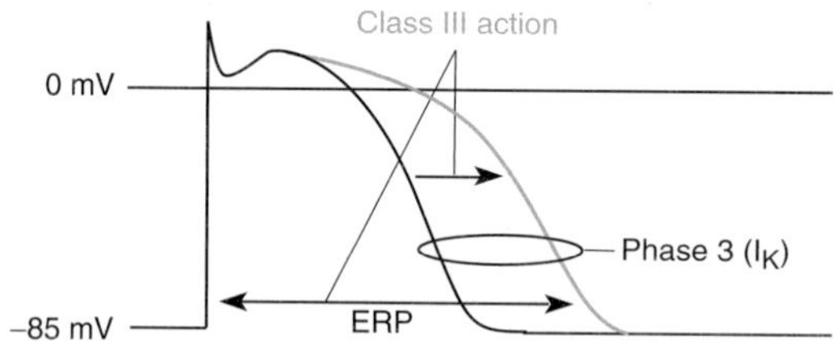

(Adapted, with permission, from Katzung BG, Trevor AJ. *Pharmacology: Examination & Board Review,* 5th ed. Stamford, CT: Appleton & Lange, 1998: 120.)

Antiarrhythmics—Ca^{2+} channel blockers (class IV)	Verapamil, diltiazem.
MECHANISM	↓ conduction velocity, ↑ ERP, ↑ PR interval. Used in prevention of nodal arrhythmias (e.g., SVT).
TOXICITY	Constipation, flushing, edema, CV effects (CHF, AV block, sinus node depression).

Other antiarrhythmics	
Adenosine	↑ K^+ out of cells → hyperpolarizing the cell + ↓ I_{Ca}. Drug of choice in diagnosing/abolishing supraventricular tachycardia. Very short acting (~ 15 sec). Toxicity includes flushing, hypotension, chest pain. Effects blocked by theophylline and caffeine.
Mg^{2+}	Effective in torsades de pointes and digoxin toxicity.

HIGH-YIELD SYSTEMS

Endocrine

"We have learned that there is an endocrinology of elation and despair, a chemistry of mystical insight, and, in relation to the autonomic nervous system, a meteorology and even . . . an astro-physics of changing moods."

—Aldous (Leonard) Huxley

"Chocolate causes certain endocrine glands to secrete hormones that affect your feelings and behavior by making you happy."

—Elaine Sherman, *Book of Divine Indulgences*

▶ ENDOCRINE–EMBRYOLOGY

Thyroid development

Thyroid diverticulum arises from floor of primitive pharynx, descends into neck. Connected to tongue by thyroglossal duct, which normally disappears but may persist as pyramidal lobe of thyroid. Foramen cecum is normal remnant of thyroglossal duct. Most common ectopic thyroid tissue site is the tongue.

Thyroglossal duct cyst presents as an anterior midline neck mass that moves with swallowing (vs. persistent cervical sinus leading to branchial cleft cyst in lateral neck).

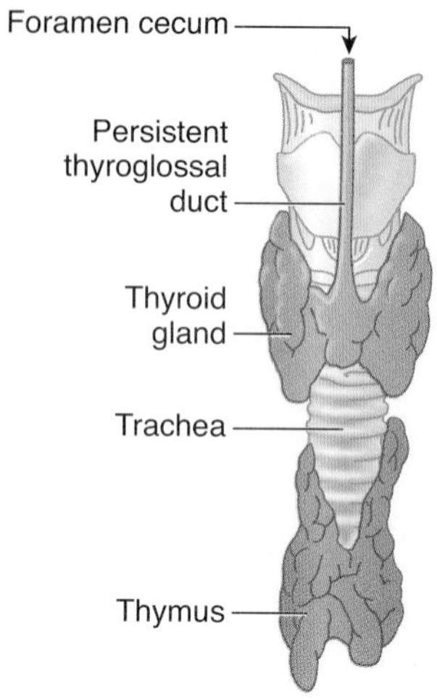
Foramen cecum
Persistent thyroglossal duct
Thyroid gland
Trachea
Thymus

Fetal adrenal gland

Consists of an outer adult zone and inner active fetal zone. Adult zone is dormant during early fetal life but begins to secrete cortisol late in gestation. Cortisol secretion is controlled by ACTH and CRH from fetal pituitary and placenta. Cortisol is responsible for fetal lung maturation and surfactant production.

▶ ENDOCRINE–ANATOMY

Adrenal cortex and medulla

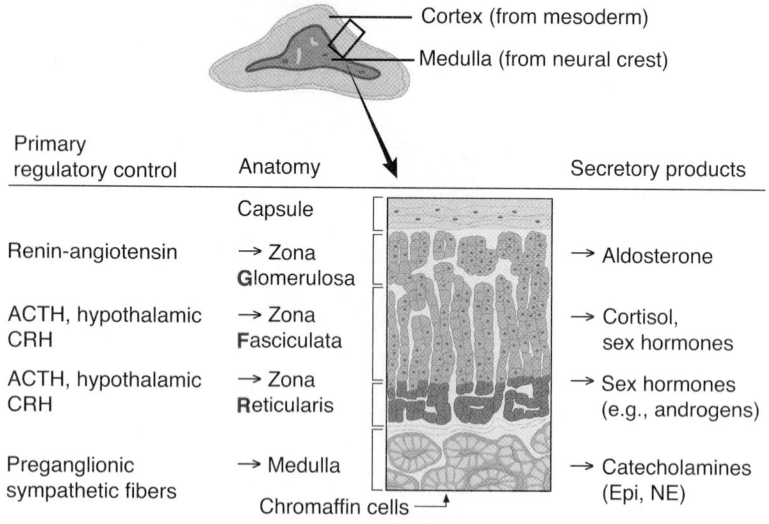
Cortex (from mesoderm)
Medulla (from neural crest)
Primary regulatory control
Anatomy
Secretory products
Capsule
Renin-angiotensin
→ Zona Glomerulosa
→ Aldosterone
ACTH, hypothalamic CRH
→ Zona Fasciculata
→ Cortisol, sex hormones
ACTH, hypothalamic CRH
→ Zona Reticularis
→ Sex hormones (e.g., androgens)
Preganglionic sympathetic fibers
→ Medulla
→ Catecholamines (Epi, NE)
Chromaffin cells

GFR corresponds with **S**alt (Na^+), **S**ugar (glucocorticoids), and **S**ex (androgens). "The deeper you go, the sweeter it gets."

Pheochromocytoma—most common tumor of the adrenal medulla in adults.
Neuroblastoma—most common tumor of the adrenal medulla in children.

Pheochromocytoma causes episodic hypertension; neuroblastoma does not.

Adrenal gland drainage

Left adrenal → left adrenal vein → left renal vein → IVC.
Right adrenal → right adrenal vein → IVC.

Same as left and right gonadal vein.

Pituitary gland

Posterior pituitary (neurohypophysis)	Secretes vasopressin (ADH) and oxytocin, made in the hypothalamus and shipped to posterior pituitary via neurophysins (carrier proteins). Derived from neuroectoderm.	
Anterior pituitary (adenohypophysis)	Secretes FSH, LH, ACTH, TSH, prolactin, GH, melanotropin (MSH). Derived from oral ectoderm (Rathke's pouch). ▪ α subunit—hormone subunit common to TSH, LH, FSH, and hCG. ▪ β subunit—determines hormone specificity.	Acidophils—GH, prolactin. **B-FLAT**: **B**asophils—**F**SH, **L**H, **A**CTH, **T**SH. **FLAT PiG**: **F**SH, **L**H, **A**CTH, **T**SH, **P**rolact**i**n, **G**H.

Endocrine pancreas cell types	Islets of Langerhans are collections of α, β, and δ endocrine cells. Islets arise from pancreatic buds. α = glucagon (peripheral); β = insulin (central); δ = somatostatin (interspersed).	**Ins**ulin (β cells) **ins**ide. 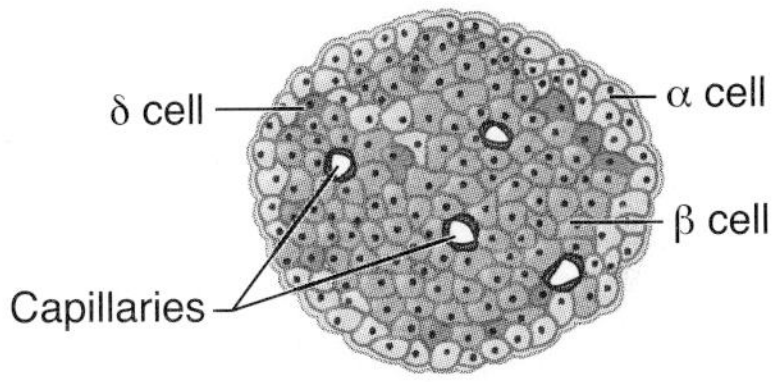

Insulin

SOURCE

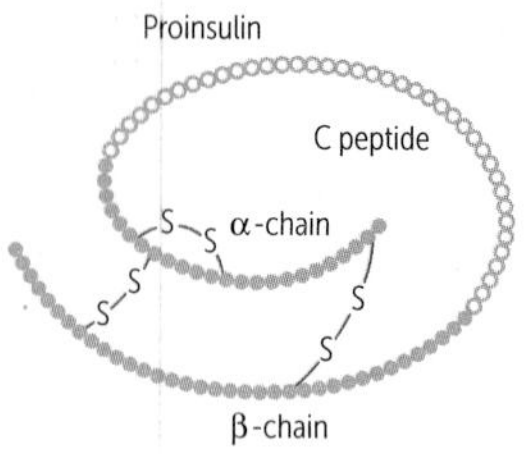

Released from cells of pancreas.

Glucose is major regulator of insulin release.

ATP generated by glucose metabolism closes K^+ channels and depolarizes β cell membrane → opens voltage-gated Ca^{2+} channels. Ca^{2+} influx stimulates insulin secretion.

Insulin moves glucose **In**to cells.

Insulin does not cross the placenta.

BRICK L (insulin-independent glucose uptake): **B**rain, **R**BCs, **I**ntestine, **C**ornea, **K**idney, **L**iver

GLUT-1 (insulin independent): RBCs, brain.

GLUT-2 (bidirectional): β islet cells, liver, kidney, small intestine.

GLUT-4 (insulin dependent): adipose tissue, skeletal muscle.

FUNCTION

Anabolic effects of insulin:

- ↑ glucose transport in skeletal muscle and adipose
- ↑ glycogen synthesis and storage
- ↑ triglyceride synthesis and storage
- ↑ Na^+ retention (kidneys)
- ↑ protein synthesis (muscles)
- ↑ cellular uptake of K^+ and amino acids
- ↓ glucagon release

REGULATION

Hyperglycemia, GH, and β_2-antagonists → ↑ insulin.

Hypoglycemia, somatostatin, and α_2-agonists → ↓ insulin.

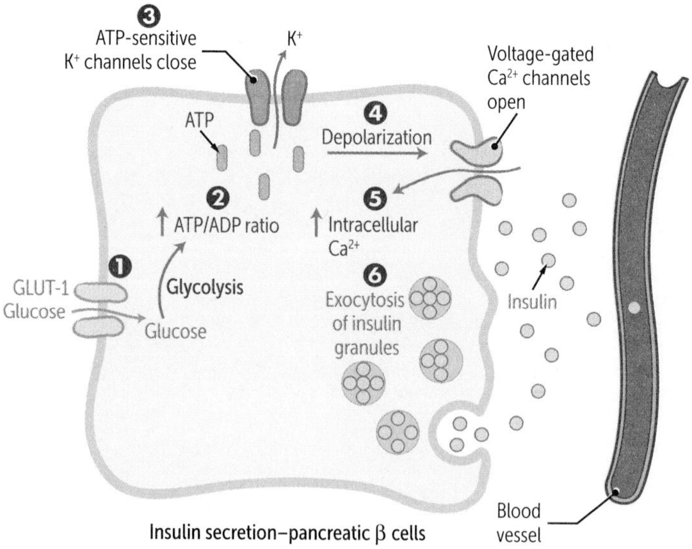

Insulin secretion—pancreatic β cells

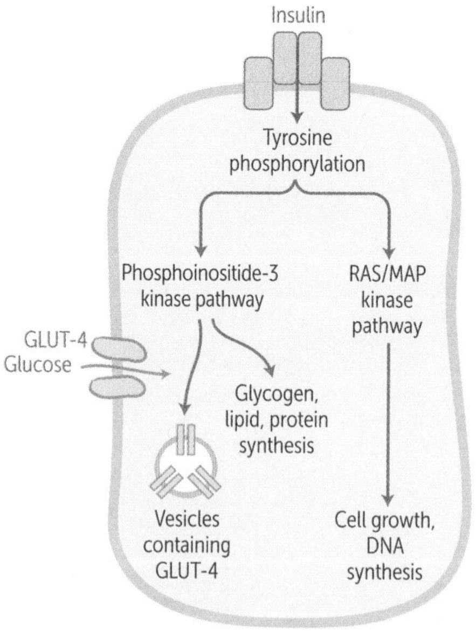

Glucose uptake

Insulin-dependent organs

Resting skeletal muscle and adipose tissue depend on insulin for ↑ glucose uptake (GLUT-4).

Brain and RBCs take up glucose independent of insulin levels (GLUT-1). Brain depends on glucose for metabolism under normal circumstances and uses ketone bodies in starvation. RBCs always depend on glucose because they have no mitochondria for aerobic metabolism.

Glucagon

SOURCE	Made by α cells of pancreas.
FUNCTION	Catabolic effects of glucagon: ▪ Glycogenolysis, gluconeogenesis ▪ Lipolysis and ketone production
REGULATION	Secreted in response to hypoglycemia. Inhibited by insulin, hyperglycemia, and somatostatin.

▸ ENDOCRINE—PHYSIOLOGY

Hypothalamic-pituitary hormone regulation

TRH —⊕→ TSH, prolactin.

Dopamine —⊖→ prolactin.

CRH —⊕→ ACTH, melanocyte-stimulating hormone, β-endorphin.

GHRH —⊕→ GH.

Somatostatin —⊖→ GH, TSH.

GnRH —⊕→ FSH, LH.

Prolactin —⊖→ GnRH.

Prolactin

SOURCE	Secreted mainly by anterior pituitary.	
FUNCTION	Stimulates milk production in breast; inhibits ovulation in females and spermatogenesis in males by inhibiting GnRH synthesis and release.	
REGULATION	Prolactin secretion from anterior pituitary is tonically inhibited by dopamine from hypothalamus. Prolactin in turn inhibits its own secretion by increasing dopamine synthesis and secretion from hypothalamus. TRH ↑ prolactin secretion.	Dopamine agonists (bromocriptine) inhibit prolactin secretion and can be used in treatment of prolactinoma. Dopamine antagonists (most antipsychotics) and estrogens (OCPs, pregnancy) stimulate prolactin secretion.

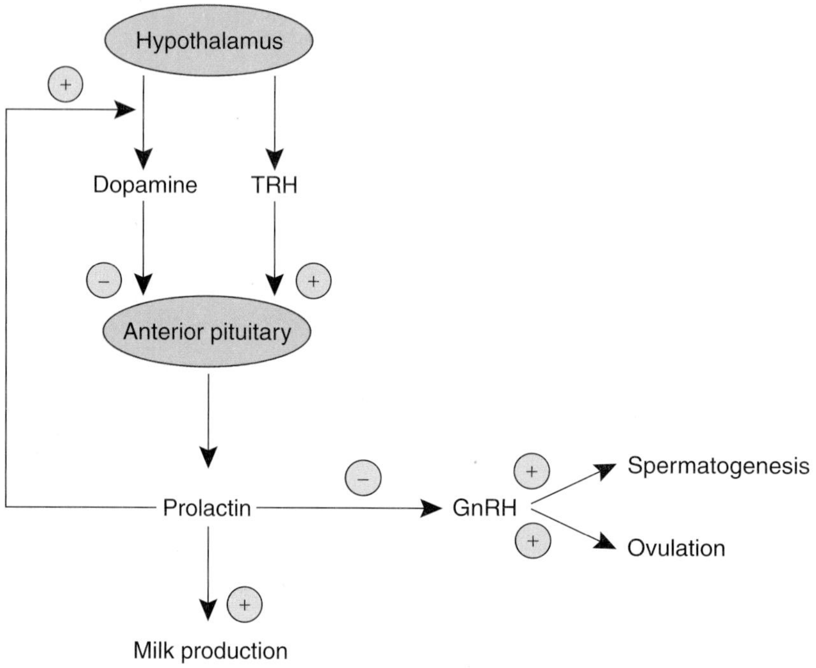

Growth hormone (somatotropin)

SOURCE	Secreted mainly by anterior pituitary.	
FUNCTION	Stimulates linear growth and muscle mass through IGF-1/somatomedin secretion. ↑ insulin resistance (diabetogenic).	
REGULATION	Released in pulses in response to GHRH. Secretion ↑ during exercise and sleep. Secretion inhibited by glucose and somatostatin.	Excess secretion of GH (e.g., pituitary adenoma) may cause acromegaly (adults) or gigantism (children).

Adrenal steroids

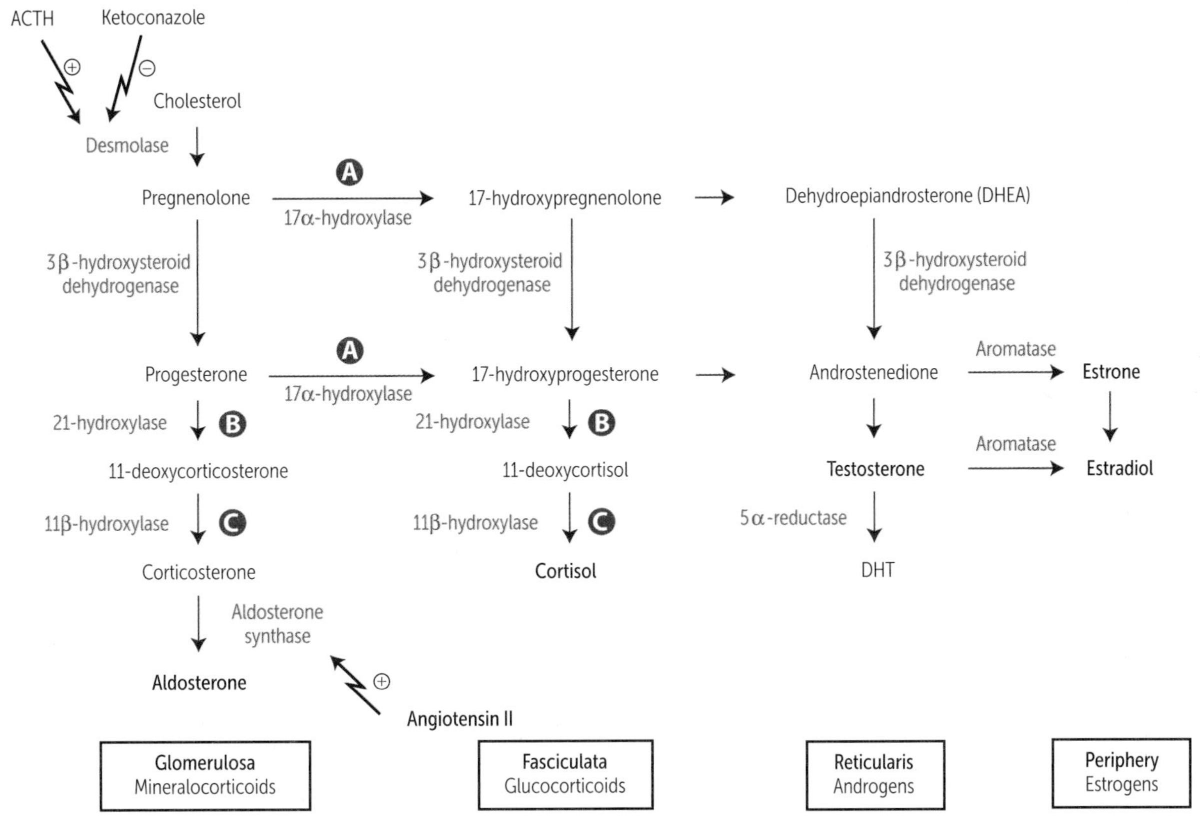

Congenital bilateral adrenal hyperplasias[a]

DEFICIENCY	MINERALOCORTICOIDS	CORTISOL	SEX HORMONES	PRESENTATION
A 17α-hydroxylase deficiency	↑	↓	↓	**Hyper**tension, hypokalemia. XY: ↓ DHT → pseudohermaphroditism (variable, ambiguous genitalia; undescended testes). XX: externally phenotypic female with normal internal sex organs, lacks 2° sex characteristics.
B 21-hydroxylase deficiency	↓	↓	↑	Most common form. **Hypo**tension, hyperkalemia, ↑ renin activity, volume depletion. Masculinization, leading to pseudohermaphroditism in females.
C 11β-hydroxylase deficiency	↓ aldosterone ↑ 11-deoxycorticosterone	↓	↑	**Hyper**tension (11-deoxycorticosterone is a mineralocorticoid and secreted in excess). Masculinization.

[a]All congenital adrenal enzyme deficiencies are characterized by an enlargement of both adrenal glands due to ↑ ACTH stimulation because of ↓ cortisol.

Cortisol

SOURCE	Adrenal zona fasciculata.	Bound to corticosteroid-binding globulin (CBG).
FUNCTION	Maintains **B**lood pressure (upregulates α_1-receptors on arterioles → ↑ sensitivity to NE and epinephrine) ↓ **B**one formation Anti-**I**nflammatory/**I**mmunosuppressive: ▪ Inhibits production of leukotrienes and prostaglandins ▪ Inhibits leukocyte adhesion → neutrophilia ▪ Blocks histamine release from mast cells ▪ Reduces eosinophils ▪ Blocks IL-2 production ↑ **I**nsulin resistance (diabetogenic) ↑ **G**luconeogenesis, lipolysis, proteolysis Inhibits fibroblasts (causes striae)	Cortisol is **BBIIG**
REGULATION	CRH (hypothalamus) stimulates ACTH release (pituitary), causing cortisol production in adrenal zona fasciculata. Excess cortisol ↓ CRH, ACTH, and cortisol secretion.	Chronic stress induces prolonged secretion.

PTH

SOURCE	Chief cells of parathyroid.	
FUNCTION	↑ bone resorption of calcium and phosphate ↑ kidney reabsorption of calcium in distal convoluted tubule ↓ reabsorption of phosphate in proximal convoluted tubule ↑ 1,25-$(OH)_2$ D_3 (calcitriol) production by stimulating kidney 1α-hydroxylase	PTH ↑ serum Ca^{2+}, ↓ serum (PO_4^{3-}), ↑ urine (PO_4^{3-}). ↑ production of M-CSF and RANK-L in osteo**blasts**, stimulating osteo**clasts**. **PTH** = **P**hosphate **T**rashing **H**ormone.
REGULATION	↓ serum Ca^{2+} → ↑ PTH secretion. ↓ serum Mg^{2+} → ↑ PTH secretion. ↓↓ serum Mg^{2+} → ↓ PTH secretion. Common causes of ↓ Mg^{2+} include diarrhea, aminoglycosides, diuretics, and alcohol abuse.	

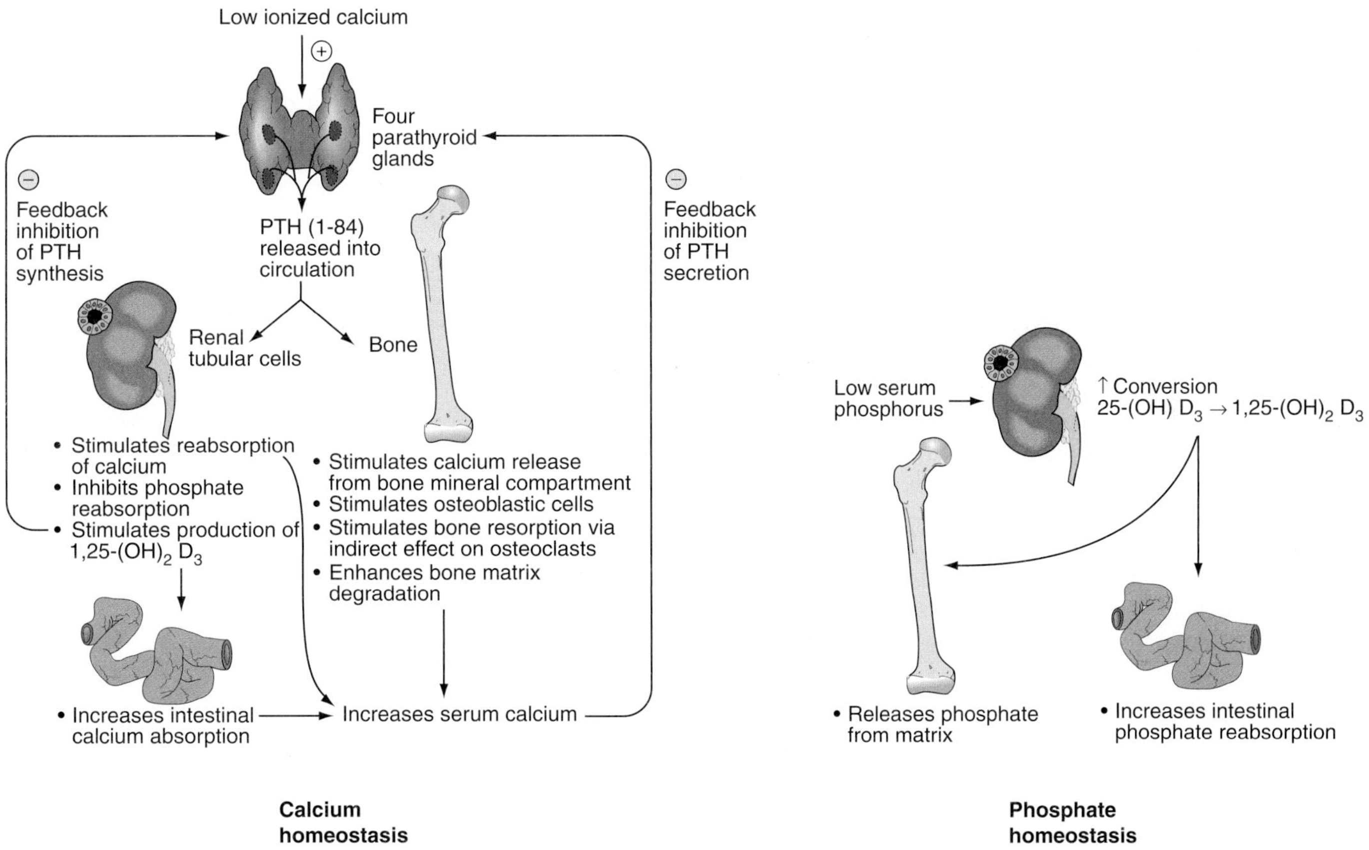

Low ionized calcium
Four parathyroid glands
Feedback inhibition of PTH synthesis
Feedback inhibition of PTH secretion
PTH (1-84) released into circulation
Renal tubular cells
Bone
• Stimulates reabsorption of calcium
• Inhibits phosphate reabsorption
• Stimulates production of 1,25-(OH)2 D3
• Stimulates calcium release from bone mineral compartment
• Stimulates osteoblastic cells
• Stimulates bone resorption via indirect effect on osteoclasts
• Enhances bone matrix degradation
• Increases intestinal calcium absorption
Increases serum calcium
Low serum phosphorus
↑ Conversion 25-(OH) D3 → 1,25-(OH)2 D3
• Releases phosphate from matrix
• Increases intestinal phosphate reabsorption
Calcium homeostasis
Phosphate homeostasis

(Adapted, with permission, from Chandrasoma P et al. *Concise Pathology,* 3rd ed. Stamford, CT: Appleton & Lange, 1998.)

Vitamin D (cholecalciferol)

SOURCE	D_3 from sun exposure in skin. D_2 ingested from plants. Both converted to 25-OH in liver and to 1,25-$(OH)_2$ (active form) in kidney.	Vitamin D deficiency causes rickets in kids and osteomalacia in adults. 24,25-$(OH)_2$ D_3 is an inactive form of vitamin D. PTH leads to ↑ Ca^{2+} reabsorption and ↓ PO_4^{3-} reabsorption in the kidney, whereas 1,25-$(OH)_2$ leads to ↑ absorption of both Ca^{2+} and PO_4^{3-} in the gut.
FUNCTION	↑ absorption of dietary Ca^{2+} and PO_4^{3-} ↑ bone resorption of Ca^{2+} and PO_4^{3-}	
REGULATION	↑ PTH, ↓ $[Ca^{2+}]$, ↓ PO_4^{3-} cause ↑ 1,25-$(OH)_2$ production. 1,25-$(OH)_2$ feedback inhibits its own production.	

Calcitonin

SOURCE	Parafollicular cells (C cells) of thyroid.	Calcitonin opposes actions of PTH. Not important in normal calcium homeostasis. Calci**ton**in **tone**s down calcium levels.
FUNCTION	↓ bone resorption of calcium.	
REGULATION	↑ serum Ca^{2+} causes calcitonin secretion.	

Signaling pathways of endocrine hormones

cAMP	**F**SH, **L**H, **A**CTH, **T**SH, **C**RH, **h**CG, **A**DH (V_2 receptor), **M**SH, **P**TH, calcitonin, GHRH, glucagon	**FLAT ChAMP**
cGMP	ANP, NO (EDRF)	Think vasodilators
IP_3	**G**nRH, **G**HRH, **O**xytocin, **A**DH (V_1 receptor), **T**RH, histamine (H_1), angiotensin II, gastrin	**GGOAT**
Steroid receptor	**V**itamin D, **E**strogen, **T**estosterone, T_3/T_4 **C**ortisol, **A**ldosterone, **P**rogesterone	**VETTT CAP**
Intrinsic tyrosine kinase	Insulin, IGF-1, FGF, PDGF, EGF	MAP kinase pathway Think growth factors
Receptor-associated tyrosine kinase	**P**rolactin, **I**mmunomodulators (e.g., cytokines IL-2, IL-6, IL-8, IFN), **G**H	JAK/STAT pathway Think acidophiles and cytokines **PIG**

Signaling pathway of steroid hormones

Steroid hormones are lipophilic and therefore must circulate bound to specific binding globulins, which ↑ their solubility.
In men, ↑ sex hormone–binding globulin (SHBG) lowers free testosterone → gynecomastia.
In women, ↓ SHBG raises free testosterone → hirsutism; SHBG levels ↑ during pregnancy.

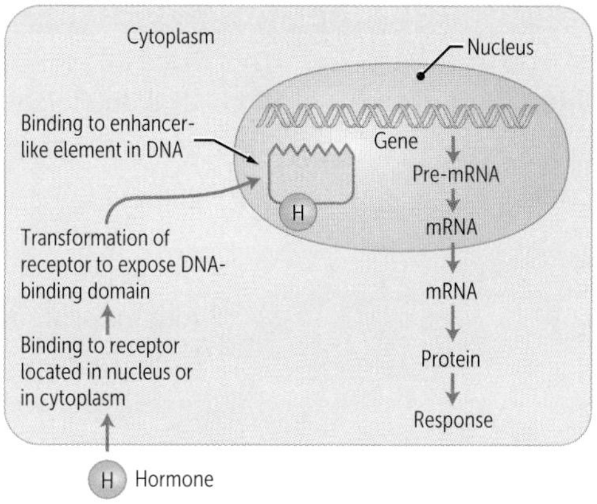

Signaling mechanism

Thyroid hormones (T_3/T_4)

Iodine-containing hormones that control the body's metabolic rate.

SOURCE	Follicles of thyroid. Most T_3 formed in target tissues.	T_3 functions—**4 B's**: **B**rain maturation **B**one growth **B**eta-adrenergic effects **B**asal metabolic rate ↑ Thyroxine-binding globulin (TBG) binds most T_3/T_4 in blood; only free hormone is active. ↓ TBG in hepatic failure; ↑ TBG in pregnancy or OCP use (estrogen ↑ TBG). T_4 is major thyroid product; converted to T_3 in peripheral tissue by 5'-deiodinase. T_3 binds receptors with greater affinity than T_4. Peroxidase is enzyme responsible for oxidation and organification of iodide as well as coupling of MIT and DIT. Propylthiouracil inhibits both peroxidase and 5'-deiodinase. Methimazole inhibits peroxidase only.
FUNCTION	Bone growth (synergism with GH) CNS maturation ↑ β_1 receptors in heart = ↑ CO, HR, SV, contractility ↑ basal metabolic rate via ↑ Na^+/K^+-ATPase activity = ↑ O_2 consumption, RR, body temperature ↑ glycogenolysis, gluconeogenesis, lipolysis	
REGULATION	TRH (hypothalamus) stimulates TSH (pituitary), which stimulates follicular cells. Negative feedback by free T_3 to anterior pituitary ↓ sensitivity to TRH. Thyroid-stimulating immunoglobulins (TSIs), like TSH, stimulates follicular cells (Graves' disease). Wolff-Chaikoff effect—excess iodine temporarily inhibits thyroid peroxidase → ↓ iodine organification → ↓ T_3/T_4 production.	

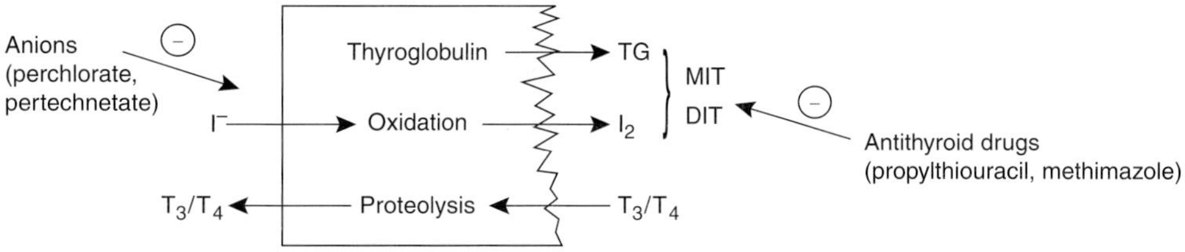

▸ ENDOCRINE–PATHOLOGY

Cushing's syndrome

↑ cortisol due to a variety of causes.
Exogenous (iatrogenic) steroids—#1 cause; ↓ ACTH.
Endogenous causes:

- Cushing's disease (70%)—due to ACTH secretion from pituitary adenoma; ↑ ACTH
- Ectopic ACTH (15%)—from nonpituitary tissue making ACTH (e.g., small cell lung cancer, bronchial carcinoids); ↑ ACTH
- Adrenal (15%)—adenoma A, carcinoma, nodular adrenal hyperplasia; ↓ ACTH

Findings: hypertension, weight gain, moon facies, truncal obesity, buffalo hump, hyperglycemia (insulin resistance), skin changes (thinning, striae), osteoporosis, amenorrhea, and immune suppression B.

Effect of dexamethasone suppression test on cortisol

	CORTISOL LEVEL WITH LOW-DOSE "DEX"	CORTISOL LEVEL WITH HIGH-DOSE "DEX"
Normal	Suppressed	Suppressed
ACTH-pituitary tumor	Remains elevated	Suppressed
Ectopic ACTH-producing tumor	Remains elevated	Remains elevated
Cortisol-producing tumor	Remains elevated	Remains elevated

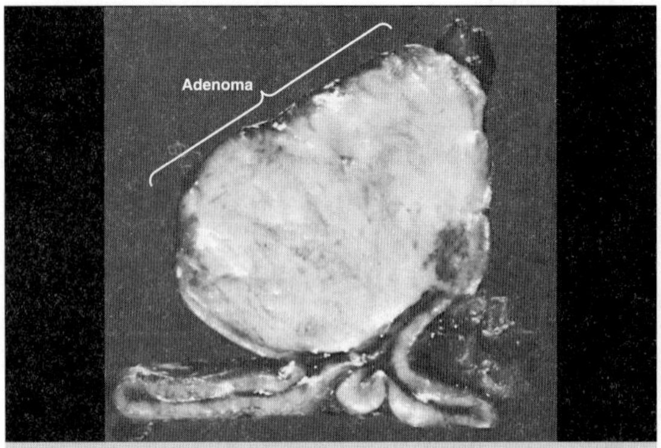

A **Adrenocortical adenoma.** This can also present as primary aldosteronism (Conn's syndrome).

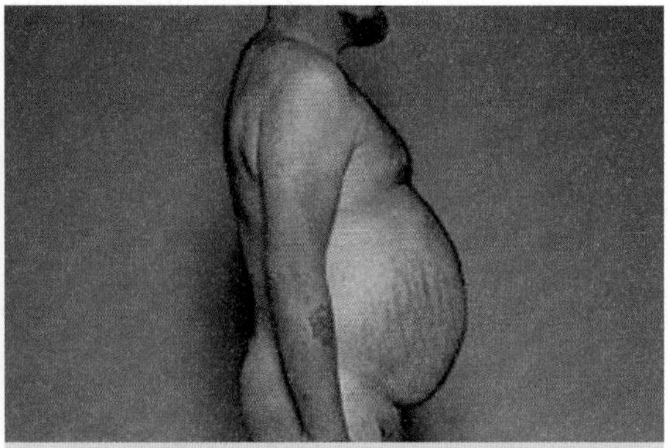

B **Cushing's disease.** Note the truncal obesity and abdominal striae.

Hyperaldosteronism

Primary	Caused by adrenal hyperplasia or an aldosterone-secreting adrenal adenoma (Conn's syndrome), resulting in hypertension, hypokalemia, metabolic alkalosis, and **low** plasma renin. May be bilateral or unilateral.	Treatment: surgery to remove the tumor and/or spironolactone, a K^+-sparing diuretic that works by acting as an aldosterone antagonist.
Secondary	Renal perception of low intravascular volume results in an overactive renin-angiotensin system. Due to renal artery stenosis, chronic renal failure, CHF, cirrhosis, or nephrotic syndrome. Associated with **high** plasma renin.	Treatment: spironolactone.

Addison's disease

Chronic 1° adrenal insufficiency due to adrenal atrophy or destruction by disease (e.g., autoimmune, TB, metastasis). Deficiency of aldosterone and cortisol, causing hypotension (hyponatremic volume contraction), hyperkalemia, acidosis, and skin hyperpigmentation (due to MSH, a by-product of ↑ ACTH production from POMC). Characterized by **A**drenal **A**trophy and **A**bsence of hormone production; involves **A**ll **3** cortical divisions (spares medulla). Distinguish from 2° adrenal insufficiency (↓ pituitary ACTH production), which has no skin hyperpigmentation and no hyperkalemia.

Waterhouse-Friderichsen syndrome

Acute 1° adrenal insufficiency due to adrenal hemorrhage associated with *Neisseria meningitidis* septicemia, DIC, and endotoxic shock.

Pheochromocytoma

Most common tumor of the adrenal medulla in **adults**. Derived from chromaffin cells (arise from neural crest) A.

Most tumors secrete epinephrine, NE, and dopamine, which can cause episodic hypertension. Urinary VMA (a breakdown product of norepinephrine and epinephrine) and plasma catecholamines are elevated.

Associated with neurofibromatosis type 1, MEN types 2A and 2B.

Treatment: tumor surgically removed only after effective α- and β-blockade is achieved. Irreversible α-antagonists (phenoxybenzamine) must be given first to avoid a hypertensive crisis. β-blockers are then given to slow the heart rate.

Episodic hyperadrenergic symptoms (**5 P's**):
- Pressure (elevated blood pressure)
- Pain (headache)
- Perspiration
- Palpitations (tachycardia)
- Pallor

Rule of 10's:
- 10% malignant
- 10% bilateral
- 10% extra-adrenal
- 10% calcify
- 10% kids

Symptoms occur in "spells"—relapse and remit.

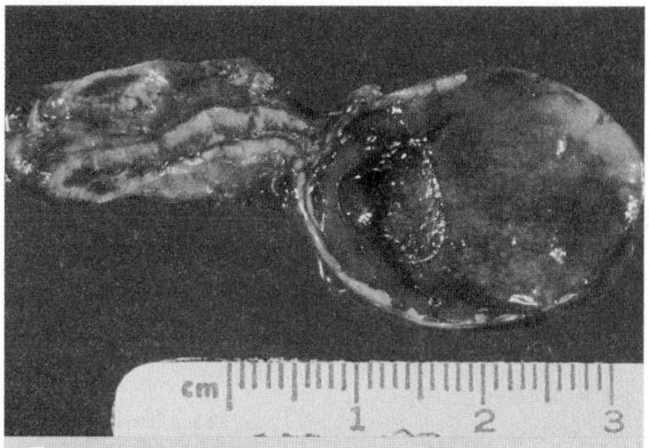
A Pheochromocytoma (in adrenal gland).

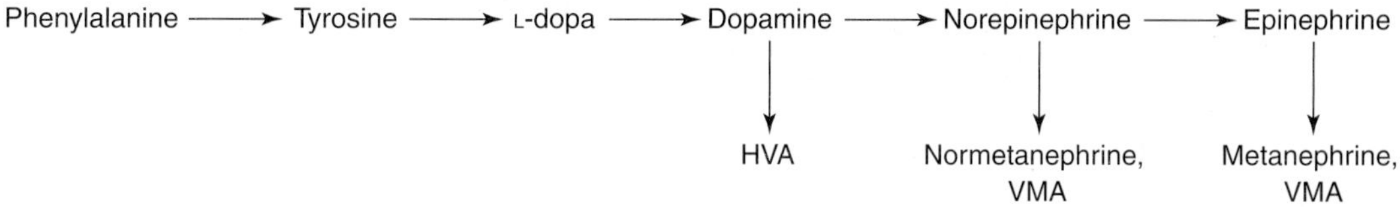
Phenylalanine
Tyrosine
L-dopa
Dopamine
Norepinephrine
Epinephrine
HVA
Normetanephrine, VMA
Metanephrine, VMA

Neuroblastoma

The most common tumor of the adrenal medulla in **children**. Can occur anywhere along the sympathetic chain. Homovanillic acid (HVA), a breakdown product of dopamine, elevated in urine. Less likely to develop hypertension. Overexpression of N-*myc* oncogene associated with rapid tumor progression.

Hypothyroidism vs. hyperthyroidism

	Hypothyroidism	Hyperthyroidism
SIGNS/SYMPTOMS	Cold intolerance (↓ heat production)	Heat intolerance (↑ heat production)
	Weight gain, ↓ appetite	Weight loss, ↑ appetite
	Hypoactivity, lethargy, fatigue, weakness	Hyperactivity
	Constipation	Diarrhea
	↓ reflexes	↑ reflexes
	Myxedema (facial/periorbital)	Pretibial myxedema (Graves' disease)
	Dry, cool skin; coarse, brittle hair	Warm, moist skin; fine hair
	Bradycardia, dyspnea on exertion	Chest pain, palpitations, arrhythmias, ↑ β-adrenergic receptors
LAB FINDINGS	↑ TSH (sensitive test for 1° hypothyroidism)	↓ TSH (if 1°)
	↓ free T_4	↑ free or total T_4
		↑ free or total T_3

Hypothyroidism

Hashimoto's thyroiditis	Most common cause of hypothyroidism; an autoimmune disorder (thyroid peroxidase, antithyroglobulin antibodies). Associated with HLA-DR5. ↑ risk of non-Hodgkin's lymphoma. Histology: Hürthle cells, lymphocytic infiltrate with germinal centers. Findings: moderately enlarged, **nontender** thyroid.	May be hyperthyroid early in course (thyrotoxicosis during follicular rupture).
Cretinism	Due to severe fetal hypothyroidism. Endemic cretinism occurs wherever endemic goiter is prevalent (lack of dietary iodine); sporadic cretinism is caused by defect in T_4 formation or developmental failure in thyroid formation. Findings: **P**ot-bellied, **P**ale, **P**uffy-faced child with **P**rotruding umbilicus and **P**rotuberant tongue.	**5 P's**
Subacute thyroiditis (de Quervain's)	Self-limited hypothyroidism often following a flu-like illness. Histology: granulomatous inflammation. Findings: ↑ ESR, jaw pain, early inflammation, very **tender** thyroid.	May be hyperthyroid early in course.
Riedel's thyroiditis	Thyroid replaced by fibrous tissue (hypothyroid). Findings: fixed, hard (rock-like), and **painless** goiter.	Considered a manifestation of IgG_4-related systemic disease.
Other causes	Congenital hypothyroidism, iodine deficiency, goitrogens, Wolff-Chaikoff effect, painless thyroiditis.	

Hyperthyroidism

Toxic multinodular goiter	Focal patches of hyperfunctioning follicular cells working independently of TSH due to mutation in TSH receptor A. ↑ release of T_3 and T_4. Hot nodules are rarely malignant. Jod-Basedow phenomenon—thyrotoxicosis if a patient with iodine deficiency goiter is made iodine replete.
Graves' disease	An autoimmune hyperthyroidism with thyroid-stimulating immunoglobulins. Ophthalmopathy (proptosis, EOM swelling) B, pretibial myxedema, ↑ in connective tissue deposition, diffuse goiter. Often presents during stress (e.g., childbirth).
Thyroid storm	Stress-induced catecholamine surge leading to death by arrhythmia. Seen as a serious complication of Graves' and other hyperthyroid disorders. May see ↑ ALP due to ↑ bone turnover.

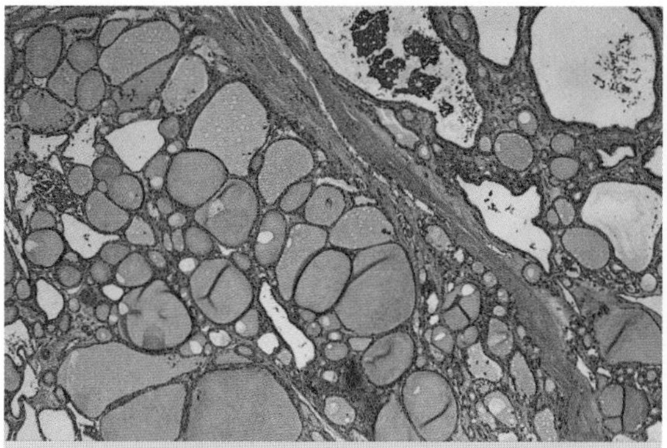

A **Multinodular goiter.** Note follicles distended with colloid and lined by flattened epithelium with areas of fibrosis and hemorrhage.

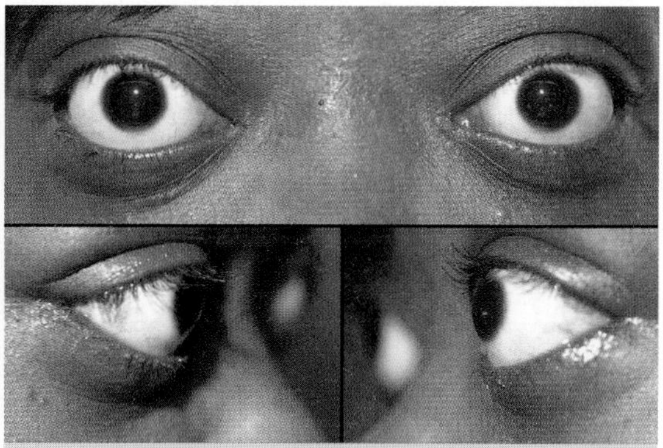

B **Graves' disease (exophthalmos).** Patient with bilateral proptosis and eyelid retraction. Visible sclera causes appearance of a "stare".

Thyroid cancer

Papillary carcinoma—most common, excellent prognosis, empty-appearing nuclei (Orphan Annie's eyes) A, psammoma bodies, nuclear grooves. ↑ risk with childhood irradiation.

Follicular carcinoma—good prognosis, uniform follicles.

Medullary carcinoma—from parafollicular "C cells"; produces calcitonin, sheets of cells in amyloid stroma. Associated with MEN types 2A and 2B.

Undifferentiated/anaplastic—older patients; very poor prognosis.

Lymphoma—associated with Hashimoto's thyroiditis.

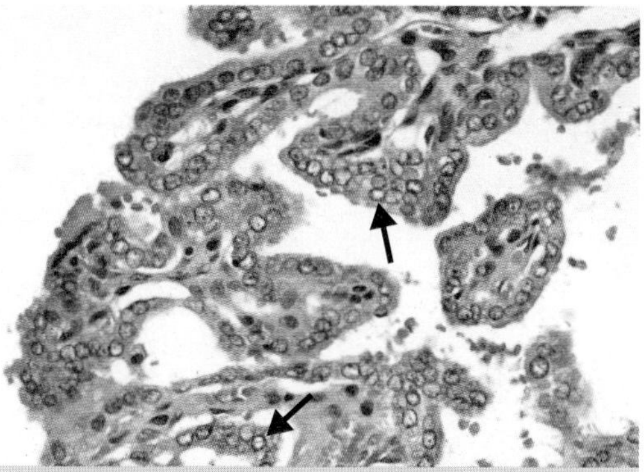

A **Thyroid papillary carcinoma.** Note classic nuclear chromatin clearing ("Orphan Annie's eyes," arrows).

Hyperparathyroidism

Primary	Usually an adenoma. **Hypercalcemia**, hypercalciuria (renal **stones**), hypophosphatemia, ↑ PTH, ↑ alkaline phosphatase, ↑ cAMP in urine. Often asymptomatic, or may present with weakness and constipation ("**groans**").	**Osteitis fibrosa cystica**—cystic **bone** spaces filled with brown fibrous tissue (bone pain). "**Stones, bones, and groans.**"
Secondary	2° hyperplasia due to ↓ gut Ca^{2+} absorption and ↑ phosphate, most often in chronic renal disease (causes hypovitaminosis D → ↓ Ca^{2+} absorption). **Hypocalcemia**, hyperphosphatemia in chronic renal failure (hypophospatemia with most other causes), ↑ alkaline phosphatase, ↑ PTH.	**Renal osteodystrophy**—bone lesions due to 2° or 3° hyperparathyroidism due in turn to renal disease.
Tertiary	Refractory (autonomous) hyperparathyroidism resulting from chronic renal disease. ↑↑ PTH, ↑ Ca^{2+}.	

Hypoparathyroidism

Due to accidental surgical excision (thyroid surgery), autoimmune destruction, or DiGeorge syndrome. Findings: hypocalcemia, tetany.

Chvostek's sign—tapping of facial nerve → contraction of facial muscles.

Trousseau's sign—occlusion of brachial artery with BP cuff → carpal spasm.

Pseudohypoparathyroidism (Albright's hereditary osteodystrophy)—autosomal-dominant kidney unresponsiveness to PTH. Hypocalcemia, shortened 4th/5th digits, short stature.

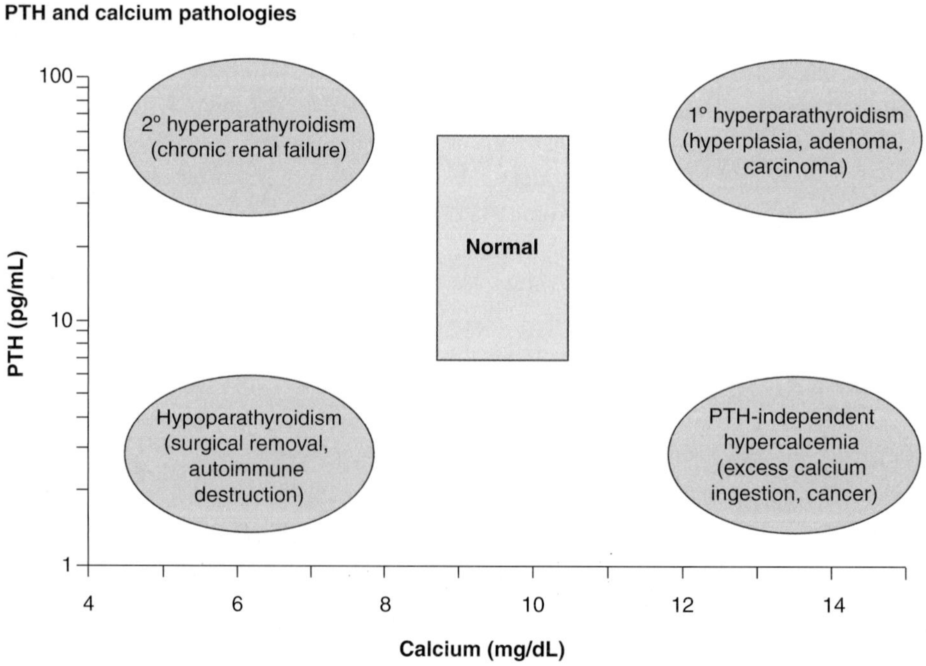

Pituitary adenoma

Most commonly prolactinoma. Findings: amenorrhea, galactorrhea, low libido, infertility (↓ GnRH). Can impinge on optic chiasm → bitemporal hemianopia. Treatment: dopamine agonists (bromocriptine or cabergoline) cause shrinkage of prolactinomas.

Acromegaly

Excess GH in adults. Typically caused by pituitary adenoma.

FINDINGS	Large tongue with deep furrows, deep voice, large hands and feet, coarse facial features, impaired glucose tolerance (insulin resistance).	↑ GH in children → gigantism (↑ linear bone growth).
DIAGNOSIS	↑ serum IGF-1; failure to suppress serum GH following oral glucose tolerance test; pituitary mass seen on brain MRI.	
TREATMENT	Pituitary adenoma resection followed by somatostatin analog if not cured.	

Diabetes insipidus

Characterized by intense thirst and polyuria together with an inability to concentrate urine owing to lack of ADH (central DI—pituitary tumor, trauma, surgery, histiocytosis X) or to a lack of renal response to ADH (nephrogenic DI—hereditary or 2° to hypercalcemia, lithium, demeclocycline [ADH antagonist]).

FINDINGS	Urine specific gravity < 1.006; serum osmolality > 290 mOsm/L.
DIAGNOSIS	Water deprivation test—urine osmolality doesn't ↑. Response to desmopressin distinguishes central DI from nephrogenic DI.
TREATMENT	Adequate fluid intake. For central DI—intranasal desmopressin (ADH analog). For nephrogenic DI—hydrochlorothiazide, indomethacin, or amiloride.

SIADH

Syndrome of inappropriate antidiuretic hormone secretion:
- Excessive water retention
- Hyponatremia with continued urinary Na^+ excretion
- Urine osmolarity > serum osmolarity

Body responds with ↓ aldosterone (hyponatremia) to maintain near-normal volume status. Very low serum sodium levels can lead to seizures (correct slowly).

Causes include:
- Ectopic ADH (small cell lung cancer)
- CNS disorders/head trauma
- Pulmonary disease
- Drugs (e.g., cyclophosphamide)

Treatment: fluid restriction, IV saline, conivaptan, tolvaptan, demeclocycline.

Hypopituitarism

Undersecretion of pituitary hormones due to:
- Nonsecreting pituitary adenoma, craniopharyngioma
- **Sheehan's syndrome** (ischemic infarct of pituitary following postpartum bleeding; usually presents with failure to lactate)
- **Empty sella syndrome** (atrophy or compression of pituitary, often idiopathic, common in obese women)
- Brain injury, hemorrhage
- Radiation

Treatment: substitution therapy (corticosteroids, thyroxine, sex steroids, human growth hormone).

Diabetes mellitus

ACUTE MANIFESTATIONS

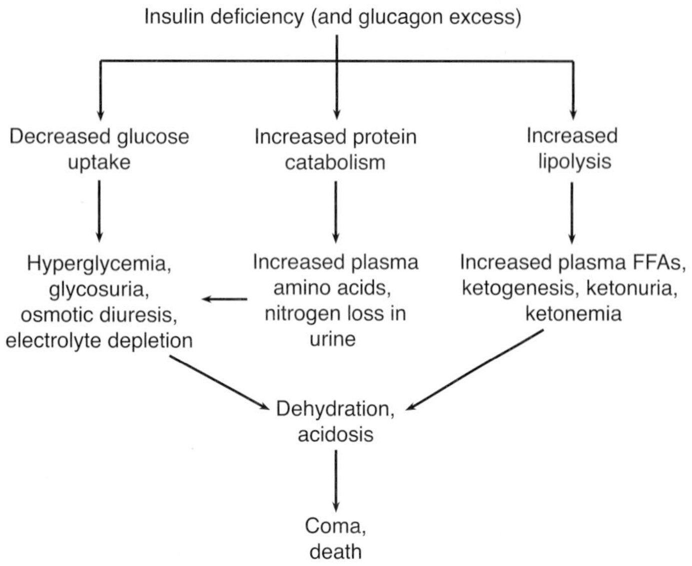
Insulin deficiency (and glucagon excess)
Decreased glucose uptake
Increased protein catabolism
Increased lipolysis
Hyperglycemia, glycosuria, osmotic diuresis, electrolyte depletion
Increased plasma amino acids, nitrogen loss in urine
Increased plasma FFAs, ketogenesis, ketonuria, ketonemia
Dehydration, acidosis
Coma, death

Polydipsia, polyuria, polyphagia, weight loss, DKA (type 1), hyperosmolar coma (type 2), unopposed secretion of GH and epinephrine (exacerbating hyperglycemia).

CHRONIC MANIFESTATIONS

Nonenzymatic glycosylation:
- Small vessel disease (diffuse thickening of basement membrane) → retinopathy (hemorrhage, exudates, microaneurysms, vessel proliferation) A, glaucoma, nephropathy (nodular sclerosis, progressive proteinuria, chronic renal failure, arteriosclerosis leading to hypertension, Kimmelstiel-Wilson nodules)
- Large vessel atherosclerosis, CAD, peripheral vascular occlusive disease, and gangrene → limb loss, cerebrovascular disease

Osmotic damage (sorbitol accumulation in organs with aldose reductase):
- Neuropathy (motor, sensory, and autonomic degeneration)
- Cataracts

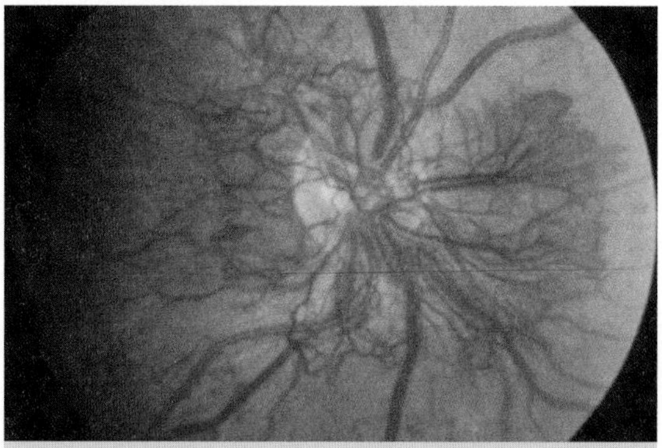

A **Diabetic retinopathy.** Note microhemorrhages and vessel proliferation.

TESTS

Fasting serum glucose, oral glucose tolerance test, HbA_{1c} (reflects average blood glucose over prior 3 months).

Type 1 vs. type 2 diabetes mellitus

Variable	Type 1	Type 2
1° DEFECT	Autoimmune destruction of β cells	↑ resistance to insulin, progressive pancreatic β-cell failure
INSULIN NECESSARY IN TREATMENT	Always	Sometimes
AGE (EXCEPTIONS COMMONLY OCCUR)	< 30	> 40
ASSOCIATION WITH OBESITY	No	Yes
GENETIC PREDISPOSITION	Relatively weak (50% concordance in identical twins), polygenic	Relatively strong (90% concordance in identical twins), polygenic
ASSOCIATION WITH HLA SYSTEM	Yes (HLA-DR3 and 4)	No
GLUCOSE INTOLERANCE	Severe	Mild to moderate
INSULIN SENSITIVITY	High	Low
KETOACIDOSIS	Common	Rare
β-CELL NUMBERS IN THE ISLETS	↓	Variable (with amyloid deposits)
SERUM INSULIN LEVEL	↓	Variable
CLASSIC SYMPTOMS OF POLYURIA, POLYDIPSIA, POLYPHAGIA, WEIGHT LOSS	Common	Sometimes
HISTOLOGY	Islet leukocytic infiltrate	Islet amyloid (AIAPP) deposit

Diabetic ketoacidosis	One of the most important complications of diabetes (usually type 1). Usually due to ↑ insulin requirements from ↑ stress (e.g., infection). Excess fat breakdown and ↑ ketogenesis from ↑ free fatty acids, which are then made into ketone bodies (β-hydroxybutyrate > acetoacetate).
SIGNS/SYMPTOMS	Kussmaul respirations (rapid/deep breathing), nausea/vomiting, abdominal pain, psychosis/delirium, dehydration. Fruity breath odor (due to exhaled acetone).
LABS	Hyperglycemia, ↑ H^+, ↓ HCO_3^- (anion gap metabolic acidosis), ↑ blood ketone levels, leukocytosis. Hyperkalemia, but depleted intracellular K^+ due to transcellular shift from ↓ insulin.
COMPLICATIONS	Life-threatening mucormycosis, *Rhizopus* infection, cerebral edema, cardiac arrhythmias, heart failure.
TREATMENT	IV fluids, IV insulin, and K^+ (to replete intracellular stores); glucose if necessary to prevent hypoglycemia.

Carcinoid syndrome

Rare syndrome caused by carcinoid tumors (neuroendocrine cells), especially metastatic small bowel tumors, which secrete high levels of serotonin (5-HT). Not seen if tumor is limited to GI tract (5-HT undergoes first-pass metabolism in liver). Results in recurrent diarrhea, cutaneous flushing, asthmatic wheezing, and right-sided valvular disease. ↑ 5-HIAA in urine, niacin deficiency.

Treatment: somatostatin analog (e.g., octreotide).

Rule of 1/3s:
- **1/3** metastasize
- **1/3** present with 2nd malignancy
- **1/3** multiple

Most common tumor of appendix.

Zollinger-Ellison syndrome

Gastrin-secreting tumor of pancreas or duodenum. Stomach shows rugal thickening with acid hypersecretion. Causes recurrent ulcers. May be associated with MEN type 1.

Multiple endocrine neoplasias (MEN)

SUBTYPE	CHARACTERISTICS	COMMENTS
MEN 1 (Wermer's syndrome)	Parathyroid tumors Pituitary tumors (prolactin or GH) Pancreatic endocrine tumors—Zollinger-Ellison syndrome, insulinomas, VIPomas, glucagonomas (rare) Commonly presents with kidney stones and stomach ulcers	MEN 1 = **3 P's** (from cephalad to caudad: **P**ituitary, **P**arathyroid, and **P**ancreas; remember by drawing a diamond). MEN 2A = **2 P's** (**P**arathyroids and **P**heochromocytoma; remember by drawing a square). MEN 2B = **1 P** (**P**heochromocytoma; remember by drawing a triangle). All MEN syndromes have autosomal-dominant inheritance. Associated with *ret* gene mutation in MEN types 2A and 2B.
MEN 2A (Sipple's syndrome)	Medullary thyroid carcinoma (secretes calcitonin) Pheochromocytoma Parathyroid tumors	
MEN 2B	Medullary thyroid carcinoma (secretes calcitonin) Pheochromocytoma Oral/intestinal ganglioneuromatosis (associated with marfanoid habitus)	

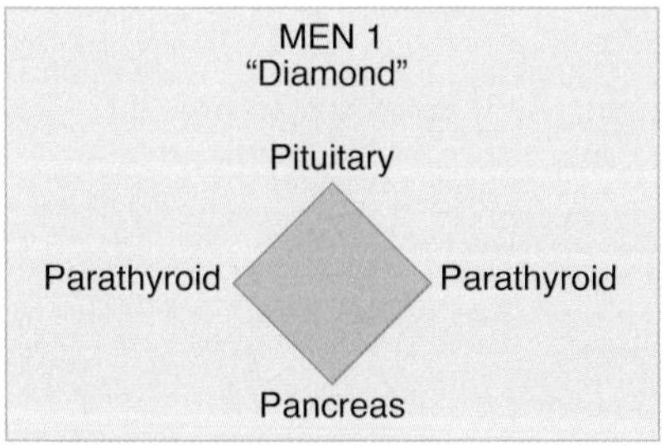

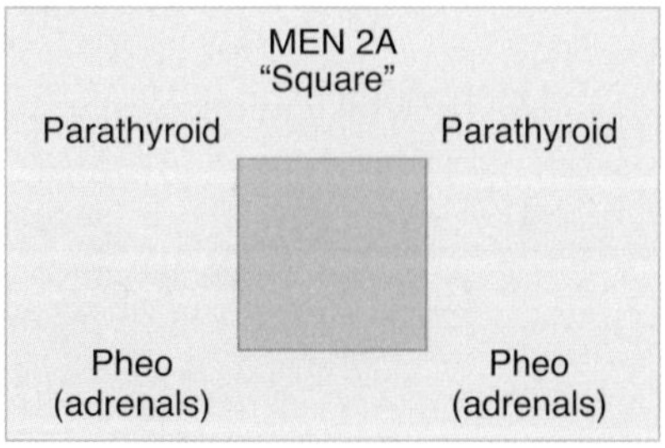

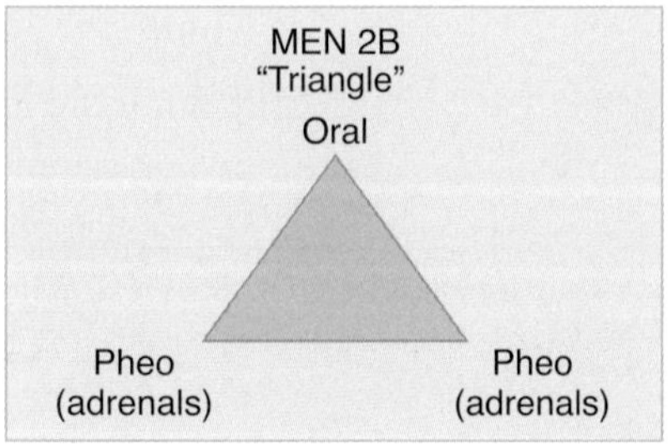

▶ ENDOCRINE—PHARMACOLOGY

Diabetes drugs

Treatment strategy for type 1 DM—low-sugar diet, insulin replacement.
Treatment strategy for type 2 DM—dietary modification and exercise for weight loss; oral hypoglycemics and insulin replacement.

DRUG CLASSES	ACTION	CLINICAL USE	TOXICITIES
Insulin: Lispro (rapid-acting) Aspart (rapid-acting) Glulisine (rapid-acting) Regular (short-acting) NPH (intermediate) Glargine (long-acting) Detemir (long-acting)	Bind insulin receptor (tyrosine kinase activity). Liver: ↑ glucose stored as glycogen. Muscle: ↑ glycogen and protein synthesis, K^+ uptake. Fat: aids TG storage.	Type 1 DM, type 2 DM, gestational diabetes, life-threatening hyperkalemia, and stress-induced hyperglycemia.	Hypoglycemia, very rarely hypersensitivity reactions.
Biguanides: Metformin	Exact mechanism is unknown. ↓ gluconeogenesis, ↑ glycolysis, ↑ peripheral glucose uptake (insulin sensitivity).	Oral. First-line therapy in type 2 DM. Can be used in patients without islet function.	GI upset; most serious adverse effect is lactic acidosis (thus contraindicated in renal failure).
Sulfonylureas: First generation: Tolbutamide Chlorpropamide Second generation: Glyburide Glimepiride Glipizide	Close K^+ channel in β-cell membrane, so cell depolarizes → triggering of insulin release via ↑ Ca^{2+} influx.	Stimulate release of endogenous insulin in type 2 DM. Require some islet function, so useless in type 1 DM.	First generation: disulfiram-like effects. Second generation: hypoglycemia.
Glitazones/ thiazolidinediones: Pioglitazone Rosiglitazone	↑ insulin sensitivity in peripheral tissue. Binds to PPAR-γ nuclear transcription regulator.[a]	Used as monotherapy in type 2 DM or combined with above agents.	Weight gain, edema. Hepatotoxicity, heart failure.
α-glucosidase inhibitors: Acarbose Miglitol	Inhibit intestinal brush-border α-glucosidases. Delayed sugar hydrolysis and glucose absorption → ↓ postprandial hyperglycemia.	Used as monotherapy in type 2 DM or in combination with above agents.	GI disturbances.
Amylin analogs: Pramlintide	↓ glucagon.	Type 1 and type 2 DM.	Hypoglycemia, nausea, diarrhea.
GLP-1 analogs: Exenatide Liraglutide	↑ insulin, ↓ glucagon release.	Type 2 DM.	Nausea, vomiting; pancreatitis.
DPP-4 inhibitors: Linagliptin Saxagliptin Sitagliptin	↑ insulin, ↓ glucagon release.	Type 2 DM.	Mild urinary or respiratory infections.

[a]Genes activated by PPAR-γ regulate fatty acid storage and glucose metabolism. Activation of PPAR-γ ↑ insulin sensitivity and levels of adiponectin.

Propylthiouracil, methimazole

MECHANISM	Block peroxidase, thereby inhibiting organification of iodide and coupling of thyroid hormone synthesis. Propylthiouracil also blocks 5'-deiodinase, which ↓ peripheral conversion of T_4 to T_3.
CLINICAL USE	Hyperthyroidism.
TOXICITY	Skin rash, agranulocytosis (rare), aplastic anemia, hepatotoxicity (propylthiouracil). Methimazole is a possible teratogen.

Levothyroxine, triiodothyronine

MECHANISM	Thyroxine replacement.
CLINICAL USE	Hypothyroidism, myxedema.
TOXICITY	Tachycardia, heat intolerance, tremors, arrhythmias.

Hypothalamic/pituitary drugs

DRUG	CLINICAL USE
GH	GH deficiency, Turner syndrome.
Somatostatin (octreotide)	Acromegaly, carcinoid, gastrinoma, glucagonoma, esophageal varices.
Oxytocin	Stimulates labor, uterine contractions, milk let-down; controls uterine hemorrhage.
ADH (desmopressin)	Pituitary (central, not nephrogenic) DI.

Demeclocycline

MECHANISM	ADH antagonist (member of the tetracycline family).
CLINICAL USE	SIADH.
TOXICITY	Nephrogenic DI, photosensitivity, abnormalities of bone and teeth.

Glucocorticoids

Glucocorticoids	Hydrocortisone, prednisone, triamcinolone, dexamethasone, beclomethasone.
MECHANISM	↓ the production of leukotrienes and prostaglandins by inhibiting phospholipase A_2 and expression of COX-2.
CLINICAL USE	Addison's disease, inflammation, immune suppression, asthma.
TOXICITY	Iatrogenic Cushing's syndrome—buffalo hump, moon facies, truncal obesity, muscle wasting, thin skin, easy bruisability, osteoporosis, adrenocortical atrophy, peptic ulcers, diabetes (if chronic). Adrenal insufficiency when drug stopped abruptly after chronic use.

HIGH-YIELD SYSTEMS

Gastrointestinal

"A good set of bowels is worth more to a man than any quantity of brains."
—Josh Billings

"Man should strive to have his intestines relaxed all the days of his life."
—Moses Maimonides

"The colon is the playing field for all human emotions."
—Cyrus Kapadia, MD

▸ GASTROINTESTINAL–EMBRYOLOGY

GI embryology

Foregut—pharynx to duodenum.
Midgut—duodenum to transverse colon.
Hindgut—distal transverse colon to rectum.
Developmental defects of anterior abdominal wall due to failure of:
- Rostral fold closure: sternal defects
- Lateral fold closure: omphalocele, gastroschisis
- Caudal fold closure: bladder exstrophy

Duodenal atresia—failure to recanalize (trisomy 21).
Jejunal, ileal, colonic atresia—due to vascular accident (apple peel atresia).
Midgut development:
- 6th week—midgut herniates through umbilical ring
- 10th week—returns to abdominal cavity + rotates around SMA

Pathology—malrotation of midgut, omphalocele, intestinal atresia or stenosis, volvulus.

Gastroschisis—extrusion of abdominal contents through abdominal folds; not covered by peritoneum.
Omphalocele—persistence of herniation of abdominal contents into umbilical cord, covered by peritoneum A.

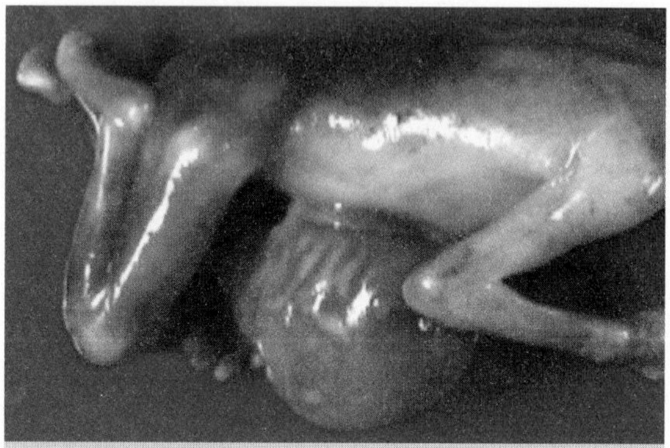

A **Omphalocele.** Note protruding intestine covered in peritoneum. Rx

Tracheoesophageal anomalies

Esophageal atresia (EA) with distal tracheoesophageal fistula (TEF) is the most common (85%). Results in drooling, choking, and vomiting with first feeding. TEF allows air to enter stomach (visible on CXR). Cyanosis is secondary to laryngospasm (to avoid reflux-related aspiration). Clinical test: failure to pass NG tube into stomach.
In H-type it is a fistula alone. In pure atresia (isolated) EA the CXR shows gasless abdomen.

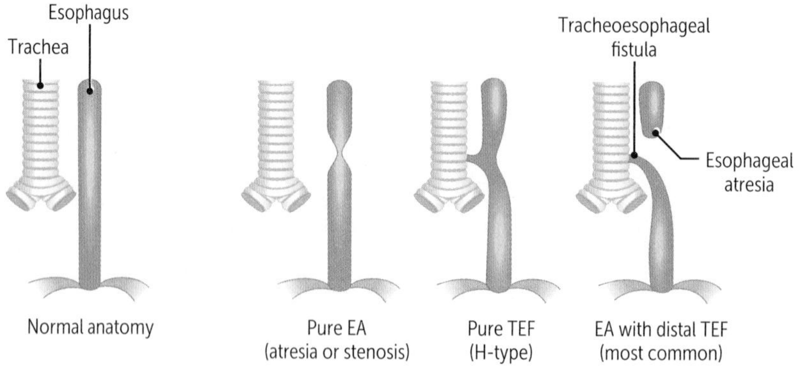
Esophagus
Trachea
Tracheoesophageal fistula
Esophageal atresia
Normal anatomy
Pure EA (atresia or stenosis)
Pure TEF (H-type)
EA with distal TEF (most common)

Congenital pyloric stenosis

Hypertrophy of the pylorus causes obstruction. Palpable "olive" mass in epigastric region and nonbilious projectile vomiting at ≈ 2 weeks of age. Treatment is surgical incision. Occurs in 1/600 live births, more often in firstborn males.

Pancreas and spleen embryology

Pancreas—derived from foregut. Ventral pancreatic buds contribute to the pancreatic head and main pancreatic duct. The uncinate process is formed by the ventral bud alone. The dorsal pancreatic bud becomes everything else (body, tail, isthmus, and accessory pancreatic duct).

Annular pancreas—ventral pancreatic bud abnormally encircles 2nd part of duodenum; forms a ring of pancreatic tissue that may cause duodenal narrowing.

Pancreas divisum—ventral and dorsal parts fail to fuse at 8 weeks.

Spleen—arises in mesentery of stomach (hence is mesodermal) but is supplied by foregut (celiac artery).

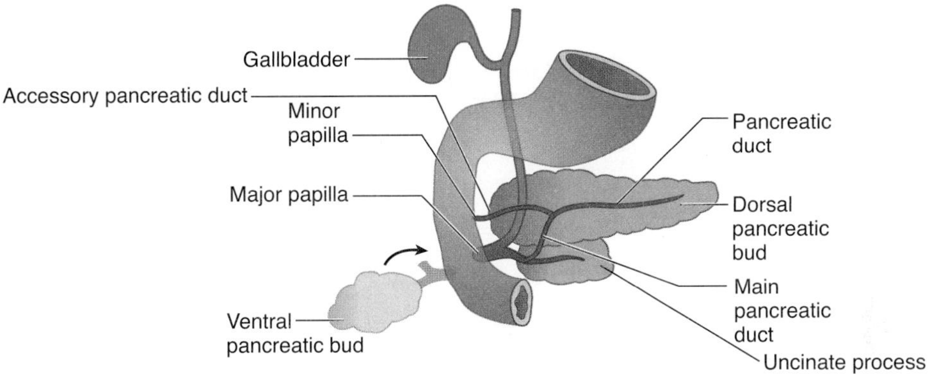

▸ GASTROINTESTINAL—ANATOMY

Retroperitoneal structures

Retroperitoneal structures include GI structures that lack a mesentery and non-GI structures. Injuries to retroperitoneal structures can cause blood or gas accumulation in retroperitoneal space.

SAD PUCKER:
- Suprarenal (adrenal) gland [not shown]
- Aorta and IVC
- Duodenum (2nd and 3rd parts)
- Pancreas (except tail)
- Ureters [not shown]
- Colon (descending and ascending)
- Kidneys
- Esophagus (lower $^2/_3$) [not shown]
- Rectum (lower $^2/_3$) [not shown]

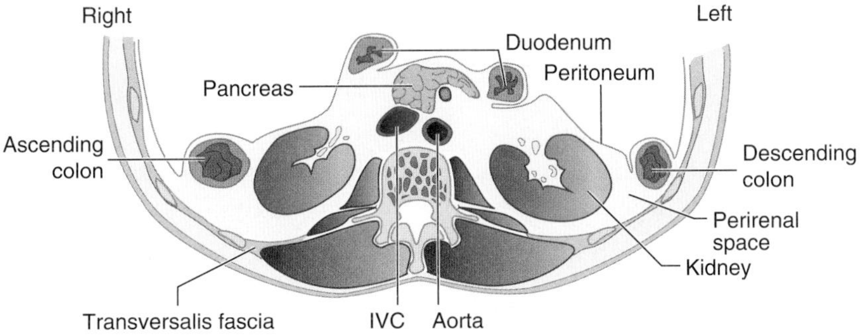

Important GI ligaments

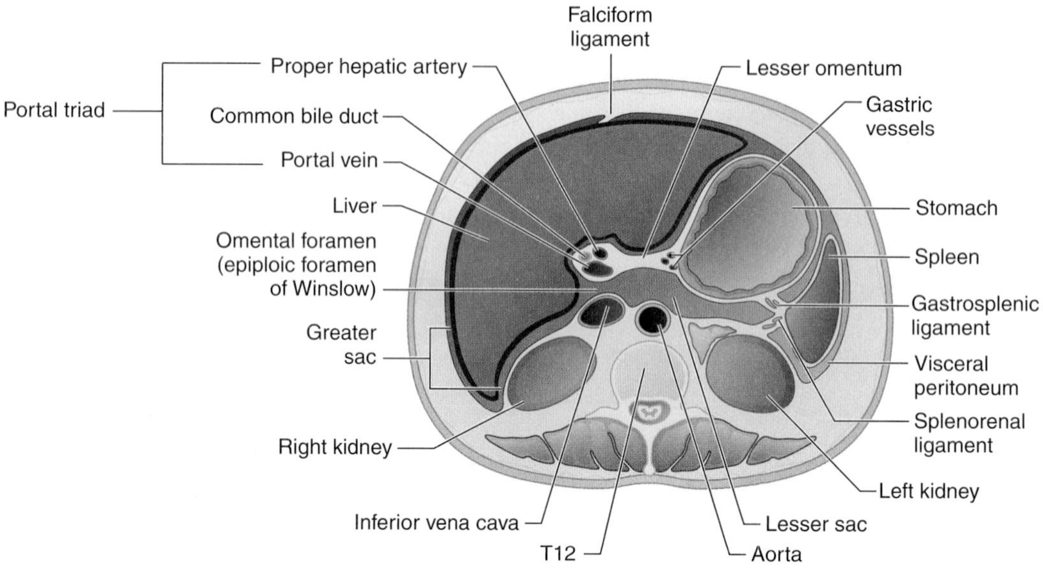

LIGAMENT	CONNECTS	STRUCTURES CONTAINED	NOTES
Falciform	Liver to anterior abdominal wall	Ligamentum teres hepatis (derivative of fetal umbilical vein)	Derivative of ventral mesentery
Hepatoduodenal	Liver to duodenum	Portal triad: hepatic artery, portal vein, common bile duct	Pringle maneuver—ligament may be compressed between thumb and index finger placed in omental foramen to control bleeding Connects greater and lesser sacs
Gastrohepatic (not shown)	Liver to lesser curvature of stomach	Gastric arteries	Separates greater and lesser sacs on the right May be cut during surgery to access lesser sac
Gastrocolic (not shown)	Greater curvature and transverse colon	Gastroepiploic arteries	Part of greater omentum
Gastrosplenic	Greater curvature and spleen	Short gastrics, left gastroepiploic vessels	Separates greater and lesser sacs on the left
Splenorenal	Spleen to posterior abdominal wall	Splenic artery and vein, tail of pancreas	

Digestive tract anatomy

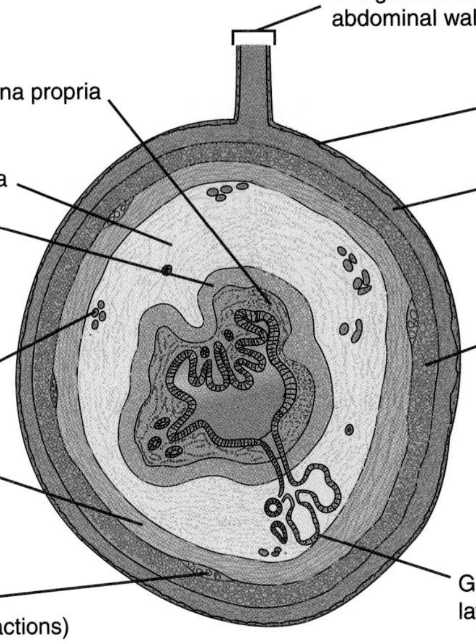

Layers of gut wall (inside to outside—**MSMS**):

- **M**ucosa—epithelium (absorption), lamina propria (support), muscularis mucosa (motility)
- **S**ubmucosa—includes **S**ubmucosal nerve plexus (Meissner's)
- **M**uscularis externa—includes **M**yenteric nerve plexus (Auerbach's)
- **S**erosa (when intraperitoneal)/adventitia (when retroperitoneal)

Ulcers can extend into submucosa, inner or outer muscular layer. Erosions are in the mucosa only.

Frequencies of basal electric rhythm (slow waves):

- Stomach—3 waves/min
- Duodenum—12 waves/min
- Ileum—8–9 waves/min

Digestive tract histology

ORGAN	HISTOLOGY
Esophagus	Nonkeratinized stratified squamous epithelium.
Stomach	Gastric glands.
Duodenum	Villi and microvilli ↑ absorptive surface. Brunner's glands (submucosa) and crypts of Lieberkühn.
Jejunum	Plicae circulares and crypts of Lieberkühn.
Ileum	Peyer's patches (lamina propria, submucosa), plicae circulares (proximal ileum), and crypts of Lieberkühn. Largest number of goblet cells in the small intestine.
Colon	Colon has crypts but no villi, numerous goblet cells.

Abdominal aorta and branches

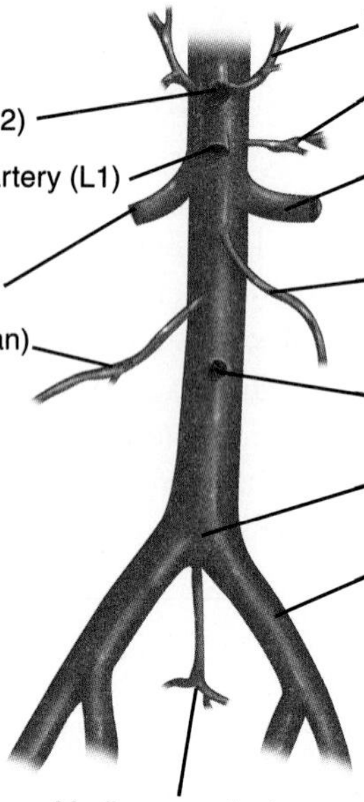
Left inferior phrenic artery
Left middle suprarenal artery
Celiac trunk (T12)
Superior mesenteric artery (L1)
Left renal artery (L1)
Right renal artery
Left testicular (ovarian) artery
Right testicular (ovarian) artery
Inferior mesenteric artery (L3)
Bifurcation of abdominal aorta (L4)
Left common iliac artery
Median sacral artery

Arteries supplying GI structures branch **anteriorly.** Arteries supplying non-GI structures branch **laterally.**

Superior mesenteric artery (SMA) syndrome occurs when the transverse portion (third segment) of the duodenum is entrapped between SMA and aorta, causing intestinal obstruction.

GI blood supply and innervation

EMBRYONIC GUT REGION	ARTERY	PARASYMPATHETIC INNERVATION	VERTEBRAL LEVEL	STRUCTURES SUPPLIED
Foregut	Celiac	Vagus	T12/L1	Stomach to proximal duodenum; liver, gallbladder, pancreas, spleen (mesoderm)
Midgut	SMA	Vagus	L1	Distal duodenum to proximal $^2/_3$ of transverse colon
Hindgut	IMA	Pelvic	L3	Distal $^1/_3$ of transverse colon to upper portion of rectum; splenic flexure is a watershed region

Celiac trunk

Branches of celiac trunk: common hepatic, splenic, left gastric. These constitute the main blood supply of the stomach.

Short gastrics have poor anastomoses if splenic artery is blocked.

Strong anastomoses exist between:

- Left and right gastroepiploics
- Left and right gastrics

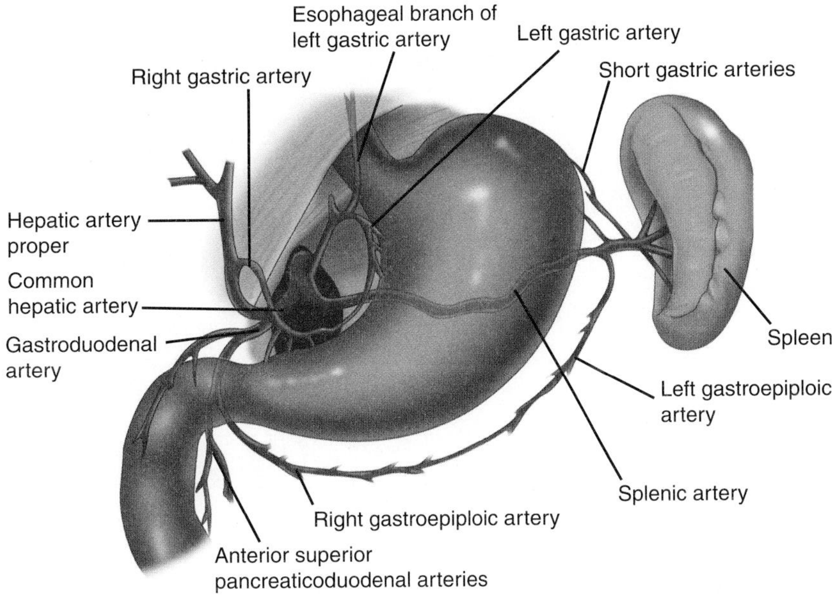
Esophageal branch of left gastric artery
Left gastric artery
Right gastric artery
Short gastric arteries
Hepatic artery proper
Common hepatic artery
Gastroduodenal artery
Spleen
Left gastroepiploic artery
Splenic artery
Right gastroepiploic artery
Anterior superior pancreaticoduodenal arteries

Collateral circulation

If branches off of the abdominal aorta are blocked, these arterial anastomoses (origin) compensate:

- Superior epigastric (internal thoracic/mammary) ↔ inferior epigastric (external iliac)
- Superior pancreaticoduodenal (celiac trunk) ↔ inferior pancreaticoduodenal (SMA)
- Middle colic (SMA) ↔ left colic (IMA)
- Superior rectal (IMA) ↔ middle and inferior rectal (internal iliac)

Portosystemic anastomoses

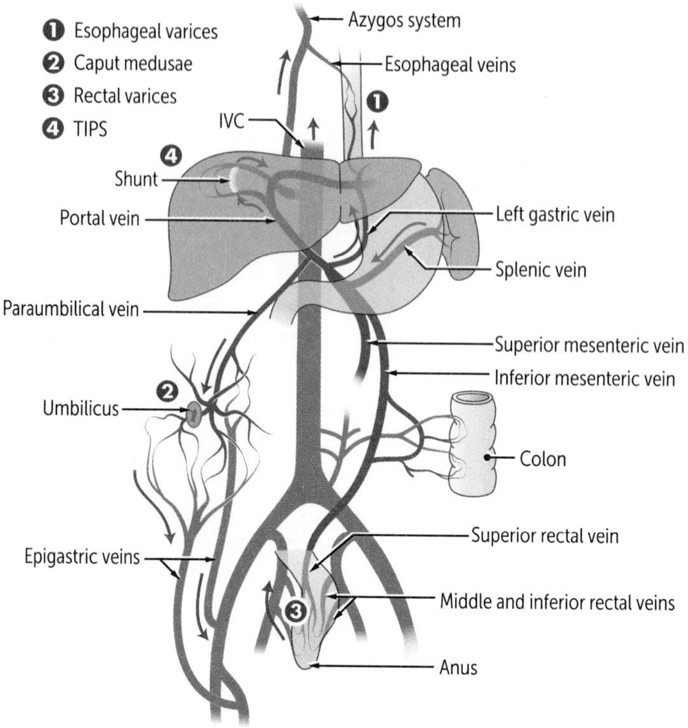

SITE OF ANASTOMOSIS	CLINICAL SIGN	PORTAL ↔ SYSTEMIC
❶ Esophag**us**	Esophageal varices	Left gastric ↔ esophageal
❷ Umbilicus	**Caput** medusae	Paraumbilical ↔ superficial and inferior epigastric below the umbilicus, and superior epigastric and lateral thoracic above the umbilicus.
❸ **Rectum**	Internal hemorrhoids	Superior rectal ↔ middle and inferior rectal

Varices of **gut, butt,** and **caput** (medusae) are commonly seen with portal hypertension.

Treatment with a transjugular intrahepatic portosystemic shunt (TIPS) ❹ between the portal vein and hepatic vein percutaneously relieves portal hypertension by shunting blood to the systemic circulation.

Pectinate (dentate) line Formed where endoderm (hindgut) meets ectoderm.

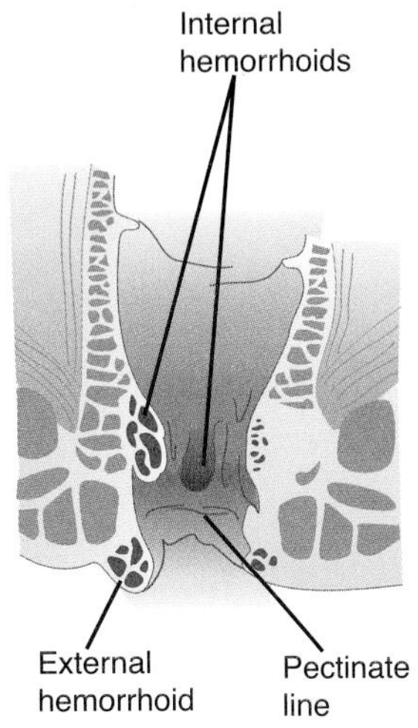
Internal hemorrhoids
External hemorrhoid
Pectinate line

Above pectinate line—internal hemorrhoids, adenocarcinoma. Arterial supply from superior rectal artery (branch of IMA). Venous drainage is to superior rectal vein → inferior mesenteric vein → portal system.

Internal hemorrhoids receive visceral innervation and are therefore **not painful**.
Lymphatic drainage to deep nodes.

Below pectinate line—external hemorrhoids, squamous cell carcinoma. Arterial supply from inferior rectal artery (branch of internal pudendal artery). Venous drainage to inferior rectal vein → internal pudendal vein → internal iliac vein → IVC.

External hemorrhoids receive somatic innervation (inferior rectal branch of pudendal nerve) and are therefore **painful**.
Lymphatic drainage to superficial inguinal nodes.

Liver anatomy Apical surface of hepatocytes faces bile canaliculi. Basolateral surface faces sinusoids.

Zone I: periportal zone:
- Affected 1st by viral hepatitis

Zone II: intermediate zone.
Zone III: pericentral vein (centrilobular) zone:
- Affected 1st by ischemia
- Contains P-450 system
- Most sensitive to toxic injury
- Site of alcoholic hepatitis

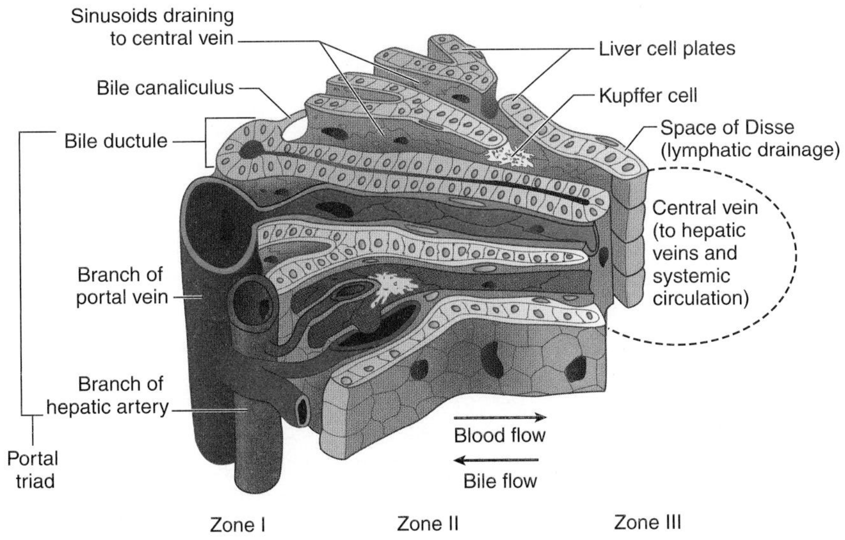
Sinusoids draining to central vein
Bile canaliculus
Bile ductule
Branch of portal vein
Branch of hepatic artery
Portal triad
Liver cell plates
Kupffer cell
Space of Disse (lymphatic drainage)
Central vein (to hepatic veins and systemic circulation)
Blood flow
Bile flow
Zone I
Zone II
Zone III

Biliary structures

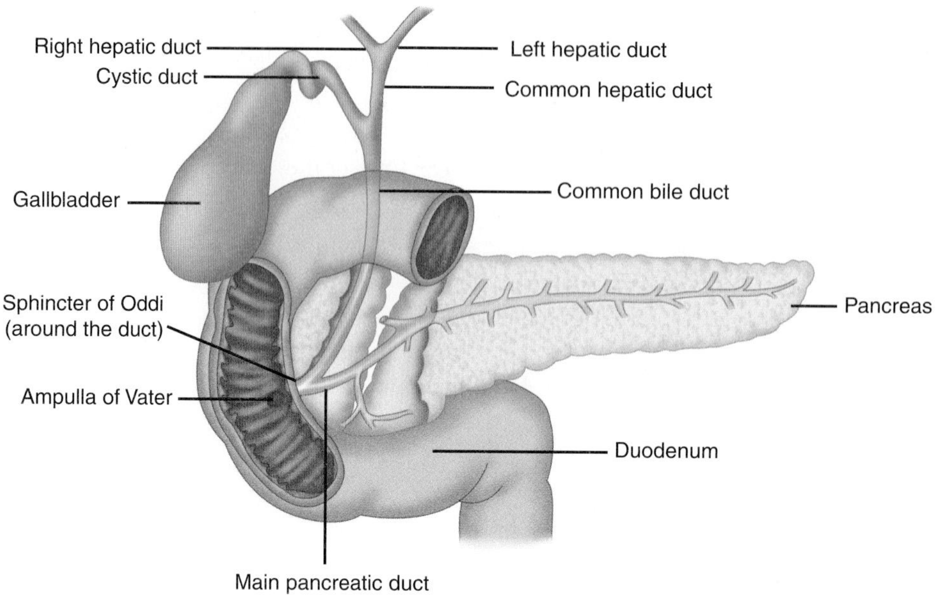

Right hepatic duct
Cystic duct
Left hepatic duct
Common hepatic duct
Gallbladder
Common bile duct
Sphincter of Oddi (around the duct)
Pancreas
Ampulla of Vater
Duodenum
Main pancreatic duct

Gallstones that reach the common channel at ampulla of Vater can block both the bile and pancreatic ducts.
Tumors that arise in the head of the pancreas (near the duodenum) can cause obstruction of the common bile duct.

Femoral region

ORGANIZATION	**Lateral to medial:** Nerve-Artery-Vein-Empty space-Lymphatics.	You go from **lateral to medial** to find your **NAVEL**.
Femoral triangle	Contains femoral vein, artery, nerve.	**Venous** near the **penis**.
Femoral sheath	Fascial tube 3–4 cm below inguinal ligament. Contains femoral vein, artery, and canal (deep inguinal lymph nodes) but not femoral nerve.	

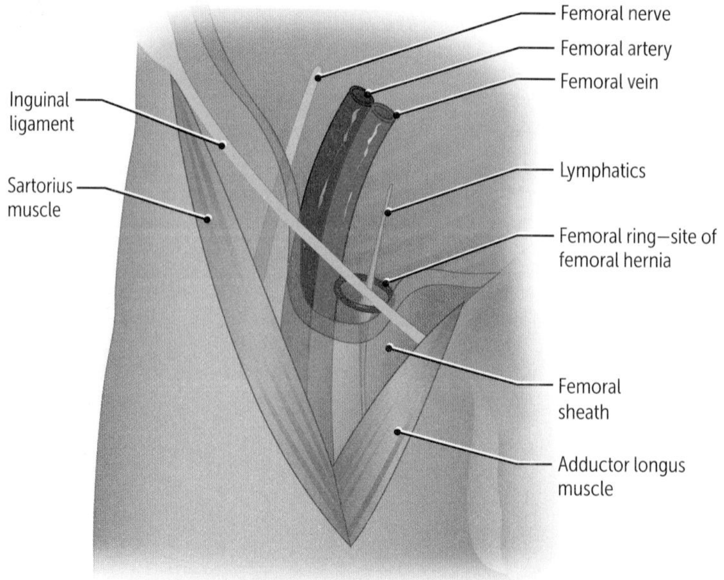

Femoral nerve
Femoral artery
Femoral vein
Inguinal ligament
Sartorius muscle
Lymphatics
Femoral ring—site of femoral hernia
Femoral sheath
Adductor longus muscle

Inguinal canal

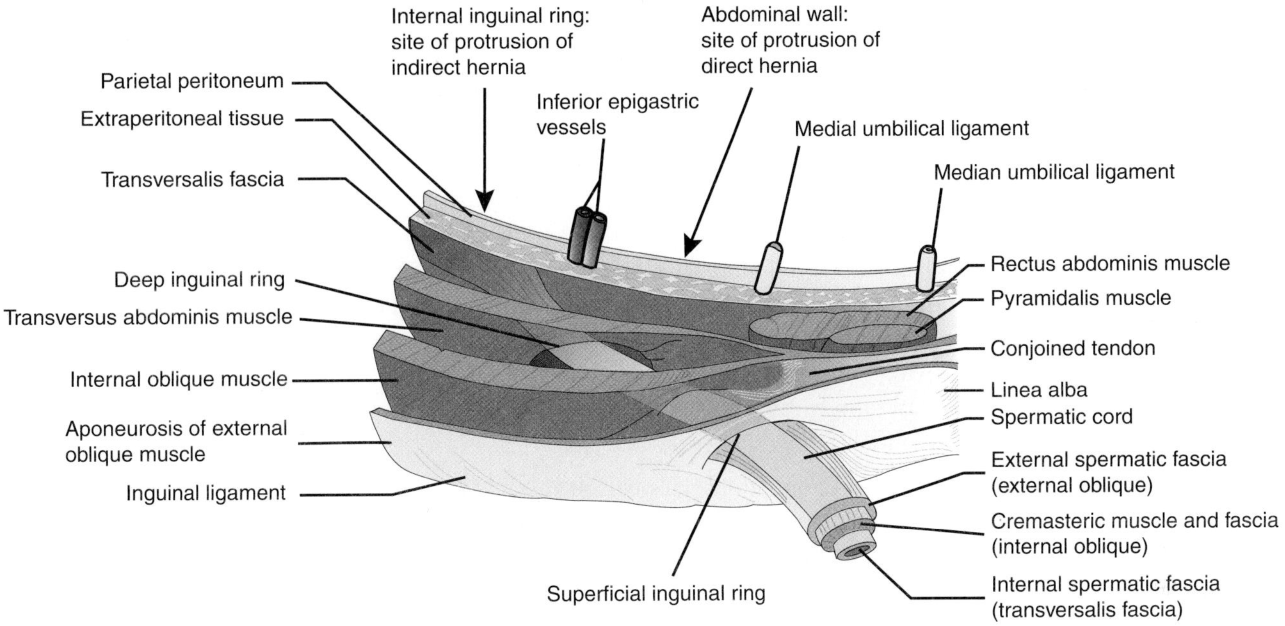

Internal inguinal ring: site of protrusion of indirect hernia
Abdominal wall: site of protrusion of direct hernia
Parietal peritoneum
Extraperitoneal tissue
Transversalis fascia
Inferior epigastric vessels
Medial umbilical ligament
Median umbilical ligament
Deep inguinal ring
Transversus abdominis muscle
Internal oblique muscle
Aponeurosis of external oblique muscle
Inguinal ligament
Rectus abdominis muscle
Pyramidalis muscle
Conjoined tendon
Linea alba
Spermatic cord
External spermatic fascia (external oblique)
Cremasteric muscle and fascia (internal oblique)
Internal spermatic fascia (transversalis fascia)
Superficial inguinal ring

Hernias	A protrusion of peritoneum through an opening, usually a site of weakness.	
Diaphragmatic hernia	Abdominal structures enter the thorax; may occur in infants as a result of defective development of pleuroperitoneal membrane. Most commonly a **hiatal hernia**, in which stomach herniates upward through the esophageal hiatus of the diaphragm.	**Sliding hiatal hernia** is most common. GE junction is displaced ↑; "hourglass stomach." **Paraesophageal hernia**—GE junction is normal. Fundus protrudes into the thorax.
Indirect inguinal hernia	Goes through the **in**ternal (deep) inguinal ring, external (superficial) inguinal ring, and **in**to the scrotum. Enters internal inguinal ring lateral to inferior epigastric artery. Occurs in **in**fants owing to failure of processus vaginalis to close (can form hydrocele). Much more common in males.	An indirect inguinal hernia follows the path of descent of the testes. Covered by all 3 layers of spermatic fascia.
Direct inguinal hernia	Protrudes through the inguinal (Hesselbach's) triangle. Bulges directly through abdominal wall medial to inferior epigastric artery. Goes through the external (superficial) inguinal ring only. Covered by external spermatic fascia. Usually in older men.	**MD**s don't **LI**e: **M**edial to inferior epigastric artery = **D**irect hernia. **L**ateral to inferior epigastric artery = **I**ndirect hernia.
Femoral hernia	Protrudes below inguinal ligament through femoral canal below and lateral to pubic tubercle. More common in women.	Leading cause of bowel incarceration.

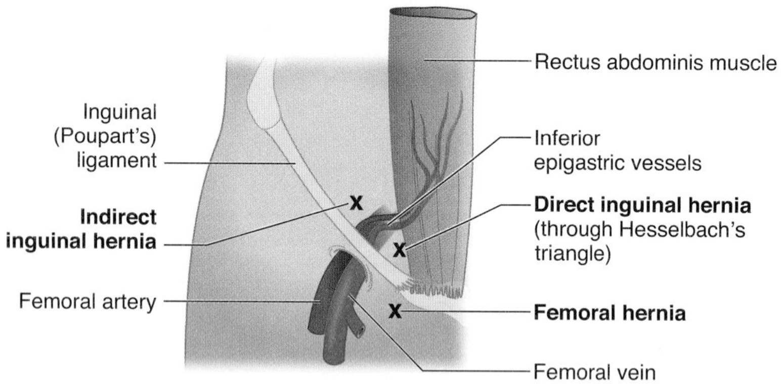
Rectus abdominis muscle
Inguinal (Poupart's) ligament
Inferior epigastric vessels
Indirect inguinal hernia
Direct inguinal hernia (through Hesselbach's triangle)
X
X
X
Femoral artery
Femoral hernia
Femoral vein

Hesselbach's triangle:
- Inferior epigastric vessels
- Lateral border of rectus abdominis
- Inguinal ligament

▶ GASTROINTESTINAL–PHYSIOLOGY

GI hormones

HORMONE	SOURCE	ACTION	REGULATION	NOTES
Gastrin	G cells (antrum of stomach)	↑ gastric H^+ secretion ↑ growth of gastric mucosa ↑ gastric motility	↑ by stomach distention/alkalinization, amino acids, peptides, vagal stimulation ↓ by stomach pH < 1.5	↑↑ in Zollinger-Ellison syndrome. ↑ by chronic PPI use. Phenylalanine and tryptophan are potent stimulators.
Cholecystokinin	I cells (duodenum, jejunum)	↑ pancreatic secretion ↑ gallbladder contraction ↓ gastric emptying ↑ sphincter of Oddi relaxation	↑ by fatty acids, amino acids	CCK acts on neural muscarinic pathways to cause pancreatic secretion.
Secretin	S cells (duodenum)	↑ pancreatic HCO_3^- secretion ↓ gastric acid secretion ↑ bile secretion	↑ by acid, fatty acids in lumen of duodenum	↑ HCO_3^- neutralizes gastric acid in duodenum, allowing pancreatic enzymes to function.
Somatostatin	D cells (pancreatic islets, GI mucosa)	↓ gastric acid and pepsinogen secretion ↓ pancreatic and small intestine fluid secretion ↓ gallbladder contraction ↓ insulin and glucagon release	↑ by acid ↓ by vagal stimulation	Inhibitory hormone. Antigrowth hormone effects (inhibits digestion and absorption of substances needed for growth).
Glucose-dependent insulinotropic peptide	K cells (duodenum, jejunum)	Exocrine: ↓ gastric H^+ secretion Endocrine: ↑ insulin release	↑ by fatty acids, amino acids, oral glucose	Also known as gastric inhibitory peptide (GIP). An oral glucose load is used more rapidly than the equivalent given by IV due to GIP secretion.
Vasoactive intestinal polypeptide (VIP)	Parasympathetic ganglia in sphincters, gallbladder, small intestine	↑ intestinal water and electrolyte secretion ↑ relaxation of intestinal smooth muscle and sphincters	↑ by distention and vagal stimulation ↓ by adrenergic input	VIPoma—non-α, non-β islet cell pancreatic tumor that secretes VIP. Copious **W**atery **D**iarrhea, **H**ypokalemia, and **A**chlorhydria (**WDHA** syndrome).
Nitric oxide		↑ smooth muscle relaxation, including lower esophageal sphincter		Loss of NO secretion is implicated in ↑ lower esophageal tone of achalasia.
Motilin	Small intestine	Produces migrating motor complexes (MMCs)	↑ in fasting state	Motilin receptor agonists (such as erythromycin) are used to stimulate intestinal peristalsis.

GI secretory products

PRODUCT	SOURCE	ACTION	REGULATION	NOTES
Intrinsic factor	Parietal cells (stomach)	Vitamin B_{12}–binding protein (required for B_{12} uptake in terminal ileum)		Autoimmune destruction of parietal cells → chronic gastritis and pernicious anemia.
Gastric acid	Parietal cells (stomach)	↓ stomach pH	↑ by histamine, ACh, gastrin ↓ by somatostatin, GIP, prostaglandin, secretin	Gastrinoma: gastrin-secreting tumor that causes continuous high levels of acid secretion and ulcers.
Pepsin	Chief cells (stomach)	Protein digestion	↑ by vagal stimulation, local acid	Inactive pepsinogen → pepsin by H^+.
HCO_3^-	Mucosal cells (stomach, duodenum, salivary glands, pancreas) and Brunner's glands (duodenum)	Neutralizes acid	↑ by pancreatic and biliary secretion with secretin	HCO_3^- is trapped in mucus that covers the gastric epithelium.

Saliva

Secretion from parotid, submandibular, and sublingual glands is stimulated by sympathetic and parasympathetic activity. Amylase digests starch, HCO_3^- neutralizes bacterial acids, mucins lubricate food. Normally hypotonic because of absorption but more isotonic with higher flow rates (less time for absorption).

Locations of GI secretory cells

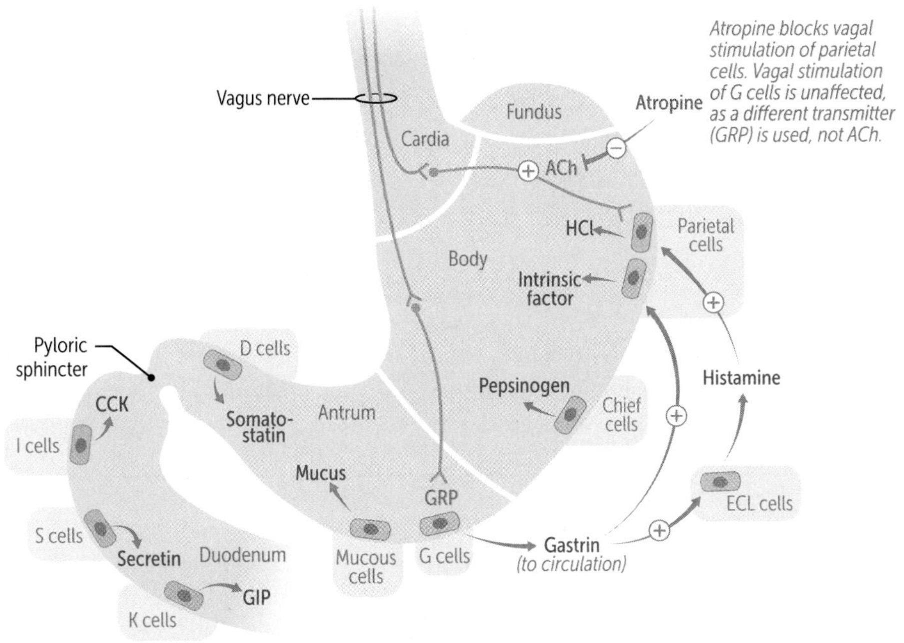

Gastrin ↑ acid secretion primarily through its effects on ECL cells (leading to histamine release) rather than through its direct effect on parietal cells.

Gastric parietal cell

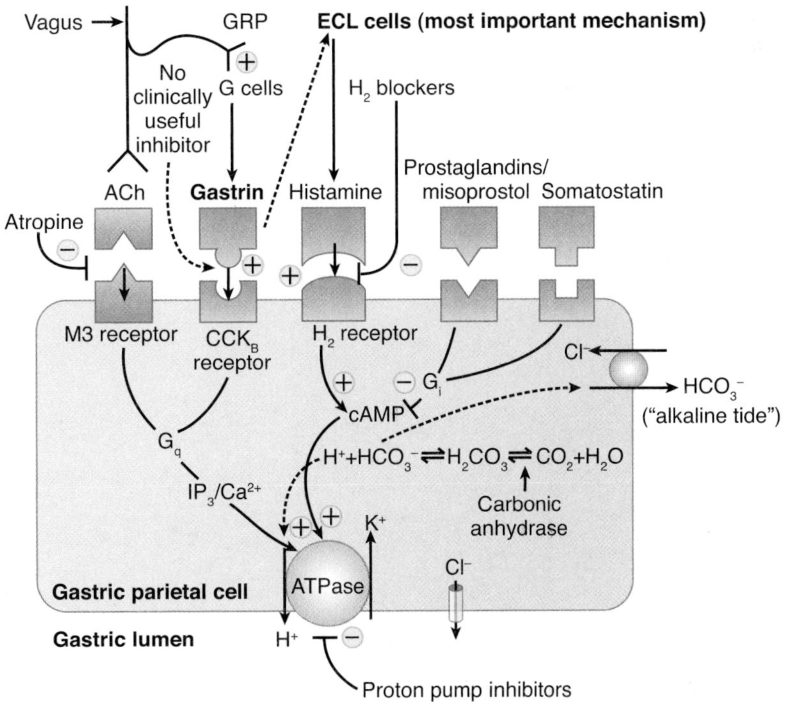

Brunner's glands	Located in duodenal submucosa. Secrete alkaline mucus. Hypertrophy seen in peptic ulcer disease.

Pancreatic secretions Isotonic fluid; low flow → high Cl^-, high flow → high HCO_3^-.

ENZYME	ROLE	NOTES
α-amylase	Starch digestion	Secreted in active form
Lipase, phospholipase A, colipase	Fat digestion	
Proteases	Protein digestion	Includes trypsin, chymotrypsin, elastase, carboxypeptidases Secreted as proenzymes also known as zymogens
Trypsinogen	Converted to active enzyme trypsin → activation of other proenzymes and creation of more trypsinogen (positive feedback loop)	Converted to trypsin by enterokinase/enteropeptidase, an enzyme secreted from duodenal mucosa

Carbohydrate digestion

Salivary amylase	Starts digestion, hydrolyzes α-1,4 linkages to yield disaccharides (maltose and α-limit dextrins).
Pancreatic amylase	Highest concentration in duodenal lumen, hydrolyzes starch to oligosaccharides and disaccharides.
Oligosaccharide hydrolases	At brush border of intestine, the rate-limiting step in carbohydrate digestion, produce monosaccharides from oligo- and disaccharides.

Carbohydrate absorption

Only monosaccharides (glucose, galactose, fructose) are absorbed by enterocytes. Glucose and galactose are taken up by SGLT1 (Na^+ dependent). Fructose is taken up by facilitated diffusion by GLUT-5. All are transported to blood by GLUT-2.

D-xylose absorption test: distinguishes GI mucosal damage from other causes of malabsorption.

Vitamin/mineral absorption

Iron	Absorbed as Fe^{2+} in duodenum.
Folate	Absorbed in jejunum.
B_{12}	Absorbed in terminal ileum along with bile acids, requires intrinsic factor.

Peyer's patches

Unencapsulated lymphoid tissue A found in lamina propria and submucosa of ileum. Contain specialized M cells that take up antigen.

B cells stimulated in germinal centers of Peyer's patches differentiate into IgA-secreting plasma cells, which ultimately reside in lamina propria. IgA receives protective secretory component and is then transported across the epithelium to the gut to deal with intraluminal antigen.

Think of **IgA**, the **I**ntra-gut **A**ntibody. And always say "secretory IgA."

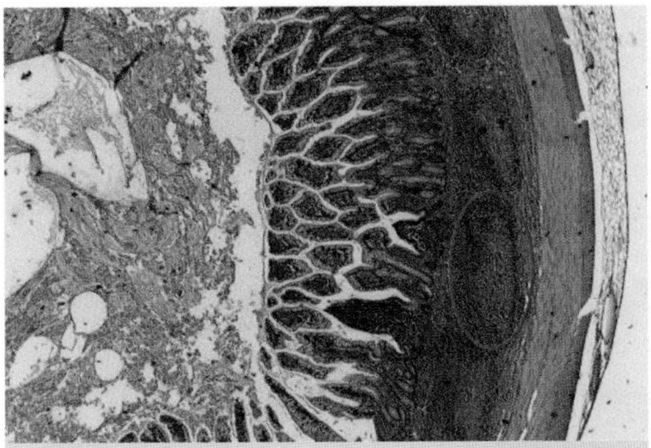

A **Peyer's patches.** Seen in cross-section of ileum (oval).

Bile

Composed of bile salts (bile acids conjugated to glycine or taurine, making them water soluble), phospholipids, cholesterol, bilirubin, water, and ions. Cholesterol 7α-hydroxylase catalyzes rate-limiting step.

Functions:
- Digestion and absorption of lipids and fat-soluble vitamins
- Cholesterol excretion (body's only means of eliminating cholesterol)
- Antimicrobial activity (via membrane disruption)

Bilirubin

Product of heme metabolism. Bilirubin is removed from blood by liver, conjugated with glucuronate, and excreted in bile.

Direct bilirubin—conjugated with glucuronic acid; water soluble.

Indirect bilirubin—unconjugated; water insoluble.

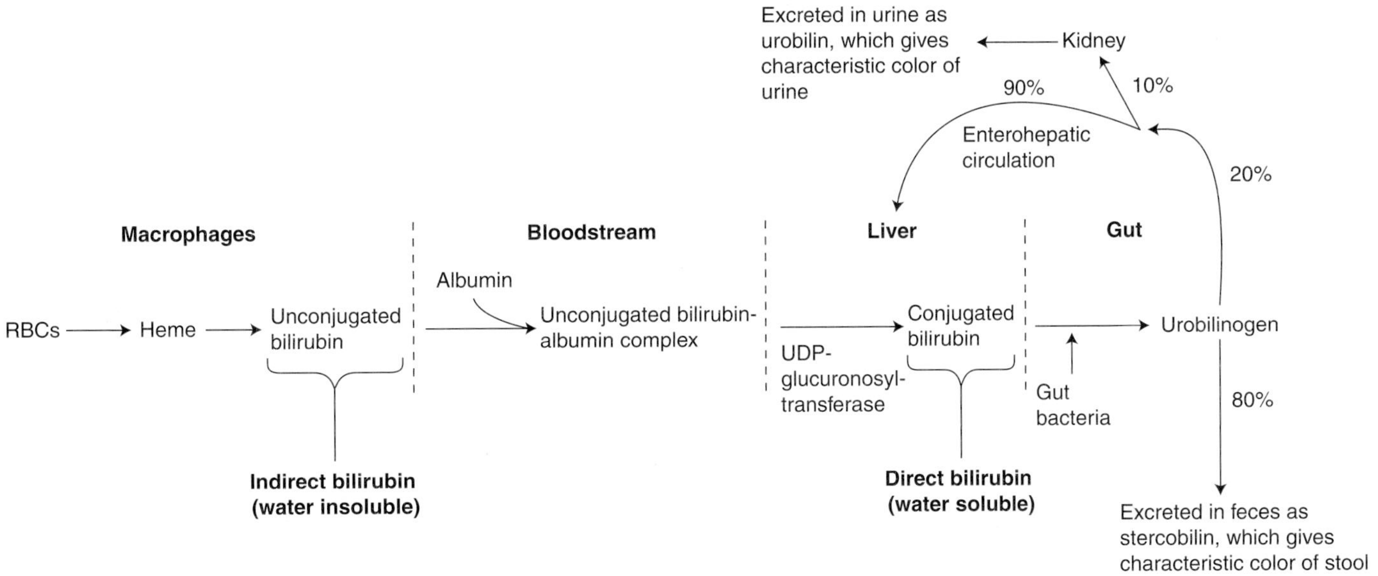

▸ GASTROINTESTINAL–PATHOLOGY

Salivary gland tumors

Generally benign and occur in parotid gland:
- **Pleomorphic adenoma** (benign mixed tumor) is the most common salivary gland tumor. Presents as a painless, mobile mass. It is composed of cartilage and epithelium and recurs frequently.
- **Warthin's tumor** (papillary cystadenoma lymphomatosum) is a benign cystic tumor with germinal centers.
- **Mucoepidermoid carcinoma** is the most common malignant tumor and has mucinous and squamous components. It presents as a painful mass because of common involvement of the facial nerve.

Achalasia

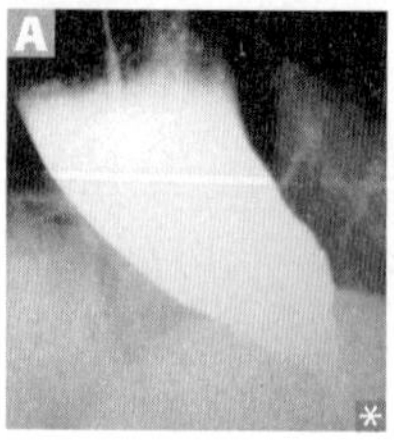

Failure of relaxation of lower esophageal sphincter (LES) due to loss of myenteric (Auerbach's) plexus. High LES opening pressure and uncoordinated peristalsis → progressive dysphagia to solids and liquids (vs. obstruction—solids only). Barium swallow shows dilated esophagus with an area of distal stenosis. Associated with an ↑ risk of esophageal squamous cell carcinoma.

A-*chalasia* = absence of relaxation.
"Bird's beak" on barium swallow A.
2° achalasia may arise from Chagas' disease.
Scleroderma (CREST syndrome) is associated with esophageal dysmotility involving low pressure proximal to LES.

Esophageal pathologies

Gastroesophageal reflux disease (GERD)	Commonly presents as heartburn and regurgitation upon lying down. May also present with nocturnal cough and dyspnea, adult-onset asthma. Decrease in LES tone.
Esophageal varices	Painless bleeding of dilated submucosal veins in lower ⅓ of esophagus secondary to portal hypertension.
Esophagitis	Associated with reflux, infection (*Candida:* white pseudomembrane; HSV-1: punched-out ulcers; CMV: linear ulcers), or chemical ingestion.
Mallory-Weiss syndrome	Mucosal lacerations at the gastroesophageal junction due to severe vomiting. Leads to hematemesis. Usually found in alcoholics and bulimics.
BoerHaave Syndrome	Transmural esophageal rupture due to violent retching. "Been-Heaving Syndrome."
Esophageal strictures	Associated with lye ingestion and acid reflux.
Plummer-Vinson syndrome	Triad of: ▪ Dysphagia (due to esophageal webs) ▪ Glossitis ▪ Iron deficiency anemia

Barrett's esophagus

Glandular metaplasia—replacement of nonkeratinized (stratified) squamous epithelium with intestinal (nonciliated columnar) epithelium in the distal esophagus A. Due to chronic acid reflux (GERD). Associated with esophagitis, esophageal ulcers, and increased risk of esophageal adenocarcinoma.

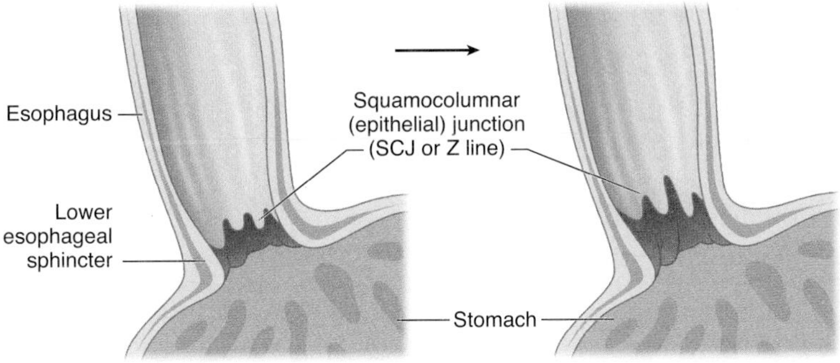
Esophagus
Squamocolumnar (epithelial) junction (SCJ or Z line)
Lower esophageal sphincter
Stomach

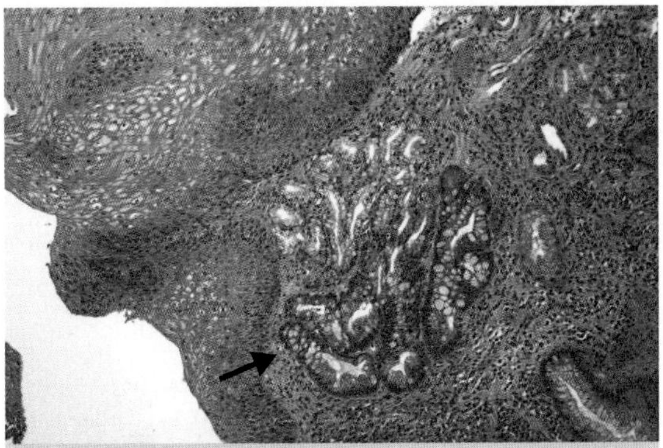

A **Barrett's esophagus.** Characterized by metaplastic columnar epithelium with goblet cells (arrow).

Esophageal cancer

Can be squamous cell carcinoma or adenocarcinoma. Typically presents with progressive dysphagia (first solids, then liquids) and weight loss; poor prognosis. Risk factors include:

- Achalasia
- Alcohol—squamous
- Barrett's esophagus—adeno
- Cigarettes—both
- Diverticula (e.g., Zenker's)—squamous
- Esophageal web—squamous
- Familial
- Fat (obesity)—adeno
- GERD—adeno
- Hot liquids—squamous

AABCDEFFGH.

Worldwide, squamous cell is more common.

In the United States, adenocarcinoma is more common.

Squamous cell—upper $^2/_3$.

Adenocarcinoma—lower $^1/_3$.

Malabsorption syndromes	Can cause diarrhea, steatorrhea, weight loss, weakness, and vitamin and mineral deficiencies.	These Will Cause Devastating Absorption Problems.
Tropical sprue	Unknown cause, but responds to antibiotics. Similar to celiac sprue, can affect entire small bowel.	
Whipple's disease	Infection with *Tropheryma whipplei* (gram positive); PAS-positive **foamy** macrophages in intestinal lamina propria, mesenteric nodes. Cardiac symptoms, Arthralgias, and Neurologic symptoms are common. Most often occurs in older men.	**Foamy Whipped** cream in a **CAN**.
Celiac sprue	Autoantibodies to gluten (gliadin) in wheat and other grains. Primarily affects distal duodenum or proximal jejunum. Histology shows loss of villi.	
Disaccharidase deficiency	Most common is lactase deficiency → milk intolerance. Normal-appearing villi. Osmotic diarrhea. Since lactase is located at tips of intestinal villi, self-limited lactase deficiency can occur following injury (e.g., viral diarrhea).	Lactose tolerance test: positive for lactase deficiency if: ▪ Administration of lactose produces symptoms, and ▪ Glucose rises < 20 mg/dL
Abetalipoproteinemia	↓ synthesis of apolipoprotein B → inability to generate chylomicrons → ↓ secretion of cholesterol, VLDL into bloodstream → fat accumulation in enterocytes. Presents in early childhood with malabsorption and neurologic manifestations.	
Pancreatic insufficiency	Due to cystic fibrosis, obstructing cancer, and chronic pancreatitis. Causes malabsorption of fat and fat-soluble vitamins (vitamins A, D, E, K).	↑ neutral fat in stool

Celiac sprue

Autoimmune-mediated intolerance of gliadin (wheat) leading to steatorrhea. Associated with HLA-DQ2, HLA-DQ8, and people of northern European descent. Findings include anti-endomysial, anti-tissue transglutaminase, and anti-gliadin antibodies; blunting of villi; and lymphocytes in the lamina propria A. ↓ mucosal absorption that primarily affects jejunum. Serum levels of tissue transglutaminase antibodies are used for screening. Associated with dermatitis herpetiformis. Moderately ↑ risk of malignancy (e.g., T-cell lymphoma).

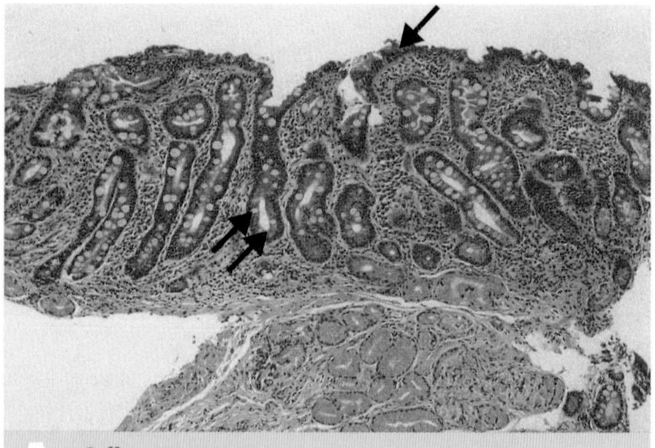

A **Celiac sprue.** Blunting of villi (single arrow) and crypt hyperplasia (double arrows).

Gastritis

Acute gastritis (erosive)	Disruption of mucosal barrier → inflammation. Can be caused by stress, NSAIDs (↓ PGE_1 → ↓ gastric mucosa protection), alcohol, uremia, burns (**Curling**'s ulcer—↓ plasma volume → sloughing of gastric mucosa), and brain injury (**Cushing**'s ulcer—↑ vagal stimulation → ↑ ACh → ↑ H^+ production).	Burned by the **Curling** iron. Always **Cush**ion the brain. Especially common among alcoholics and patients taking daily NSAIDs (e.g., patients with rheumatoid arthritis).
Chronic gastritis (nonerosive)		
Type A (fundus/body)	Autoimmune disorder characterized by **A**utoantibodies to parietal cells, pernicious **A**nemia, and **A**chlorhydria. Associated with other autoimmune disorders.	Think **ABBA**: Pernicious **A**nemia affects gastric **B**ody. *H. pylori* **B**acterium affects **A**ntrum.
Type B (antrum)	Most common type. Caused by *H. pylori* infection. ↑ risk of MALT lymphoma.	

Ménétrier's disease

Gastric hypertrophy with protein loss, parietal cell atrophy, and ↑ mucous cells. Precancerous. Rugae of stomach are so hypertrophied that they look like brain gyri.

Stomach cancer

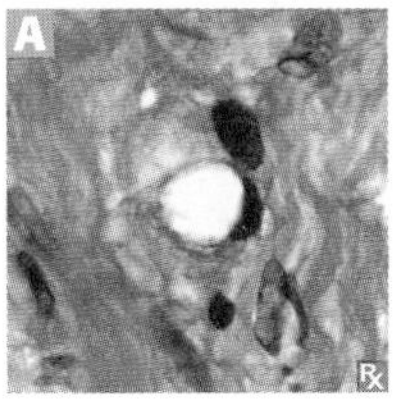

Almost always adenocarcinoma. Early aggressive local spread and node/liver metastases. Often presents with acanthosis nigricans.

- **Intestinal**—associated with *H. pylori* infection, dietary nitrosamines (smoked foods), achlorhydria, chronic gastritis, type A blood. Commonly on lesser curvature; looks like ulcer with raised margins.
- **Diffuse**—not associated with *H. pylori*; signet ring cells A; stomach wall grossly thickened and leathery (linitis plastica).

Virchow's node—involvement of left supraclavicular node by metastasis from stomach.

Krukenberg's tumor—bilateral metastases to ovaries. Abundant mucus, signet ring cells.

Sister Mary Joseph's nodule—subcutaneous periumbilical metastasis.

Peptic ulcer disease

	Gastric ulcer	Duodenal ulcer
Pain	Can be **G**reater with meals—weight loss	**D**ecreases with meals—weight gain
H. pylori infection	In 70%	In almost 100%
Causes	↓ mucosal protection against gastric acid; NSAID use also implicated	↓ mucosal protection or ↑ gastric acid secretion (e.g., Zollinger-Ellison syndrome)
Risk of carcinoma	Increased	Generally benign
Other	Often occurs in older patients	Hypertrophy of Brunner's glands

Ulcer complications

Hemorrhage	Gastric, duodenal (posterior > anterior).	Ruptured gastric ulcer on the lesser curvature of the stomach → bleeding from left gastric artery. An ulcer on the posterior wall of the duodenum → bleeding from gastroduodenal artery.
Perforation	Duodenal (anterior > posterior).	

Inflammatory bowel disease

	Crohn's disease	Ulcerative colitis
POSSIBLE ETIOLOGY	Disordered response to intestinal bacteria.	Autoimmune.
LOCATION	Any portion of the GI tract, usually the terminal ileum and colon. **Skip** lesions, **rec**tal sparing.	Colitis = colon inflammation. Continuous colonic lesions, always with rectal involvement.
GROSS MORPHOLOGY	Transmural inflammation. **Cobblestone** mucosa, creeping **fat**, bowel wall thickening ("string sign" on barium swallow x-ray A), linear ulcers, fissures, fistulas.	Mucosal and submucosal inflammation only. Friable mucosal pseudopolyps with freely hanging mesentery B. Loss of haustra → "lead pipe" appearance on imaging.
MICROSCOPIC MORPHOLOGY	Noncaseating **gran**ulomas and lymphoid aggregates (Th_1 mediated).	Crypt abscesses and ulcers, bleeding, no granulomas (Th_2 mediated).
COMPLICATIONS	Strictures, fistulas, perianal disease, malabsorption, nutritional depletion, colorectal cancer.	Malnutrition, sclerosing cholangitis, toxic megacolon, colorectal carcinoma (worse with right-sided colitis or pancolitis).
INTESTINAL MANIFESTATION	Diarrhea that may or may not be bloody.	Bloody diarrhea.
EXTRAINTESTINAL MANIFESTATIONS	Migratory polyarthritis, erythema nodosum, ankylosing spondylitis, uveitis, kidney stones.	Pyoderma gangrenosum, 1° sclerosing cholangitis, ankylosing spondylitis, uveitis.
TREATMENT	Corticosteroids, azathioprine, methotrexate, infliximab, adalimumab.	ASA preparations (sulfasalazine), 6-mercaptopurine, infliximab, colectomy.

For **Crohn's**, think of a **fat gran**ny and an old **crone skipping** down a **cobblestone** road away from the **wreck** (rectal sparing).

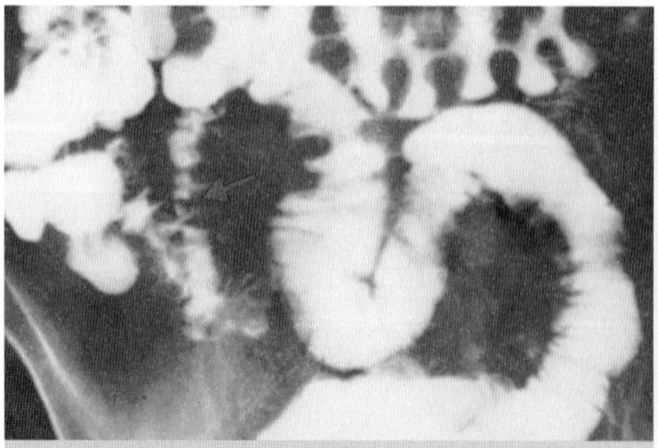

A **Crohn's disease.** Note "string sign" lesion (arrow).

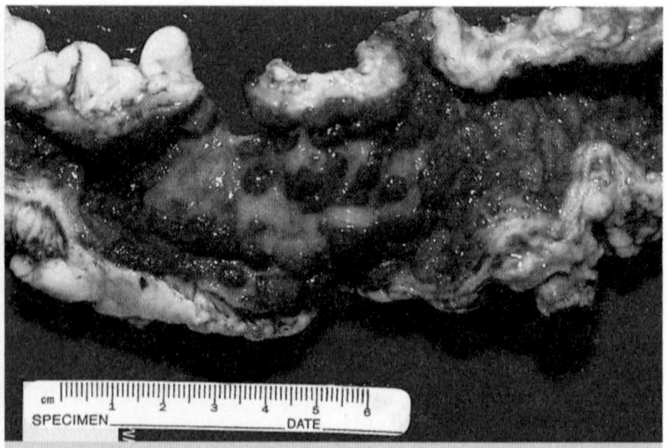

B **Ulcerative colitis.** Note pseudopolyps.

Irritable bowel syndrome

Recurrent abdominal pain associated with ≥ 2 of the following:
- Pain improves with defecation
- Change in stool frequency
- Change in appearance of stool

No structural abnormalities. Most common in middle-aged women. Chronic symptoms. May present with diarrhea, constipation, or alternating symptoms. Pathophysiology is multifaceted. Treat symptoms.

Appendicitis

Acute inflammation of the appendix due to obstruction by fecalith (in adults) or lymphoid hyperplasia (in children).

Initial diffuse periumbilical pain migrates to McBurney's point (⅓ the distance from anterior superior iliac spine to umbilicus). Nausea, fever; may perforate → peritonitis.

Differential: diverticulitis (elderly), ectopic pregnancy (use β-hCG to rule out).

Treatment: appendectomy.

Diverticular disease

Diverticulum	Blind pouch protruding from the alimentary tract that communicates with the lumen of the gut. Most diverticula (esophagus, stomach, duodenum, colon) are acquired and are termed "false" in that they lack or have an attenuated muscularis externa. Most often in sigmoid colon.	"True" diverticulum—all 3 gut wall layers outpouch (e.g., Meckel's). "False" diverticulum or pseudodiverticulum—only mucosa and submucosa outpouch. Occur especially where vasa recta perforate muscularis externa.
Diverticulosis	Many false diverticula. Common (in ~50% of people > 60 years). Caused by ↑ intraluminal pressure and focal weakness in colonic wall. Associated with low-fiber diets. Most often in sigmoid colon.	Often asymptomatic or associated with vague discomfort. A common cause of hematochezia. Complications include diverticulitis, fistulas.
Diverticulitis	Inflammation of diverticula classically causing LLQ pain, fever, leukocytosis. May perforate → peritonitis, abscess formation, or bowel stenosis. Give antibiotics.	Stool occult blood is common +/– hematochezia.May also cause colovesical fistula (fistula with bladder) → pneumaturia. Sometimes called "left-sided appendicitis" due to overlapping clinical presentation.

Zenker's diverticulum

False diverticulum. Herniation of mucosal tissue at Killian's triangle between the thyropharyngeal and cricopharyngeal parts of the inferior pharyngeal constrictor. Presenting symptoms: halitosis (due to trapped food particles), dysphagia, obstruction.

Meckel's diverticulum

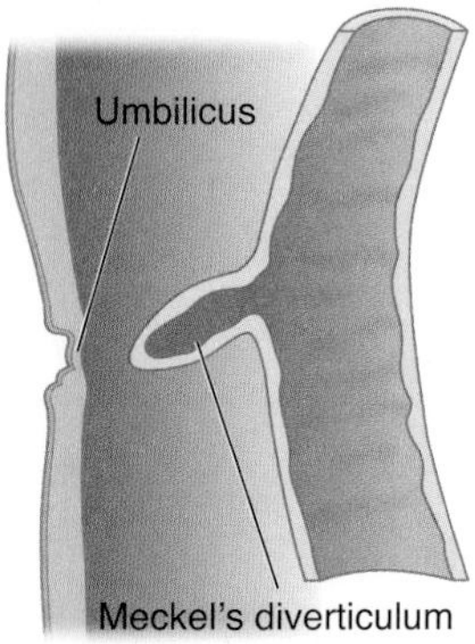

True diverticulum. Persistence of the vitelline duct. May contain ectopic acid–secreting gastric mucosa and/or pancreatic tissue. Most common congenital anomaly of the GI tract. Can cause melena, RLQ pain, intussusception, volvulus, or obstruction near the terminal ileum. Contrast with omphalomesenteric cyst = cystic dilation of vitelline duct.

Diagnosis: pertechnetate study for ectopic uptake.

The **five 2's**:
- 2 inches long.
- 2 feet from the ileocecal valve.
- 2% of population.
- Commonly presents in first 2 years of life.
- May have 2 types of epithelia (gastric/pancreatic).

Intussusception and volvulus

Intussusception

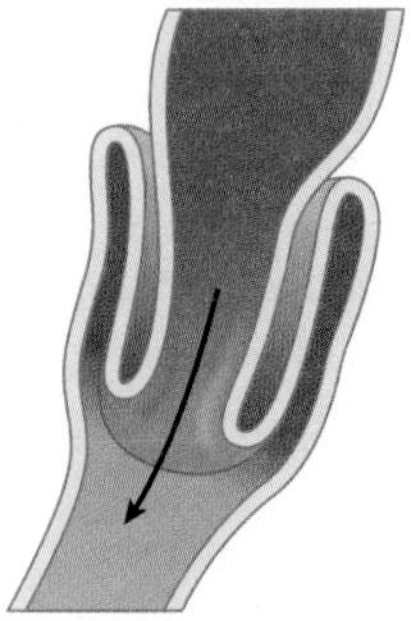

"Telescoping" of 1 bowel segment into distal segment, commonly at ileocecal junction; can cause "currant jelly" stools and compromise blood supply. Unusual in adults (associated with intraluminal mass or tumor). Majority of cases occur in children (usually idiopathic; may be viral [adenovirus]). Abdominal emergency in early childhood.

Volvulus

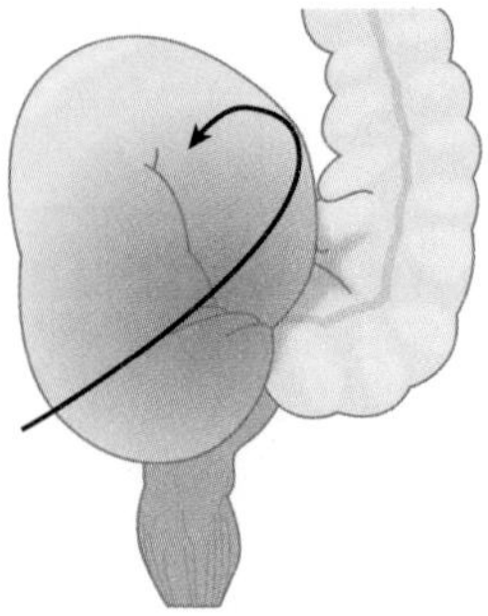

Twisting of portion of bowel around its mesentery; can lead to obstruction and infarction. May occur at cecum and sigmoid colon, where there is redundant mesentery. Usually in elderly.

Hirschsprung's disease

Congenital megacolon characterized by lack of ganglion cells/enteric nervous plexuses (Auerbach's and Meissner's plexuses) in segment on intestinal biopsy. Due to failure of neural crest cell migration.

Presents as chronic constipation early in life. Dilated portion of the colon proximal to the aganglionic segment, resulting in a "transition zone." Involves rectum. Usually failure to pass meconium.

Think of Hirsch**sprung**'s as a giant spring that has **sprung** in the colon. Risk ↑ with Down syndrome.

Diagnosed by rectal suction biopsy.

Treatment: resection.

Other intestinal disorders

Duodenal atresia	Causes early bilious vomiting with proximal stomach distention ("double bubble" on X-ray) because of failure of recanalization of small bowel. Associated with Down syndrome.
Meconium ileus	In cystic fibrosis, meconium plug obstructs intestine, preventing stool passage at birth.
Necrotizing enterocolitis	Necrosis of intestinal mucosa and possible perforation. Colon is usually involved, but can involve entire GI tract. In neonates, more common in preemies (↓ immunity).
Ischemic colitis	Reduction in intestinal blood flow causes ischemia (pain out of proportion with physical findings). Pain after eating → weight loss. Commonly occurs at splenic flexure and distal colon. Typically affects elderly.
Adhesion	Fibrous band of scar tissue; commonly forms after surgery; most common cause of small bowel obstruction. Can have well-demarcated necrotic zones.
Angiodysplasia	Tortuous dilation of vessels → hematochezia. Most often found in cecum, terminal ileum, and ascending colon. More common in older patients. Confirmed by angiography.

Colonic polyps

Masses protruding into gut lumen → sawtooth appearance. 90% are non-neoplastic. Often rectosigmoid. Can be tubular A or villous B.

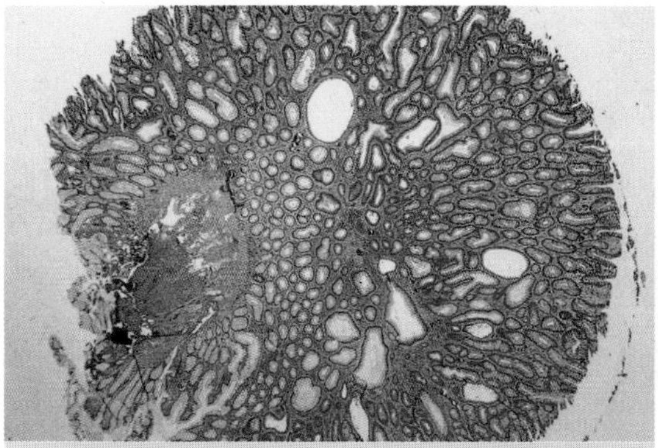

A **Tubular adenoma.** Smaller, more rounded, and more likely to be benign.

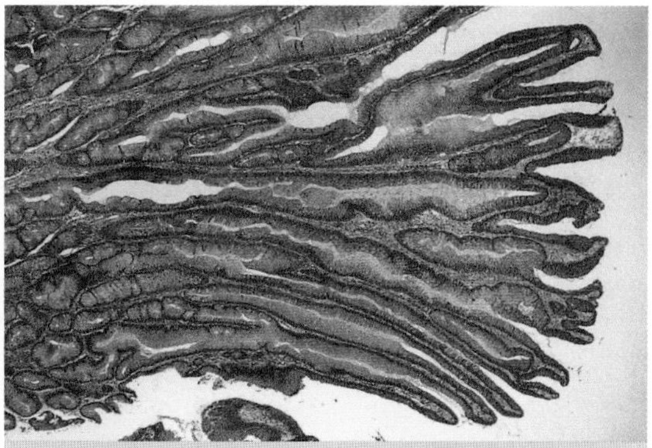

B **Villous adenoma.** Note long, finger-like projections.

Adenomatous	Adenomatous polyps are precancerous. Malignant risk is associated with ↑ size, villous histology, ↑ epithelial dysplasia. Precursor to colorectal cancer (CRC). The more villous the polyp, the more likely it is to be malignant (**villous** = **villainous**). Polyp symptoms—often asymptomatic, lower GI bleed, partial obstruction, secretory diarrhea.
Hyperplastic	Most common non-neoplastic polyp in colon (> 50% found in rectosigmoid colon).
Juvenile	Mostly sporadic lesions in children < 5 years of age. 80% in rectum. If single, no malignant potential. Juvenile polyposis syndrome—multiple juvenile polyps in GI tract, ↑ risk of adenocarcinoma.
Peutz-Jeghers	Single polyps are not malignant. Peutz-Jeghers syndrome—autosomal-dominant syndrome featuring multiple nonmalignant hamartomas throughout GI tract, along with hyperpigmented mouth, lips, hands, genitalia. Associated with ↑ risk of CRC and other visceral malignancies.

Colorectal cancer

EPIDEMIOLOGY	3rd most common cancer; 3rd most deadly in United States. Most patients are > 50 years of age. ~ 25% have a family history.
GENETICS	**Familial adenomatous polyposis (FAP)**—autosomal-dominant mutation of *APC* gene on chromosome 5q. 2-hit hypothesis. 100% progress to CRC. Thousands of polyps; pancolonic; always involves rectum. **Gardner's syndrome**—FAP + osseous and soft tissue tumors, congenital hypertrophy of retinal pigment epithelium. **Turcot's syndrome**—FAP + malignant CNS tumor. **Turc**ot = **Turb**an. **Hereditary nonpolyposis colorectal cancer (HNPCC/Lynch syndrome)**—autosomal-dominant mutation of DNA mismatch repair genes. ~ 80% progress to CRC. Proximal colon is always involved.
ADDITIONAL RISK FACTORS	IBD, tobacco use, large villous adenomas, juvenile polyposis syndrome, Peutz-Jeghers syndrome.
PRESENTATION	Rectosigmoid > ascending > descending. Ascending—exophytic mass, iron deficiency anemia, weight loss. Descending—infiltrating mass, partial obstruction, colicky pain, hematochezia. Rarely presents as *Streptococcus bovis* bacteremia.
DIAGNOSIS	Iron deficiency anemia in males (especially > 50 years of age) and postmenopausal females raises suspicion. Screen patients > 50 years of age with colonoscopy or stool occult blood test. "Apple core" lesion seen on barium enema x-ray A. CEA tumor marker: good for monitoring recurrence, not useful for screening.

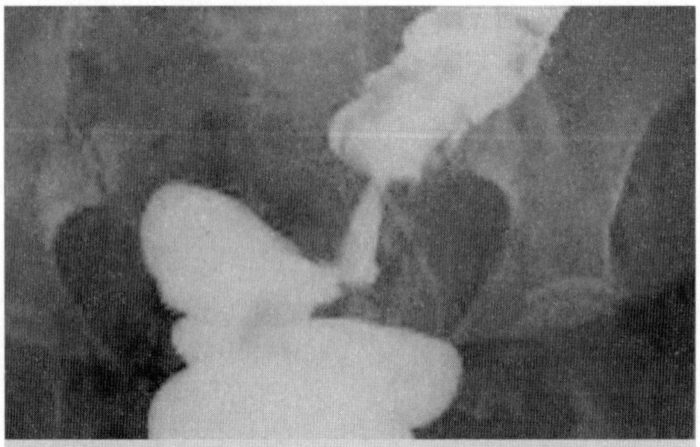

A **"Apple core" lesion.** Seen here in the sigmoid colon.

Molecular pathogenesis of CRC

There are 2 molecular pathways that lead to CRC:

- Microsatellite instability pathway (15%): DNA mismatch repair gene mutations → sporadic and HNPCC syndrome. Mutations accumulate, but no defined morphologic correlates.
- APC/β-catenin (chromosomal instability) pathway (85%):

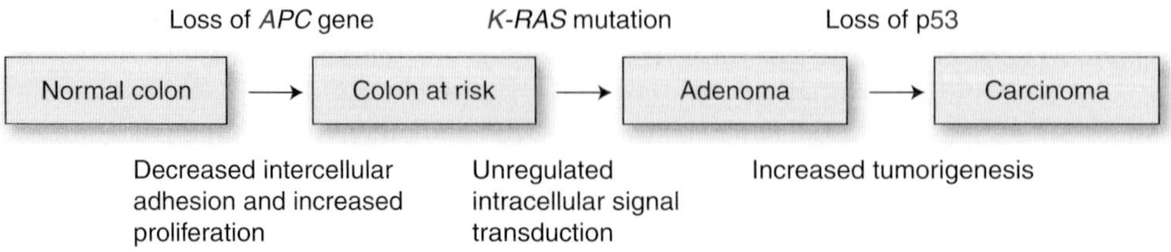
Loss of *APC* gene
K-RAS mutation
Loss of p53
Normal colon
Colon at risk
Adenoma
Carcinoma
Decreased intercellular adhesion and increased proliferation
Unregulated intracellular signal transduction
Increased tumorigenesis

Order of gene events—**AK-53**.

Carcinoid tumor

Tumor of neuroendocrine cells. Constitute 50% of small bowel tumors. Most common sites are the appendix, ileum, and rectum. Most common malignancy in the small intestine. "Dense core bodies" seen on EM. Often produce 5-HT, which can lead to carcinoid syndrome. Classic symptoms: wheezing, right-sided heart murmurs, diarrhea, flushing. If tumor is confined to GI system, no carcinoid syndrome is observed, since liver metabolizes 5-HT. If tumor or metastases (usually to liver) exist outside GI system, carcinoid syndrome is observed. Thus, tumor location determines whether the syndrome appears. Treatment: resection, octreotide, somatostatin.

Cirrhosis and portal hypertension

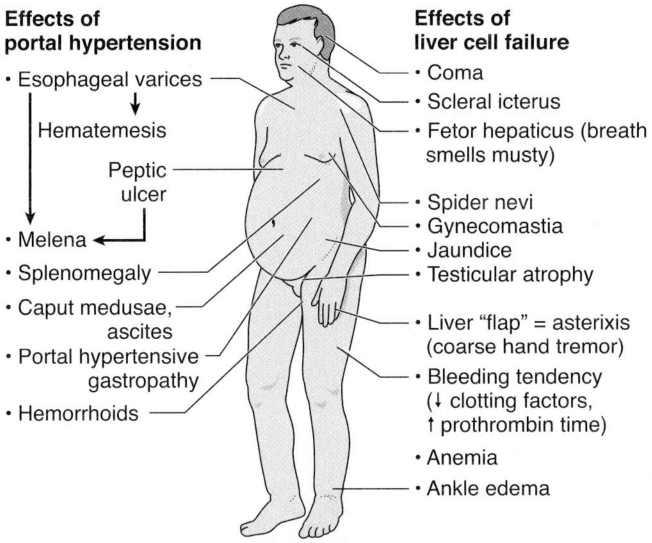

Effects of portal hypertension
• Esophageal varices
Hematemesis
Peptic ulcer
• Melena
• Splenomegaly
• Caput medusae, ascites
• Portal hypertensive gastropathy
• Hemorrhoids
Effects of liver cell failure
• Coma
• Scleral icterus
• Fetor hepaticus (breath smells musty)
• Spider nevi
• Gynecomastia
• Jaundice
• Testicular atrophy
• Liver "flap" = asterixis (coarse hand tremor)
• Bleeding tendency (↓ clotting factors, ↑ prothrombin time)
• Anemia
• Ankle edema

Cirrhosis—diffuse fibrosis and nodular regeneration destroys normal architecture of liver A B; ↑ risk for hepatocellular carcinoma.

Etiologies—alcohol (60–70%), viral hepatitis, biliary disease, hemochromatosis.

Portosystemic shunts partially alleviate portal hypertension:
- Esophageal varices
- Caput medusae

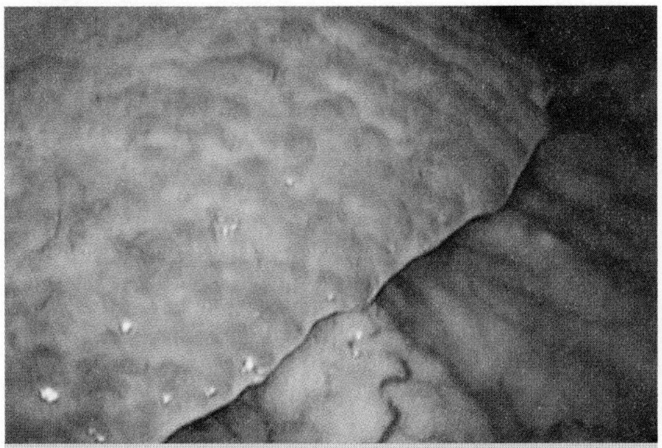

A **Cirrhosis, gross.** With regenerating macronodules.

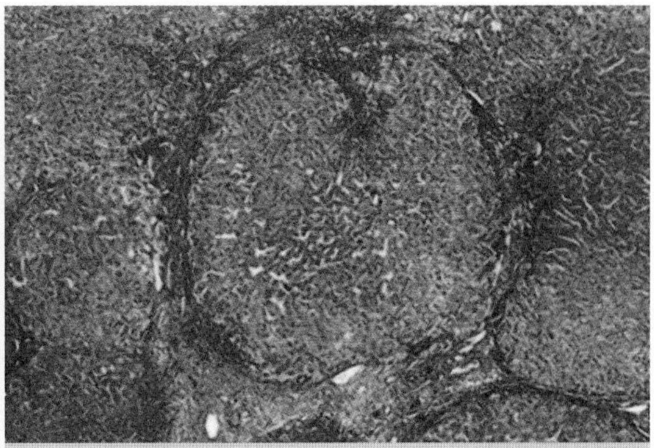

B **Cirrhosis, microscopic.** Typical regenerative nodules and bridging fibrosis.

Serum markers of liver and pancreas pathology

SERUM MARKER	MAJOR DIAGNOSTIC USE
Aminotransferases (AST and ALT) (often called "liver enzymes")	Viral hepatitis (ALT > AST) Alcoholic hepatitis (AST > ALT)
Alkaline phosphatase (ALP)	Obstructive liver disease (hepatocellular carcinoma), bone disease, bile duct disease
γ-glutamyl transpeptidase (GGT)	↑ in various liver and biliary diseases like ALP, but **not** in bone disease.
Amylase	Acute pancreatitis, mumps
Lipase	Acute pancreatitis
Ceruloplasmin	↓ in Wilson's disease

Reye's syndrome

Rare, often fatal childhood hepatoencephalopathy. Findings: mitochondrial abnormalities, fatty liver (microvesicular fatty change), hypoglycemia, vomiting, hepatomegaly, coma. Associated with viral infection (especially VZV and influenza B) that has been treated with aspirin. Mechanism: aspirin metabolites ↓ β-oxidation by reversible inhibition of mitochondrial enzyme. Avoid aspirin in children, except in those with Kawasaki's disease.

Alcoholic liver disease

Hepatic steatosis

Short-term change with moderate alcohol intake.

Macrovesicular fatty change that may be reversible with alcohol cessation A.

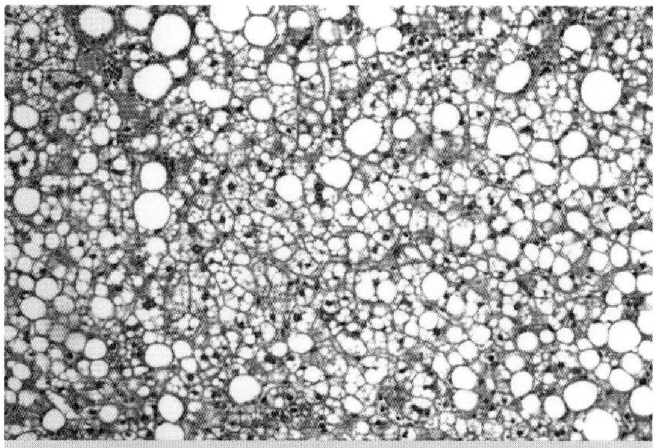

A **Macrovesicular steatosis.** Hepatocytes filled with fat droplets.

Alcoholic hepatitis

Requires sustained, long-term consumption. Swollen and necrotic hepatocytes with neutrophilic infiltration. Mallory bodies (intracytoplasmic eosinophilic inclusions) are present.

Make a to**AST** with alcohol: **AST** > ALT (ratio usually > 1.5).

Alcoholic cirrhosis

Final and irreversible form. Micronodular, irregularly shrunken liver with "hobnail" appearance. Sclerosis around central vein (zone III). Has manifestations of chronic liver disease (e.g., jaundice, hypoalbuminemia).

Hepatocellular carcinoma/hepatoma	Most common 1° malignant tumor of the liver in adults. ↑ incidence is associated with hepatitis B and C, Wilson's disease, hemochromatosis, α_1-antitrypsin deficiency, alcoholic cirrhosis, and carcinogens (e.g., aflatoxin from *Aspergillus*). Findings: jaundice, tender hepatomegaly, ascites, polycythemia, and hypoglycemia.	Commonly spread by hematogenous dissemination. ↑ α-fetoprotein. May lead to Budd-Chiari syndrome.

Other liver tumors

Cavernous hemangioma	Common, benign liver tumor; typically occurs at age 30–50 years. Biopsy contraindicated because of risk of hemorrhage.
Hepatic adenoma	Benign liver tumor, often related to oral contraceptive or steroid use; can regress spontaneously.
Angiosarcoma	Malignant tumor of endothelial origin; associated with exposure to arsenic, polyvinyl chloride.

Nutmeg liver

Due to backup of blood into liver. Commonly caused by right-sided heart failure and Budd-Chiari syndrome. The liver appears mottled like a nutmeg. If the condition persists, centrilobular congestion and necrosis can result in cardiac cirrhosis.

Budd-Chiari syndrome

Occlusion of IVC or hepatic veins with centrilobular congestion and necrosis, leading to congestive liver disease (hepatomegaly, ascites, abdominal pain, and eventual liver failure). May develop varices and have visible abdominal and back veins. Absence of JVD. Associated with hypercoagulable state, polycythemia vera, pregnancy, and hepatocellular carcinoma.

α_1-antitrypsin deficiency

Misfolded gene product protein aggregates in hepatocellular ER → cirrhosis with PAS-positive globules in liver. In lungs, lack of functioning enzyme → ↓ elastic tissue → panacinar emphysema. Codominant trait.

Jaundice

Yellow skin and/or sclerae resulting from elevated bilirubin. Caused by:
- Direct hepatocellular injury
- Obstruction to bile flow
- Hemolysis

JAUNDICE TYPE	HYPERBILIRUBINEMIA	URINE BILIRUBIN	URINE UROBILINOGEN
Hepatocellular	Direct/indirect	↑	Normal/↓
Obstructive	Direct	↑	↓
Hemolytic	Indirect	Absent (acholuria)	↑

Physiologic neonatal jaundice

At birth, immature UDP-glucuronyl transferase → unconjugated hyperbilirubinemia → jaundice/kernicterus.

Treatment: phototherapy (converts UCB to water-soluble form).

Hereditary hyperbilirubinemias

Gilbert's syndrome	Mildly ↓ UDP-glucuronyl transferase or ↓ bilirubin uptake. Asymptomatic. Elevated unconjugated bilirubin without overt hemolysis. Bilirubin increases with fasting and stress.	No clinical consequences.
Crigler-Najjar syndrome, type I	Absent UDP-glucuronyl transferase. Presents early in life; patients die within a few years. Findings: jaundice, kernicterus (bilirubin deposition in brain), ↑ unconjugated bilirubin. Treatment: plasmapheresis and phototherapy.	Type II is less severe and responds to phenobarbital, which ↑ liver enzyme synthesis.
Dubin-Johnson syndrome	Conjugated hyperbilirubinemia due to defective liver excretion. Grossly black liver. Benign.	Rotor's syndrome is similar but even milder and does not cause black liver.

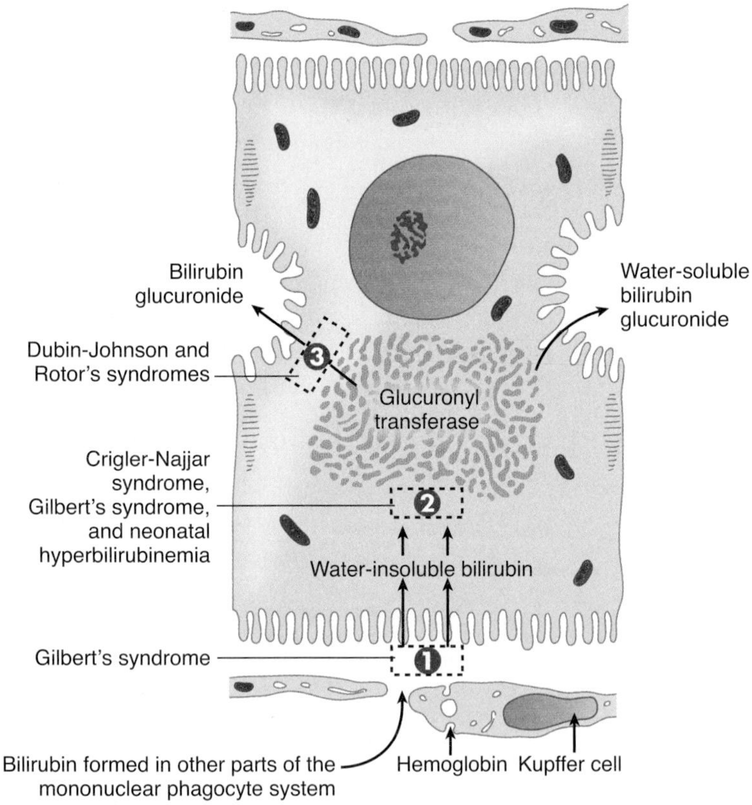
Bilirubin glucuronide
Water-soluble bilirubin glucuronide
Dubin-Johnson and Rotor's syndromes
3
Glucuronyl transferase
Crigler-Najjar syndrome, Gilbert's syndrome, and neonatal hyperbilirubinemia
2
Water-insoluble bilirubin
Gilbert's syndrome
1
Bilirubin formed in other parts of the mononuclear phagocyte system
Hemoglobin
Kupffer cell

(Adapted, with permission, from Junqueira LC, Carneiro J. *Basic Histology,* 11th ed. New York: McGraw-Hill, 2005: 335.)

❶ **Gilbert's** = problem with bilirubin uptake → unconjugated bilirubinemia

❷ **Crigler-Najjar** = problem with bilirubin conjugation → unconjugated bilirubinemia

❸ **Dubin-Johnson** = problem with excretion of conjugated bilirubin → conjugated bilirubinemia

Wilson's disease (hepatolenticular degeneration)

Inadequate hepatic copper excretion and failure of copper to enter circulation as ceruloplasmin. Leads to **copper** accumulation, especially in liver, brain, cornea, kidneys, and joints.

Characterized by:

- **C**eruloplasmin ↓, **C**irrhosis, **C**orneal deposits (Kayser-Fleischer rings) A, **C**opper accumulation, **C**arcinoma (hepatocellular)
- **H**emolytic anemia
- **B**asal ganglia degeneration (parkinsonian symptoms)
- **A**sterixis
- **D**ementia, **D**yskinesia, **D**ysarthria

Treat with penicillamine. Autosomal-recessive inheritance (chromosome 13). Copper is normally excreted into bile by hepatocyte copper transporting ATPase (*ATP7B* gene).

"Copper is **H**ella **BAD**."

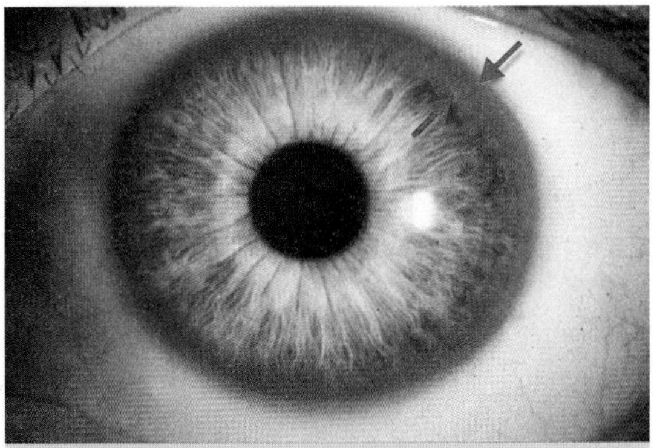

A **Kayser-Fleischer ring.** Note golden brown corneal ring (arrows).

Hemochromatosis

Hemosiderosis is the deposition of hemosiderin (iron); hemochromatosis is the disease caused by this iron deposition. Classic triad of micronodular **C**irrhosis, **D**iabetes mellitus, and skin pigmentation → "bronze" diabetes. Results in CHF, testicular atrophy in males, and ↑ risk of hepatocellular carcinoma. Disease may be 1° (autosomal recessive) or 2° to chronic transfusion therapy (e.g., β-thalassemia major). ↑ ferritin, ↑ iron, ↓ TIBC → ↑ transferrin saturation.

Hemochromatosis **C**an **C**ause **D**eposits.

Total body iron may reach 50 g, enough to set off metal detectors at airports.

Primary hemochromatosis due to C282Y or H63D mutation on *HFE* gene. Associated with HLA-A3.

Treatment of hereditary hemochromatosis: repeated phlebotomy, deferasirox, deferoxamine.

Biliary tract disease

	Secondary biliary cirrhosis	Primary biliary cirrhosis	Primary sclerosing cholangitis
PATHOPHYSIOLOGY/ PATHOLOGY	Extrahepatic biliary obstruction (gallstone, biliary stricture, chronic pancreatitis, carcinoma of the pancreatic head) → ↑ pressure in intrahepatic ducts → injury/ fibrosis and bile stasis.	Autoimmune reaction → lymphocytic infiltrate + granulomas.	Unknown cause of concentric "onion skin" bile duct fibrosis → alternating strictures and dilation with "beading" of intra- and extrahepatic bile ducts on ERCP.
PRESENTATION	Pruritus, jaundice, dark urine, light stools, hepatosplenomegaly.	Same.	Same.
LABS	↑ conjugated bilirubin, ↑ cholesterol, ↑ alkaline phosphatase.	Same.	Same.
ADDITIONAL INFORMATION	Complicated by ascending cholangitis.	↑ serum mitochondrial antibodies, including IgM. Associated with other autoimmune conditions (e.g., CREST, rheumatoid arthritis, celiac disease).	Hypergammaglobulinemia (IgM). Associated with ulcerative colitis. Can lead to 2° biliary cirrhosis.

Gallstones (cholelithiasis)

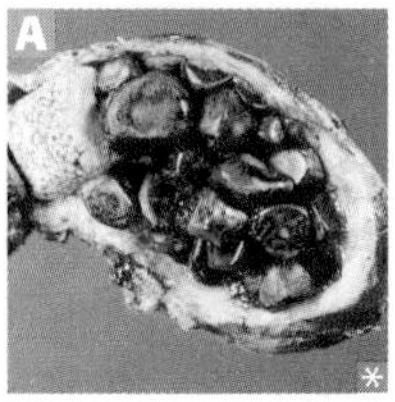

↑ cholesterol and/or bilirubin, ↓ bile salts, and gallbladder stasis all cause stones A.

2 types of stones:

- Cholesterol stones (radiolucent with 10–20% opaque due to calcifications)—80% of stones. Associated with obesity, Crohn's disease, cystic fibrosis, advanced age, clofibrate, estrogens, multiparity, rapid weight loss, and Native American origin.
- Pigment stones (radiopaque)—seen in patients with chronic hemolysis, alcoholic cirrhosis, advanced age, and biliary infection. Black—hemolysis; brown—infection.

Most often causes cholecystitis; also ascending cholangitis, acute pancreatitis, bile stasis.

Can also lead to **biliary colic**—neurohormonal activation (e.g., by CCK after a fatty meal) triggers contraction of the gallbladder, forcing a stone into the cystic duct. May present without pain (e.g., in diabetics).

Can cause fistula between gallbladder and small intestine, leading to air in the biliary tree. If gallstone obstructs ileocecal valve (gallstone ileus), air can be seen in biliary tree on imaging.

Diagnose with ultrasound, radionuclide biliary scan (HIDA). Treat with cholecystectomy.

Risk factors (**4 F's**):

1. **F**emale
2. **F**at
3. **F**ertile (pregnant)
4. **F**orty

Charcot's triad of cholangitis:

- Jaundice
- Fever
- RUQ pain

Positive Murphy's sign—inspiratory arrest on deep RUQ palpation due to pain.

Cholecystitis

Inflammation of gallbladder. Usually from gallstones; rarely ischemia or infectious (CMV). ↑ alkaline phosphatase if bile duct becomes involved (e.g., ascending cholangitis).

Acute pancreatitis

Autodigestion of pancreas by pancreatic enzymes.

Causes: idiopathic, **G**allstones, **E**thanol, **T**rauma, **S**teroids, **M**umps, **A**utoimmune disease, **S**corpion sting, **H**ypercalcemia/**H**ypertriglyceridemia (> 1000), **E**RCP, **D**rugs (e.g., sulfa drugs).

Clinical presentation: epigastric abdominal pain radiating to back, anorexia, nausea.

Labs: elevated amylase, lipase (higher specificity).

Can lead to DIC, ARDS, diffuse fat necrosis, hypocalcemia (Ca^{2+} collects in pancreatic calcium soap deposits), pseudocyst formation, hemorrhage, infection, and multiorgan failure.

Complication: pancreatic pseudocyst (lined by granulation tissue, not epithelium; can rupture and hemorrhage).

GET SMASHED.

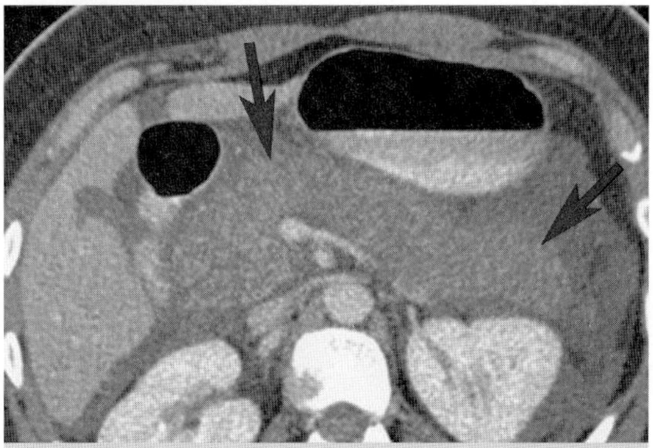

A **Acute pancreatitis.** With peri-pancreatic edema (arrows).

Chronic pancreatitis	Chronic inflammation, atrophy, calcification of the pancreas. Major causes are alcohol abuse and idiopathic. Can lead to pancreatic insufficiency → steatorrhea, fat-soluble vitamin deficiency, diabetes mellitus, and ↑ risk of pancreatic adenocarcinoma. Amylase and lipase are less elevated (compared to levels in acute pancreatitis).
Pancreatic adenocarcinoma	Prognosis averages 6 months or less; very aggressive tumor arising from pancreatic ducts; usually already metastasized at presentation; tumors more common in pancreatic head (→ obstructive jaundice). Associated with CA-19-9 tumor marker (also CEA, less specific). Risk factors: ▪ Tobacco use (but not EtOH) ▪ Chronic pancreatitis (especially > 20 years) ▪ Age > 50 years ▪ Jewish and African-American males Often presents with: ▪ Abdominal pain radiating to back ▪ Weight loss (due to malabsorption and anorexia) ▪ Migratory thrombophlebitis—redness and tenderness on palpation of extremities (**Trousseau's syndrome**) ▪ Obstructive jaundice with palpable, nontender gallbladder (Courvoisier's sign) Treatment: Whipple procedure, chemotherapy, radiation therapy.

▸ GASTROINTESTINAL–PHARMACOLOGY

GI therapy

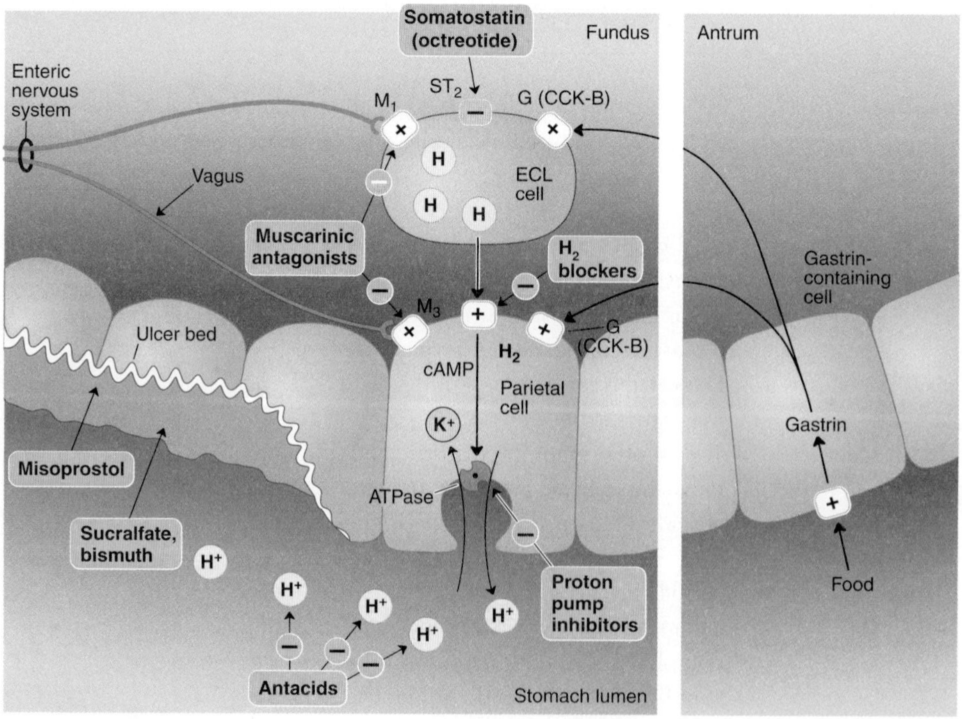

(Adapted, with permission, from Katzung BG, Trevor AJ. *USMLE Road Map: Pharmacology,* 1st ed. New York: McGraw-Hill, 2003: 159.)

H_2 blockers	Cimetidine, ranitidine, famotidine, nizatidine.	Take H_2 blockers before you **dine**. Think "**table for 2**" to remember H_2.
MECHANISM	Reversible block of histamine H_2-receptors → ↓ H^+ secretion by parietal cells.	
CLINICAL USE	Peptic ulcer, gastritis, mild esophageal reflux.	
TOXICITY	Cimetidine is a potent inhibitor of cytochrome P-450 (multiple drug interactions); it also has antiandrogenic effects (prolactin release, gynecomastia, impotence, ↓ libido in males); can cross blood-brain barrier (confusion, dizziness, headaches) and placenta. Both cimetidine and ranitidine ↓ renal excretion of creatinine. Other H_2 blockers are relatively free of these effects.	

Proton pump inhibitors	Omeprazole, lansoprazole, esomeprazole, pantoprazole, dexlansoprazole.
MECHANISM	Irreversibly inhibit H^+/K^+ ATPase in stomach parietal cells.
CLINICAL USE	Peptic ulcer, gastritis, esophageal reflux, Zollinger-Ellison syndrome.
TOXICITY	Increased risk of *C. difficile* infection, pneumonia. Hip fractures, ↓ serum Mg^{2+} with long-term use.

Bismuth, sucralfate	
MECHANISM	Bind to ulcer base, providing physical protection and allowing HCO_3^- secretion to reestablish pH gradient in the mucous layer.
CLINICAL USE	↑ ulcer healing, traveler's diarrhea.

Misoprostol	
MECHANISM	A PGE_1 analog. ↑ production and secretion of gastric mucous barrier, ↓ acid production.
CLINICAL USE	Prevention of NSAID-induced peptic ulcers; maintenance of a patent ductus arteriosus. Also used to induce labor (ripens cervix).
TOXICITY	Diarrhea. Contraindicated in women of childbearing potential (abortifacient).

Octreotide	
MECHANISM	Long-acting somatostatin analog.
CLINICAL USE	Acute variceal bleeds, acromegaly, VIPoma, and carcinoid tumors.
TOXICITY	Nausea, cramps, steatorrhea.

Antacid use	Can affect absorption, bioavailability, or urinary excretion of other drugs by altering gastric and urinary pH or by delaying gastric emptying. All can cause hypokalemia. Overuse can also cause the following problems.	
Aluminum hydroxide	Constipation and hypophosphatemia; proximal muscle weakness, osteodystrophy, seizures	**Aluminimum** amount of feces.
Magnesium hydroxide	Diarrhea, hyporeflexia, hypotension, cardiac arrest	**Mg** = **M**ust **g**o to the bathroom.
Calcium carbonate	Hypercalcemia, rebound acid ↑	Can chelate and ↓ effectiveness of other drugs (e.g., tetracycline).

Osmotic laxatives	Magnesium hydroxide, magnesium citrate, polyethylene glycol, lactulose.
MECHANISM	Provide osmotic load to draw water out. Lactulose also treats hepatic encephalopathy since gut flora degrade it into metabolites (lactic acid and acetic acid) that promote nitrogen excretion as NH_4^+.
CLINICAL USE	Constipation.
TOXICITY	Diarrhea, dehydration; may be abused by bulimics.

Infliximab	
MECHANISM	Monoclonal antibody to TNF-α.
CLINICAL USE	Crohn's disease, ulcerative colitis, rheumatoid arthritis.
TOXICITY	Infection (including reactivation of latent TB), fever, hypotension.

Sulfasalazine	
MECHANISM	A combination of sulfapyridine (antibacterial) and 5-aminosalicylic acid (anti-inflammatory). Activated by colonic bacteria.
CLINICAL USE	Ulcerative colitis, Crohn's disease.
TOXICITY	Malaise, nausea, sulfonamide toxicity, reversible oligospermia.

Ondansetron		
MECHANISM	$5\text{-}HT_3$ antagonist. Powerful central-acting antiemetic.	At a party but feeling queasy? Keep **on dancing** with **ondans**etron!
CLINICAL USE	Control vomiting postoperatively and in patients undergoing cancer chemotherapy.	
TOXICITY	Headache, constipation.	

Metoclopramide	
MECHANISM	D_2 receptor antagonist. ↑ resting tone, contractility, LES tone, motility. Does not influence colon transport time.
CLINICAL USE	Diabetic and post-surgery gastroparesis, antiemetic.
TOXICITY	↑ parkinsonian effects. Restlessness, drowsiness, fatigue, depression, nausea, diarrhea. Drug interaction with digoxin and diabetic agents. Contraindicated in patients with small bowel obstruction or Parkinson's disease.

HIGH-YIELD SYSTEMS

Hematology and Oncology

"Of all that is written, I love only what a person has written with his own blood."

—Friedrich Nietzsche

"I used to get stressed out, but my cancer has put everything into perspective."

—Delta Goodrem

"The best blood will at some time get into a fool or a mosquito."

—Austin O'Malley

Study tip: When reviewing oncologic drugs, focus on mechanisms and side effects, rather than details of clinical uses, which may be lower yield.

▶ HEMATOLOGY AND ONCOLOGY—ANATOMY

Erythrocyte

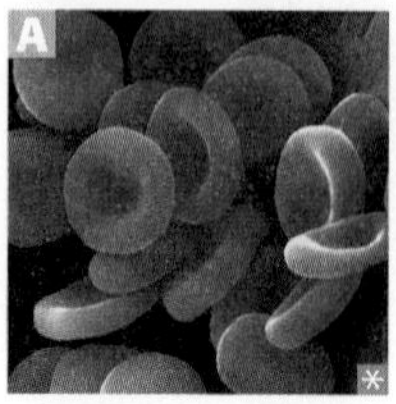

Carries O_2 to tissues and CO_2 to lungs. Anucleate and biconcave A, with large surface area-to-volume ratio for rapid gas exchange. Life span of 120 days. Source of energy is glucose (90% used in glycolysis, 10% used in HMP shunt). Membrane contains chloride-HCO_3^- antiporter, which allows RBCs to sequester HCO_3^- and transport CO_2 from the periphery to the lungs for elimination.

Eryth = red; *cyte* = cell.

Erythrocytosis = polycythemia = ↑ hematocrit.
Anisocytosis = varying sizes.
Poikilocytosis = varying shapes.

Reticulocyte = immature erythrocyte, marker of erythroid proliferation.

Platelet (thrombocyte)

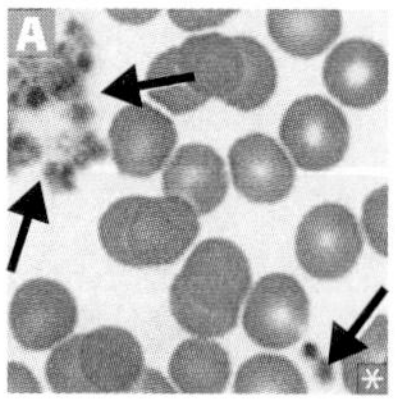

Involved in 1° hemostasis. Small cytoplasmic fragment derived from megakaryocytes A. Life span of 8–10 days. When activated by endothelial injury, aggregates with other platelets and interacts with fibrin to form platelet plug. Contains dense granules (ADP, calcium) and α granules (vWF, fibrinogen). Approximately ⅓ of platelet pool is stored in the spleen.

Thrombocytopenia or platelet dysfunction results in petechiae.
vWF receptor: GpIb.
Fibrinogen receptor: GpIIb/IIIa.

Leukocyte

Divided into granulocytes (neutrophil, eosinophil, basophil) and mononuclear cells (monocytes, lymphocytes). Responsible for defense against infections. Normally 4000–10,000 cells/mm^3.

Leuk = white; *cyte* = cell.

Blood cell differentiation

WBC differential from highest to lowest (per USMLE):
- Neutrophils (54–62%)
- Lymphocytes (25–33%)
- Monocytes (3–7%)
- Eosinophils (1–3%)
- Basophils (0–0.75%)

Neutrophils **L**ike **M**aking **E**verything **B**etter.

Neutrophil 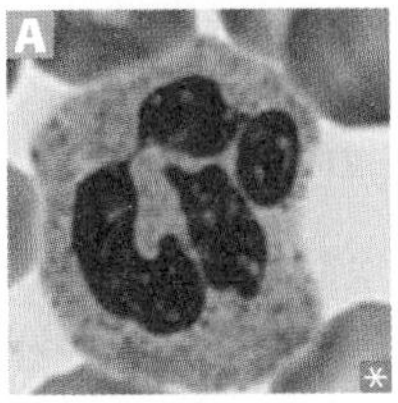	Acute inflammatory response cell. Increased in bacterial infections. Phagocytic. Multilobed nucleus A. Small, more numerous specific granules contain alkaline phosphatase, collagenase, lysozyme, and lactoferrin. Larger, less numerous azurophilic granules (lysosomes) contain acid phosphatase, peroxidase, and β-glucuronidase.	Hypersegmented polys (5 or more lobes) are seen in vitamin B_{12}/ folate deficiency. ↑ band cells (immature neutrophils) reflect states of increased myeloid proliferation (bacterial infections, CML).
Monocyte 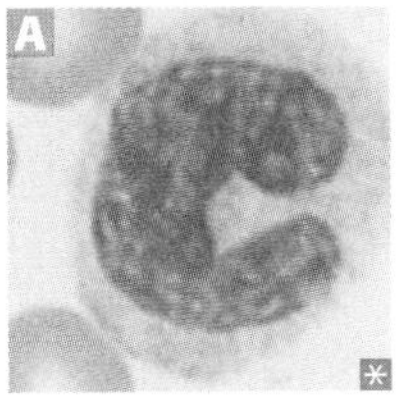	Differentiates into macrophages in tissues. Large, kidney-shaped nucleus A. Extensive "frosted glass" cytoplasm.	*Mono* = one (nucleus); *cyte* = cell. Monocyte: in the blood.
Macrophage 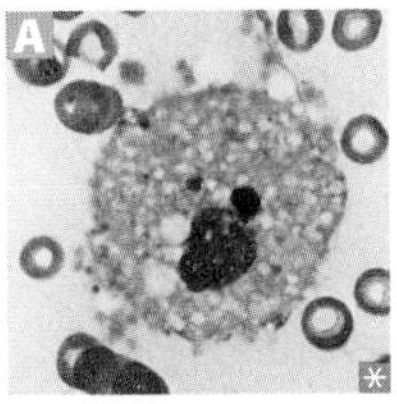	Phagocytoses bacteria, cell debris, and senescent RBCs and scavenges damaged cells and tissues A. Long life in tissues. Macrophages differentiate from circulating blood monocytes. Activated by γ-interferon. Can function as antigen-presenting cell via MHC II. CD14 is a cell surface marker for macrophages.	*Macro* = large; *phage* = eater. Macrophage: in the tissue.
Eosinophil 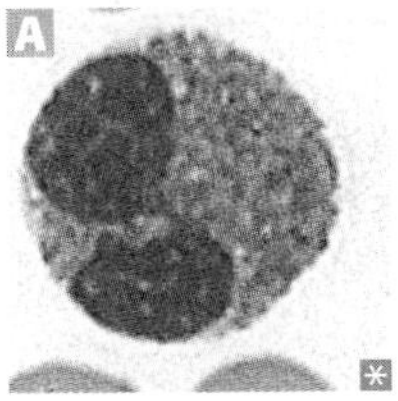	Defends against helminthic infections (major basic protein). Bilobate nucleus A. Packed with large eosinophilic granules of uniform size. Highly phagocytic for antigen-antibody complexes. Produces histaminase and arylsulfatase (helps limit reaction following mast cell degranulation).	*Eosin* = a dye; *philic* = loving. Causes of eosinophilia = **NAACP**: **N**eoplastic **A**sthma **A**llergic processes **C**ollagen vascular diseases **P**arasites (invasive)
Basophil 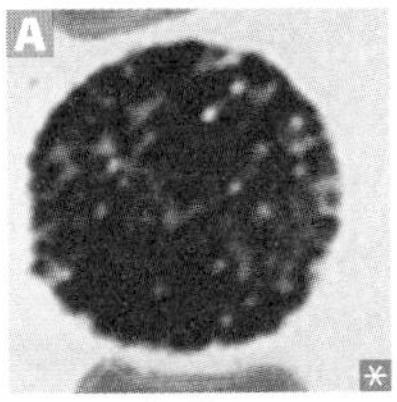	Mediates allergic reaction. Densely basophilic granules A containing heparin (anticoagulant), histamine (vasodilator), and leukotrienes (LTD_4).	Basophilic—staining readily with **basic** stains.

Mast cell 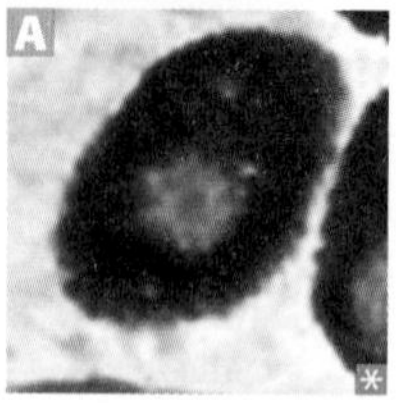	Mediates allergic reaction in local tissues. Mast cells resemble basophils structurally and functionally but are not the same cell type A. Can bind the Fc portion of IgE to membrane. IgE cross-links upon antigen binding, causing degranulation, which releases histamine, heparin, and eosinophil chemotactic factors.	Involved in type I hypersensitivity reactions. Cromolyn sodium prevents mast cell degranulation (used for asthma prophylaxis).
Dendritic cells 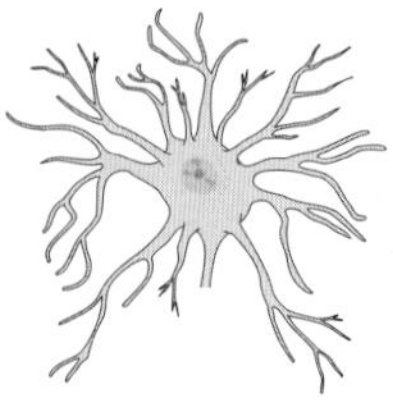	Highly phagocytic antigen-presenting cells (APCs). Function as link between innate and adaptive immune system. Express MHC class II and Fc receptor on surface. Called Langerhans cells in the skin.	
Lymphocyte 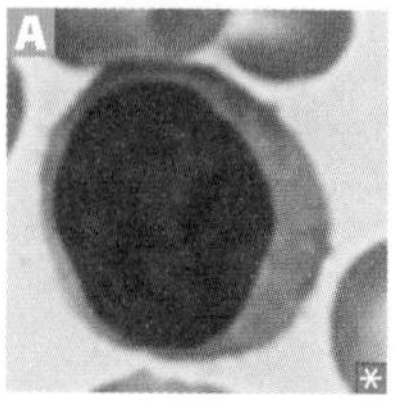	Mediates adaptive immunity. Divided into B cells and T cells. Round, densely staining nucleus with small amount of pale cytoplasm A.	
B lymphocyte 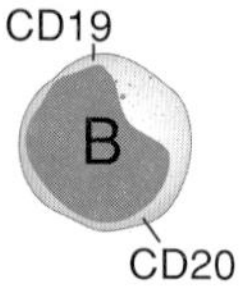	Part of humoral immune response. Arises from stem cells in bone marrow. Matures in marrow. Migrates to peripheral lymphoid tissue (follicles of lymph nodes, white pulp of spleen, unencapsulated lymphoid tissue). When antigen is encountered, B cells differentiate into plasma cells that produce antibodies, and memory cells. Can function as an APC via MHC II.	B = Bone marrow.
Plasma cell 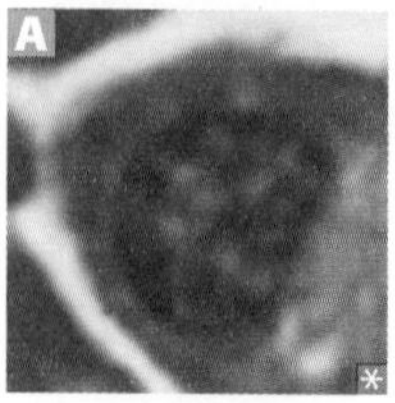	Produces large amounts of antibody specific to a particular antigen. Off-center nucleus, clock-face chromatin distribution, abundant RER, and well-developed Golgi apparatus A.	Multiple myeloma is a plasma cell cancer.

T lymphocyte 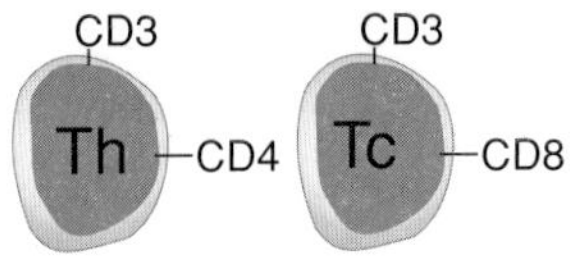	Mediates cellular immune response. Originates from stem cells in the bone marrow, but matures in the thymus. T cells differentiate into cytotoxic T cells (express CD8, recognize MHC I), helper T cells (express CD4, recognize MHC II), and regulatory T cells. CD28 (costimulatory signal) necessary for T-cell activation. The majority of circulating lymphocytes are T cells (80%).	**T** is for **T**hymus. **CD** is for **C**luster of **D**ifferentiation. **MHC × CD = 8** (e.g., MHC 2 × CD4 = 8, and MHC 1 × CD8 = 8).

▸ HEMATOLOGY AND ONCOLOGY—PHYSIOLOGY

Blood groups

A	A antigen on RBC surface and anti-B antibody in plasma.	Incompatible blood transfusions can cause immunologic response, hemolysis, renal failure, shock, and death. Note: anti-A and anti-B antibodies—IgM (do not cross placenta); anti-Rh—IgG (cross placenta).
B	B antigen on RBC surface and anti-A antibody in plasma.	
AB	A and B antigens on RBC surface; no antibodies in plasma; "universal recipient" of RBCs, "universal donor" of plasma.	
O	Neither A nor B antigen on RBC surface; both antibodies in plasma; "universal donor" of RBCs, "universal recipient" of plasma.	
Rh	Rh antigen on RBC surface. Rh– mothers exposed to fetal Rh+ blood (often during delivery) may make anti-Rh IgG. In subsequent pregnancies, anti-Rh IgG crosses the placenta, causing hemolytic disease of the newborn (erythroblastosis fetalis) in the next fetus that is Rh+.	Treatment: Rho(D) immune globulin for mother at first delivery to prevent initial sensitization of Rh– mother to Rh antigen.

Coagulation, complement, and kinin pathways

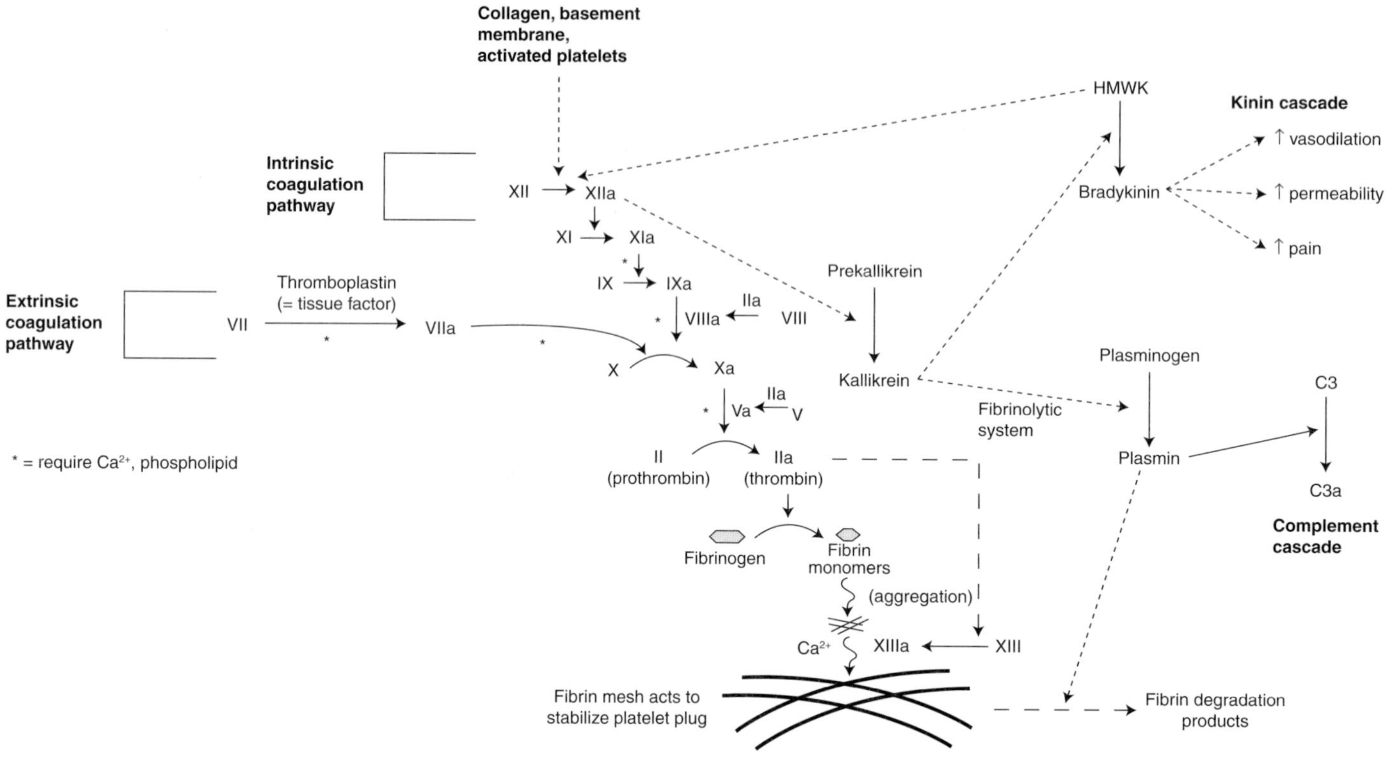

Note. Kallikrein activates bradykinin; ACE inactivates bradykinin.

Hemophilia A: deficiency of factor VIII.
Hemophilia B: deficiency of factor IX.

Coagulation cascade components

Procoagulation

Oxidized vitamin K —(epoxide reductase)→ reduced vitamin K —(acts as cofactor)→ + precursors of II, VII, IX, X, C, S → mature II, VII, IX, X, C, S

Warfarin inhibits epoxide reductase. Neonates lack enteric bacteria, which produce vitamin K.

Vitamin K deficiency: ↓ synthesis of factors II, VII, IX, X, protein C, protein S.

vWF carries/protects VIII.

Anticoagulation

Protein C —(thrombomodulin (endothelial cells))→ activated protein C —(Protein S)→ cleaves and inactivates Va, VIIIa

Plasminogen —(tPA)→ plasmin → cleavage of fibrin mesh

Antithrombin inhibits activated forms of factors II, VII, IX, X, XI, XII.

Heparin activates antithrombin.

Factor V Leiden mutation produces a factor V resistant to inhibition by activated protein C.

tPA is used clinically as a thrombolytic.

Platelet plug formation

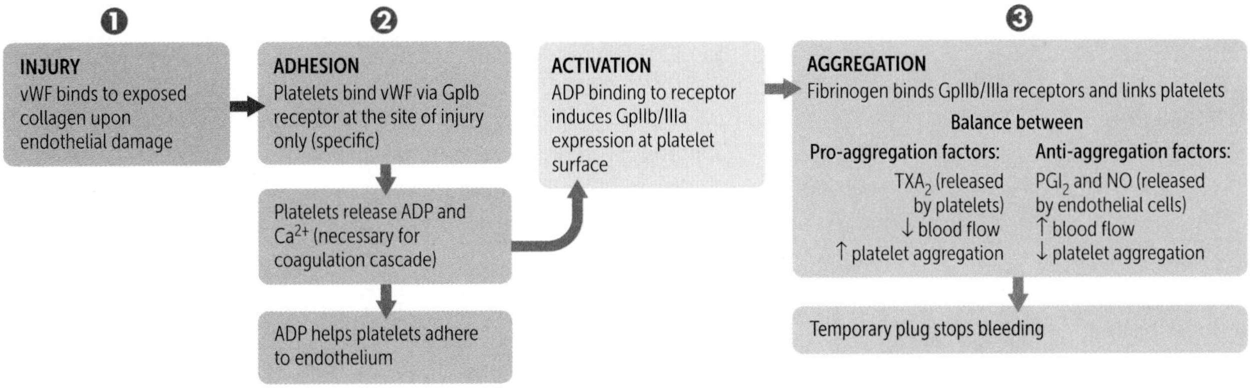

❶
INJURY
vWF binds to exposed collagen upon endothelial damage
❷
ADHESION
Platelets bind vWF via GpIb receptor at the site of injury only (specific)
Platelets release ADP and Ca^{2+} (necessary for coagulation cascade)
ADP helps platelets adhere to endothelium
ACTIVATION
ADP binding to receptor induces GpIIb/IIIa expression at platelet surface
❸
AGGREGATION
Fibrinogen binds GpIIb/IIIa receptors and links platelets
Balance between
Pro-aggregation factors:
TXA_2 (released by platelets)
↓ blood flow
↑ platelet aggregation
Anti-aggregation factors:
PGI_2 and NO (released by endothelial cells)
↑ blood flow
↓ platelet aggregation
Temporary plug stops bleeding

Thrombogenesis

Formation of insoluble fibrin mesh.

Aspirin inhibits cyclooxygenase (TXA_2 synthesis).

Ticlopidine and clopidogrel inhibit ADP-induced expression of GpIIb/IIIa.

Abciximab inhibits GpIIb/IIIa directly.

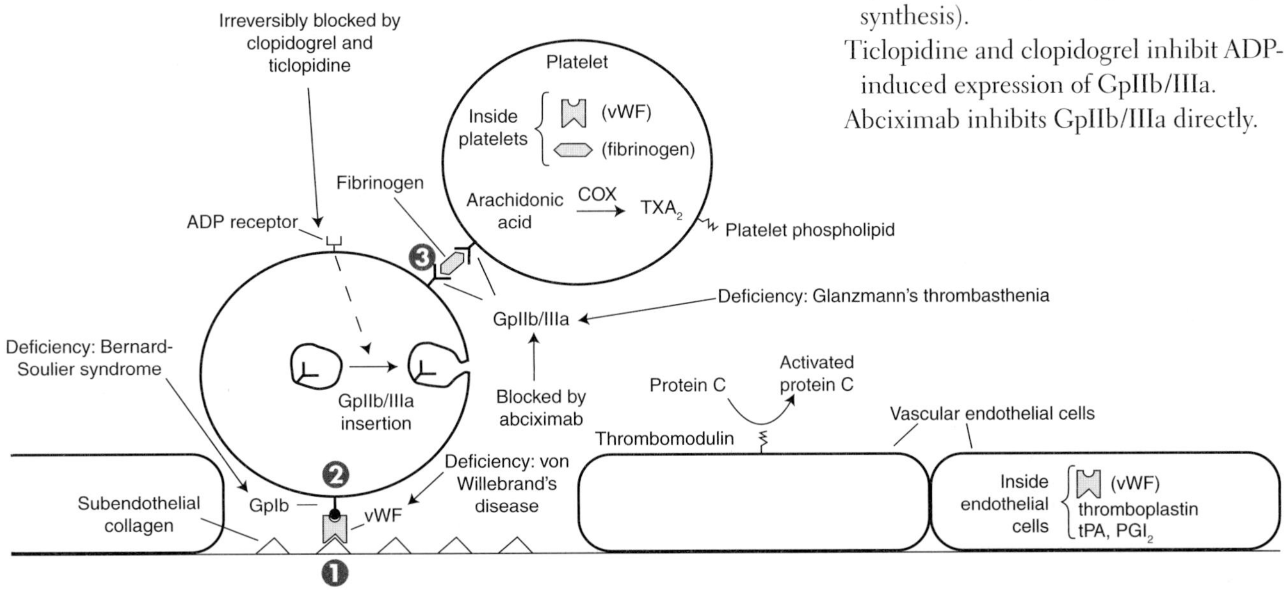

Irreversibly blocked by clopidogrel and ticlopidine
Platelet
Inside platelets
(vWF)
(fibrinogen)
Fibrinogen
Arachidonic acid
COX
TXA_2
Platelet phospholipid
ADP receptor
❸
GpIIb/IIIa
Deficiency: Glanzmann's thrombasthenia
Deficiency: Bernard-Soulier syndrome
GpIIb/IIIa insertion
Blocked by abciximab
Protein C
Activated protein C
Vascular endothelial cells
Thrombomodulin
Deficiency: von Willebrand's disease
❷
Subendothelial collagen
GpIb
vWF
Inside endothelial cells
(vWF)
thromboplastin
tPA, PGI_2
❶

Erythrocyte sedimentation rate

Acute-phase reactants in plasma (e.g., fibrinogen) can cause RBC aggregation, thereby ↑ RBC sedimentation rate (RBC aggregates have a higher density than plasma).

↑ ESR → infections, autoimmune diseases (e.g., SLE, rheumatoid arthritis, temporal arteritis), malignant neoplasms, GI disease (ulcerative colitis), pregnancy.

↓ ESR → polycythemia, sickle cell anemia, congestive heart failure, microcytosis, hypofibrinogenemia.

▶ HEMATOLOGY AND ONCOLOGY–PATHOLOGY

Pathologic RBC forms

TYPE	EXAMPLE	ASSOCIATED PATHOLOGY	NOTES
Acanthocyte (spur cell)	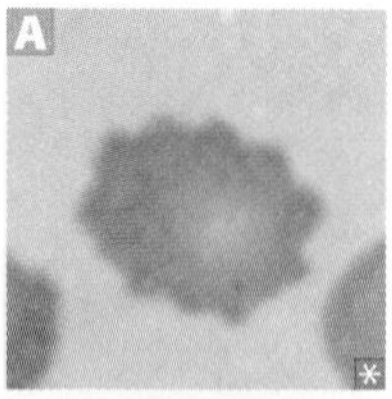	Liver disease, abetalipoproteinemia (states of cholesterol dysregulation).	*Acantho* = spiny.
Basophilic stippling	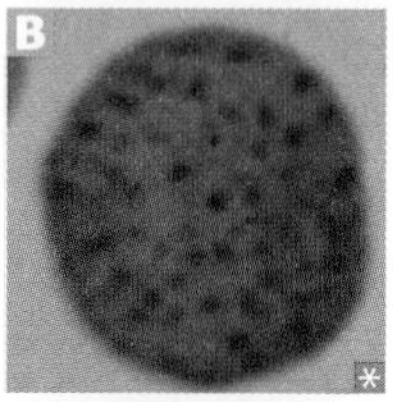	Thalassemias, Anemia of chronic disease, Lead poisoning.	**Bas**te the ox **TAiL**.
Bite cell	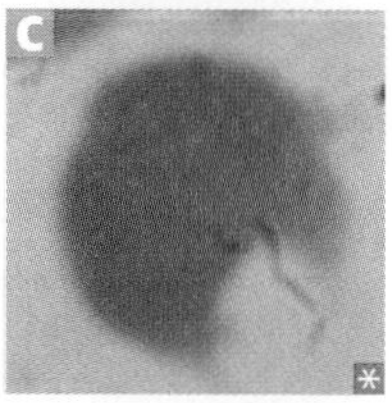	G6PD deficiency.	
Elliptocyte	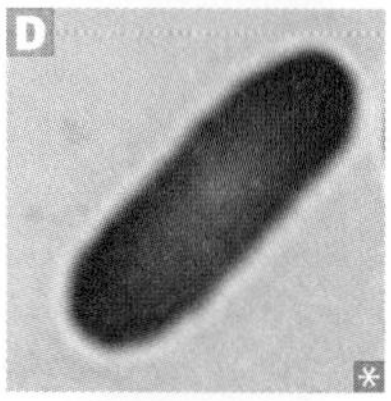	Hereditary elliptocytosis.	
Macro-ovalocyte	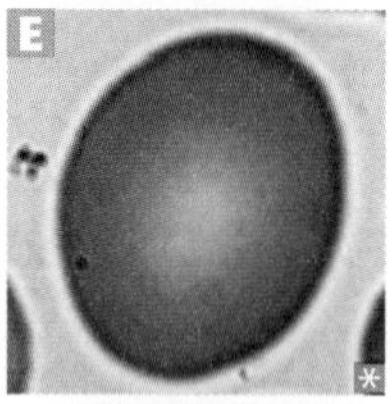	Megaloblastic anemia (also hypersegmented PMNs), marrow failure.	
Ringed sideroblasts	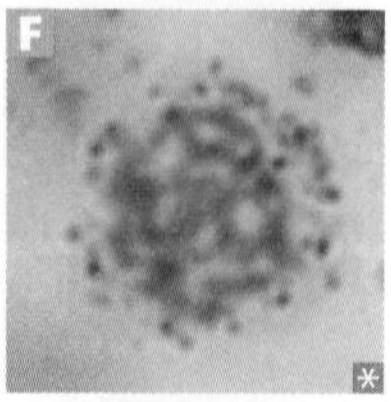	Sideroblastic anemia. Excess iron in mitochondria = pathologic.	
Schistocyte, helmet cell	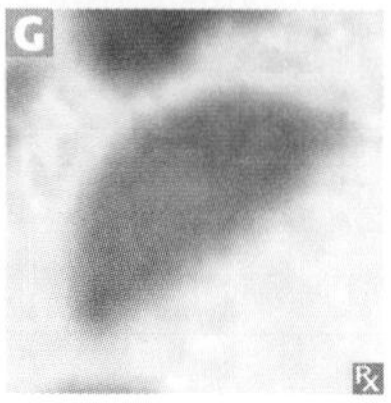	DIC, TTP/HUS, traumatic hemolysis (i.e., metal heart valve prosthesis).	

Pathologic RBC forms *(continued)*

TYPE	EXAMPLE	ASSOCIATED PATHOLOGY	NOTES
Sickle cell	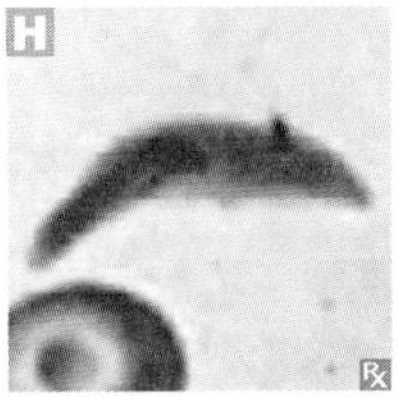	Sickle cell anemia.	
Spherocyte	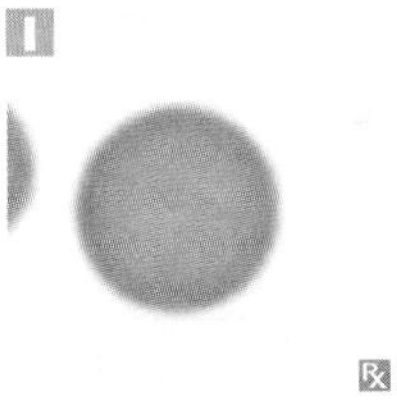	Hereditary spherocytosis, autoimmune hemolysis.	
Teardrop cell	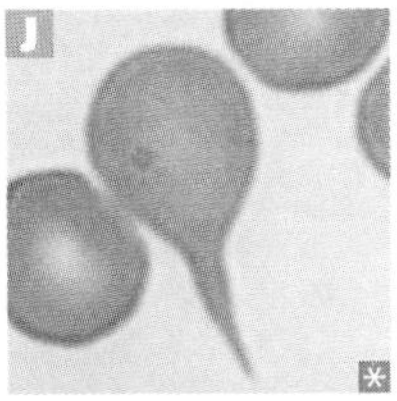	Bone marrow infiltration (e.g., myelofibrosis).	RBC "sheds a **tear**" because it's been forced out of its home in the bone marrow.
Target cell	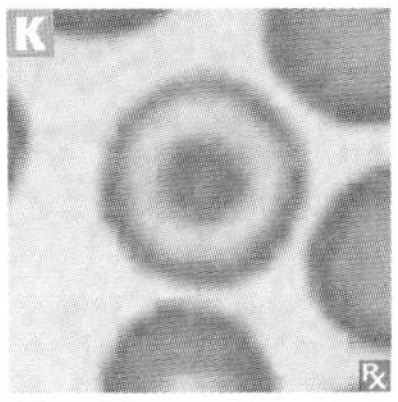	**H**bC disease, **A**splenia, **L**iver disease, **T**halassemia.	"**HALT**," said the hunter to his **target**.

Other RBC pathologies

TYPE	EXAMPLE	PROCESS	ASSOCIATED PATHOLOGY
Heinz bodies	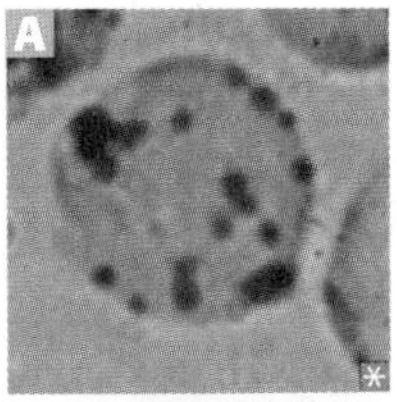	Oxidation of iron from ferrous to ferric form leads to denatured hemoglobin precipitation and damage to RBC membrane → formation of bite cells.	Seen in G6PD deficiency; Heinz body–like inclusions seen in α-thalassemia.
Howell-Jolly bodies	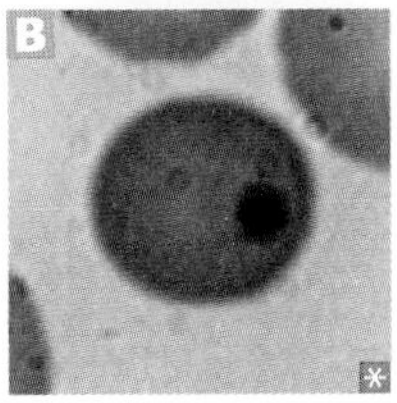	Basophilic nuclear remnants found in RBCs. Howell-Jolly bodies are normally removed from RBCs by splenic macrophages.	Seen in patients with functional hyposplenia or asplenia, or after mothball ingestion (naphthalene).

Anemias

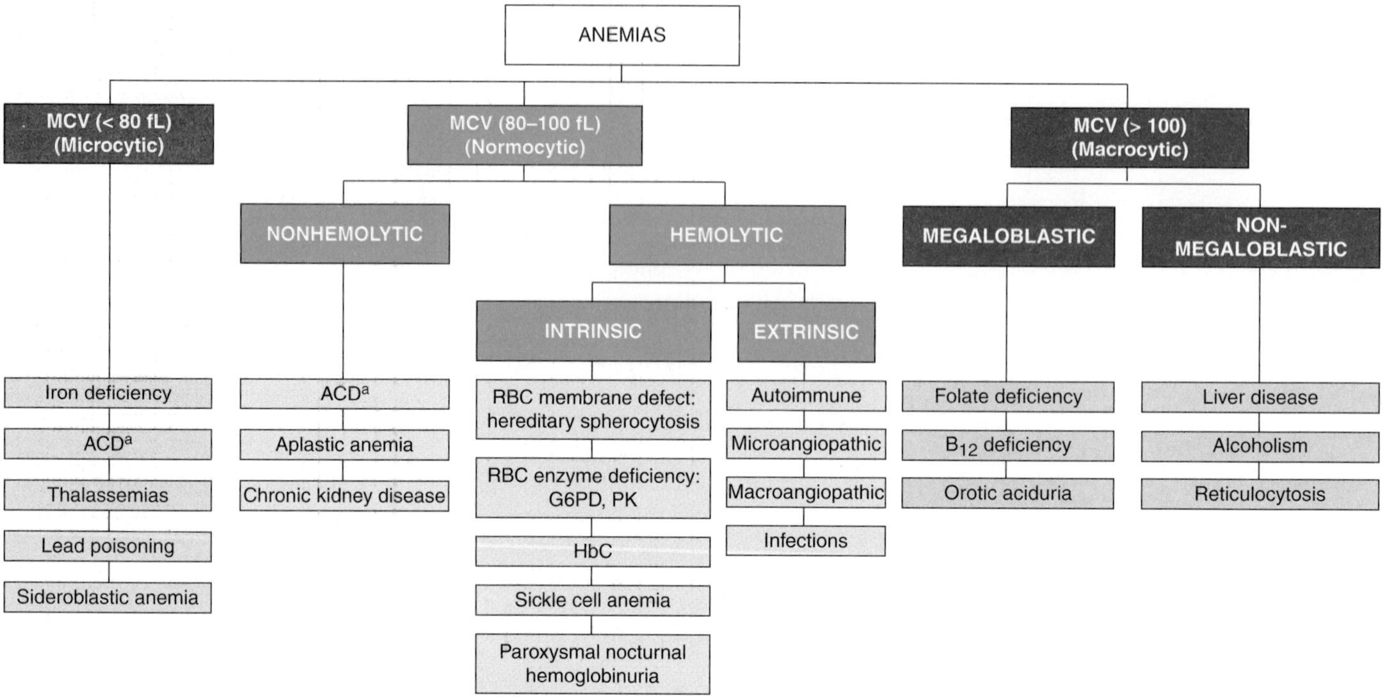

[a]ACD may first present as a normocytic anemia and then progress to a microcytic anemia.

Microcytic, hypochromic (MCV < 80 fL) anemia

	DESCRIPTION	FINDINGS
Iron deficiency	↓ iron due to chronic bleeding (GI loss, menorrhagia), malnutrition/absorption disorders or ↑ demand (e.g., pregnancy) → ↓ final step in heme synthesis.	↓ iron, ↑ TIBC, ↓ ferritin. Microcytosis and hypochromia A. May manifest as **Plummer-Vinson syndrome** (triad of iron deficiency anemia, esophageal webs, and atrophic glossitis). 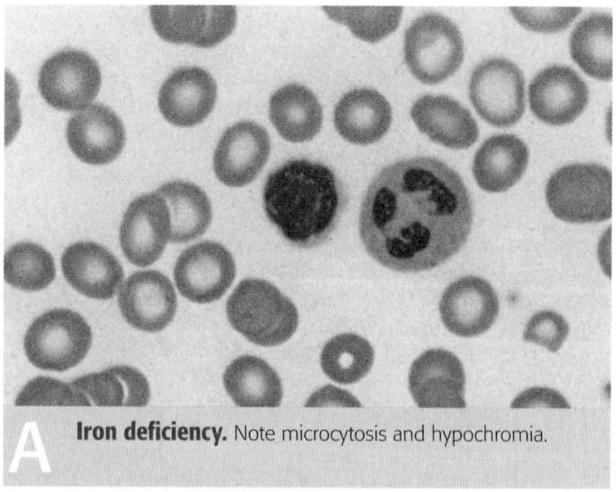 A **Iron deficiency.** Note microcytosis and hypochromia.
α-thalassemia	Defect: α-globin gene mutations → ↓ α-globin synthesis. *cis* deletion prevalent in Asian populations; *trans* deletion prevalent in African populations.	4 gene deletion: No α-globin. Excess γ-globin forms γ_4 (Hb Barts). Incompatible with life (causes hydrops fetalis). 3 gene deletion: HbH disease. Very little α-globin. Excess β-globin forms β_4 (HbH). 1–2 gene deletion: no clinically significant anemia.

Microcytic, hypochromic (MCV < 80 fL) anemia *(continued)*

	DESCRIPTION	FINDINGS
β-thalassemia	Point mutations in splice sites and promoter sequences → ↓ β-globin synthesis. Prevalent in Mediterranean populations. 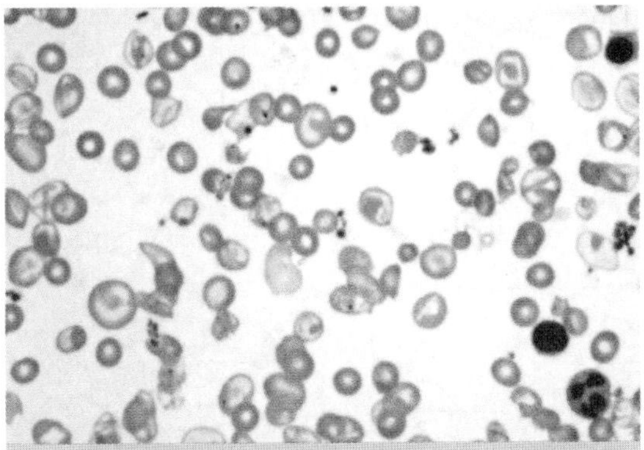 **B** **β-thalassemia major.** Note anisocytosis, poikilocytosis, microcytosis, hypochromia, target cells, and schistocytes.	β-thalassemia minor (heterozygote): ▪ β chain is underproduced ▪ Usually asymptomatic ▪ Diagnosis confirmed by ↑ HbA2 (> 3.5%) on electrophoresis β-thalassemia major (homozygote): ▪ β chain is absent → severe anemia B requiring blood transfusion (2° hemochromatosis) ▪ Marrow expansion ("crew cut" on skull x-ray) → skeletal deformities. "Chipmunk" facies Major → ↑ HbF ($\alpha_2\gamma_2$). HbS/β-thalassemia heterozygote: mild to moderate sickle cell disease depending on amount of β-globin production.
Lead poisoning	Lead inhibits ferrochelatase and ALA dehydratase → ↓ heme synthesis. Also inhibits rRNA degradation, causing RBCs to retain aggregrates of rRNA (basophilic stippling). High risk in houses with chipped paint.	LEAD: Lead Lines on gingivae (Burton's lines) and on metaphyses of long bones on x-ray. Encephalopathy and Erythrocyte basophilic stippling. Abdominal colic and sideroblastic Anemia. Drops—wrist and foot drop. Dimercaprol and EDTA are 1st line of treatment. Succimer used for chelation for kids (It "sucks" to be a kid who eats lead).
Sideroblastic anemia	Defect in heme synthesis. Hereditary: X-linked defect in δ-ALA synthase gene. Reversible etiologies: alcohol, lead, and isoniazid.	Ringed sideroblasts (with iron-laden mitochondria). ↑ iron, normal TIBC, ↑ ferritin. Treatment: pyridoxine (B_6, cofactor for δ-ALA synthase).

Macrocytic (MCV > 100 fL) anemia

	DESCRIPTION	FINDINGS
Megaloblastic anemia	Impaired DNA synthesis → maturation of nucleus delayed relative to maturation of cytoplasm. Ineffective erythropoiesis → pancytopenia.	
Folate deficiency	Etiologies: malnutrition (e.g., alcoholics), malabsorption, antifolates (e.g., methotrexate, trimethoprim, phenytoin), ↑ requirement (e.g., hemolytic anemia, pregnancy).	Hypersegmented neutrophils, glossitis, ↓ folate, ↑ homocysteine but normal methylmalonic acid.
B_{12} deficiency (cobalamin)	Etiologies: insufficient intake (e.g., strict vegans), malabsorption (e.g., Crohn's disease), pernicious anemia, *Diphyllobothrium latum* (fish tapeworm), proton pump inhibitors.	Hypersegmented neutrophils, glossitis, ↓ B_{12}, ↑ homocysteine, ↑ methylmalonic acid. **Neurologic symptoms:** subacute combined degeneration (due to involvement of B_{12} in fatty acid pathways and myelin synthesis): ▪ Peripheral neuropathy with sensorimotor dysfunction ▪ Posterior columns (vibration/proprioception) ▪ Lateral corticospinal (spasticity) ▪ Dementia
Orotic aciduria	Genetic mutation in enzyme that synthesizes uridine from orotic acid. Presents in children as megaloblastic anemia that cannot be cured by folate or B_{12}.	Hypersegmented neutrophils, glossitis, orotic acid in urine. Treatment: uridine monophosphate to bypass mutated enzyme.
Nonmegaloblastic macrocytic anemias	Macrocytic anemia in which DNA synthesis is unimpaired. Causes: Liver disease; alcoholism; reticulocytosis → ↑ MCV; drugs (5-FU, AZT, hydroxyurea).	Macrocytosis and bone marrow suppression can occur in the absence of folate/B_{12} deficiency.

Normocytic, normochromic anemia	Normocytic, normochromic anemias are classified as nonhemolytic or hemolytic. The hemolytic anemias are further classified according to the cause of the hemolysis (intrinsic vs. extrinsic to the RBC) and by the location of the hemolysis (intravascular vs. extravascular).
Intravascular hemolysis	Findings: ↓ haptoglobin, ↑ LDH, hemoglobin in urine (e.g., paroxysmal nocturnal hemoglobinuria, mechanical destruction [aortic stenosis, prosthetic valve]).
Extravascular hemolysis	Findings: macrophage in spleen clears RBC. ↑ LDH plus ↑ UCB, which causes jaundice (e.g., hereditary spherocytosis).

Nonhemolytic, normocytic anemia

	DESCRIPTION	FINDINGS
Anemia of chronic disease (ACD)	Inflammation → ↑ hepcidin (released by liver, binds ferroportin on intestinal mucosal cells and macrophages thus inhibiting iron transport) → ↓ release of iron from macrophages.	↓ iron, ↓ TIBC, ↑ ferritin. Can become microcytic, hypochromic
Aplastic anemia	Caused by failure or destruction of myeloid stem cells due to: ▪ Radiation and drugs (benzene, chloramphenicol, alkylating agents, antimetabolites) ▪ Viral agents (parvovirus B19, EBV, HIV, HCV) ▪ Fanconi's anemia (DNA repair defect) ▪ Idiopathic (immune mediated, 1° stem cell defect); may follow acute hepatitis	Pancytopenia characterized by severe anemia, leukopenia, and thrombocytopenia. Normal cell morphology, but hypocellular bone marrow with fatty infiltration (dry bone marrow tap). Symptoms: fatigue, malaise, pallor, purpura, mucosal bleeding, petechiae, infection. Treatment: withdrawal of offending agent, immunosuppressive regimens (antithymocyte globulin, cyclosporine), allogeneic bone marrow transplantation, RBC and platelet transfusion, G-CSF, or GM-CSF.
Chronic kidney disease	↓ erythropoietin → ↓ hematopoiesis.	

Intrinsic hemolytic normocytic anemia

E = extravascular; I = intravascular.

	DESCRIPTION	FINDINGS
Hereditary spherocytosis (E)	Defect in proteins interacting with RBC membrane skeleton and plasma membrane (e.g., ankyrin, band 3, protein 4.2, spectrin). Less membrane causes small and round RBCs with no central pallor (↑ MCHC, ↑ red cell distribution width) → premature removal of RBCs by spleen.	Splenomegaly, aplastic crisis (Parvovirus B19 infection). Labs: positive osmotic fragility test. Normal to ↓ MCV with abundance of cells; masks microcytia. Treatment: splenectomy.
G6PD deficiency (I/E)	X-linked. Defect in G6PD → ↓ glutathione → ↑ RBC susceptibility to oxidant stress. Hemolytic anemia following oxidant stress (e.g., sulfa drugs, infections, fava beans). RBCs primarily destroyed extravascularly.	Back pain, hemoglobinuria a few days later. Labs: blood smear shows RBCs with Heinz bodies and bite cells.
Pyruvate kinase deficiency (E)	Autosomal recessive. Defect in pyruvate kinase → ↓ ATP → rigid RBCs.	Hemolytic anemia in a newborn.
HbC defect (E)	Glutamic acid-to-lysine mutation at residue 6 in β-globin.	Patients with HbSC (1 of each mutant gene) have milder disease than have HbSS patients.
Paroxysmal nocturnal hemoglobinuria (I)	↑ complement-mediated RBC lysis (impaired synthesis of GPI anchor or decay-accelerating factor that protect RBC membrane from complement). Acquired mutation in a hematopoietic stem cell.	PNH triad: hemolytic anemia, pancytopenia, and venous thrombosis. Labs: CD55/59 ⊖ RBCs on flow cytometry. Treatment: eculizumab.
Sickle cell anemia (E)	HbS point mutation causes a single amino acid replacement in β chain (substitution of glutamic acid with valine) at position 6. Pathogenesis: low O_2 or dehydration precipitates sickling (deoxygenated HbS polymerizes), which results in anemia and vaso-occlusive disease. Newborns are initially asymptomatic because of ↑ HbF and ↓ HbS. Heterozygotes (sickle cell trait) have resistance to malaria. 8% of African Americans carry the HbS trait. 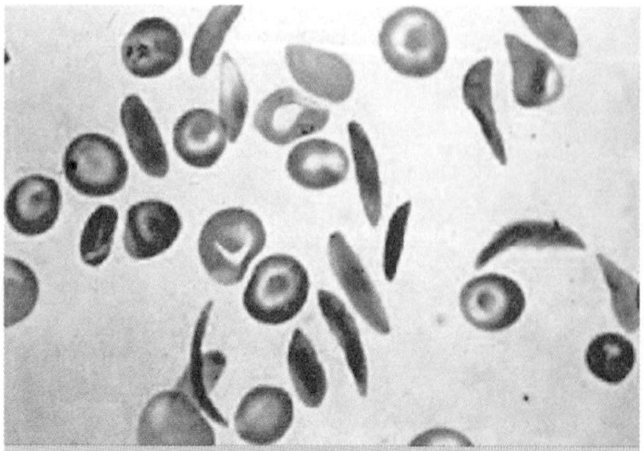 A Sickle cell disease.	Sickled cells are crescent-shaped RBCs A. "Crew cut" on skull x-ray due to marrow expansion from ↑ erythropoiesis (also in thalassemias). Complications in homozygotes (sickle cell disease): ▪ Aplastic crisis (due to parvovirus B19) ▪ Autosplenectomy (Howell-Jolly bodies) → ↑ risk of infection with encapsulated organisms; functional splenic dysfunction occurs in early childhood ▪ Splenic sequestration crisis ▪ *Salmonella* osteomyelitis ▪ Painful crisis (vaso-occlusive): dactylitis (painful hand swelling), acute chest syndrome, avascular necrosis ▪ Renal papillary necrosis (due to low O_2 in papilla) and microhematuria (medullary infarcts) Treatment: hydroxyurea (↑ HbF) and bone marrow transplantation.

Extrinsic hemolytic normocytic anemia

	DESCRIPTION	FINDINGS
Autoimmune hemolytic anemia	Warm agglutinin (IgG)—chronic anemia seen in SLE, CLL, or with certain drugs (e.g., α-methyldopa) ("**warm** weather is **GG**Great"). Cold agglutinin (IgM)—acute anemia triggered by cold; seen in CLL, *Mycoplasma pneumonia* infections, or infectious mononucleosis ("**cold** ice cream—yu**MMM**"). Many warm and cold AIHA are idiopathic in etiology.	Autoimmune hemolytic anemias are usually Coombs' positive. Direct Coombs' test—anti-Ig antibody added to patient's serum. RBCs agglutinate if RBCs are coated with Ig. Indirect Coombs' test—normal RBCs added to patient's serum agglutinate if serum has anti-RBC surface Ig.
Microangiopathic anemia	Pathogenesis: RBCs are damaged when passing through obstructed or narrowed vessel lumina. Seen in DIC, TTP-HUS, SLE, and malignant hypertension.	Schistocytes (helmet cells) are seen on blood smear due to mechanical destruction of RBCs.
Macroangiopathic anemia	Prosthetic heart valves and aortic stenosis may also cause hemolytic anemia 2° to mechanical destruction.	Schistocytes on peripheral blood smear.
Infections	↑ destruction of RBCs (e.g., malaria, *Babesia*).	

Lab values in anemia

	Iron deficiency	**Chronic disease**	**Hemo-chromatosis**	**Pregnancy/ OCP use**
Serum iron	↓ (1°)	↓	↑ (1°)	—
Transferrin or TIBC (indirectly measures transferrin)	↑	↓[a]	↓	↑ (1°)[b]
Ferritin	↓	↑ (1°)	↑	—
% transferrin saturation (serum iron/TIBC)	↓↓	—	↑↑	↓

Transferrin—transports iron in blood.
Ferritin—1° iron storage protein of body.

[a] Evolutionary reasoning—pathogens use circulating iron to thrive. The body has adapted a system in which iron is stored within the cells of the body and prevents pathogens from acquiring circulating iron.

[b] Transferrin production is ↑ in pregnancy and by oral contraceptives.

Heme synthesis, porphyrias, and lead poisoning

The porphyrias are hereditary or acquired conditions of defective heme synthesis that lead to the accumulation of heme precursors. Lead inhibits specific enzymes needed in heme synthesis, leading to a similar condition.

CONDITION	AFFECTED ENZYME	ACCUMULATED SUBSTRATE	PRESENTING SYMPTOMS
Lead poisoning	Ferrochelatase and ALA dehydratase	Protoporphyrin, δ-ALA (blood)	Microcytic anemia, GI and kidney disease. Children—exposure to lead paint → mental deterioration. Adults—environmental exposure (battery/ammunition/radiator factory) → headache, memory loss, demyelination.
Acute intermittent porphyria	Porphobilinogen deaminase	Porphobilinogen, δ-ALA, uroporphyrin (urine)	Symptoms (5 P's): ▪ Painful abdomen ▪ Port wine–colored urine ▪ Polyneuropathy ▪ Psychological disturbances ▪ Precipitated by drugs Treatment: glucose and heme, which inhibit ALA synthase.
Porphyria cutanea tarda	Uroporphyrinogen decarboxylase	Uroporphyrin (tea-colored urine)	Blistering cutaneous photosensitivity. Most common porphyria.

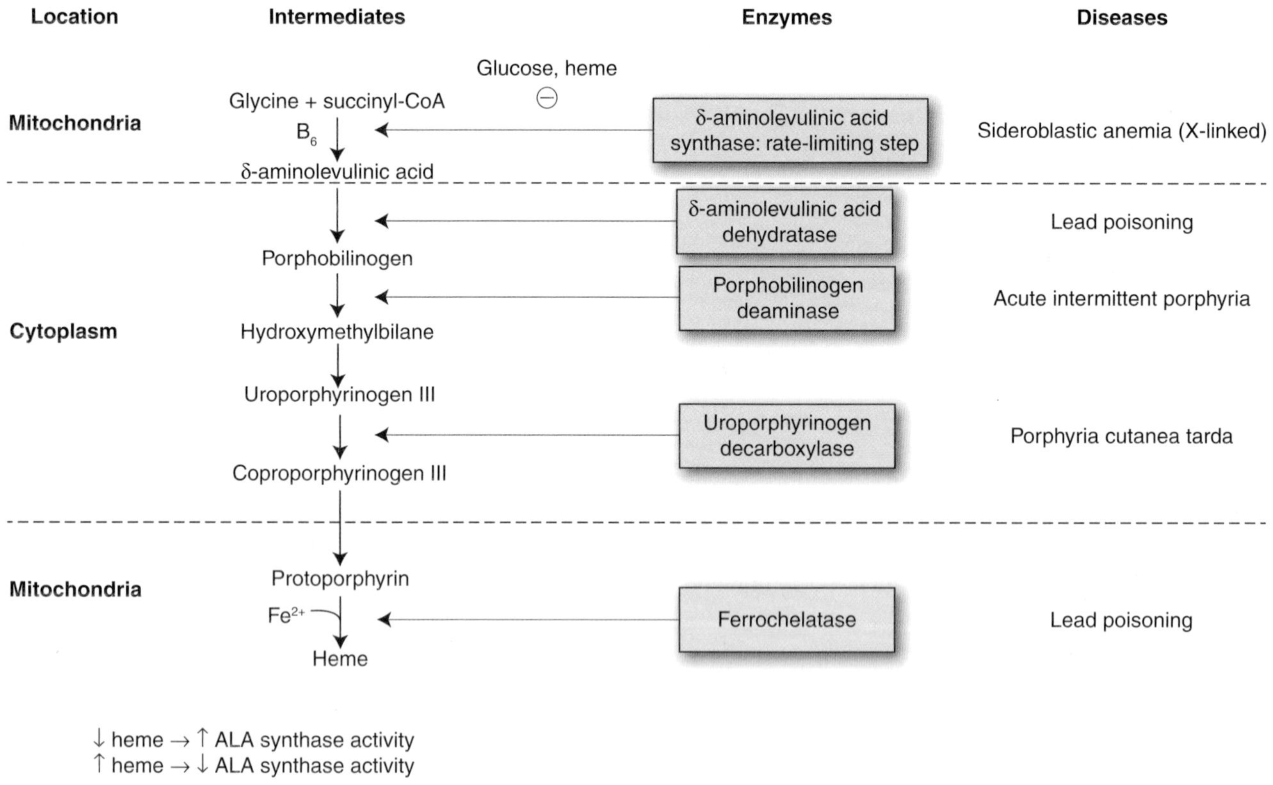
Location
Intermediates
Enzymes
Diseases
Glucose, heme
Mitochondria
Glycine + succinyl-CoA
B6
δ-aminolevulinic acid
δ-aminolevulinic acid synthase: rate-limiting step
Sideroblastic anemia (X-linked)
δ-aminolevulinic acid dehydratase
Lead poisoning
Porphobilinogen
Porphobilinogen deaminase
Acute intermittent porphyria
Cytoplasm
Hydroxymethylbilane
Uroporphyrinogen III
Uroporphyrinogen decarboxylase
Porphyria cutanea tarda
Coproporphyrinogen III
Mitochondria
Protoporphyrin
Fe2+
Heme
Ferrochelatase
Lead poisoning
↓ heme → ↑ ALA synthase activity
↑ heme → ↓ ALA synthase activity

Coagulation disorders

PT—tests function of common and extrinsic pathway (factors I, II, V, VII, and X). Defect → ↑ PT.
PTT—tests function of common and intrinsic pathway (all factors except VII and XIII). Defect → ↑ PTT.

DISORDER	PT	PTT	MECHANISM AND COMMENTS
Hemophilia A or B	—	↑	Intrinsic pathway coagulation defect. ▪ A: deficiency of factor VIII → ↑ PTT. ▪ B: deficiency of factor IX → ↑ PTT. Macrohemorrhage in hemophilia—hemarthroses (bleeding into joints), easy bruising, ↑ PTT.
Vitamin K deficiency	↑	↑	General coagulation defect. ↓ synthesis of factors II, VII, IX, X, protein C, protein S.

Platelet disorders

Defects in platelet plug formation → ↑ bleeding time (BT).
Platelet abnormalities → microhemorrhage: mucous membrane bleeding, epistaxis, petechiae, purpura, ↑ bleeding time, possible ↓ platelet count (PC).

DISORDER	PC	BT	MECHANISM AND COMMENTS
Bernard-Soulier syndrome	↓	↑	Defect in platelet plug formation. ↓ GpIb → defect in platelet-to-vWF adhesion.
Glanzmann's thrombasthenia	–	↑	Defect in platelet plug formation. ↓ GpIIb/IIIa → defect in platelet-to-platelet aggregation. Labs: blood smear shows no platelet clumping.
Idiopathic thrombocytopenic purpura (ITP)	↓	↑	Defect: anti-GpIIb/IIIa antibodies → splenic macrophage consumption of platelet/antibody complex. ↓ platelet survival. Labs: ↑ megakaryocytes.
Thrombotic thrombocytopenic purpura (TTP)	↓	↑	Deficiency of ADAMTS 13 (vWF metalloprotease) → ↓ degradation of vWF multimers. Pathogenesis: ↑ large vWF multimers → ↑ platelet aggregation and thrombosis. ↓ platelet survival. Labs: schistocytes, ↑ LDH. Symptoms: pentad of neurologic and renal symptoms, fever, thrombocytopenia, and microangiopathic hemolytic anemia.

Mixed platelet and coagulation disorders

DISORDER	PC	BT	PT	PTT	MECHANISM AND COMMENTS
von Willebrand's disease	—	↑	—	— or ↑	Intrinsic pathway coagulation defect: ↓ vWF → normal or ↑ PTT (depends on severity; vWF acts to carry/protect factor VIII). Defect in platelet plug formation: ↓ vWF → defect in platelet-to-vWF adhesion. Mild but most common inherited bleeding disorder. Autosomal dominant. Diagnosed in most cases by ristocetin cofactor assay. Treatment: DDAVP (desmopressin), which releases vWF stored in endothelium.
DIC	↓	↑	↑	↑	Widespread activation of clotting leads to a deficiency in clotting factors, which creates a bleeding state. Causes: **S**epsis (gram-negative), **T**rauma, **O**bstetric complications, acute **P**ancreatitis, **M**alignancy, **N**ephrotic syndrome, **T**ransfusion (**STOP M**aking **N**ew **T**hrombi). Labs: schistocytes, ↑ fibrin split products (D-dimers), ↓ fibrinogen, ↓ factors V and VIII.

Hereditary thrombosis syndromes leading to hypercoagulability

DISEASE	DESCRIPTION
Factor V Leiden	Production of mutant factor V that is resistant to degradation by activated protein C. Most common cause of inherited hypercoagulability in whites.
Prothrombin gene mutation	Mutation in 3′ untranslated region → ↑ production of prothrombin → ↑ plasma levels and venous clots.
Antithrombin deficiency	Inherited deficiency of antithrombin; ↑ in PTT is blunted after heparin administration.
Protein C or S deficiency	↓ ability to inactivate factors V and VIII. ↑ risk of thrombotic skin necrosis with hemorrhage following administration of warfarin.

Blood transfusion therapy

COMPONENT	DOSAGE EFFECT	CLINICAL USE
Packed RBCs	↑ Hb and O_2 carrying capacity	Acute blood loss, severe anemia
Platelets	↑ platelet count (↑ ~5,000/mm^3/unit)	Stop significant bleeding (thrombocytopenia, qualitative platelet defects)
Fresh frozen plasma	↑ coagulation factor levels	DIC, cirrhosis, warfarin overdose
Cryoprecipitate	Contains fibrinogen, factor VIII, factor XIII, vWF, and fibronectin	Treat coagulation factor deficiencies involving fibrinogen and factor VIII

Blood transfusion risks include infection transmission (low), transfusion reactions, iron overload, hypocalcemia (citrate is a calcium chelator), and hyperkalemia (RBCs may lyse in old blood units).

Leukemia vs. lymphoma

Leukemia	Lymphoid or myeloid neoplasms with widespread involvement of bone marrow. Tumor cells are usually found in peripheral blood.
Lymphoma	Discrete tumor masses arising from lymph nodes. Presentations often blur definitions.

Leukemoid reaction

Acute inflammatory response to infection. ↑ WBC count with ↑ neutrophils and neutrophil precursors such as band cells (left shift); ↑ leukocyte alkaline phosphatase. Contrast with CML (also ↑ WBC count with left shift, but ↓ leukocyte alkaline phosphatase).

Hodgkin's vs. non-Hodgkin's lymphoma

Hodgkin's	Non-Hodgkin's
Localized, single group of nodes; extranodal rare; contiguous spread (stage is strongest predictor of prognosis)	Multiple, peripheral nodes; extranodal involvement common; noncontiguous spread
Characterized by Reed-Sternberg cells	Majority involve B cells (except those of lymphoblastic T-cell origin)
Bimodal distribution–young adulthood and > 55 years; more common in men except for nodular sclerosing type	Peak incidence for certain subtypes at 20–40 years of age
50% of cases associated with EBV	May be associated with HIV and immunosuppression
Constitutional ("B") signs/symptoms—low-grade fever, night sweats, weight loss	Fewer constitutional signs/symptoms

Reed-Sternberg cells

Distinctive tumor giant cell seen in Hodgkin's disease; binucleate or bilobed with the 2 halves as mirror images ("owl's eyes" A). RS cells are CD30+ and CD15+ B-cell origin. Necessary but not sufficient for a diagnosis of Hodgkin's disease. Better prognosis with strong stromal or lymphocytic reaction against RS cells. Nodular sclerosing form most common (affects women and men equally) with best prognosis. Lymphocyte mixed or depleted forms have poor prognosis.

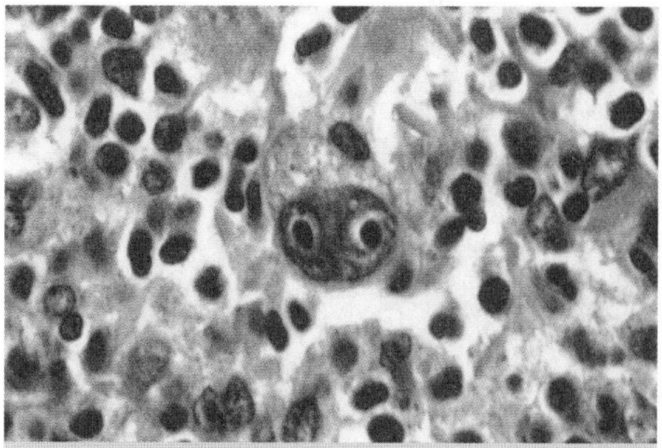

A Reed-Sternberg cell.

Non-Hodgkin's lymphoma

TYPE	OCCURS IN	GENETICS	COMMENTS
Neoplasms of mature B cells			
Burkitt's lymphoma 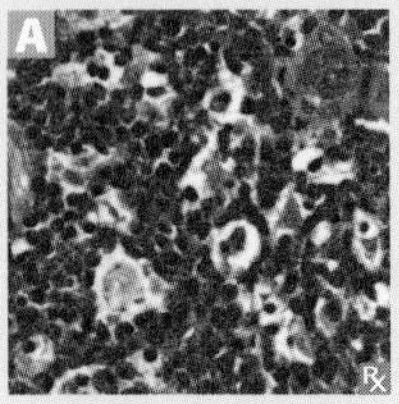	Adolescents or young adults 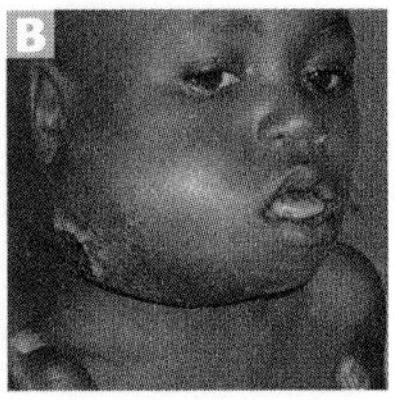	t(8;14)—translocation of c-*myc* (8) and heavy-chain Ig (14)	"Starry sky" appearance A, sheets of lymphocytes with interspersed macrophages. Associated with EBV. Jaw lesion B in endemic form in Africa; pelvis or abdomen in sporadic form.
Diffuse large B-cell lymphoma	Usually older adults, but 20% in children		Most common adult NHL. May be mature T cell in origin (20%).
Mantle cell lymphoma	Older males	t(11;14)—translocation of cyclin D1 (11) and heavy-chain Ig (14)	Poor prognosis, CD5+.
Follicular lymphoma	Adults	t(14;18)—translocation of heavy-chain Ig (14) and *bcl*-2 (18)	Difficult to cure; indolent course; *bcl*-2 inhibits apoptosis.
Neoplasms of mature T cells			
Adult T-cell lymphoma	Adults	Caused by HTLV-1	Adults present with cutaneous lesions; especially affects populations in Japan, West Africa, and the Caribbean. Aggressive.
Mycosis fungoides/ Sézary syndrome	Adults		Adults present with cutaneous patches/nodules. CD4+, indolent course.

Multiple myeloma

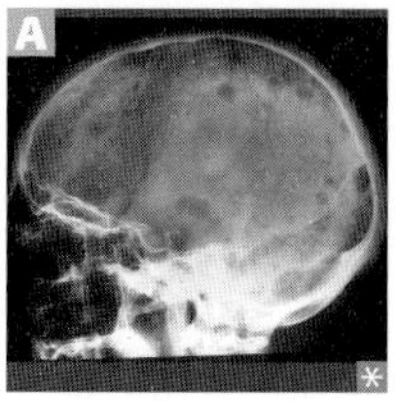

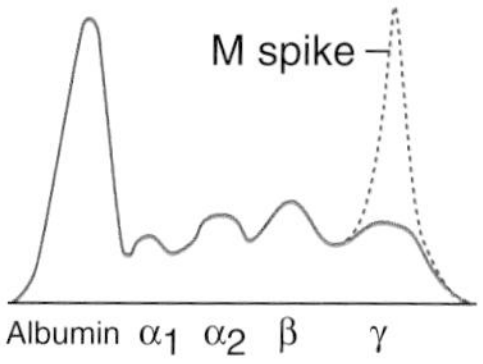

Monoclonal plasma cell ("fried egg" appearance) cancer that arises in the marrow and produces large amounts of IgG (55%) or IgA (25%). Most common 1° tumor arising within bone in the elderly (> 40–50 years of age).

Associated with:

- ↑ susceptibility to infection
- Primary amyloidosis (AL)
- Punched-out lytic bone lesions on x-ray A
- M spike on protein electrophoresis
- Ig light chains in urine (Bence Jones protein)
- Rouleaux formation (RBCs stacked like poker chips in blood smear)

Numerous plasma cells with "clock face" chromatin and intracytoplasmic inclusions containing immunoglobulin B.

Distinguish from Waldenström's macroglobulinemia → M spike = IgM (→ hyperviscosity symptoms); no lytic bone lesions.

Think **CRAB**:
- Hyper**C**alcemia
- **R**enal insufficiency
- **A**nemia
- **B**one lytic lesions/**B**ack pain

Multiple **M**yeloma: **M**onoclonal **M** protein spike

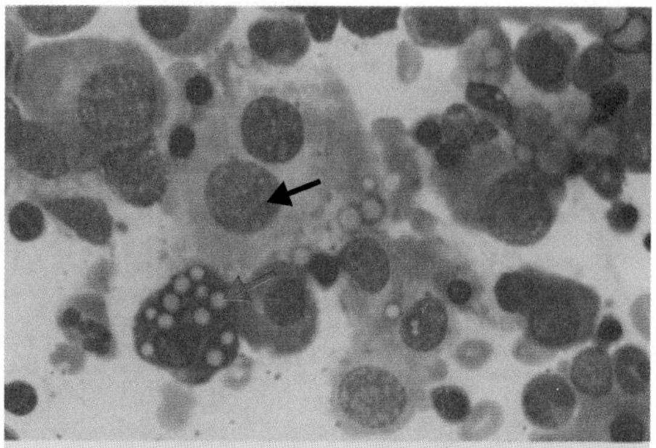

B **Multiple myeloma smear.** "Clock face" chromatin (black arrow) and whitish intracytoplasmic inclusions containing immunoglobulin (red arrow).

MGUS

Monoclonal gammopathy of undetermined significance (MGUS) is a monoclonal expansion of plasma cells with M spike. Asymptomatic precursor to multiple myeloma. Patients with MGUS develop multiple myeloma at a rate of 1–2% per year.

Leukemias

Unregulated growth of leukocytes in bone marrow → ↑ or ↓ number of circulating leukocytes in blood and marrow failure → anemia (↓ RBCs), infections (↓ mature WBCs), and hemorrhage (↓ platelets); leukemic cell infiltrates in liver, spleen, and lymph nodes are possible.

TYPE	PERIPHERAL BLOOD SMEAR	COMMENTS
Lymphoid neoplasms		
Acute lymphoblastic leukemia/ lymphoma (ALL)	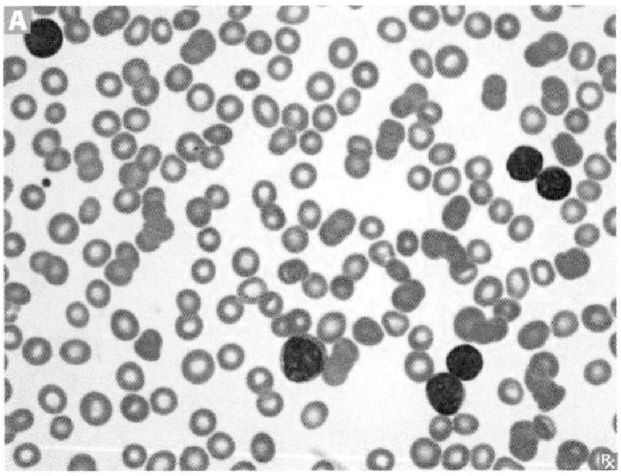	Age: < 15 years. T-cell ALL can present as mediastinal mass (leukemic infiltration of the thymus). Peripheral blood and bone marrow have ↑↑↑ lymphoblasts A. TdT+ (marker of pre-T and pre-B cells), CALLA+. Most responsive to therapy. May spread to CNS and testes. t(12;21) → better prognosis.
Small lymphocytic lymphoma (SLL)/ chronic lymphocytic leukemia (CLL)	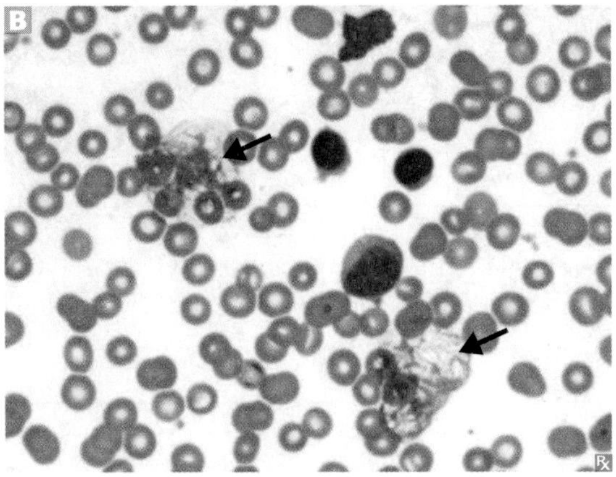	Age: > 60 years. Often asymptomatic; smudge cells in peripheral blood smear B; autoimmune hemolytic anemia. SLL same as CLL except CLL has ↑ peripheral blood lymphocytosis or bone marrow involvement.
Hairy cell leukemia	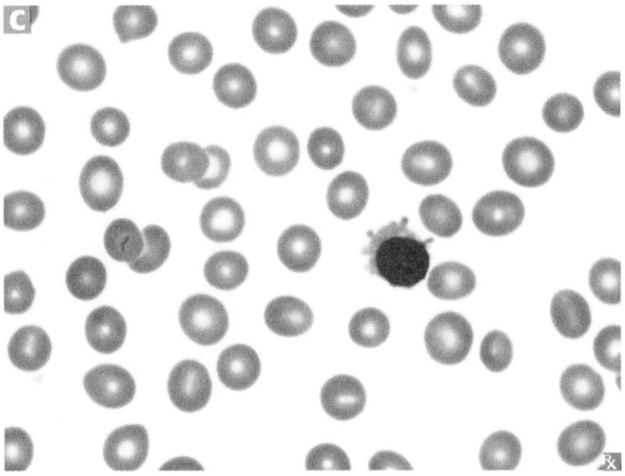	Age: Adults. Mature B-cell tumor in the elderly. Cells have filamentous, hair-like projections C. Stains TRAP (tartrate-resistant acid phosphatase) positive. Treatment: cladribine, an adenosine analog.

Leukemias *(continued)*

TYPE	PERIPHERAL BLOOD SMEAR	COMMENTS
Myeloid neoplasms		
Acute myelogenous leukemia (AML)	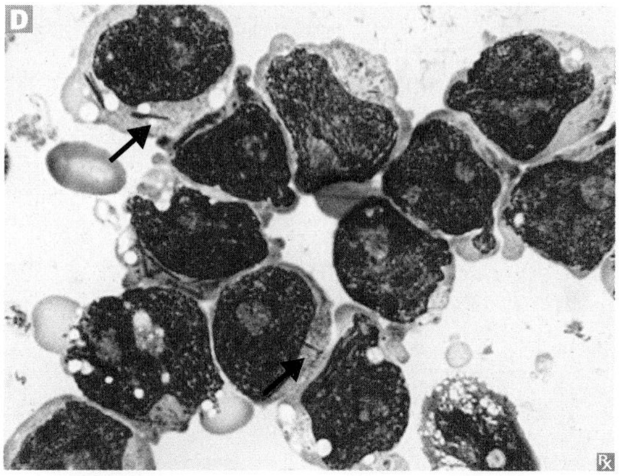	Age: median onset 65 years. Auer rods D; ↑↑↑ circulating myeloblasts on peripheral smear; adults. t(15;17) → M3 AML subtype responds to all-*trans* retinoic acid (vitamin A), inducing differentiation of myeloblasts; DIC is a common presentation in M3 AML.
Chronic myelogenous leukemia (CML)	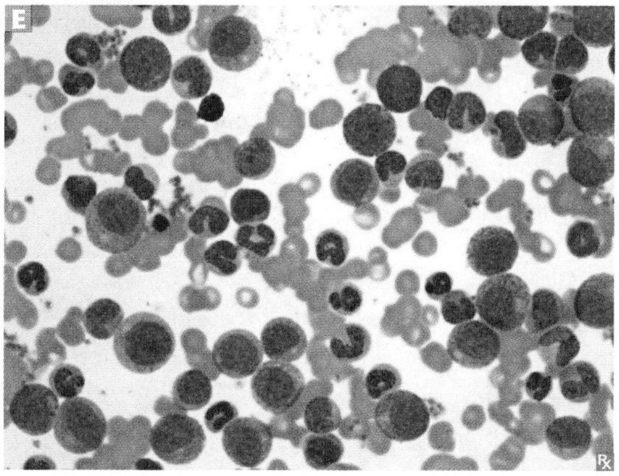	Age: highest incidence at 30–60 years. Defined by the Philadelphia chromosome (t[9;22], *bcr-abl*); myeloid stem cell proliferation; presents with ↑ neutrophils, metamyelocytes, basophils E; splenomegaly; may accelerate and transform to AML or ALL ("blast crisis"). Very low leukocyte alkaline phosphatase as a result of immature granulocytes (vs. leukemoid reaction—mature cells). Responds to imatinib (a small-molecule inhibitor of the *bcr-abl* tyrosine kinase).

Auer bodies (rods) Peroxidase-positive cytoplasmic inclusions in granulocytes and myeloblasts. Commonly seen in acute promyelocytic leukemia (M3). Treatment of AML M3 can release Auer rods → DIC.

Chromosomal translocations

TRANSLOCATION	ASSOCIATED DISORDER	
t(9;22) (**Philadelphia** chromosome)	CML (*bcr-abl* hybrid)	**Philadelphia** CreaML cheese.
t(8;14)	Burkitt's lymphoma (c-*myc* activation)	
t(11;14)	Mantle cell lymphoma (cyclin D1 activation)	
t(14;18)	Follicular lymphomas (*bcl*-2 activation)	
t(15;17)	M3 type of AML (responsive to all-*trans* retinoic acid)	

Langerhans cell histiocytosis

Proliferative disorders of dendritic (Langerhans) cells from monocyte lineage. Presents in a child as lytic bone lesions and skin rash. Cells are functionally immature and do not efficiently stimulate T lymphocytes via antigen presentation. Cells express S-100 (neural crest origin) and CD1a. Birbeck granules ("tennis rackets" on EM) are characteristic A.

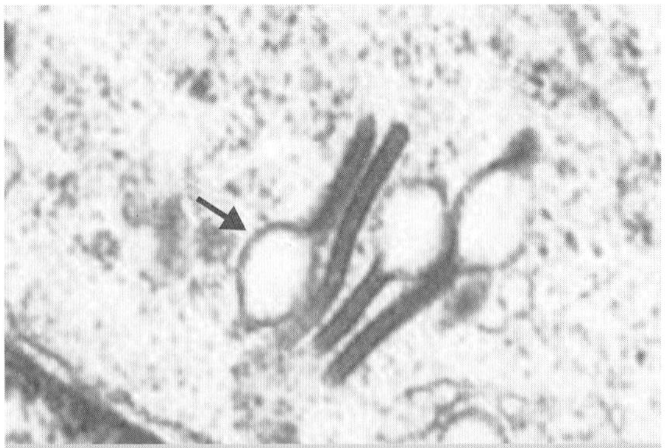

A Birbeck granules.

Chronic myeloproliferative disorders

	RBCS	WBCS	PLATELETS	PHILADELPHIA CHROMOSOME	*JAK2* MUTATIONS
Polycythemia vera	↑	↑	↑	Negative	Positive
Essential thrombocytosis	–	–	↑	Negative	Positive (30–50%)
Myelofibrosis	↓	Variable	Variable	Negative	Positive (30–50%)
CML	↓	↑	↑	Positive	Negative

The myelofibroproliferative disorders represent an often-overlapping spectrum, but the classic findings are described below. *JAK2* is involved in hematopoietic growth factor signaling. Mutations are implicated in myeloproliferative disorders other than CML.

Polycythemia vera	Abnormal clone of hematopoietic stem cells with constitutively active JAK2 receptors, proliferate without EPO stimulation. Often presents as intense itching after hot shower.
Essential thrombocytosis	Similar to polycythemia vera, but specific for megakaryocytes.
Myelofibrosis	Fibrotic obliteration of bone marrow. Teardrop cell. "Bone marrow is crying because it's fibrosed."
CML	*bcr-abl* transformation leads to ↑ cell division and inhibition of apoptosis.

Polycythemia

	PLASMA VOLUME	RBC MASS	O_2 SATURATION	ASSOCIATED DISEASES
Relative	↓	–	–	
Appropriate absolute	–	↑	↓	Lung disease, congenital heart disease, high altitude.
Inappropriate absolute	–	↑	–	Renal cell carcinoma, Wilms' tumor, cyst, hepatocellular carcinoma, hydronephrosis. Due to ectopic erythropoietin.
Polycythemia vera	↑	↑↑	–	

▸ HEMATOLOGY AND ONCOLOGY—PHARMACOLOGY

Heparin

MECHANISM	Cofactor for the activation of antithrombin, ↓ thrombin, and ↓ factor Xa. Short half-life.
CLINICAL USE	Immediate anticoagulation for pulmonary embolism, acute coronary syndrome, MI, DVT. Used during pregnancy (does not cross placenta). Follow PTT.
TOXICITY	Bleeding, thrombocytopenia (HIT), osteoporosis, drug-drug interactions. For rapid reversal (antidote), use protamine sulfate (positively charged molecule that binds negatively charged heparin).
NOTES	Low-molecular-weight heparins (e.g., enoxaparin, dalteparin) act more on factor Xa, have better bioavailability and 2–4 times longer half-life. Can be administered subcutaneously and without laboratory monitoring. Not easily reversible. **Heparin-induced thrombocytopenia** (HIT)—development of IgG antibodies against heparin bound to platelet factor 4 (PF4). Antibody-heparin-PF4 complex activates platelets → thrombosis and thrombocytopenia.

Lepirudin, bivalirudin Derivatives of hirudin, the anticoagulant used by leeches; inhibit thrombin. Used as an alternative to heparin for anticoagulating patients with HIT.

Warfarin (Coumadin)

MECHANISM	Interferes with normal synthesis and γ-carboxylation of vitamin K–dependent clotting factors II, VII, IX, and X and proteins C and S. Metabolized by the cytochrome P-450 pathway. In laboratory assay, has effect on **EX**trinsic pathway and ↑ **PT**. Long half-life.	The **EX**-**P**residen**T** went to **war**(farin).
CLINICAL USE	Chronic anticoagulation (after STEMI, venous thromboembolism prophylaxis, and prevention of stroke in atrial fibrillation). Not used in pregnant women (because warfarin, unlike heparin, can cross the placenta). Follow PT/INR values.	
TOXICITY	Bleeding, teratogenic, skin/tissue necrosis, drug-drug interactions.	For reversal of warfarin overdose, give vitamin K. For rapid reversal of severe warfarin overdose, give fresh frozen plasma.

Heparin vs. warfarin

	Heparin	Warfarin
STRUCTURE	Large anionic, acidic polymer	Small lipid-soluble molecule
ROUTE OF ADMINISTRATION	Parenteral (IV, SC)	Oral
SITE OF ACTION	Blood	Liver
ONSET OF ACTION	Rapid (seconds)	Slow, limited by half-lives of normal clotting factors
MECHANISM OF ACTION	Activates antithrombin, which ↓ the action of IIa (thrombin) and factor Xa	Impairs the synthesis of vitamin K–dependent clotting factors II, VII, IX, and X (vitamin K antagonist)
DURATION OF ACTION	Acute (hours)	Chronic (days)
INHIBITS COAGULATION IN VITRO	Yes	No
TREATMENT OF ACUTE OVERDOSE	Protamine sulfate	IV vitamin K and fresh frozen plasma
MONITORING	PTT (intrinsic pathway)	PT/INR (extrinsic pathway)
CROSSES PLACENTA	No	Yes (teratogenic)

Thrombolytics	Alteplase (tPA), reteplase (rPA), tenecteplase (TNK-tPA).
MECHANISM	Directly or indirectly aid conversion of plasminogen to plasmin, which cleaves thrombin and fibrin clots. ↑ PT, ↑ PTT, no change in platelet count.
CLINICAL USE	Early MI, early ischemic stroke, direct thrombolysis of severe pulmonary embolism.
TOXICITY	Bleeding. Contraindicated in patients with active bleeding, history of intracranial bleeding, recent surgery, known bleeding diatheses, or severe hypertension. Treat toxicity with aminocaproic acid, an inhibitor of fibrinolysis.

Aspirin (ASA)	
MECHANISM	Irreversibly inhibits cyclooxygenase (both COX-1 and COX-2) enzyme by covalent acetylation. Platelets cannot synthesize new enzyme, so effect lasts until new platelets are produced: ↑ bleeding time, ↓ TXA_2 and prostaglandins. No effect on PT or PTT.
CLINICAL USE	Antipyretic, analgesic, anti-inflammatory, antiplatelet (↓ aggregation).
TOXICITY	Gastric ulceration, tinnitus (CN VIII). Chronic use can lead to acute renal failure, interstitial nephritis, and upper GI bleeding. Reye's syndrome in children with viral infection. Overdose causes respiratory alkalosis and metabolic acidosis.

ADP receptor inhibitors	Clopidogrel, ticlopidine, prasugrel, ticagrelor.
MECHANISM	Inhibit platelet aggregation by irreversibly blocking ADP receptors. Inhibit fibrinogen binding by preventing glycoprotein IIb/IIIa from binding to fibrinogen.
CLINICAL USE	Acute coronary syndrome; coronary stenting. ↓ incidence or recurrence of thrombotic stroke.
TOXICITY	Neutropenia (ticlopidine).

Cilostazol, dipyridamole

MECHANISM	Phosphodiesterase III inhibitor; ↑ cAMP in platelets, thus inhibiting platelet aggregation; vasodilators.
CLINICAL USE	Intermittent claudication, coronary vasodilation, prevention of stroke or TIAs (combined with aspirin), angina prophylaxis.
TOXICITY	Nausea, headache, facial flushing, hypotension, abdominal pain.

GP IIb/IIIa inhibitors	Abciximab, eptifibatide, tirofiban.
MECHANISM	Bind to the glycoprotein receptor IIb/IIIa on activated platelets, preventing aggregation. Abciximab is made from monoclonal antibody Fab fragments.
CLINICAL USE	Acute coronary syndromes, percutaneous transluminal coronary angioplasty.
TOXICITY	Bleeding, thrombocytopenia.

Cancer drugs—cell cycle

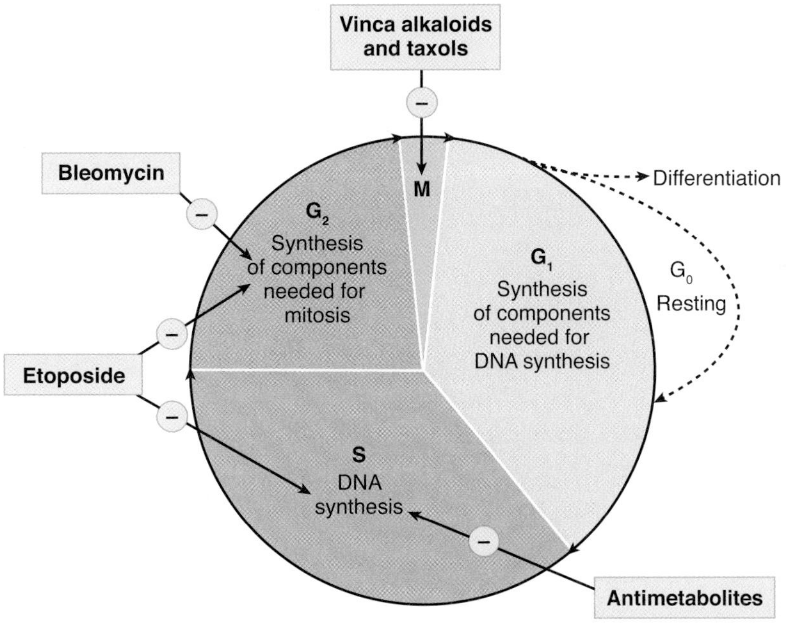

(Adapted, with permission, from Katzung BG, Trevor AJ. *USMLE Road Map: Pharmacology,* 1st ed. New York: McGraw-Hill, 2003: 133.)

Antineoplastics

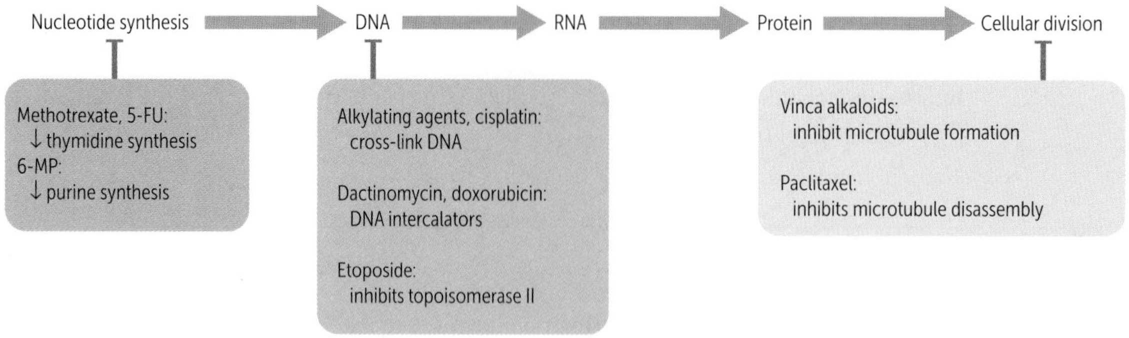

Antimetabolites

DRUG	MECHANISM[a]	CLINICAL USE	TOXICITY
Methotrexate (MTX)	Folic acid analog that inhibits dihydrofolate reductase → ↓ dTMP → ↓ DNA and ↓ protein synthesis.	Cancers: leukemias, lymphomas, choriocarcinoma, sarcomas. Non-neoplastic: abortion, ectopic pregnancy, rheumatoid arthritis, psoriasis.	Myelosuppression, which is reversible with leucovorin (folinic acid) "rescue." Macrovesicular fatty change in liver. Mucositis. Teratogenic.
5-fluorouracil (5-FU)	Pyrimidine analog bioactivated to 5F-dUMP, which covalently complexes folic acid. This complex inhibits thymidylate synthase → ↓ dTMP → ↓ DNA and ↓ protein synthesis.	Colon cancer, basal cell carcinoma (topical).	Myelosuppression, which is not reversible with leucovorin. Overdose: "rescue" with thymidine. Photosensitivity.
Cytarabine (arabinofuranosyl cytidine)	Pyrimidine analog → inhibition of DNA polymerase.	Leukemias, lymphomas.	Leukopenia, thrombocytopenia, megaloblastic anemia.
Azathioprine **6-mercaptopurine (6-MP)** **6-thioguanine (6-TG)**	Purine (thiol) analogs → ↓ de novo purine synthesis. Activated by HGPRT.	Leukemias.	Bone marrow, GI, liver. Metabolized by xanthine oxidase; thus ↑ toxicity with allopurinol.

[a]All are S-phase specific.

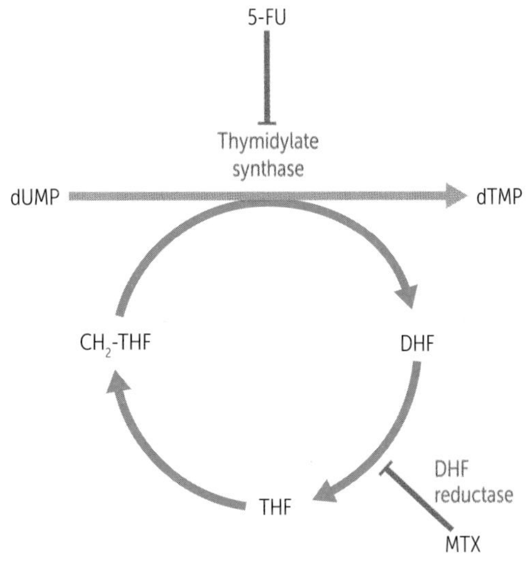

Antitumor antibiotics

DRUG	MECHANISM	CLINICAL USE	TOXICITY
Dactinomycin (actinomycin D)	Intercalates in DNA.	Wilms' tumor, Ewing's sarcoma, rhabdomyosarcoma. Used for childhood tumors ("children **act** out").	Myelosuppression.
Doxorubicin (Adriamycin), daunorubicin	Generate free radicals. Noncovalently intercalate in DNA → breaks in DNA → ↓ replication.	Solid tumors, leukemias, lymphomas.	Cardiotoxicity (dilated cardiomyopathy), myelosuppression, alopecia. Toxic to tissues following extravasation. Dexrazoxane (iron chelating agent), used to prevent cardiotoxicity.
Bleomycin	Induces free radical formation, which causes breaks in DNA strands.	Testicular cancer, Hodgkin's lymphoma.	Pulmonary fibrosis, skin changes. Minimal myelosuppression.

Alkylating agents

DRUG	MECHANISM	CLINICAL USE	TOXICITY
Cyclophosphamide, ifosfamide	Covalently X-link (interstrand) DNA at guanine N-7. Require bioactivation by liver.	Solid tumors, leukemia, lymphomas, and some brain cancers.	Myelosuppression; hemorrhagic cystitis, partially prevented with mesna (thiol group of mesna binds toxic metabolite).
Nitrosoureas (carmustine, lomustine, semustine, streptozocin)	Require bioactivation. Cross blood-brain barrier → CNS.	Brain tumors (including glioblastoma multiforme).	CNS toxicity (dizziness, ataxia).
Busulfan	Alkylates DNA.	CML. Also used to ablate patient's bone marrow before bone marrow transplantation.	Pulmonary fibrosis, hyperpigmentation.

Microtubule inhibitors

DRUG	MECHANISM	CLINICAL USE	TOXICITY
Vincristine, vinblastine	Alkaloids that bind to tubulin in M phase and block polymerization of microtubules so that mitotic spindle cannot form. "Microtubules are the **vines** of your cells."	Solid tumors, leukemias, and lymphomas.	Vincristine—neurotoxicity (areflexia, peripheral neuritis), paralytic ileus. Vin**blast**ine **blasts** **b**one marrow (suppression).
Paclitaxel, other taxols	Hyperstabilize polymerized microtubules in M phase so that mitotic spindle cannot break down (anaphase cannot occur). "It is **tax**ing to stay polymerized."	Ovarian and breast carcinomas.	Myelosuppression and hypersensitivity.

Cisplatin, carboplatin

MECHANISM	Cross-link DNA.
CLINICAL USE	Testicular, bladder, ovary, and lung carcinomas.
TOXICITY	Nephrotoxicity and acoustic nerve damage. Prevent nephrotoxicity with amifostine (free radical scavenger) and chloride diuresis.

Etoposide, teniposide

MECHANISM	Inhibit topoisomerase II → ↑ DNA degradation.
CLINICAL USE	Solid tumors, leukemias, lymphomas.
TOXICITY	Myelosuppression, GI irritation, alopecia.

Hydroxyurea

MECHANISM	Inhibits ribonucleotide reductase → ↓ DNA Synthesis (S-phase specific).
CLINICAL USE	Melanoma, CML, sickle cell disease (↑ HbF).
TOXICITY	Bone marrow suppression, GI upset.

Prednisone, prednisolone

MECHANISM	May trigger apoptosis. May even work on nondividing cells.
CLINICAL USE	Most commonly used glucocorticoid in cancer chemotherapy. Used in CLL, non-Hodgkin's lymphomas (part of combination chemotherapy regimen). Also used as an immunosuppressant (e.g., autoimmune diseases).
TOXICITY	Cushing-like symptoms; immunosuppression, cataracts, acne, osteoporosis, hypertension, peptic ulcers, hyperglycemia, psychosis.

Tamoxifen, raloxifene

MECHANISM	SERMs—receptor antagonists in breast and agonists in bone. Block the binding of estrogen to estrogen receptor–positive cells.
CLINICAL USE	Breast cancer treatment and prevention. Also useful to prevent osteoporosis.
TOXICITY	Tamoxifen—partial agonist in endometrium, which ↑ the risk of endometrial cancer; "hot flashes." Raloxifene—no ↑ in endometrial carcinoma because it is an endometrial antagonist.

Trastuzumab (Herceptin)

MECHANISM	Monoclonal antibody against HER-2 *(c-erbB2)*, a tyrosine kinase. Helps kill breast cancer cells that overexpress HER-2, possibly through antibody-dependent cytotoxicity.
CLINICAL USE	HER-2–positive breast cancer.
TOXICITY	Cardiotoxicity.

Imatinib (Gleevec)

MECHANISM	Philadelphia chromosome *bcr-abl* tyrosine kinase inhibitor.
CLINICAL USE	CML, GI stromal tumors.
TOXICITY	Fluid retention.

Rituximab

MECHANISM	Monoclonal antibody against CD20, which is found on most B-cell neoplasms.
CLINICAL USE	Non-Hodgkin's lymphoma, rheumatoid arthritis (with methotrexate).

Vemurafenib

MECHANISM	Small molecule inhibitor of forms of the B-Raf kinase with the V600E mutation.
CLINICAL USE	Metastatic melanoma.

Bevacizumab

MECHANISM	Monoclonal antibody against VEGF. Inhibits angiogenesis.
CLINICAL USE	Solid tumors.

Common chemotoxicities

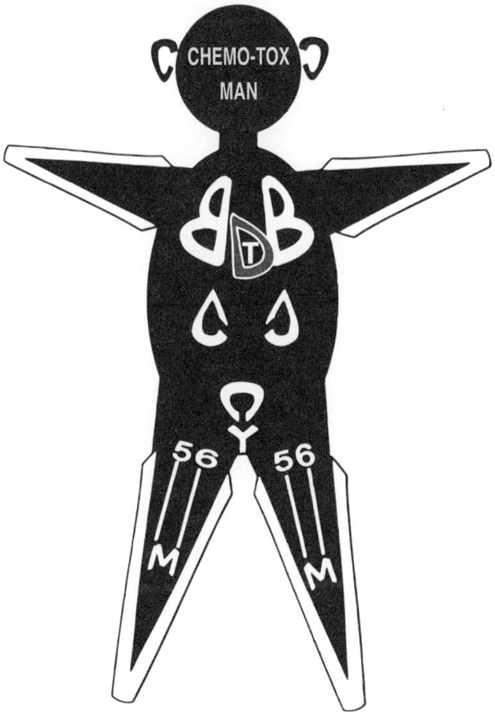

Cisplatin/Carboplatin → acoustic nerve damage (and nephrotoxicity)

Vincristine → peripheral neuropathy
Bleomycin, Busulfan → pulmonary fibrosis
Doxorubicin → cardiotoxicity
Trastuzumab → cardiotoxicity
Cisplatin/Carboplatin → nephrotoxic (and acoustic nerve damage)

CYclophosphamide → hemorrhagic cystitis

5-FU → myelosuppression
6-MP → myelosuppression

Methotrexate → myelosuppression

NOTES

HIGH-YIELD SYSTEMS

Musculoskeletal, Skin, and Connective Tissue

"Rigid, the skeleton of habit alone upholds the human frame."

—Virginia Woolf

"Beauty may be skin deep, but ugly goes clear to the bone."

—Redd Foxx

"The function of muscle is to pull and not to push, except in the case of the genitals and the tongue."

—Leonardo da Vinci

▶ MUSCULOSKELETAL, SKIN, AND CONNECTIVE TISSUE—ANATOMY AND PHYSIOLOGY

Epidermis layers

From surface to base:
- Stratum **C**orneum (keratin)
- Stratum **L**ucidum
- Stratum **G**ranulosum
- Stratum **S**pinosum (spines = desmosomes)
- Stratum **B**asale (stem cell site)

Californians **L**ike **G**irls in **S**tring **B**ikinis.

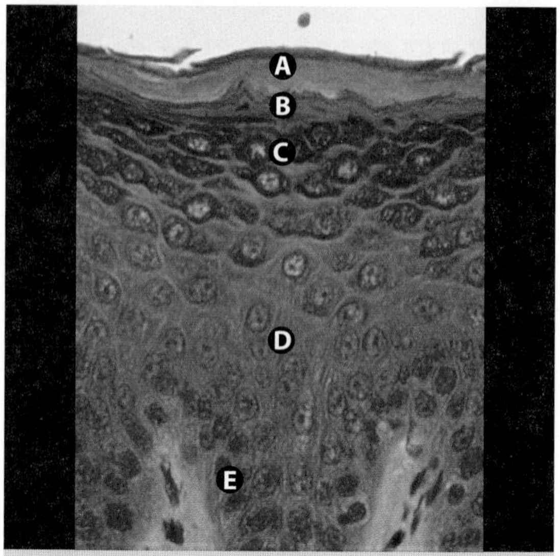
A
B
C
D
E

A **Epidermis layers.** A, Stratum corneum; B, stratum lucidum; C, stratum granulosum; D, stratum spinosum; E, stratum basale.

Epidermal appendages

Sebaceous gland	Holocrine secretion of sebum. Associated with hair follicle.
Eccrine gland	Secretes sweat. Found throughout the body ("**E**ccrine glands are **E**verywhere").
Apocrine gland	Secretes milky viscous fluid. Found in the axillae, genitalia, and areolae. Does not become functional until puberty. Malodorous because of bacterial action.

Epithelial cell junctions

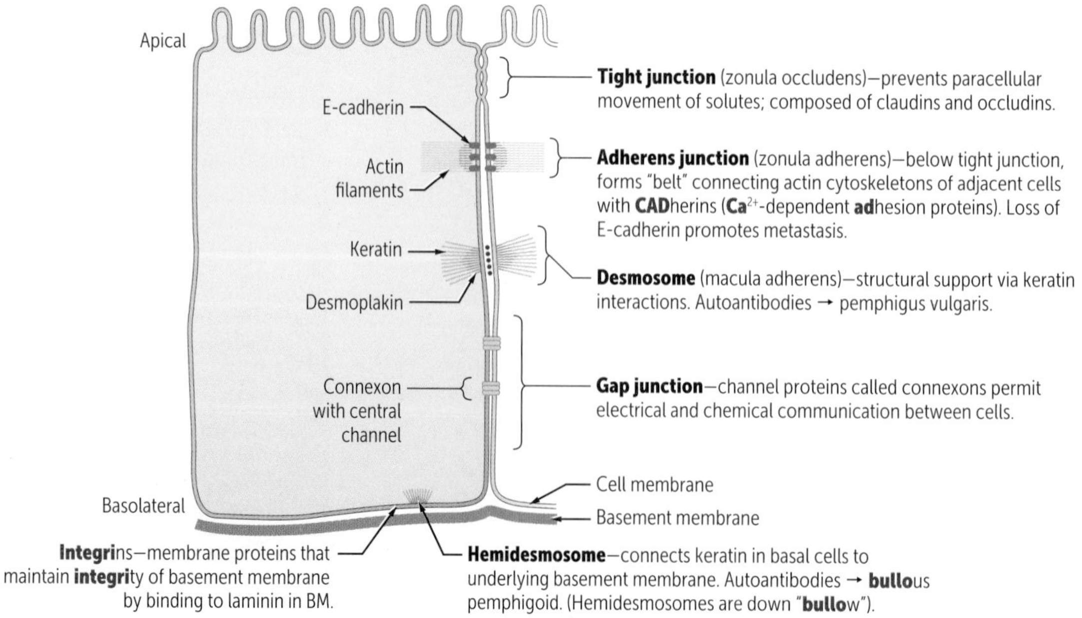
Apical
E-cadherin
Actin filaments
Keratin
Desmoplakin
Connexon with central channel
Basolateral
Tight junction (zonula occludens)—prevents paracellular movement of solutes; composed of claudins and occludins.
Adherens junction (zonula adherens)—below tight junction, forms "belt" connecting actin cytoskeletons of adjacent cells with **CAD**herins (**Ca**$^{2+}$-dependent **ad**hesion proteins). Loss of E-cadherin promotes metastasis.
Desmosome (macula adherens)—structural support via keratin interactions. Autoantibodies → pemphigus vulgaris.
Gap junction—channel proteins called connexons permit electrical and chemical communication between cells.
Cell membrane
Basement membrane
Integrins—membrane proteins that maintain **integri**ty of basement membrane by binding to laminin in BM.
Hemidesmosome—connects keratin in basal cells to underlying basement membrane. Autoantibodies → **bullo**us pemphigoid. (Hemidesmosomes are down "**bullo**w").

Unhappy triad/ knee injury

Common injury in contact sports: lateral force applied to a planted leg. Triad includes tear of the ACL, MCL, and meniscus (classically medial, but lateral more common). Often requires surgical ACL reconstruction.
"Anterior" and "posterior" in ACL and PCL refer to sites of tibial attachment.

Positive anterior drawer sign = ACL tear
Abnormal passive abduction = MCL tear

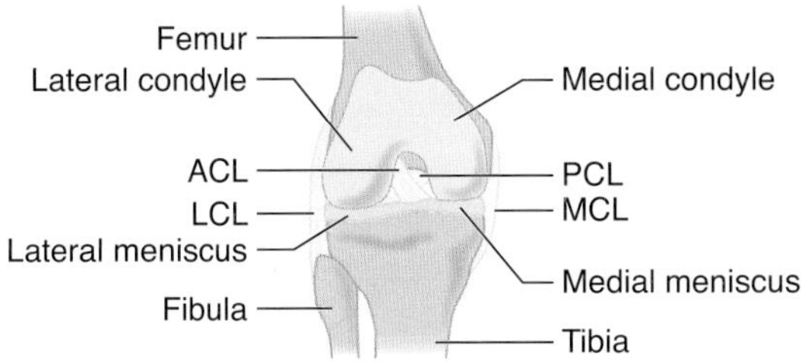
Femur
Lateral condyle
Medial condyle
ACL
PCL
LCL
MCL
Lateral meniscus
Medial meniscus
Fibula
Tibia

Clinically important landmarks

Pudendal nerve block (to relieve pain of delivery)—ischial spine.
Appendix—2/3 of the way from the umbilicus to the anterior superior iliac spine (McBurney's point).
Lumbar puncture—iliac crest.

Rotator cuff muscles

Shoulder muscles that form the rotator cuff:
- Supraspinatus—abducts arm initially (before deltoid); most common rotator cuff injury.
- Infraspinatus—laterally rotates arm; pitching injury.
- Teres minor—adducts and laterally rotates arm.
- Subscapularis—medially rotates and adducts arm.

Innervated by C5-C6.

SItS (small t is for teres minor).

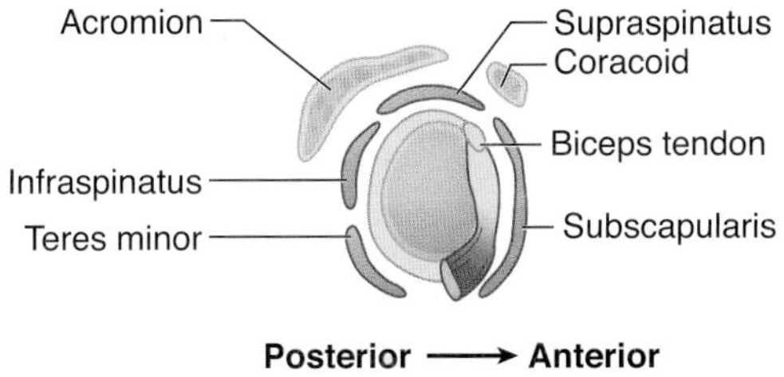
Acromion
Supraspinatus
Coracoid
Biceps tendon
Infraspinatus
Subscapularis
Teres minor
Posterior → Anterior

Wrist bones

Scaphoid, Lunate, Triquetrum, Pisiform, Hamate, Capitate, Trapezoid, Trapezium A. (So Long To Pinky, Here Comes The Thumb).
Scaphoid is most commonly fractured carpal and is prone to avascular necrosis owing to retrograde blood supply.
Dislocation of lunate may cause acute carpal tunnel syndrome.

Carpal tunnel syndrome: entrapment of median nerve in carpal tunnel; nerve compression → paresthesia, pain, and numbness in distribution of median nerve.

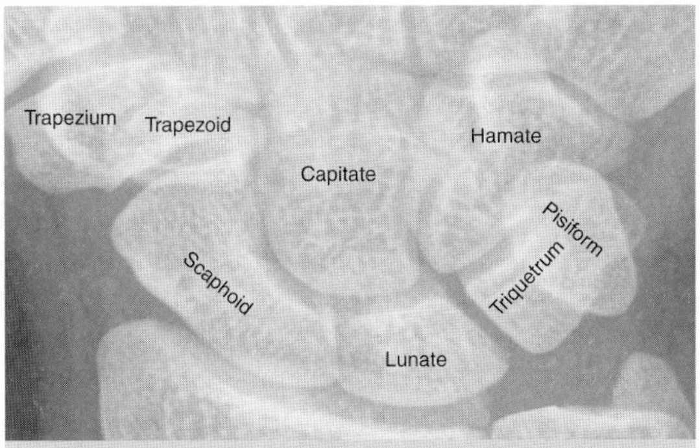
Trapezium
Trapezoid
Hamate
Capitate
Pisiform
Scaphoid
Triquetrum
Lunate

A Wrist bones.

Upper extremity innervation

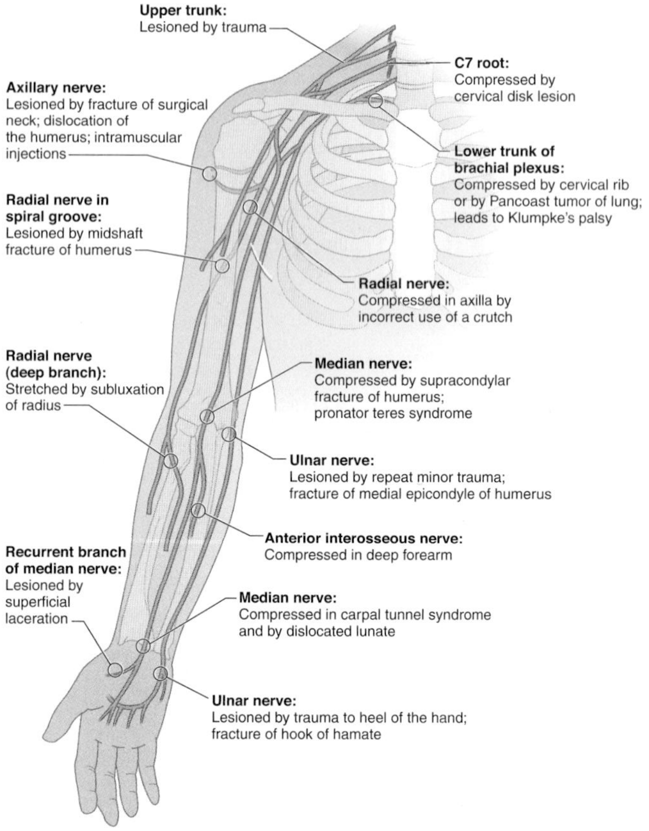

Upper trunk:
Lesioned by trauma
C7 root:
Compressed by cervical disk lesion
Axillary nerve:
Lesioned by fracture of surgical neck; dislocation of the humerus; intramuscular injections
Lower trunk of brachial plexus:
Compressed by cervical rib or by Pancoast tumor of lung; leads to Klumpke's palsy
Radial nerve in spiral groove:
Lesioned by midshaft fracture of humerus
Radial nerve:
Compressed in axilla by incorrect use of a crutch
Radial nerve (deep branch):
Stretched by subluxation of radius
Median nerve:
Compressed by supracondylar fracture of humerus; pronator teres syndrome
Ulnar nerve:
Lesioned by repeat minor trauma; fracture of medial epicondyle of humerus
Anterior interosseous nerve:
Compressed in deep forearm
Recurrent branch of median nerve:
Lesioned by superficial laceration
Median nerve:
Compressed in carpal tunnel syndrome and by dislocated lunate
Ulnar nerve:
Lesioned by trauma to heel of the hand; fracture of hook of hamate

A. Upper limb nerve routes and common lesions

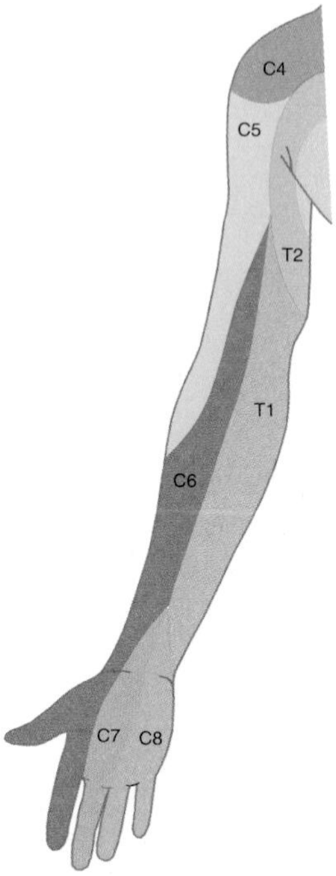

C4
C5
T2
T1
C6
C7
C8

B. Dermatomes of the upper limb/hand

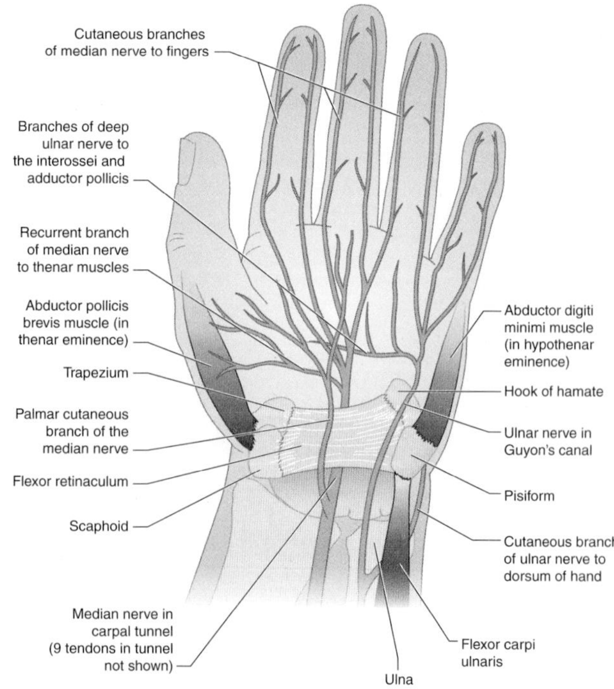

Cutaneous branches of median nerve to fingers
Branches of deep ulnar nerve to the interossei and adductor pollicis
Recurrent branch of median nerve to thenar muscles
Abductor pollicis brevis muscle (in thenar eminence)
Trapezium
Palmar cutaneous branch of the median nerve
Flexor retinaculum
Scaphoid
Median nerve in carpal tunnel (9 tendons in tunnel not shown)
Abductor digiti minimi muscle (in hypothenar eminence)
Hook of hamate
Ulnar nerve in Guyon's canal
Pisiform
Cutaneous branch of ulnar nerve to dorsum of hand
Flexor carpi ulnaris
Ulna

C. Innervation of the hand

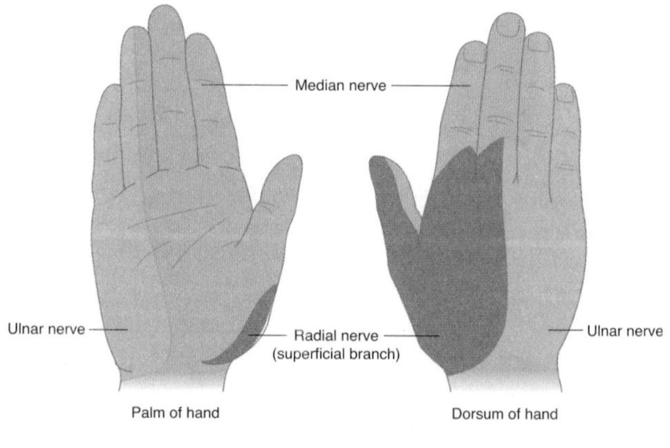

Median nerve
Ulnar nerve
Radial nerve (superficial branch)
Ulnar nerve
Palm of hand
Dorsum of hand

D. Cutaneous innervation of the hand

(Adapted, with permission, from White JS. *USMLE Road Map: Gross Anatomy,* 2nd ed. New York: McGraw-Hill, 2005: 145–147.)

Brachial plexus lesions

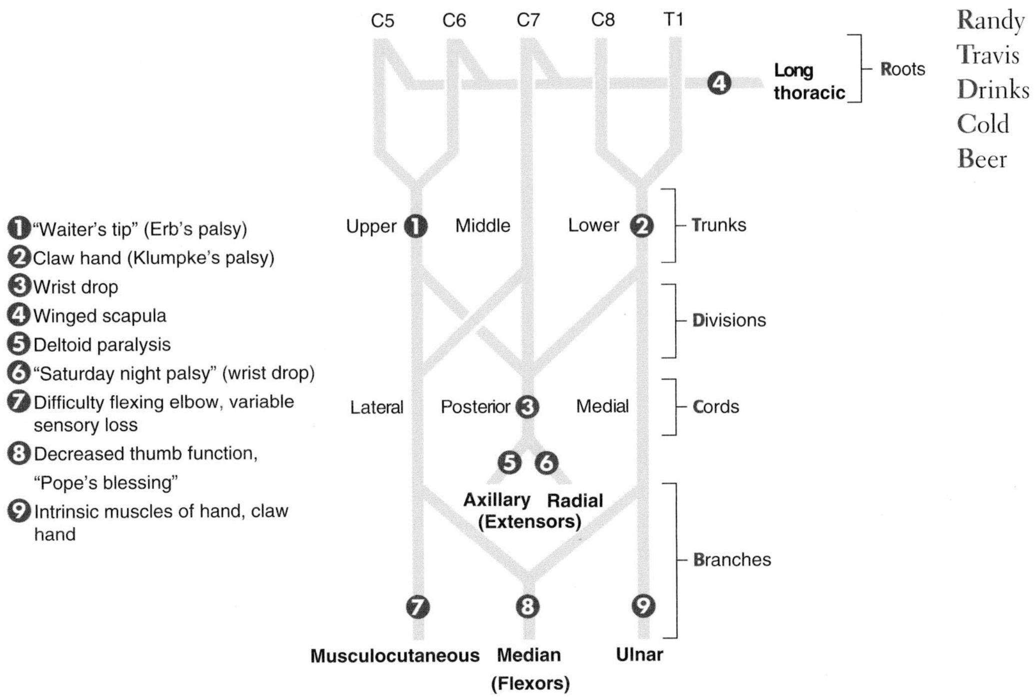

C5 C6 C7 C8 T1
Long thoracic
Roots
Randy
Travis
Drinks
Cold
Beer
❶ "Waiter's tip" (Erb's palsy)
❷ Claw hand (Klumpke's palsy)
❸ Wrist drop
❹ Winged scapula
❺ Deltoid paralysis
❻ "Saturday night palsy" (wrist drop)
❼ Difficulty flexing elbow, variable sensory loss
❽ Decreased thumb function, "Pope's blessing"
❾ Intrinsic muscles of hand, claw hand
Upper ❶
Middle
Lower ❷
Trunks
Divisions
Lateral
Posterior ❸
Medial
Cords
❺ ❻
Axillary Radial
(Extensors)
Branches
❼ ❽ ❾
Musculocutaneous
Median
(Flexors)
Ulnar

Clavicle fracture is relatively common—brachial plexus is protected from injury by subclavius muscle.

Upper extremity nerves

NERVE	TYPICAL INJURY	MOTOR DEFICIT	SENSORY DEFICIT	SIGN
Axillary (C5, C6)	Fractured surgical neck of humerus, dislocation of humeral head	Deltoid—arm abduction at shoulder	Over deltoid muscle	Atrophied deltoid
Radial (C5–T1)	Fracture at midshaft of humerus; "Saturday night palsy" (extended compression of axilla by back of chair or crutches)	"BEST extensors"—Brachioradialis, Extensors of wrist and fingers, Supinator, Triceps	Posterior arm and dorsal hand and thumb	Wrist drop
Median (C5–C8, T1)	Fracture of supracondylar humerus (proximal lesion)	Opposition of thumb Lateral finger flexion Wrist flexion	Dorsal and palmar aspects of lateral 3½ fingers, thenar eminence	"Ape hand"; "Pope's blessing" (hand)
Ulnar (C8, T1)	Fracture of medial epicondyle of humerus, "funny bone" (proximal lesion)	Medial finger flexion Wrist flexion	Medial 1½ fingers, hypothenar eminence	Radial deviation of wrist upon wrist flexion
Musculocutaneous (C5–C7)	Upper trunk compression	Biceps, brachialis, coracobrachialis Flexion of arm at elbow	Lateral forearm	

Note: Always consider the lesion location; generally, muscles innervated by nerve branches distal to the lesion will be affected. Note that this table is highly simplified. Distal median and ulnar lesions discussed later.

Erb-Duchenne palsy ("waiter's tip")

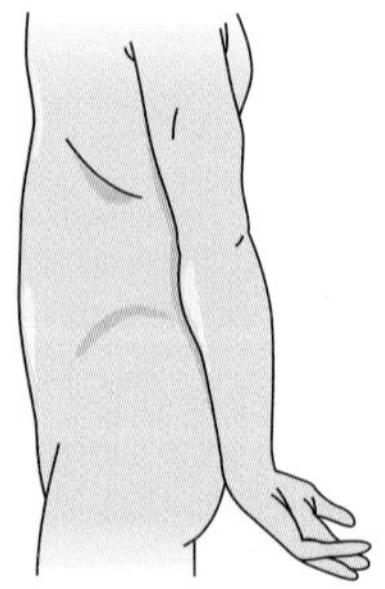

Traction or tear of the upper trunk of the brachial plexus (C5 and C6 roots); seen in infants following trauma during delivery.

Findings: limb hangs by side (paralysis of abductors), medially rotated (paralysis of lateral rotators), forearm is pronated (loss of biceps).

"Waiter's tip" owing to appearance of arm.

Klumpke's palsy and thoracic outlet syndrome

An embryologic or childbirth defect affecting inferior trunk of brachial plexus (C8, T1); a cervical rib can compress subclavian artery and inferior trunk, resulting in thoracic outlet syndrome:

- Atrophy of the thenar and hypothenar eminences
- Atrophy of the interosseous muscles
- Sensory deficits on the medial side of the forearm and hand
- Disappearance of the radial pulse upon moving the head toward the ipsilateral side

Distortions of the hand	"Clawing" is easily conceptualized as loss of the lumbricals, which flex the MCP joints and extend both the DIP and PIP joints.
Ulnar claw	Can be caused by long-standing injury to ulnar nerve at hook of hamate (e.g., by falling onto outstretched hand). Distal ulnar nerve lesion → loss of medial lumbrical function → inability to extend 4th and 5th digits ("clawing") when trying to open the hand.
Median claw	Can be caused by carpal tunnel syndrome or dislocated lunate. Distal median nerve lesion (after branch containing C5–C7 branches off to feed forearm flexors) → loss of lateral lumbrical function; 2nd and 3rd digits are clawed upon attempted finger extension.
"Pope's blessing"	Proximal median nerve lesion causes loss of lateral finger flexion and thumb opposition. When asked to make fist, 2nd and 3rd digits remain extended and thumb remains unopposed, which looks like the hand of benediction or "Pope's blessing."
"Ape hand"	Proximal median nerve lesion → loss of opponens pollicis muscle function → unopposable thumb (inability to abduct thumb), hence "ape hand."
Klumpke's total claw	Lesion of lower trunk (C8, T1) of brachial plexus → loss of function of all lumbricals; forearm finger flexors (fed by part of median nerve with C5–C7) and finger extensors (fed by radial nerve) are unopposed → clawing of all digits.

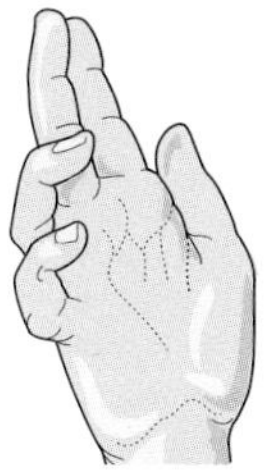

Distal ulnar claw
Claw hand of 4th and 5th digits when straightening fingers

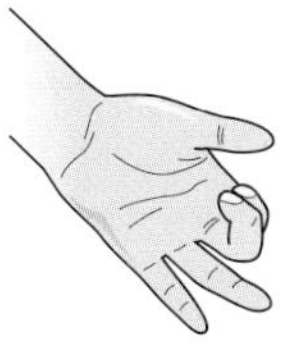

Median claw
Claw hand of 2nd and 3rd digits when straightening fingers

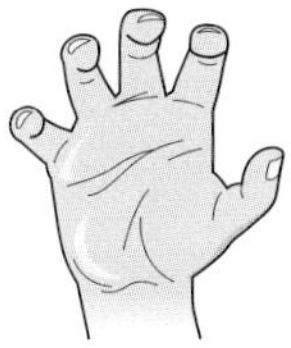

Klumpke's total claw hand
Lower trunk (C8, T1) lesion

Long thoracic nerve (C5–C7)

Serratus anterior—anchors scapula to thoracic cage. Used for abduction above horizontal position. Can be injured in mastectomy → winged scapula and ipsilateral lymphedema.

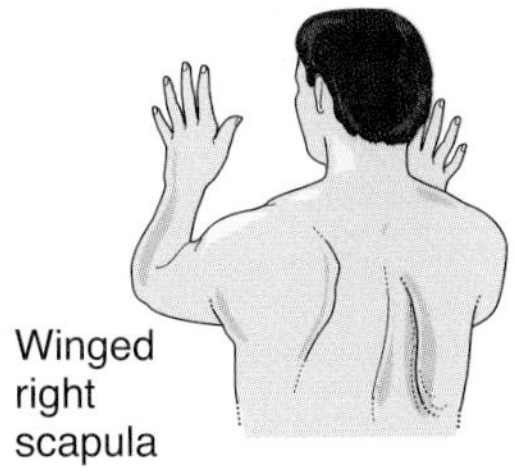
Winged
right
scapula

Hand muscles

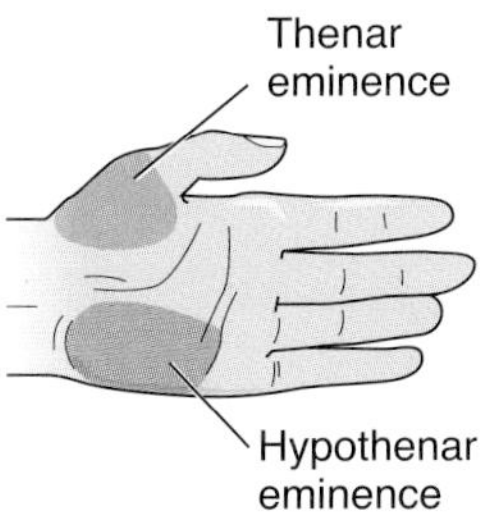
Thenar
eminence
Hypothenar
eminence

Thenar (median)—Opponens pollicis, Abductor pollicis brevis, Flexor pollicis brevis.
Hypothenar (ulnar)—Opponens digiti minimi, Abductor digiti minimi, Flexor digiti minimi.

Both groups perform the same functions: Oppose, Abduct, and Flex (OAF).

Dorsal interosseous muscles—abduct the fingers.
Palmar interosseous muscles—adduct the fingers.

DAB = Dorsals ABduct.
PAD = Palmars ADduct.

Lumbrical muscles—flex at the MCP joint, extend PIP and DIP joints.

Lower extremity nerves

NERVE	CAUSE OF INJURY	MOTOR DEFICIT	SENSORY DEFICIT
Obturator (L2–L4)	Anterior hip dislocation	Thigh adduction	Medial thigh
Femoral (L2–L4)	Pelvic fracture	Thigh flexion and leg extension	Anterior thigh and medial leg
Common peroneal (L4–S2)	Trauma or compression of lateral aspect of leg or fibula neck fracture	Foot eversion and dorsiflexion; toe extension; foot drop, foot slap, steppage gait	Anterolateral leg and dorsal aspect of foot
Tibial (L4–S3)	Knee trauma	Foot inversion and plantarflexion; toe flexion	Sole of foot
Superior gluteal (L4–S1)	Posterior hip dislocation or polio	Thigh abduction (positive Trendelenburg sign—contralateral hip drops when standing on leg ipsilateral to site of lesion)	
Inferior gluteal (L5–S2)	Posterior hip dislocation	Can't jump, climb stairs, or rise from seated position; can't push inferiorly (downward)	

PED = **P**eroneal **E**verts and **D**orsiflexes; if injured, foot drop**PED**.

TIP = **T**ibial **I**nverts and **P**lantarflexes; if injured, can't stand on **TIP**toes.

Sciatic nerve (L4–S3)—posterior thigh, splits into common peroneal and tibial nerve.

Muscle conduction to contraction

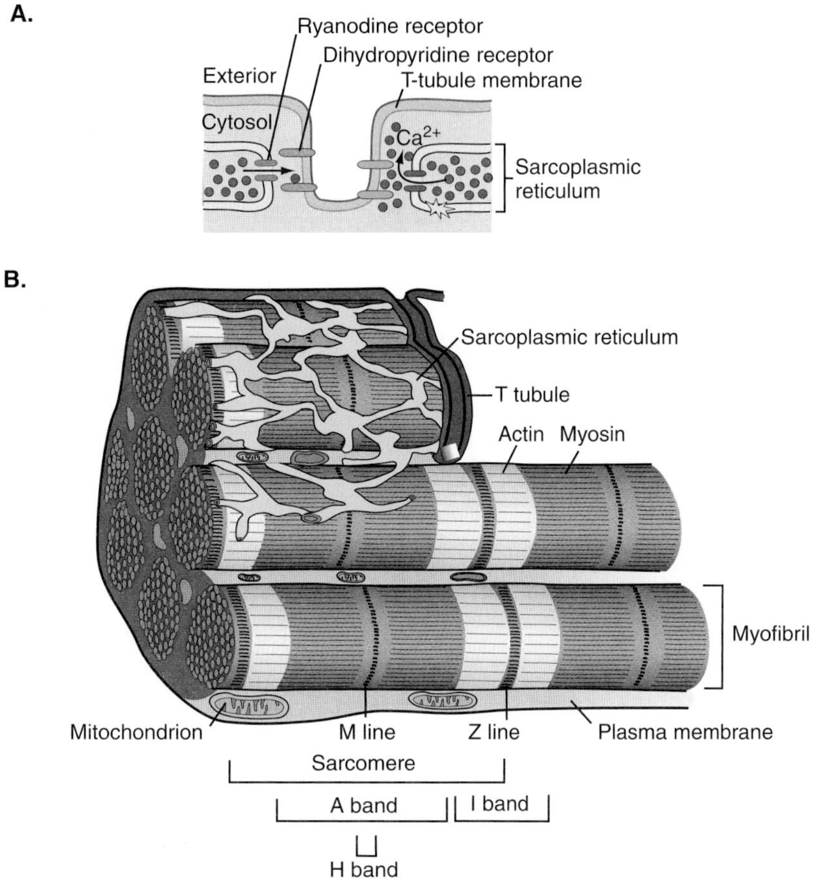

(Reproduced, with permission, from USMLE-Rx.com.)

Muscle contraction

1. Action potential depolarization opens presynaptic voltage-gated Ca^{2+} channels, inducing neurotransmitter release.
2. Postsynaptic ligand binding leads to muscle cell depolarization in the motor end plate.
3. Depolarization travels along muscle cell and down the T tubule.
4. Depolarization of the voltage-sensitive dihydropyridine receptor, mechanically coupled to the ryanodine receptor on the sarcoplasmic reticulum, induces a conformational change causing Ca^{2+} release from sarcoplasmic reticulum.
5. Released Ca^{2+} binds to troponin C, causing a conformational change that moves tropomyosin out of the myosin-binding groove on actin filaments.
6. Myosin releases bound ADP and is displaced on the actin filament (power stroke). Contraction results in shortening of **H** and **I** bands and between **Z** lines (**HIZ** shrinkage), but the A band remains the same length (**A** band is **A**lways the same length).

Types of muscle fibers

Type 1 muscle	Slow twitch; **red** fibers resulting from ↑ mitochondria and myoglobin concentration (↑ **oxidative** phosphorylation) → sustained contraction.	Think "**1 slow red ox**."
Type 2 muscle	Fast twitch; white fibers resulting from ↓ mitochondria and myoglobin concentration (↑ anaerobic glycolysis); weight training results in hypertrophy of fast-twitch muscle fibers.	

Skeletal and cardiac muscle contraction

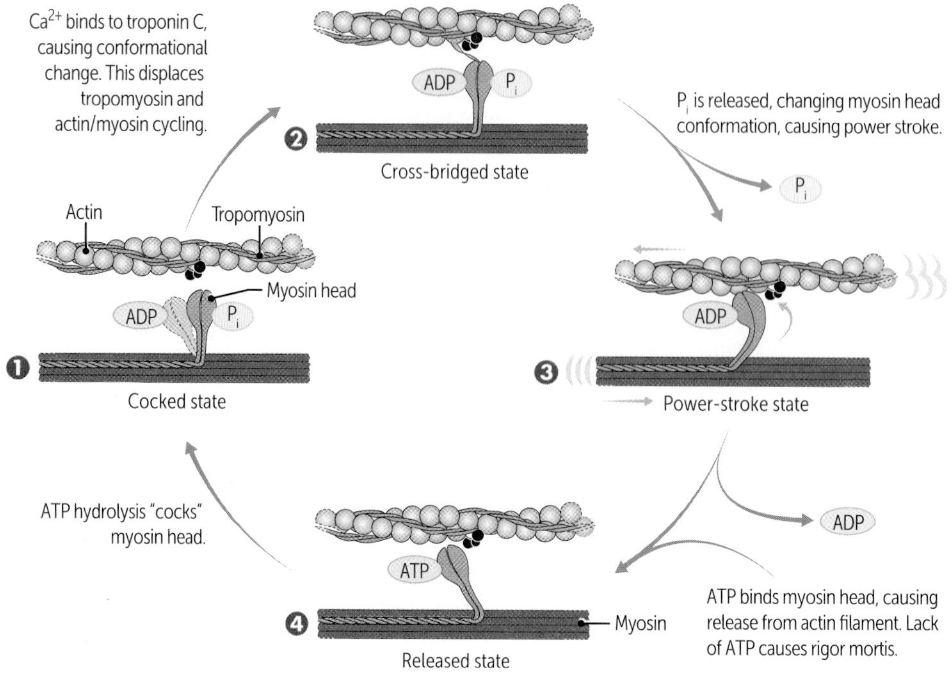

Ca2+ binds to troponin C, causing conformational change. This displaces tropomyosin and actin/myosin cycling.
ADP
Pi
2
Cross-bridged state
Pi is released, changing myosin head conformation, causing power stroke.
Pi
Actin
Tropomyosin
Myosin head
ADP
Pi
1
Cocked state
ADP
3
Power-stroke state
ATP hydrolysis "cocks" myosin head.
ADP
ATP
4
Myosin
Released state
ATP binds myosin head, causing release from actin filament. Lack of ATP causes rigor mortis.

Bone formation

Endochondral ossification	Bones of axial and appendicular skeleton, and base of the skull. Cartilaginous model of bone is first made by chondrocytes. Osteoclasts and osteoblasts later replace with woven bone and then remodel to lamellar bone. In adults, woven bone occurs after fractures and in Paget's disease.
Membranous ossification	Bones of calvarium and facial bones. Woven bone formed directly without cartilage. Later remodeled to lamellar bone.

Cell biology of bone

Osteoblasts	Build bone by secreting collagen and catalyzing mineralization. Differentiate from mesenchymal stem cells in periosteum.
Osteoclasts	Multinucleated cells that dissolve bone by secreting acid and collagenases. Differentiate from monocytes/macrophages.
Parathyroid hormone	At low, intermittent levels, exerts anabolic effects (building bone) on osteoblasts and osteoclasts (indirect). Chronic high PTH levels (primary hyperparathyroidism) cause catabolic effects (osteitis fibrosa cystica).
Estrogen	Estrogen inhibits apoptosis in bone-forming osteoblasts and induces apoptosis in bone-resorbing osteoclasts. Under estrogen deficiency (surgical or postmenopausal), excess remodeling cycles and bone resorption lead to osteoporosis.

▸ MUSCULOSKELETAL, SKIN, AND CONNECTIVE TISSUE—PATHOLOGY

Achondroplasia

Failure of longitudinal bone growth (endochondral ossification) → short limbs. Membranous ossification is not affected → large head relative to limbs. Constitutive activation of fibroblast growth factor receptor (FGFR3) actually inhibits chondrocyte proliferation. > 85% of mutations occur sporadically and are associated with advanced paternal age, but the condition also demonstrates autosomal-dominant inheritance. Common cause of dwarfism. Normal life span and fertility.

Osteoporosis

Trabecular (spongy) bone loses mass and interconnections despite normal bone mineralization and lab values (serum Ca^{2+} and PO_4^{3-}).

Can lead to **vertebral crush fractures**—acute back pain, loss of height, kyphosis.

Type I

Postmenopausal: ↑ bone resorption due to ↓ estrogen levels.

Femoral neck fracture, distal radius (Colles') fractures.

Type II

Senile osteoporosis: affects men and women > 70 years of age.

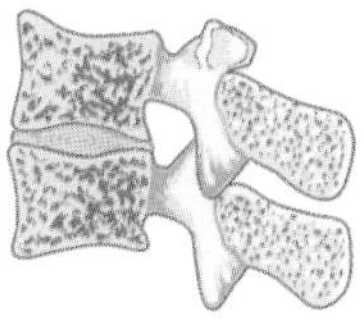

Mild compression fracture

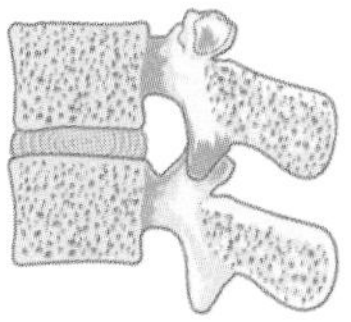

Normal vertebrae

Prophylaxis: regular weight-bearing exercise and adequate calcium and vitamin D intake throughout adulthood.

Treatment: estrogen (SERMs) and/or calcitonin; bisphosphonates or pulsatile PTH for severe cases. Glucocorticoids are contraindicated.

Osteopetrosis (marble bone disease)

Failure of normal bone resorption due to defective osteoclasts → thickened, dense bones that are prone to fracture. Bone fills marrow space, causing pancytopenia, extramedullary hematopoiesis. Mutations (e.g., carbonic anhydrase II) impair ability of osteoclast to generate acidic environment necessary for bone resorption. X-rays show bone-in-bone appearance. Can result in cranial nerve impingement and palsies as a result of narrowed foramina. Bone marrow transplant is potentially curative as osteoclasts are derived from monocytes.

Osteomalacia/rickets

Vitamin D deficiency. Osteomalacia in adults; rickets in children. Due to defective mineralization/calcification of osteoid → soft bones that bow out. ↓ vitamin D → ↓ serum calcium → ↑ PTH secretion → ↓ serum phosphate. Hyperactivity of osteoblasts → ↑ alkaline phosphatase (osteoblasts require alkaline environment).

Paget's disease of bone (osteitis deformans)

Common, localized disorder of bone remodeling caused by ↑ in both osteoblastic and osteoclastic activity. Serum calcium, phosphorus, and PTH levels are normal. ↑ ALP. Mosaic ("woven") bone pattern; long bone chalk-stick fractures. ↑ blood flow from ↑ arteriovenous shunts may cause high-output heart failure. ↑ risk of osteogenic sarcoma.

Hat size can be ↑; hearing loss is common due to auditory foramen narrowing.

Lab values in bone disorders

	SERUM Ca^{2+}	PHOSPHATE	ALP	PTH	COMMENTS
Osteoporosis	—	—	—	—	↓ bone mass
Osteopetrosis	↓	—	↑	—	Thickened, dense bones
Osteomalacia/rickets	↓	↓	↑	↑	Soft bones
Osteitis fibrosa cystica	↑	↓	↑	↑	"Brown tumors" of hyperparathyroidism
Paget's disease	—	—	↑	—	Abnormal bone architecture

Polyostotic fibrous dysplasia

Bone is replaced by fibroblasts, collagen, and irregular bony trabeculae. **McCune-Albright syndrome** is a form of polyostotic fibrous dysplasia characterized by multiple unilateral bone lesions associated with endocrine abnormalities (precocious puberty) and café-au-lait spots.

Primary bone tumors

TUMOR TYPE	EPIDEMIOLOGY/LOCATION	CHARACTERISTICS
Benign tumors		
Giant cell tumor (osteoclastoma)	20–40 years of age. Epiphyseal end of long bones.	Locally aggressive benign tumor often around the distal femur, proximal tibial region (knee). "Double bubble" or "soap bubble" appearance on x-ray. Spindle-shaped cells with multinucleated giant cells.
Osteochondroma (exostosis)	Most common benign tumor. Males < 25 years of age.	Mature bone with cartilaginous cap. Commonly originates from long metaphysis. Malignant transformation to chondrosarcoma is rare.
Malignant tumors		
Osteosarcoma (osteogenic sarcoma)	2nd most common 1° malignant bone tumor (after multiple myeloma). Male > female, 10–20 years of age (1°). Predisposing factors: Paget's disease of bone, bone infarcts, radiation, familial retinoblastoma. Metaphysis of long bones, often around distal femur, proximal tibial region (knee).	Codman's triangle (from elevation of periosteum) or sunburst pattern on x-ray. Aggressive. Treat with surgical en bloc resection (with limb salvage) and chemotherapy.
Ewing's sarcoma	Boys < 15 years of age. Commonly appears in diaphysis of long bones, pelvis, scapula, and ribs.	Anaplastic small blue cell malignant tumor. Extremely aggressive with early metastases, but responsive to chemotherapy. "**Onion** skin" appearance in bone ("going out for **Ewings** and **onion** rings"). Associated with t(**11**;**22**) translocation. **11** + **22** = **33** (Patrick **Ewing's** jersey number).
Chondrosarcoma	Men 30–60 years of age. Usually located in pelvis, spine, scapula, humerus, tibia, or femur.	Malignant cartilaginous tumor. May be of 1° origin or from osteochondroma. Expansile glistening mass within the medullary cavity.

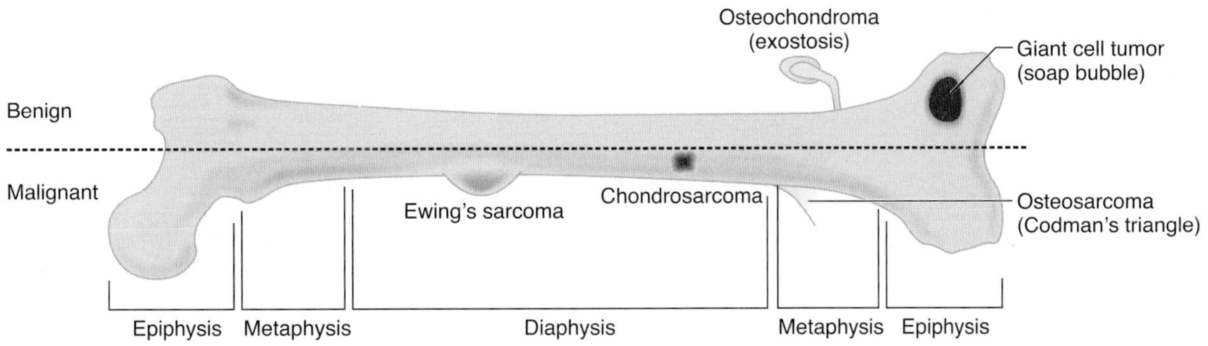

Osteoarthritis and rheumatoid arthritis

	Osteoarthritis	Rheumatoid arthritis
ETIOLOGY	Mechanical—joint wear and tear destroys articular cartilage	Autoimmune—inflammatory destruction of synovial joints. Type III hypersensitivity.
JOINT FINDINGS	Subchondral cysts, sclerosis A, osteophytes (bone spurs), eburnation (polished, ivory-like appearance of bone), Heberden's nodes (DIP), and Bouchard's nodes (PIP). No MCP involvement.	Pannus formation in joints (MCP, PIP), subcutaneous rheumatoid nodules (fibrinoid necrosis), ulnar deviation of fingers, subluxation B, Baker's cyst (in popliteal fossa). No DIP involvement.
PREDISPOSING FACTORS	Age, obesity, joint deformity	Females > males. 80% have positive rheumatoid factor (anti-IgG antibody); anti–cyclic citrullinated peptide antibody is more specific. Strong association with HLA-DR4.
CLASSIC PRESENTATION	Pain in weight-bearing joints after use (e.g., at the end of the day), improving with rest. Knee cartilage loss begins medially ("bowlegged"). Noninflammatory. No systemic symptoms.	Morning stiffness lasting > 30 minutes and improving with use, symmetric joint involvement, systemic symptoms (fever, fatigue, pleuritis, pericarditis).
TREATMENT	NSAIDs, intra-articular glucocorticoids	NSAIDs, glucocorticoids, disease-modifying agents (methotrexate, sulfasalazine, TNF-α inhibitors)

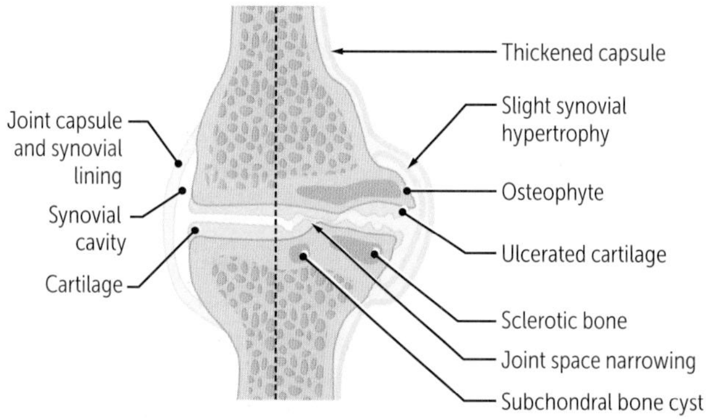
Normal
Osteoarthritis
Thickened capsule
Slight synovial hypertrophy
Joint capsule and synovial lining
Osteophyte
Synovial cavity
Ulcerated cartilage
Cartilage
Sclerotic bone
Joint space narrowing
Subchondral bone cyst

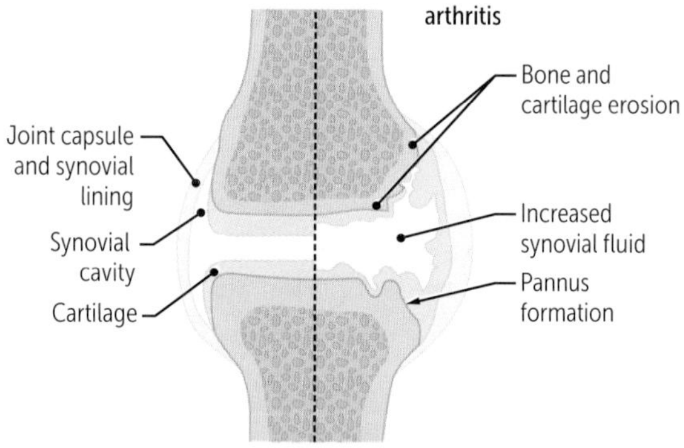
Normal
Rheumatoid arthritis
Bone and cartilage erosion
Joint capsule and synovial lining
Increased synovial fluid
Synovial cavity
Pannus formation
Cartilage

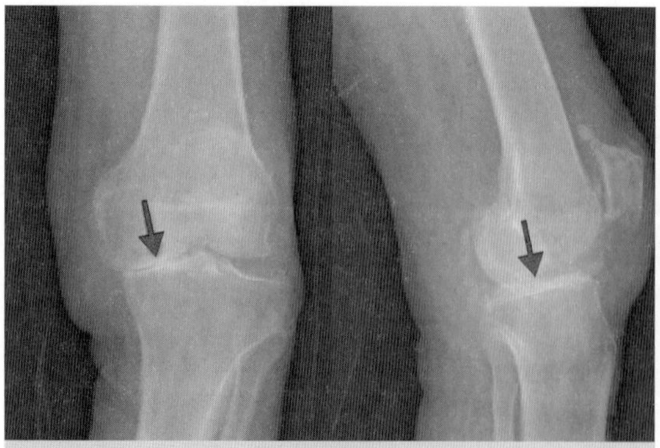

A **Osteoarthritis.** X-rays of the knee show joint space narrowing and sclerosis (arrows).

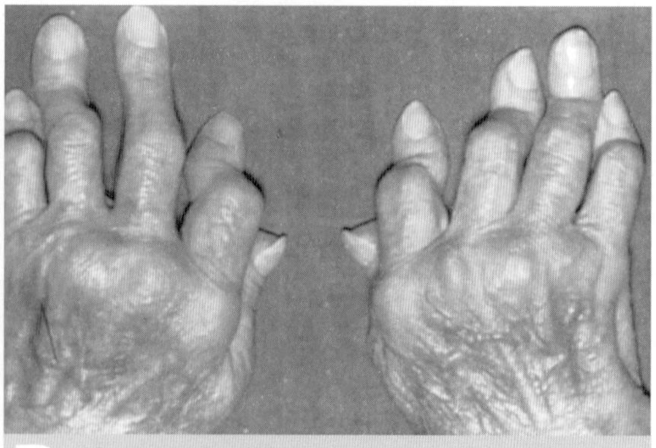

B **Rheumatoid arthritis.** Note boutonnière deformities of digits with ulnar deviation.

Sjögren's syndrome	Lymphocytic infiltration of exocrine glands, especially lacrimal and salivary. Classic triad: ▪ Xerophthalmia (dry eyes, conjunctivitis, "sand in my eyes") ▪ Xerostomia (dry mouth, dysphagia) ▪ Arthritis Parotid enlargement, ↑ risk of B-cell lymphoma, dental caries. Autoantibodies to ribonucleoprotein antigens: SS-A (Ro), SS-B (La).	Predominantly affects females between 40 and 60 years of age. Associated with rheumatoid arthritis.

Gout

FINDINGS	Precipitation of monosodium urate crystals into joints A due to hyperuricemia, which can be caused by Lesch-Nyhan syndrome, PRPP excess, ↓ excretion of uric acid (e.g., thiazide diuretics), ↑ cell turnover, or von Gierke's disease. 90% due to underexcretion; 10% due to overproduction. Crystals are needle shaped and negatively birefringent = yellow crystals under parallel light. More common in men.	
SYMPTOMS	Asymmetric joint distribution. Joint is swollen, red, and painful B. Classic manifestation is painful MTP joint of the big toe (podagra). Tophus formation (often on external ear, olecranon bursa, or Achilles tendon). Acute attack tends to occur after a large meal or alcohol consumption (alcohol metabolites compete for same excretion sites in kidney as uric acid, causing ↓ uric acid secretion and subsequent buildup in blood).	
TREATMENT	Acute: NSAIDs (e.g., indomethacin), glucocorticoids. Chronic: xanthine oxidase inhibitors (e.g., allopurinol, febuxostat).	

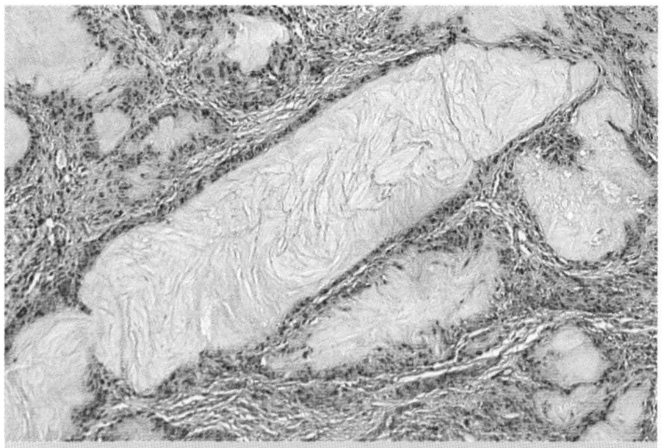

A **Tophi in joints.** Aggregates of urate crystals surrounded by inflammation.

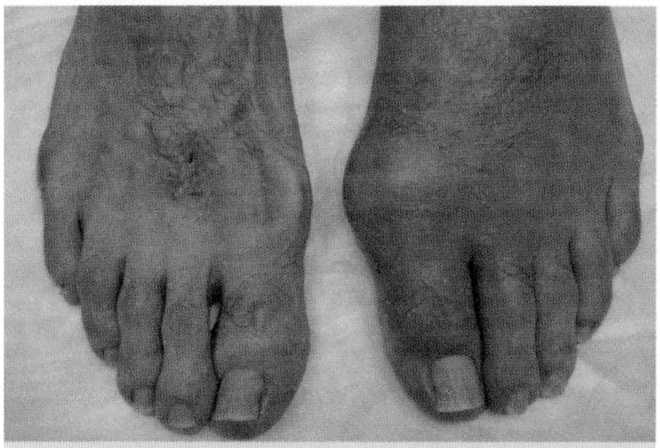

B **Gout.** Left big toe (podagra) is swollen and red.

Pseudogout	Caused by deposition of calcium pyrophosphate crystals within the joint space. Forms basophilic, rhomboid crystals that are weakly positively birefringent. Usually affects large joints (classically the knee). > 50 years old; both sexes affected equally. Treatment includes NSAIDs for sudden, severe attacks; steroids; and colchicine. Gout—crystals are yellow when parallel (‖) to the light. Pseudogout—crystals are blue when parallel (‖) to the light.

Infectious arthritis	*S. aureus*, *Streptococcus*, and *Neisseria gonorrhoeae* are common causes. Gonococcal arthritis is an STD that presents as a migratory arthritis with an asymmetric pattern. Affected joint is swollen, red, and painful. STD = Synovitis (e.g., knee), Tenosynovitis (e.g., hand), and Dermatitis (e.g., pustules).	
Osteonecrosis (avascular necrosis)	Infarction of bone and marrow. Pain associated with activity. Caused by trauma, high-dose corticosteroids, alcoholism, sickle cell. Most common site is femoral head.	
Seronegative spondyloarthropathies	Arthritis without rheumatoid factor (no anti-IgG antibody). Strong association with HLA-B27 (gene that codes for HLA MHC class I). Occurs more often in males.	PAIR
Psoriatic arthritis	Joint pain and stiffness associated with psoriasis. Asymmetric and patchy involvement. Dactylitis ("sausage fingers"), "pencil-in-cup" deformity on x-ray. Seen in fewer than ⅓ of patients with psoriasis.	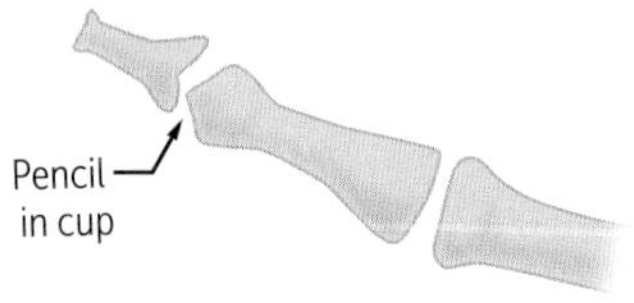
Ankylosing spondylitis	Chronic inflammatory disease of spine and sacroiliac joints → ankylosis (stiff spine due to fusion of joints), uveitis, and aortic regurgitation.	Bamboo spine (vertebral fusion).
Inflammatory bowel disease	Crohn's disease and ulcerative colitis are often accompanied by anklyosing spondylitis or peripheral arthritis.	
Reactive arthritis (Reiter's syndrome)	Classic triad: ▪ **Conjunctivitis** and anterior uveitis ▪ **Urethritis** ▪ **Arthritis**	**"Can't see, can't pee, can't climb a tree."** Post-GI or chlamydia infections.

Systemic lupus erythematosus

90% are female and between ages 14 and 45. Most common and severe in black females.

Presentation can include fever, fatigue, weight loss, Libman-Sacks endocarditis (verrucous, wart-like, sterile vegetations on both sides of valve), hilar adenopathy, and Raynaud's phenomenon.

Nephritis is common cause of death in SLE. Diffuse proliferative glomerulonephritis (if nephritic); membranous glomerulonephritis (if nephrotic).

False positives on syphilis tests (RPR/VDRL) due to antiphospholipid antibodies, which cross-react with cardiolipin used in tests. Lab tests detect presence of:

- Antinuclear antibodies (ANA)—sensitive, (primary screening) but not specific for SLE
- Antibodies to double-stranded DNA (anti-dsDNA)—very specific, poor prognosis
- Anti-Smith antibodies (anti-Sm)—very specific, but not prognostic
- Antihistone antibodies—more sensitive for drug-induced lupus

I'M DAMN SHARP:

- Immunoglobulins (anti-dsDNA, anti-Sm, antiphospholipid)
- Malar rash A
- Discoid rash
- Antinuclear antibody
- Mucositis (oropharyngeal ulcers)
- Neurologic disorders
- Serositis (pleuritis, pericarditis)
- Hematologic disorders
- Arthritis
- Renal disorders
- Photosensitivity

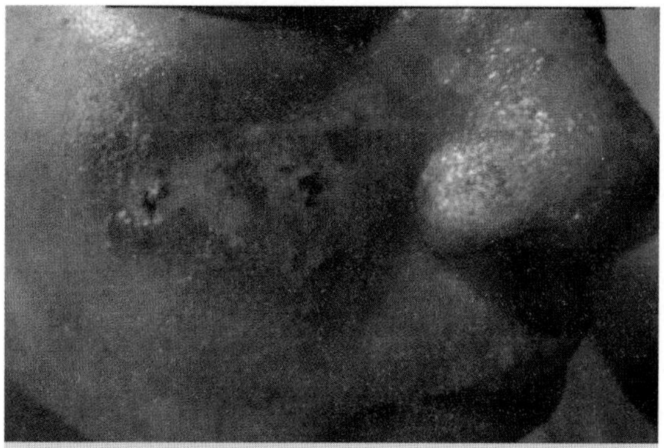

A Malar rash.

Sarcoidosis

Characterized by immune-mediated, widespread noncaseating granulomas A and elevated serum ACE levels. Common in black females. Often asymptomatic except for enlarged lymph node. Incidental findings on CXR of **bilateral hilar adenopathy** or reticular opacities.

Associated with restrictive lung disease (interstitial fibrosis), erythema nodosum, Bell's palsy, epithelial granulomas containing microscopic Schaumann and asteroid bodies, uveitis, and hypercalcemia (due to elevated 1α-hydroxylase–mediated vitamin D activation in epithelioid macrophages).

Treatment: steroids.

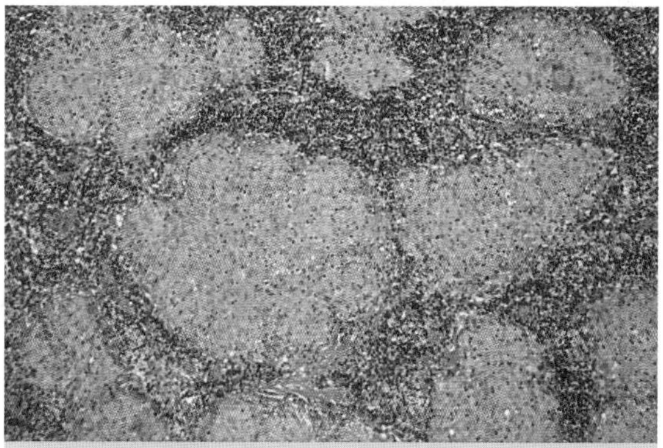

A Sarcoidosis.

Polymyalgia rheumatica

SYMPTOMS	Pain and stiffness in shoulders and hips, often with fever, malaise, and weight loss. Does not cause muscular weakness. More common in women > 50 years of age; associated with temporal (giant cell) arteritis.
FINDINGS	↑ ESR, normal CK.
TREATMENT	Rapid response to low-dose corticosteroids.

Fibromyalgia	Most commonly seen in women 20–50 years of age. Chronic, widespread musculoskeletal pain associated with stiffness, paresthesia, poor sleep, and fatigue.

Polymyositis/dermatomyositis

SYMPTOMS 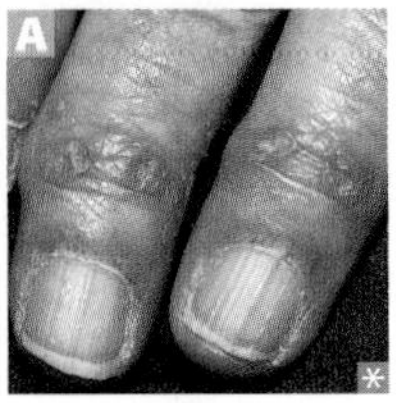	**Polymyositis**—progressive symmetric proximal muscle weakness, characterized by endomysial inflammation with CD8+ T cells. Most often involves shoulders. **Dermatomyositis**—similar to polymyositis, but also involves malar rash (similar to SLE), Gottron's papules A, heliotrope rash B, "shawl and face" rash, "mechanic's hands." ↑ risk of occult malignancy. Perimysial inflammation and atrophy with CD4+ T cells.
FINDINGS	↑ CK, positive ANA, positive anti-Jo-1 antibodies.
TREATMENT	Steroids.

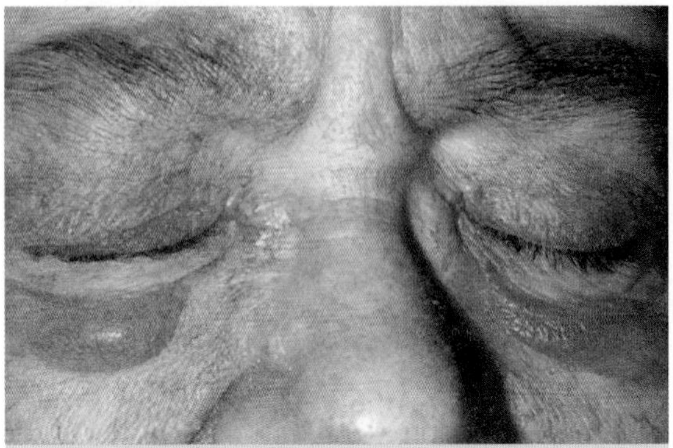

B Heliotrope rash.

Neuromuscular junction diseases

	Myasthenia gravis	Lambert-Eaton myasthenic syndrome
FREQUENCY	Most common NMJ disorder	Uncommon
PATHOPHYSIOLOGY	Autoantibodies to postsynaptic ACh receptor	Autoantibodies to presynaptic Ca^{2+} channel → ↓ ACh release
CLINICAL	Ptosis, diplopia, weakness Worsens with muscle use	Proximal muscle weakness Improves with muscle use
ASSOCIATED WITH	Thymoma, thymic hyperplasia	Small cell lung cancer
AChE INHIBITOR ADMINISTRATION	Reversal of symptoms	No effect

Myositis ossificans	Metaplasia of skeletal muscle to bone following muscular trauma A. Most often seen in upper or lower extremity. May present as suspicious "mass" at site of known trauma or as incidental finding on radiography.

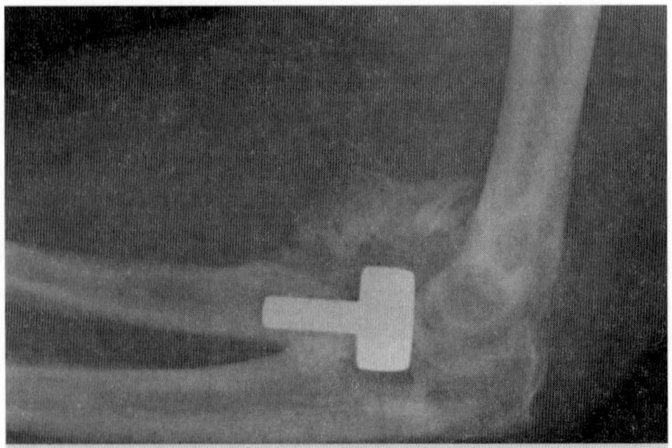

A **Myositis ossificans.** Heterotopic ossification of elbow after injury.

Scleroderma (systemic sclerosis)

Excessive fibrosis and collagen deposition throughout the body. Commonly sclerosis of skin, manifesting as puffy and taut skin A with absence of wrinkles. Also sclerosis of renal, pulmonary (most likely cause of death), cardiovascular, and GI systems. 75% female. 2 major types:

- **Diffuse scleroderma**—widespread skin involvement, rapid progression, early visceral involvement. Associated with anti-Scl-70 antibody (anti-DNA topoisomerase I antibody).
- **CREST syndrome**—Calcinosis, Raynaud's phenomenon, Esophageal dysmotility, Sclerodactyly, and Telangiectasia. Limited skin involvement, often confined to fingers and face. More benign clinical course. Associated with antiCentromere antibody (C for CREST).

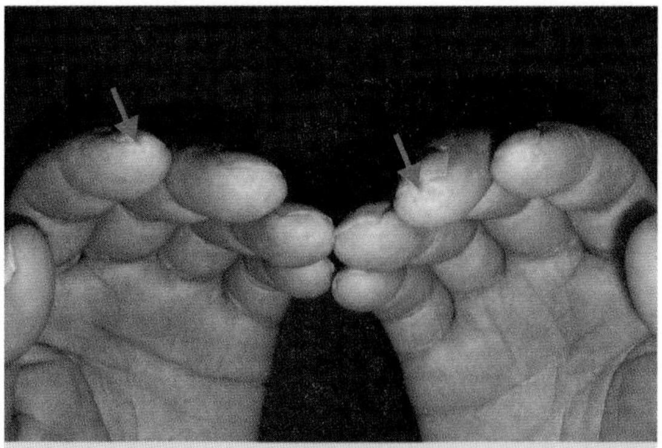

A **Scleroderma.** Note "tightening" of skin with ulceration (arrows).

Dermatologic macroscopic terms (morphology)

LESION	CHARACTERISTICS	EXAMPLES
Macule	Flat lesion with well-circumscribed change in skin color < 5 mm	Freckle, labial macule A
Patch	Macule > 5 mm	Large birthmark (congenital nevus) B
Papule	Elevated solid skin lesion < 5 mm	Mole (nevus) C, acne
Plaque	Papule > 5 mm	Psoriasis D
Vesicle	Small fluid-containing blister < 5 mm	Chickenpox (varicella), shingles (zoster) E
Bulla	Large fluid-containing blister > 5 mm	Bullous pemphigoid F
Pustule	Vesicle containing pus	Pustular psoriasis G
Wheal	Transient smooth papule or plaque	Hives (urticaria) H
Scale	Flaking off of stratum corneum	Eczema, psoriasis, SCC I
Crust	Dry exudate	Impetigo J

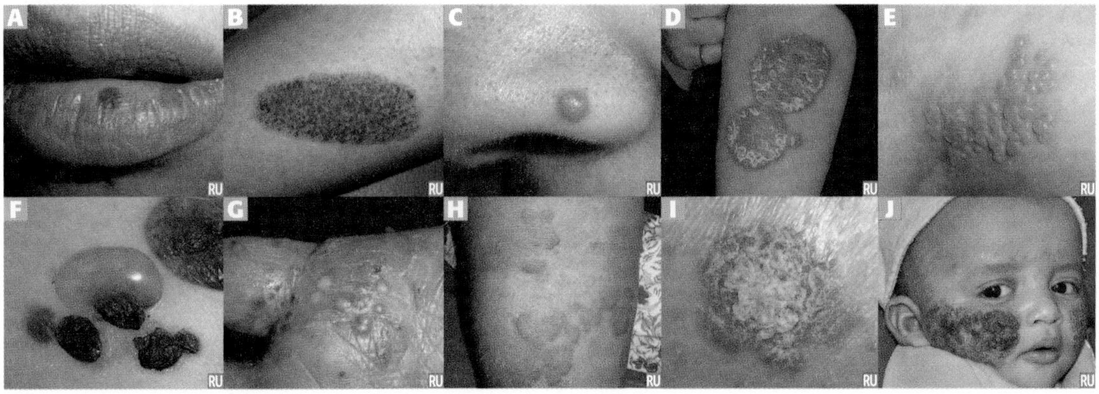

RU Courtesy of Dr. Richard P. Usatine and the *Color Atlas of Family Medicine* (www.usatinemedia.com).

Dermatologic microscopic terms

LESION	CHARACTERISTICS	EXAMPLES
Hyperkeratosis	↑ thickness of stratum corneum	Psoriasis
Parakeratosis	Hyperkeratosis with retention of nuclei in stratum corneum	Psoriasis
Acantholysis	Separation of epidermal cells	Pemphigus vulgaris
Acanthosis	Epidermal hyperplasia (↑ spinosum)	Acanthosis nigricans
Dermatitis	Inflammation of the skin	Atopic dermatitis

Pigmented skin disorders

Albinism	Normal melanocyte number with ↓ melanin production due to ↓ tyrosinase activity A. Can also be caused by failure of neural crest cell migration during development.
Melasma (chloasma)	Hyperpigmentation associated with pregnancy ("mask of pregnancy") or OCP use B.
Vitiligo	Irregular areas of complete depigmentation C. Caused by a ↓ in melanocytes.

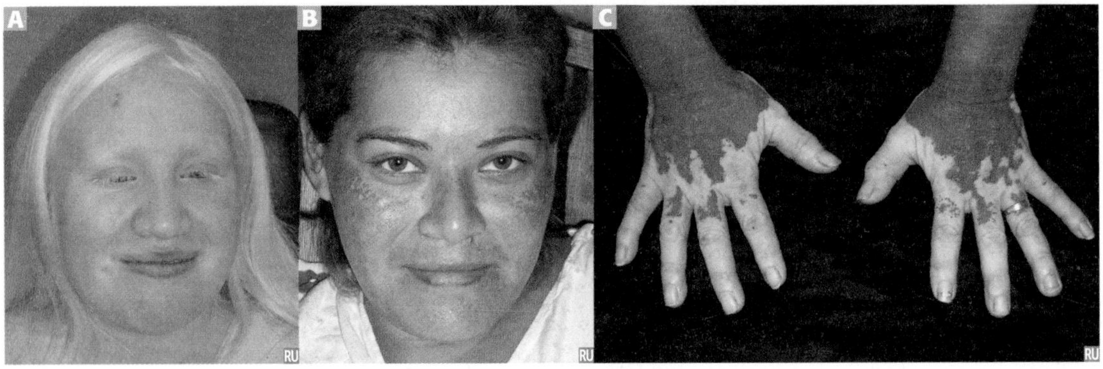

Common skin disorders

Verrucae	Warts; caused by HPV. Soft, tan-colored, cauliflower-like papules A. Epidermal hyperplasia, hyperkeratosis, koilocytosis. Condyloma acuminatum on genitals B.
Melanocytic nevus	Common mole. Benign, but melanoma can arise in congenital or atypical moles. Intradermal nevi are papular C. Junctional nevi are flat macules D.
Urticaria	Hives. Pruritic wheals that form after mast cell degranulation E.
Ephelis	Freckle. Normal number of melanocytes, ↑ melanin pigment F.
Atopic dermatitis (eczema)	Pruritic eruption, commonly on skin flexures. Often associated with other atopic diseases (asthma, allergic rhinitis). Usually starts on the face in infancy G and often appears in the antecubital fossae H thereafter.
Allergic contact dermatitis	Type IV hypersensitivity reaction that follows exposure to allergen. Lesions occur at site of contact (e.g., nickel I, poison ivy, neomycin J).
Psoriasis	Papules and plaques with silvery scaling, especially on knees and elbows. Acanthosis with parakeratotic scaling (nuclei still in stratum corneum). ↑ stratum spinosum, ↓ stratum granulosum. Auspitz sign K — pinpoint bleeding spots from exposure of dermal papillae when scales are scraped off. Can be associated with nail pitting and psoriatic arthritis L.
Seborrheic keratosis	Flat, greasy, pigmented squamous epithelial proliferation with keratin-filled cysts (horn cysts) M. Looks "stuck on" N. Lesions occur on head, trunk, and extremities. Common benign neoplasm of older persons. Leser-Trélat sign—sudden appearance of multiple seborrheic keratoses, indicating an underlying malignancy (e.g., GI, lymphoid).

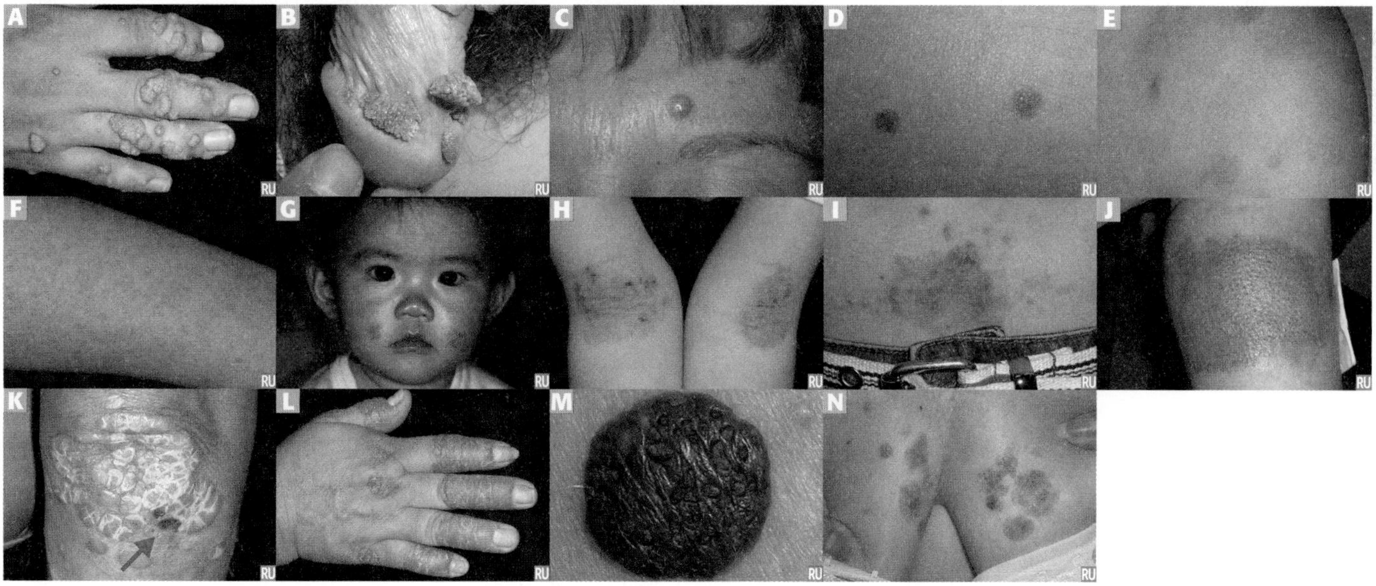

Blistering skin disorders

Pemphigus vulgaris

Potentially fatal autoimmune skin disorder with IgG antibody against desmoglein 3 (1 and/or 3), a part of the desmosomes (needed for cell adhesion). Immunofluorescence reveals antibodies around epidermal cells in a reticular or netlike pattern. Acantholysis—intraepidermal bullae causing flaccid blister A involving the skin and oral mucosa. Positive Nikolsky's sign (separation of epidermis upon manual stroking of skin).

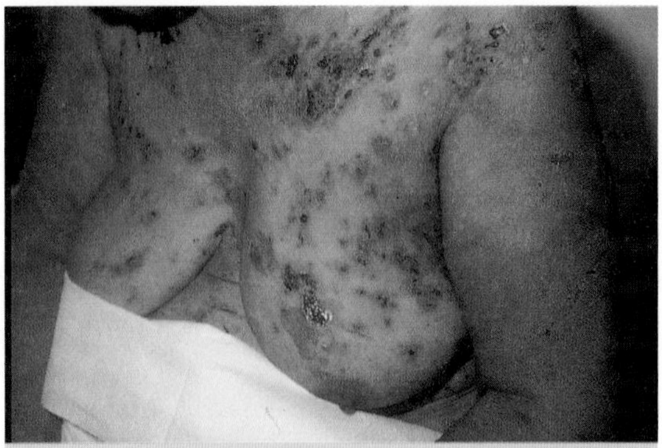

A **Pemphigus vulgaris.** Note multiple crusty and weepy erythematous erosions where blisters have broken.

Bullous pemphigoid

Autoimmune disorder with IgG antibody against hemidesmosomes (epidermal basement membrane; antibodies are "**bullow**" the epidermis); shows linear immunofluorescence. Eosinophils within tense blisters B. Similar to but less severe than pemphigus vulgaris—affects skin but spares oral mucosa. Negative Nikolsky's sign.

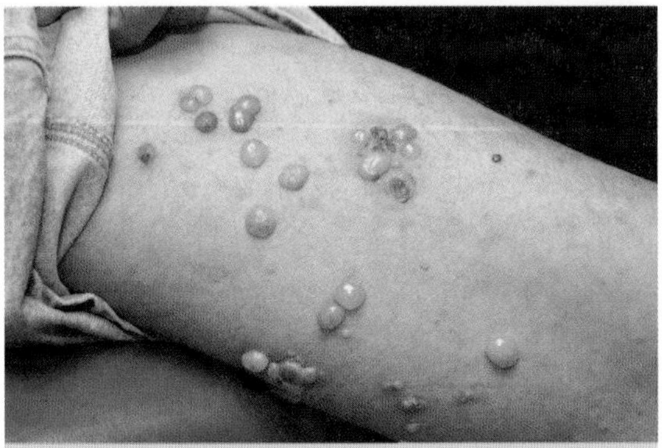

B **Bullous pemphigoid.** Note multiple intact, tense bullae.

Dermatitis herpetiformis

Pruritic papules, vesicles, and bullae C. Deposits of IgA at the tips of dermal papillae. Associated with celiac disease.

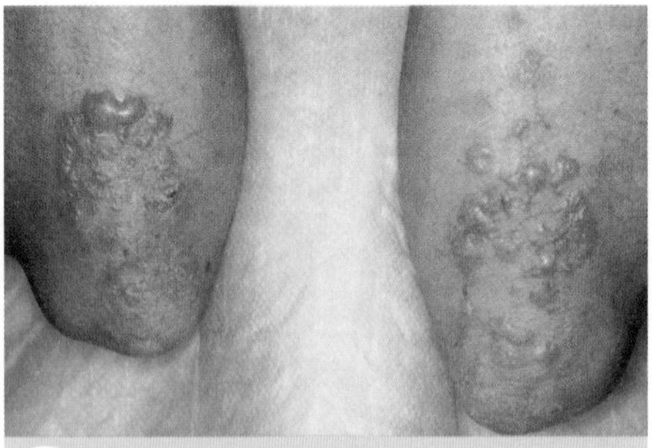

C **Dermatitis herpetiformis.** Vesicles and bullae are often found on elbows.

Blistering skin disorders *(continued)*

Erythema multiforme

Associated with infections (e.g., *Mycoplasma pneumoniae,* HSV), drugs (e.g., sulfa drugs, β-lactams, phenytoin), cancers, and autoimmune disease. Presents with multiple types of lesions—macules, papules, vesicles, and target lesions (look like targets with multiple rings and a dusky center showing epithelial disruption) D.

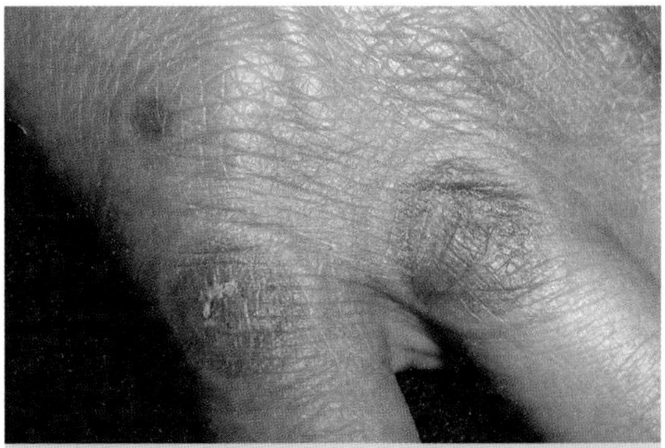

D **Erythema multiforme.** Note target lesions in patient with erythema multiforme secondary to HSV. RU

Stevens-Johnson syndrome

Characterized by fever, bulla formation and necrosis, sloughing of skin, and a high mortality rate. Typically 2 mucus membranes are involved E and skin lesions may be appear like targets as seen in erythema multiforme. Usually associated with adverse drug reaction. A more severe form of Stevens-Johnson syndrome with > 30% of the body surface area involved is toxic epidermal necrolysis F G.

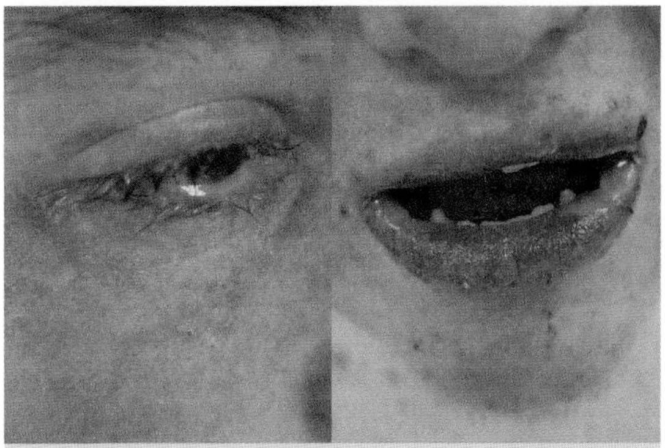

E **Stevens-Johnson syndrome.** Mucosal involvement of the eye (left RU) and lip (right RU).

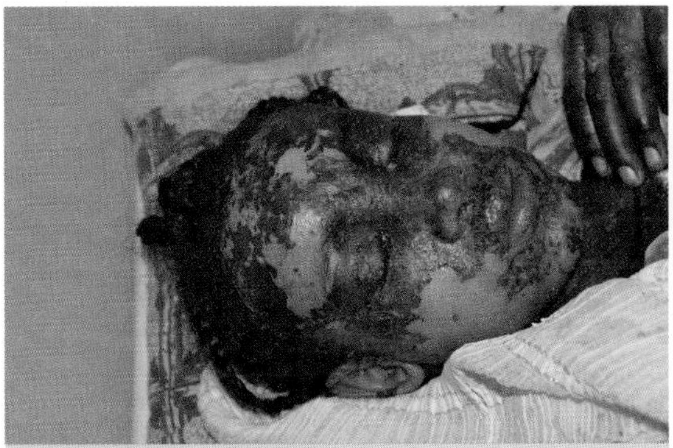

F **Toxic epidermal necrolysis.** Note sloughing of skin. RU

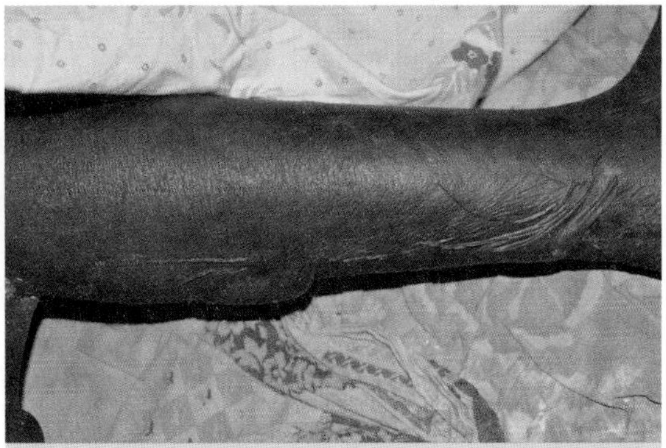

G **Toxic epidermal necrolysis.** Large bullae led to skin sloughing. RU

Miscellaneous skin disorders

Acanthosis nigricans

Epidermal hyperplasia causing symmetrical, hyperpigmented, velvety thickening of skin, especially on neck or in axilla A. Associated with hyperinsulinemia (e.g., diabetes, obesity, Cushing's syndrome) and visceral malignancy.

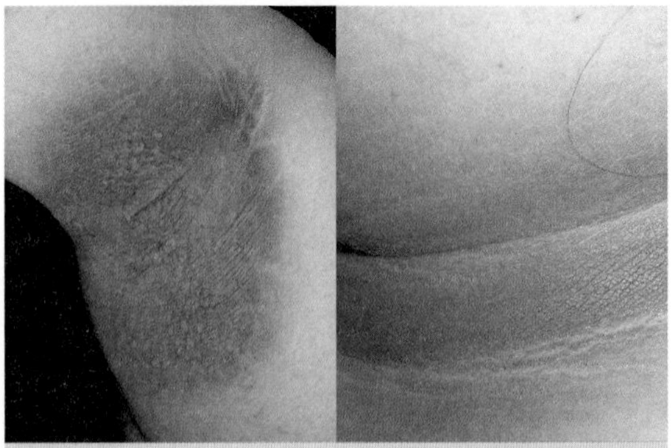

A **Acanthosis nigricans.** Note multiple skin tags on left, and velvety appearance on right.

Actinic keratosis

Premalignant lesions caused by sun exposure. Small, rough, erythematous or brownish papules or plaques B. Risk of squamous cell carcinoma is proportional to degree of epithelial dysplasia.

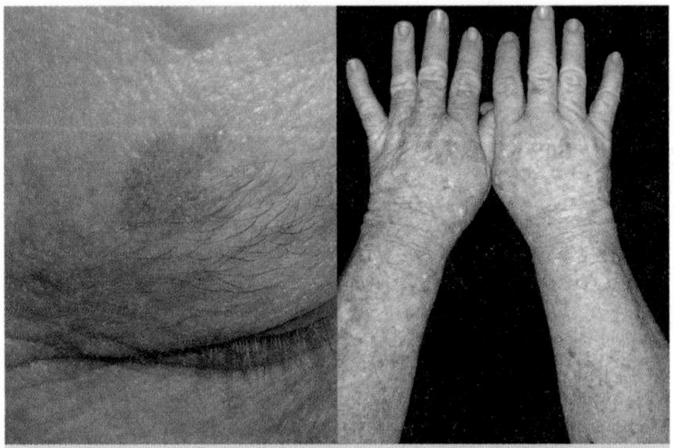

B **Actinic keratosis.** Biopsy-proven AK in case of suspected early skin cancer (left). Multiple AKs on hands and forearms (right).

Erythema nodosum

Inflammatory lesions of subcutaneous fat, usually on anterior shins. Associated with sarcoidosis, coccidioidomycosis, histoplasmosis, TB, streptococcal infections, leprosy, and Crohn's disease C.

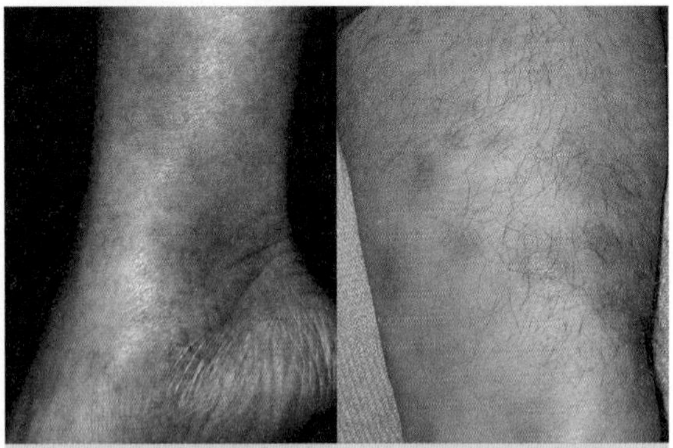

C **Erythema nodosum** Lesions on leg in patient with streptococcal infection (left) and patient with leprosy and erythema nodosum leprosum (right).

Miscellaneous skin disorders *(continued)*

Lichen Planus	Pruritic, Purple, Polygonal Planar Papules and Plaques are the 6 P's of lichen planus. D Sawtooth infiltrate of lymphocytes at dermal-epidermal junction. Associated with hepatitis C.	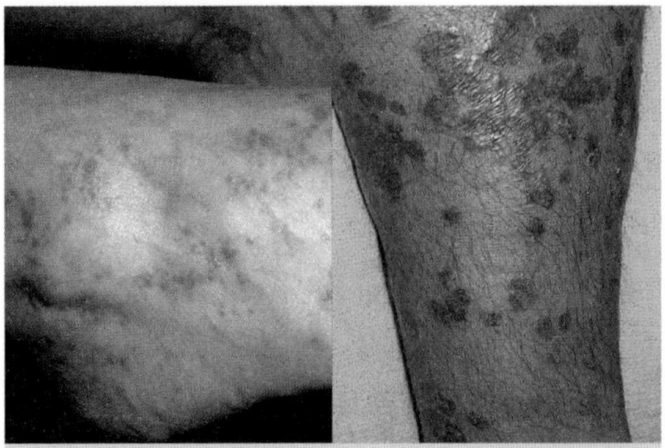 D **Lichen planus.** Appearance on light skin (left) RU and dark skin (right). RU
Pityriasis rosea	"Herald patch" followed days later by "Christmas tree" distribution E. Multiple plaques with collarette scale. Self-resolving in 6–8 weeks.	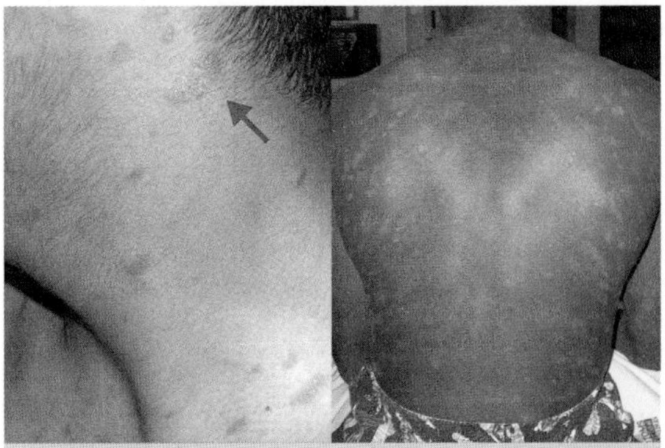 E **Pityriasis rosea.** Herald patch (left, arrow) RU and Christmas tree distribution (right). RU
Sunburn	UV irradiation causes DNA mutations, inducing apoptosis of keratinocytes. UVA is dominant in tanning and photoaging, UVB in sunburn. Can lead to impetigo F and skin cancers (basal cell carcinoma, squamous cell carcinoma, and melanoma).	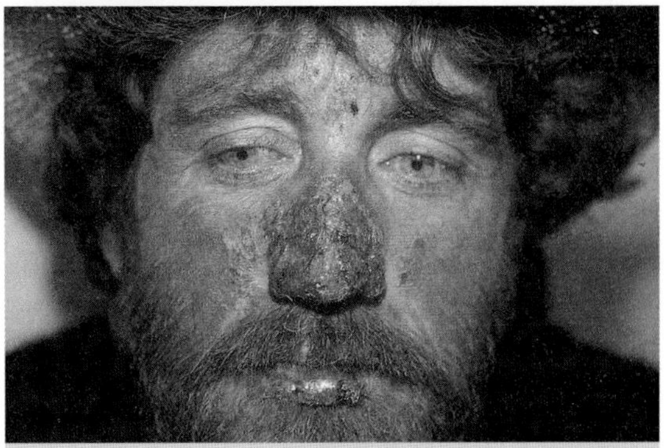 F **Sunburn.** Secondary bacterial infection led to impetigo. RU

Infectious skin disorders

Impetigo	Very superficial skin infection. Usually from S. *aureus* or S. *pyogenes*. Highly contagious. Honey-colored crusting A. Bullous impetigo B has bullae and is usually caused by S. *aureus*.
Cellulitis	Acute, painful, spreading infection of dermis and subcutaneous tissues. Usually from S. *pyogenes* or S. *aureus*. Often starts with a break in skin from trauma or another infection C.
Necrotizing fasciitis	Deeper tissue injury, usually from anaerobic bacteria or S. *pyogenes*. Results in crepitus from methane and CO_2 production. "Flesh-eating bacteria." Causes bullae and a purple color to the skin D.
Staphylococcal scalded skin syndrome (SSSS)	Exotoxin destroys keratinocyte attachments in the stratum granulosum only (vs. toxic epidermal necrolysis, which destroys the epidermal-dermal junction). Characterized by fever and generalized erythematous rash with sloughing of the upper layers of the epidermis that heals completely. Seen in newborns and children E.
Hairy leukoplakia	White, painless plaques on the tongue that cannot be scraped off. EBV mediated. Occurs in HIV-positive patients F.

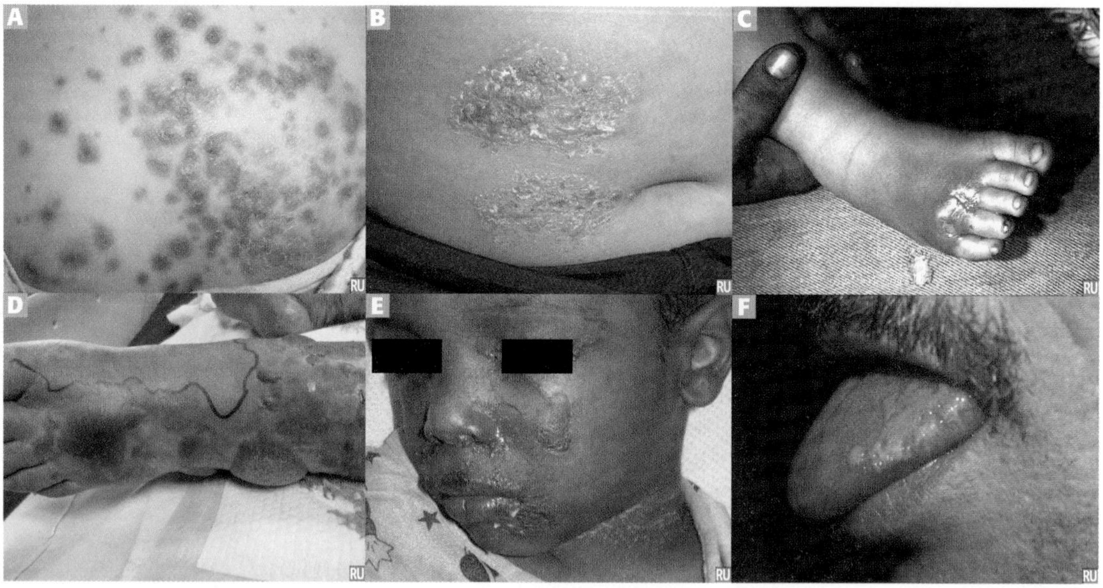

Skin cancer

Basal cell carcinoma

Most common skin cancer. Found in sun-exposed areas of body. Locally invasive, but almost never metastasizes. Pink, pearly nodules, commonly with telangiectasias, rolled borders, and central crusting or ulceration A. BCCs also appear as nonhealing ulcers with infiltrating growth B or as a scaling plaque (superficial BCC) C. Basal cell tumors have "palisading" nuclei D.

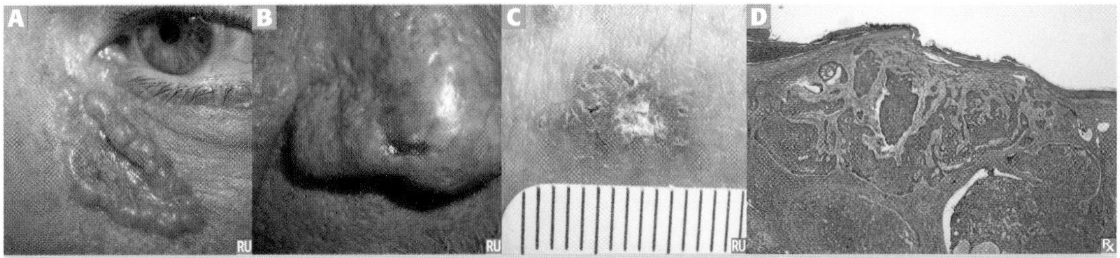

Basal cell carcinoma. Appearance includes A rolled borders, B nonhealing ulcer, or C scaling plaque. Histology D reveals nests of basaloid cells in dermis with peripheral "palisading."

Squamous cell carcinoma

Second most common skin cancer. Associated with excessive exposure to sunlight, immunosuppression, and occasionally arsenic exposure. Commonly appears on face E, lower lip F, ears, and hands. Locally invasive, but may spread to lymph nodes and will rarely metastasize. Ulcerative red lesions with frequent scale. Associated with chronic draining sinuses. Histopathology: keratin "pearls" G.

Actinic keratosis, a scaly plaque, is a precursor to squamous cell carcinoma.

Keratoacanthoma is a variant that grows rapidly (4–6 weeks) and may regress spontaneously over months H.

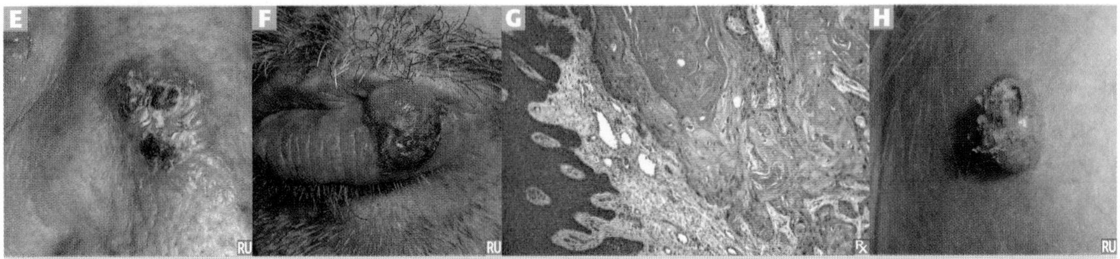

Squamous cell carcinoma. Commonly seen on faces E and lips F. Histology G reveals keratin "pearls." Keratoacanthoma H is a variant.

Melanoma

Common tumor with significant risk of metastasis. S-100 tumor marker. Associated with sunlight exposure; fair-skinned persons are at ↑ risk. Depth of tumor correlates with risk of metastasis. Look for the **ABCDE**s: **A**symmetry, **B**order irregularity, **C**olor variation, **D**iameter > 6 mm, and **E**volution over time. At least 4 different types of melanoma I J K L. Often driven by activating mutation in BRAF kinase. Primary treatment is excision with appropriately wide margins. Metastatic or unresectable melanoma in patients with *BRAF* V600E mutation may benefit from vemurafenib, a BRAF kinase inhibitor.

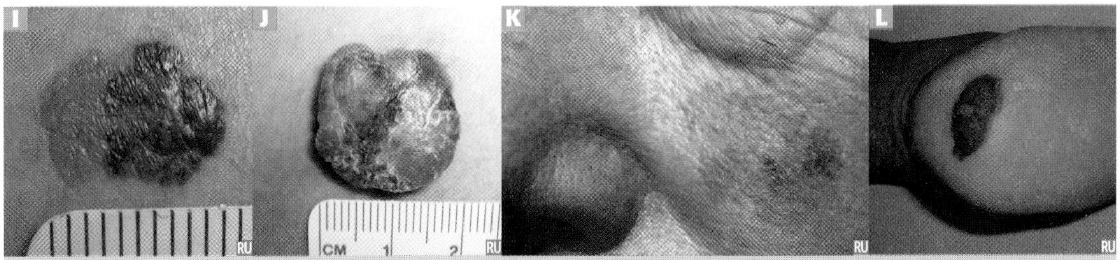

Melanoma. Multiple variants, including superficial spreading melanoma I, nodular melanoma J, lentigo maligna melanoma K, and acrolentiginous melanoma L.

▸ MUSCULOSKELETAL, SKIN, AND CONNECTIVE TISSUE–PHARMACOLOGY

Arachidonic acid products

Lipoxygenase pathway yields Leukotrienes. — L for Lipoxygenase and Leukotriene.

LTB_4 is a **neutrophil** chemotactic agent. — **Neutrophils** arrive "B4" others.

LTC_4, D_4, and E_4 function in bronchoconstriction, vasoconstriction, contraction of smooth muscle, and ↑ vascular permeability.

PGI_2 inhibits platelet aggregation and promotes vasodilation. — Platelet-Gathering Inhibitor.

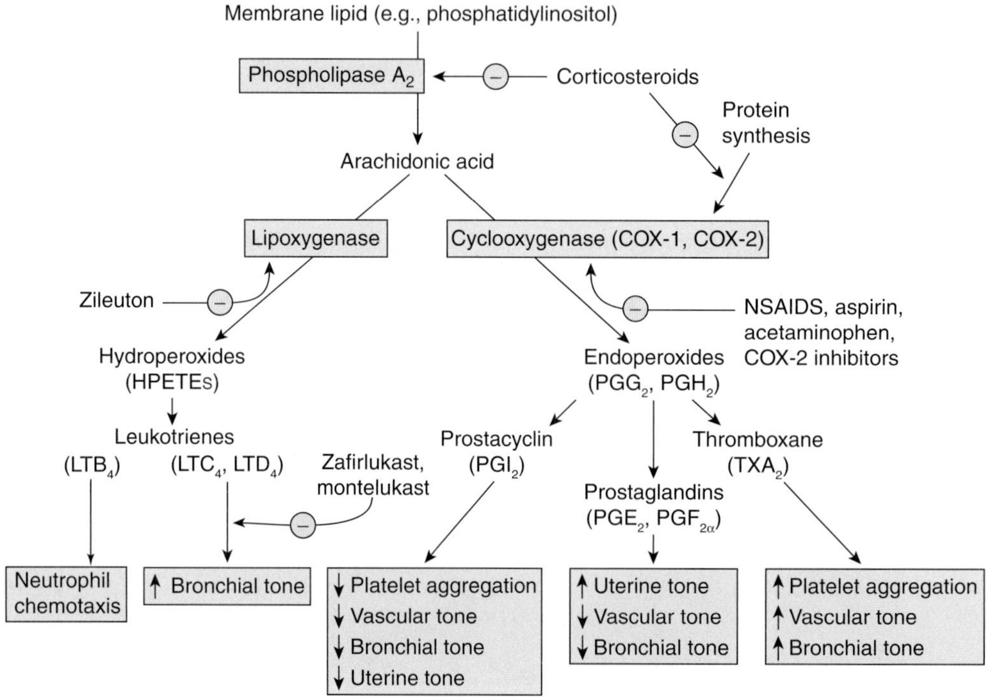

(Adapted, with permission, from Katzung BG, Trevor AJ. *Pharmacology: Examination & Board Review,* 5th ed. Stamford, CT: Appleton & Lange, 1998: 150.)

Aspirin

MECHANISM	Irreversibly inhibits cyclooxygenase (both COX-1 and COX-2) by acetylation, which ↓ synthesis of both thromboxane A_2 (TXA_2) and prostaglandins. ↑ bleeding time. No effect on PT, PTT. A type of NSAID.
CLINICAL USE	Low dose (< 300 mg/day): ↓ platelet aggregation. Intermediate dose (300–2400 mg/day): antipyretic and analgesic. High dose (2400–4000 mg/day): anti-inflammatory.
TOXICITY	Gastric ulceration, tinnitus (CN VIII). Chronic use can lead to acute renal failure, interstitial nephritis, and upper GI bleeding. Risk of Reye's syndrome in children treated with aspirin for viral infection. Also stimulates respiratory centers, causing hyperventilation and respiratory alkalosis.

NSAIDs	Ibuprofen, naproxen, indomethacin, ketorolac, diclofenac.
MECHANISM	Reversibly inhibit cyclooxygenase (both COX-1 and COX-2). Block prostaglandin (PG) synthesis.
CLINICAL USE	Antipyretic, analgesic, anti-inflammatory. Indomethacin is used to close a PDA.
TOXICITY	Interstitial nephritis, gastric ulcer (PGs protect gastric mucosa), renal ischemia (PGs vasodilate afferent arteriole).

COX-2 inhibitors (celecoxib)	
MECHANISM	Reversibly inhibit specifically the cyclooxygenase (COX) isoform 2, which is found in inflammatory cells and vascular endothelium and mediates inflammation and pain; spares COX-1, which helps maintain the gastric mucosa. Thus, should not have the corrosive effects of other NSAIDs on the GI lining. Spares platelet function as TXA_2 production is dependent on COX-1.
CLINICAL USE	Rheumatoid arthritis and osteoarthritis; patients with gastritis or ulcers.
TOXICITY	↑ risk of thrombosis. Sulfa allergy.

Acetaminophen	
MECHANISM	Reversibly inhibits cyclooxygenase, mostly in CNS. Inactivated peripherally.
CLINICAL USE	Antipyretic, analgesic, but not anti-inflammatory. Used instead of aspirin to avoid Reye's syndrome in children with viral infection.
TOXICITY	Overdose produces hepatic necrosis; acetaminophen metabolite depletes glutathione and forms toxic tissue adducts in liver. N-acetylcysteine is antidote—regenerates glutathione.

Bisphosphonates	Alendronate, other -dronates.
MECHANISM	Pyrophosphate analogs; bind hydroxyapatite in bone, inhibiting osteoclast activity.
CLINICAL USE	Osteoporosis, hypercalcemia, Paget's disease of bone.
TOXICITY	Corrosive esophagitis, osteonecrosis of the jaw.

Gout drugs

Chronic gout drugs	
Allopurinol	Inhibits xanthine oxidase, ↓ conversion of xanthine to uric acid. Also used in lymphoma and leukemia to prevent tumor lysis–associated urate nephropathy. ↑ concentrations of azathioprine and 6-MP (both normally metabolized by xanthine oxidase). Do not give salicylates; all but the highest doses depress uric acid clearance. Even high doses (5–6 g/day) have only minor uricosuric activity.
Febuxostat	Inhibits xanthine oxidase.
Probenecid	Inhibits reabsorption of uric acid in PCT (also inhibits secretion of penicillin).
Colchicine	Binds and stabilizes tubulin to inhibit polymerization, impairing leukocyte chemotaxis and degranulation. GI side effects, especially if given orally.
Acute gout drugs	
NSAIDs	Naproxen, indomethacin.
Glucocorticoids	Oral or intraarticular.

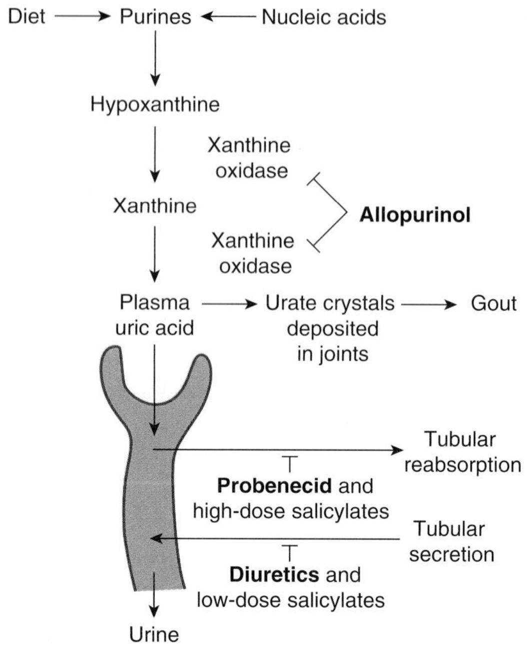
Diet
Purines
Nucleic acids
Hypoxanthine
Xanthine oxidase
Xanthine
Allopurinol
Xanthine oxidase
Plasma uric acid
Urate crystals deposited in joints
Gout
Tubular reabsorption
Probenecid and high-dose salicylates
Tubular secretion
Diuretics and low-dose salicylates
Urine

TNF-α inhibitors

All TNF-α inhibitors predispose to infection including reactivation of latent TB since TNF blockade prevents activation of macrophages and destruction of phagocytosed microbes.

DRUG	MECHANISM	CLINICAL USE
Etanercept	Fusion protein (receptor for TNF-α + IgG_1 Fc), produced by recombinant DNA. Etaner**cept** is a TNF decoy re**cept**or.	Rheumatoid arthritis, psoriasis, ankylosing spondylitis
Infliximab, adalimumab	Anti-TNF-α monoclonal antibody	Crohn's disease, rheumatoid arthritis, ankylosing spondylitis, psoriasis

Neurology

"Estimated amount of glucose used by an adult human brain each day, expressed in M&Ms: 250."

—Harper's Index

"He has two neurons held together by a spirochete."

—Anonymous

"I never came upon any of my discoveries through the process of rational thinking."

—Albert Einstein

"I like nonsense; it wakes up the brain cells."

—Dr. Seuss

▸ NEUROLOGY–EMBRYOLOGY

Neural development

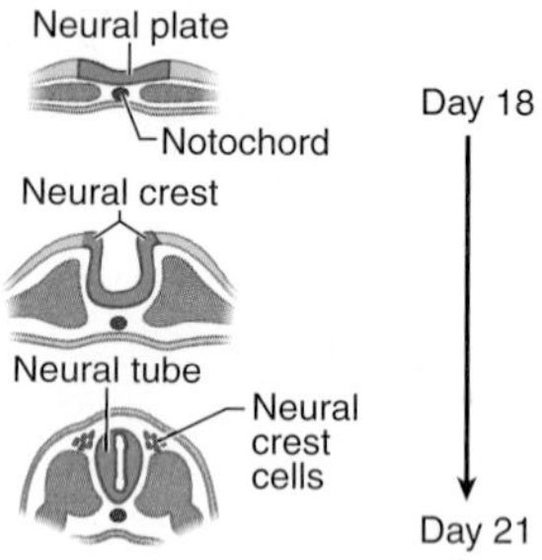
Neural plate
Notochord
Neural crest
Neural tube
Neural crest cells
Day 18
Day 21

Notochord induces overlying ectoderm to differentiate into neuroectoderm and form the neural plate.
Neural plate gives rise to the neural tube and neural crest cells.
Notochord becomes nucleus pulposus of the intervertebral disc in adults.

Alar plate (dorsal): sensory
Basal plate (ventral): motor
] Same orientation as spinal cord.

Regional specification of developing brain

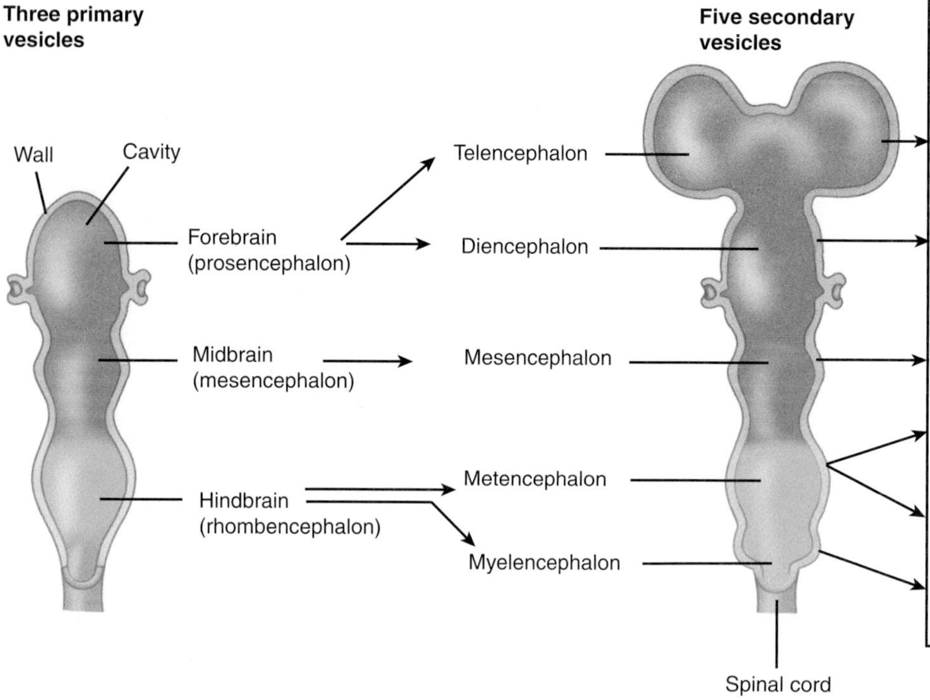
Three primary vesicles
Wall
Cavity
Forebrain (prosencephalon)
Midbrain (mesencephalon)
Hindbrain (rhombencephalon)
Telencephalon
Diencephalon
Mesencephalon
Metencephalon
Myelencephalon
Five secondary vesicles
Spinal cord

Adult derivatives of: Walls	Cavities
Cerebral hemispheres	Lateral ventricles
Thalamus	Third ventricle
Midbrain	Aqueduct
Pons	Upper part of fourth ventricle
Cerebellum	
Medulla	Lower part of fourth ventricle

Neural tube defects	Neuropores fail to fuse (4th week) → persistent connection between amniotic cavity and spinal canal. Associated with low folic acid intake before conception and during pregnancy. Elevated α-fetoprotein (AFP) in amniotic fluid and maternal serum. ↑ acetylcholinesterase (AChE) in amniotic fluid is a helpful confirmatory test (fetal AChE in CSF transudates across defect into the amniotic fluid).
Spina bifida occulta	Failure of bony spinal canal to close, but no structural herniation. Usually seen at lower vertebral levels. Dura is intact. Associated with tuft of hair or skin dimple at level of bony defect.
Meningocele	Meninges (but not the spinal cord) herniate through spinal canal defect.
Meningomyelocele	Meninges and spinal cord herniate through spinal canal defect.

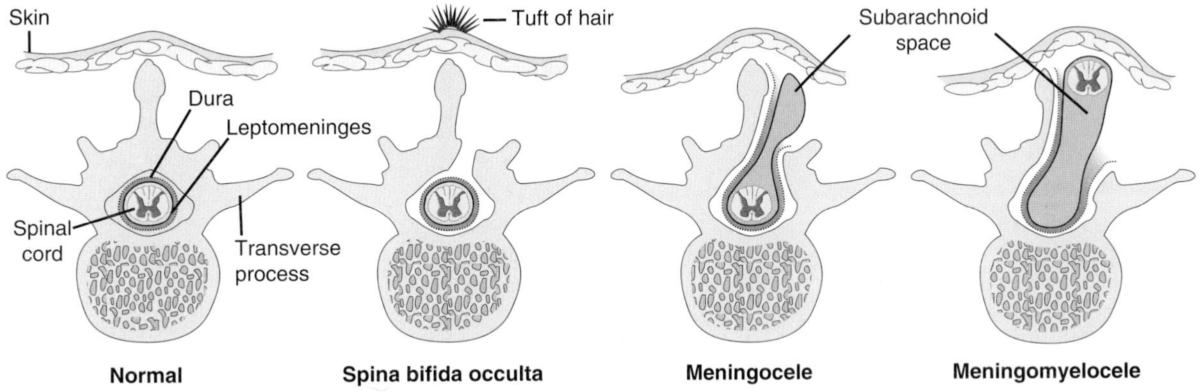

Forebrain anomalies

Anencephaly	Malformation of anterior neural tube resulting in no forebrain, open calvarium ("frog-like appearance"). Clinical findings: ↑ AFP; polyhydramnios (no swallowing center in brain). Associated with maternal diabetes (type I). Maternal folate supplementation ↓ risk.
Holoprosencephaly	Failure of left and right hemispheres to separate; usually occurs during weeks 5–6. Complex multifactorial etiology that may be related to mutations in sonic hedgehog signaling pathway. Moderate form has cleft lip/palate, most severe form results in cyclopia.

Posterior fossa malformations

Chiari II (Arnold-Chiari malformation)	Significant cerebellar tonsillar and vermian herniation through foramen magnum with aqueductal stenosis and hydrocephalus. Often presents with thoraco-lumbar myelomeningocele and paralysis below the defect.
Dandy-Walker	Agenesis of cerebellar vermis with cystic enlargement of 4th ventricle (fills the enlarged posterior fossa). Associated with hydrocephalus and spina bifida.

Syringomyelia

Cystic enlargement of central canal of spinal cord. Crossing fibers of spinothalamic tract are typically damaged first. Results in a "cape-like," bilateral loss of pain and temperature sensation in upper extremities (fine touch sensation is preserved).

Syrinx = tube, as in syringe.
Associated with Chiari I malformation (> 3–5 mm cerebellar tonsillar ectopia).
Most common at C8–T1.

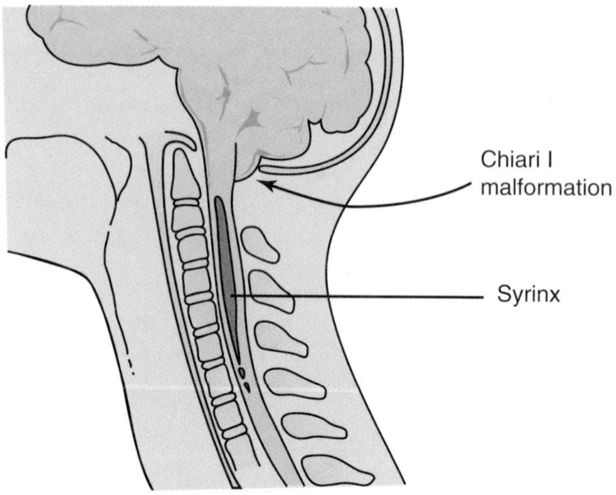

Tongue development

1st branchial arch forms anterior 2/3 (thus sensation via CN V_3, taste via CN VII).
3rd and 4th arches form posterior 1/3 (thus sensation and taste mainly via CN IX, extreme posterior via CN X).
Motor innervation is via CN XII.
Muscles of the tongue are derived from occipital myotomes.

Taste—CN VII, IX, X (solitary nucleus).
Pain—CN V_3, IX, X.
Motor—CN XII.

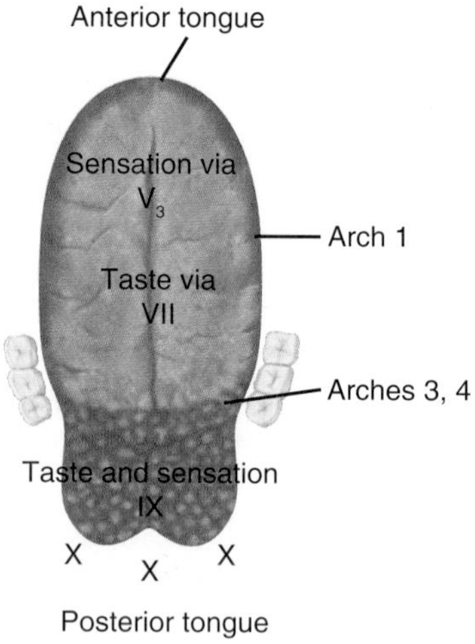

▸ NEUROLOGY—ANATOMY AND PHYSIOLOGY

CNS/PNS origins

Neuroectoderm—CNS neurons; ependymal cells (inner lining of ventricles, make CSF); oligodendroglia; astrocytes.
Neural crest—PNS neurons, Schwann cells.
Mesoderm—Microglia (like Macrophages, originate from Mesoderm).

Neurons

Signal-transmitting cells of the nervous system. Permanent cells—do not divide in adulthood (and, as a general rule, have no progenitor stem cell population).
Signal-relaying cells with dendrites (receive input), cell bodies, and axons (send output). Cell bodies and dendrites can be stained via the Nissl substance (stains RER). RER is not present in the axon.
If an axon is injured, it undergoes Wallerian degeneration—degeneration distal to the injury and axonal retraction proximally; allows for potential regeneration of axon (if in PNS).

Astrocytes

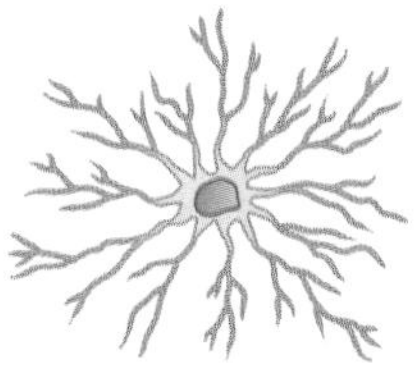

Physical support, repair, K^+ metabolism, removal of excess neurotransmitter, maintenance of blood-brain barrier. Reactive gliosis in response to injury. Astrocyte marker—GFAP.

Microglia

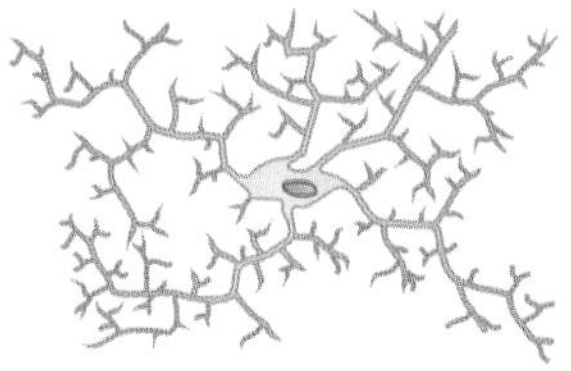

CNS phagocytes. Mesodermal origin. Not readily discernible in Nissl stains. Have small irregular nuclei and relatively little cytoplasm.
Scavenger cells of the CNS. Respond to tissue damage by differentiating into large phagocytic cells.

HIV-infected microglia fuse to form multinucleated giant cells in the CNS.

Myelin

↑ conduction velocity of signals transmitted down axons. Results in saltatory conduction of action potential between nodes of Ranvier, where there are high concentrations of Na^+ channels. CNS—oligodendrocytes; PNS—Schwann cells.

Wraps and insulates axons: ↑ space constant and ↑ conduction velocity.

Oligodendroglia

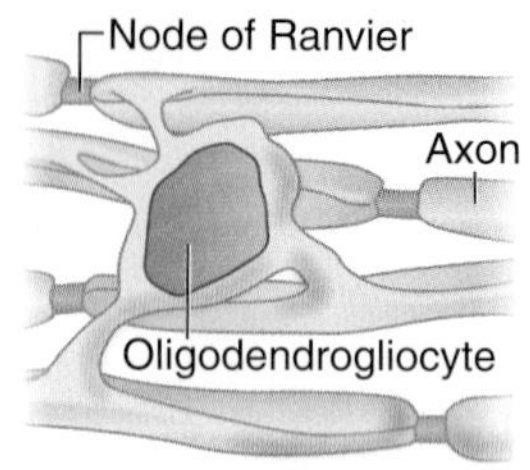

Each oligodendrocyte myelinates multiple CNS axons (up to 50 each). In Nissl stains, they appear as small nuclei with dark chromatin and little cytoplasm. Predominant type of glial cell in white matter.

These cells are destroyed in multiple sclerosis. Look like fried eggs on H&E staining.

Schwann cells

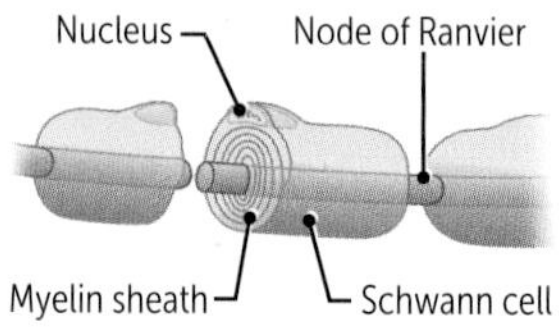

Each Schwann cell myelinates only 1 PNS axon. Also promote axonal regeneration. Derived from neural crest.

↑ conduction velocity via saltatory conduction between nodes of Ranvier, where there are high concentrations of Na^+ channels.

These cells are destroyed in Guillain-Barré syndrome.

Acoustic neuroma—type of schwannoma. Typically located in internal acoustic meatus (CN VIII).

Sensory corpuscles

RECEPTOR TYPE	DESCRIPTION	LOCATION	SENSES
Free nerve endings	C—slow, unmyelinated fibers Aδ—fast, myelinated fibers	All skin, epidermis, some viscera	Pain and temperature
Meissner's corpuscles	Large, myelinated fibers; adapt quickly	Glabrous (hairless) skin	Dynamic, fine/light touch; position sense
Pacinian corpuscles	Large, myelinated fibers	Deep skin layers, ligaments, and joints	Vibration, pressure
Merkel's discs	Large, myelinated fibers; adapt slowly	Hair follicles	Pressure, deep static touch (e.g., shapes, edges), position sense

---

Peripheral nerve

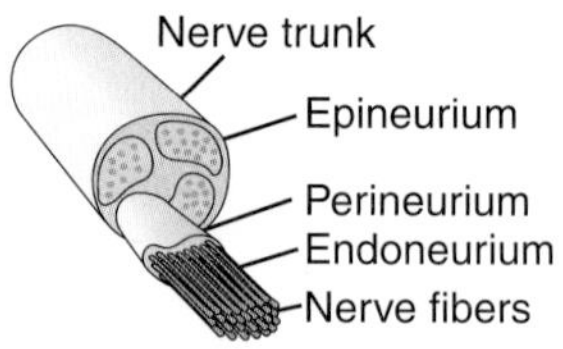

Endoneurium—invests single nerve fiber layers (inflammatory infiltrate in Guillain-Barré).

Perineurium (Permeability barrier)—surrounds a fascicle of nerve fibers. Must be rejoined in microsurgery for limb reattachment.

Epineurium—dense connective tissue that surrounds entire nerve (fascicles and blood vessels).

Endo = inner.
Peri = around.
Epi = outer.

Neurotransmitters

TYPE	CHANGE IN DISEASE	LOCATIONS OF SYNTHESIS[a]
NE	↑ in anxiety; ↓ in depression	Locus ceruleus (pons)
Dopamine	↑ in schizophrenia; ↓ in Parkinson's; ↓ in depression	Ventral tegmentum and SNc (midbrain)
5-HT	↓ in anxiety; ↓ in depression	Raphe nucleus (pons)
ACh	↓ in Alzheimer's; ↓ in Huntington's; ↑ in REM sleep	Basal nucleus of Meynert
GABA	↓ in anxiety; ↓ in Huntington's	Nucleus accumbens

[a]Locus ceruleus—stress and panic. Nucleus accumbens and septal nucleus—reward center, pleasure, addiction, fear.

Blood-brain barrier

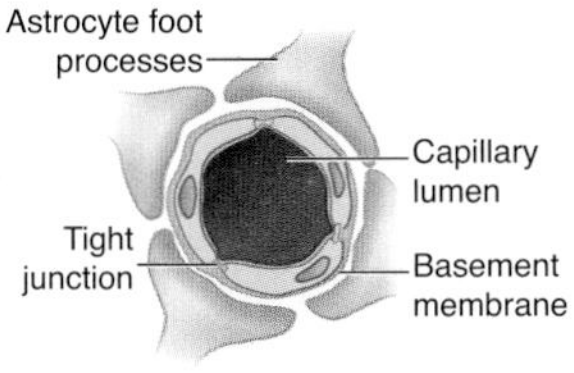
Astrocyte foot processes
Capillary lumen
Tight junction
Basement membrane

Prevents circulating blood substances from reaching the CSF/CNS. Formed by 3 structures:
- Tight junctions between nonfenestrated capillary endothelial cells
- Basement membrane
- Astrocyte foot processes

Glucose and amino acids cross slowly by carrier-mediated transport mechanism.

Nonpolar/lipid-soluble substances cross rapidly via diffusion.

A few specialized brain regions with fenestrated capillaries and no blood-brain barrier allow molecules in the blood to affect brain function (e.g., area postrema—vomiting after chemo, OVLT—osmotic sensing) or neurosecretory products to enter circulation (e.g., neurohypophysis—ADH release).

Other notable barriers include:
- Blood-testis barrier
- Maternal-fetal blood barrier of placenta

Infarction and/or neoplasm destroys endothelial cell tight junctions → vasogenic edema.

Hypothalamic inputs and outputs permeate the BBB.

Helps prevent bacterial infection from spreading into the CNS. Also restricts drug delivery to brain.

Hypothalamus	The hypothalamus wears **TAN HATS**—**T**hirst and water balance, **A**denohypophysis control (regulates anterior pituitary), **N**eurohypophysis releases hormones produced in the hypothalamus, **H**unger, **A**utonomic regulation, **T**emperature regulation, **S**exual urges. Inputs: OVLT (senses change in osmolarity), area postrema (responds to emetics)—areas not protected by BBB. Supraoptic nucleus makes ADH. Paraventricular nucleus makes oxytocin. ADH and oxytocin: made by hypothalamus but stored and released by posterior pituitary.	
Lateral area	Hunger. Destruction → anorexia, failure to thrive (infants). Inhibited by leptin.	If you zap your **lateral** nucleus, you shrink **lateral**ly.
Ventromedial area	Satiety. Destruction (e.g., craniopharyngioma) → hyperphagia. Stimulated by leptin.	If you zap your **ventromedial** nucleus, you grow **ventral**ly and **medial**ly.
Anterior hypothalamus	Cooling, parasympathetic.	Anterior nucleus = cool off (cooling, p**A**rasympathetic). **A/C = anterior cooling.**
Posterior hypothalamus	Heating, sympathetic.	Posterior nucleus = get fired up (heating, sympathetic). If you zap your posterior hypothalamus, you become a poikilotherm (cold-blooded, like a snake).
Suprachiasmatic nucleus	Circadian rhythm.	You need **sleep** to be **charismatic** (chiasmatic).

Posterior pituitary (neurohypophysis)	Receives hypothalamic axonal projections from supraoptic (ADH) and paraventricular (oxytocin) nuclei.	Oxytocin: *oxys* = quick; *tocos* = birth. **A**denohypophysis = **A**nterior pituitary.

Thalamus Major relay for all ascending sensory information except olfaction.

NUCLEUS	INPUT	INFO	DESTINATION	MNEMONIC
VPL	Spinothalamic and dorsal columns/medial lemniscus.	Pain and temperature; pressure, touch, vibration, and proprioception.	1° somatosensory cortex.	
VPM	Trigeminal and gustatory pathway.	Face sensation and taste.	1° somatosensory cortex.	**M**akeup goes on the face (VP**M**).
LGN	CN II.	Vision.	Calcarine sulcus.	**L**ateral = **L**ight.
MGN	Superior olive and inferior colliculus of tectum.	Hearing.	Auditory cortex of temporal lobe.	**M**edial = **M**usic.
VL	Basal ganglia.	Motor.	Motor cortex.	

Limbic system

Collection of neural structures involved in emotion, long-term memory, olfaction, behavior modulation, and autonomic nervous system function.

Structures include hippocampus, amygdala, fornix, mammillary bodies, and cingulate gyrus. Responsible for **F**eeding, **F**leeing, **F**ighting, **F**eeling, and **S**ex.

The famous **5 F's**.

Cerebellum

Modulates movement; aids in coordination and balance.

Input:

- Contralateral cortex via middle cerebellar peduncle.
- Ipsilateral proprioceptive information via inferior cerebellar peduncle from the spinal cord (input nerves = climbing and mossy fibers).

Output:

- Sends information to contralateral cortex to modulate movement. Output nerves = Purkinje fibers send information to deep nuclei of cerebellum, which in turn sends information to the contralateral cortex via the superior cerebellar peduncle.
- Deep nuclei (lateral → medial)—**D**entate, **E**mboliform, **G**lobose, **F**astigial ("**D**on't **E**at **G**reasy **F**oods").

Lateral—voluntary movement of extremities; when injured, propensity to fall toward injured (ipsilateral) side.

Medial—balance, truncal coordination.

Basal ganglia

Important in voluntary movements and making postural adjustments.

Receives cortical input, provides negative feedback to cortex to modulate movement.

Striatum = putamen (motor) + caudate (cognitive).

Lentiform = putamen + globus pallidus.

D_1-**R**eceptor = **D1R**ect pathway.

Indirect = **In**hibitory.

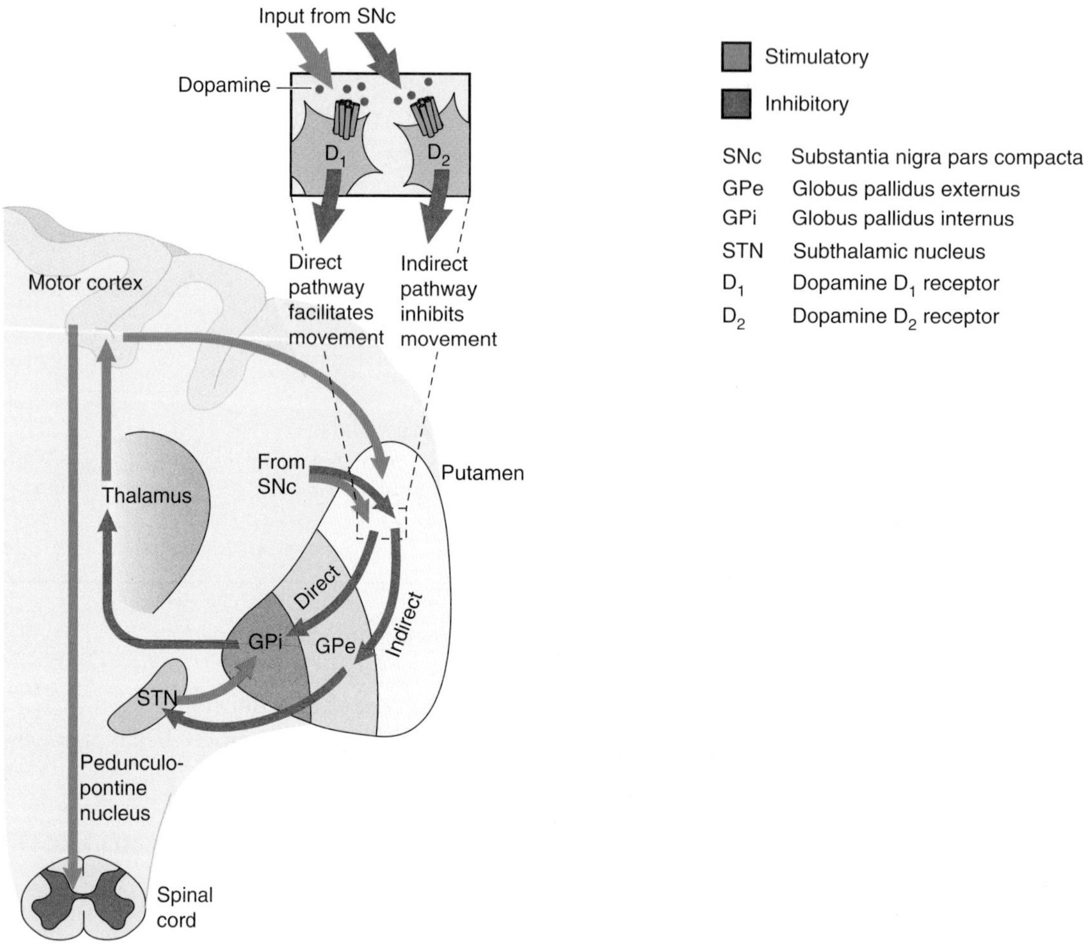

Excitatory pathway—cortical inputs stimulate the striatum, stimulating the release of GABA, which disinhibits the thalamus via the GPi/SNr (↑ motion).

Inhibitory pathway—cortical inputs stimulate the striatum, which disinhibits STN via GPe, and STN stimulates GPi/SNr to inhibit the thalamus (↓ motion).

Dopamine binds to D_1, stimulating the excitatory pathway, and to D_2, inhibiting the inhibitory pathway → ↑ motion.

Parkinson's disease

Degenerative disorder of CNS associated with Lewy bodies (composed of α-synuclein—intracellular inclusion) and loss of dopaminergic neurons (i.e., depigmentation) of the substantia nigra pars compacta.

Your body becomes a **TRAP** = **T**remor (at rest—e.g., pill-rolling tremor), cogwheel **R**igidity, **A**kinesia (or bradykinesia), and **P**ostural instability.

Huntington's disease	Autosomal-dominant trinucleotide repeat disorder. Characterized by chorea, aggression, depression, and dementia (sometimes initially mistaken for substance abuse). Neuronal death via NMDA-R binding and glutamate toxicity. Atrophy of striatal nuclei (main inhibitors of movement) can be seen on imaging.	Expansion of **CAG** repeats (anticipation). Caudate loses **ACh** and **GABA**.

Movement disorders

DISORDER	PRESENTATION	CHARACTERISTIC LESION	NOTES
Hemiballismus	Sudden, wild flailing of 1 arm +/− ipsilateral leg	Contralateral subthalamic nucleus (e.g., lacunar stroke)	"Half-of-body ballistic." Contralateral lesion.
Chorea	Sudden, jerky, purposeless movements	Basal ganglia (e.g., Huntington's)	*Chorea* = dancing.
Athetosis	Slow, writhing movements; especially seen in fingers	Basal ganglia (e.g., Huntington's)	Writhing, snake-like movement.
Myoclonus	Sudden, brief, uncontrolled muscle contraction		Jerks; hiccups; common in metabolic abnormalities such as renal and liver failure.
Dystonia	Sustained, involuntary muscle contractions		Writer's cramp; blepharospasm (sustained eyelid twitch).
Essential tremor (postural tremor)	Action tremor; exacerbated by holding posture/limb position		Genetic predisposition. Patients often self-medicated with EtOH, which ↓ tremor amplitude. Treatment: β-blockers, primidone.
Resting tremor	Uncontrolled movement of distal appendages (most noticeable in hands); tremor alleviated by intentional movement	Parkinson's disease	Occurs at rest; "pill-rolling tremor" of Parkinson's disease.
Intention tremor	Slow, zigzag motion when pointing/extending toward a target	Cerebellar dysfunction	

Cerebral cortex functions

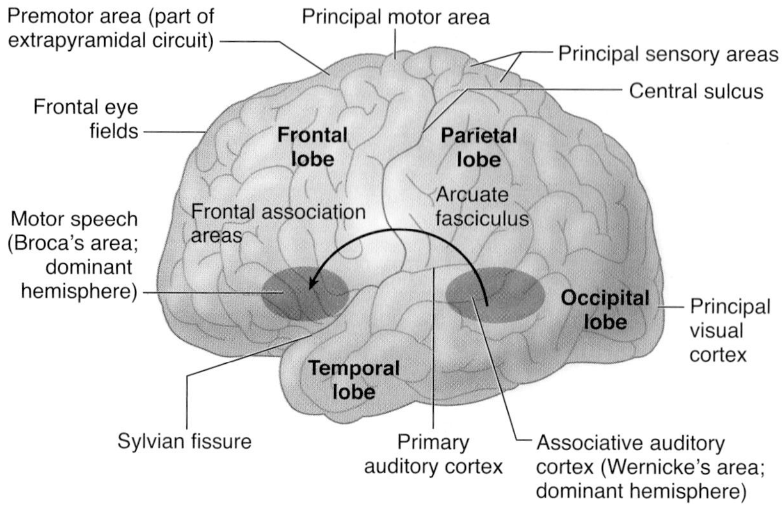

Premotor area (part of extrapyramidal circuit)
Principal motor area
Principal sensory areas
Central sulcus
Frontal eye fields
Frontal lobe
Parietal lobe
Arcuate fasciculus
Frontal association areas
Motor speech (Broca's area; dominant hemisphere)
Occipital lobe
Principal visual cortex
Temporal lobe
Sylvian fissure
Primary auditory cortex
Associative auditory cortex (Wernicke's area; dominant hemisphere)

Homunculus

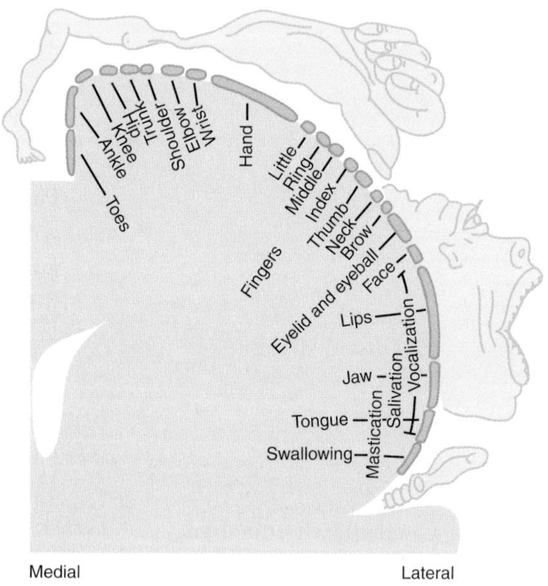

Toes
Ankle
Knee
Hip
Trunk
Shoulder
Elbow
Wrist
Hand
Little
Ring
Middle
Index
Thumb
Neck
Brow
Fingers
Eyelid and eyeball
Face
Lips
Vocalization
Jaw
Salivation
Tongue
Mastication
Swallowing
Medial
Lateral

Topographical representation of sensory and motor areas in the cerebral cortex. Used to localize lesion (e.g., in blood supply) leading to specific defects.

For example, lower extremity deficit in sensation or movement may indicate involvement of the anterior cerebral artery.

Common brain lesions

AREA OF LESION	CONSEQUENCE	NOTES
Amygdala (bilateral)	Klüver-Bucy syndrome (hyperorality, hypersexuality, disinhibited behavior)	Associated with HSV-1.
Frontal lobe	Disinhibition and deficits in concentration, orientation, and judgment; may have reemergence of primitive reflexes	
Right parietal lobe	Spatial neglect syndrome (agnosia of the contralateral side of the world)	
Reticular activating system (midbrain)	Reduced levels of arousal and wakefulness (e.g., coma)	
Mammillary bodies (bilateral)	Wernicke-Korsakoff syndrome: confusion, ophthalmoplegia, ataxia; memory loss (anterograde and retrograde amnesia), confabulation, personality changes	Associated with thiamine (B_1) deficiency and excessive EtOH use; can be precipitated by giving glucose without B_1 to a B_1-deficient patient.
Basal ganglia	May result in tremor at rest, chorea, or athetosis	Parkinson's disease.
Cerebellar hemisphere	Intention tremor, limb ataxia, and loss of balance; damage to the cerebellum results in ipsilateral deficits; fall toward side of lesion	Cerebellar hemispheres are **lateral**ly located—affect **lateral** limbs.
Cerebellar vermis	Truncal ataxia, dysarthria	Vermis is **central**ly located—affects **central** body.
Subthalamic nucleus	Contralateral hemiballismus	
Hippocampus	Anterograde amnesia—inability to make new memories	
Paramedian pontine reticular formation (PPRF)	Eyes look away from side of lesion	
Frontal eye fields	Eyes look toward lesion	

Central pontine myelinolysis

Acute paralysis, dysarthria, dysphagia, diplopia, and loss of consciousness. Can cause "locked-in syndrome." Massive axonal demyelination in pontine white matter tracts. Commonly iatrogenic, caused by overly rapid correction of Na^+ levels (hyponatremia). Arrow in axial T2-weighted MRI with FLAIR shows abnormal increased signal in central pons A.

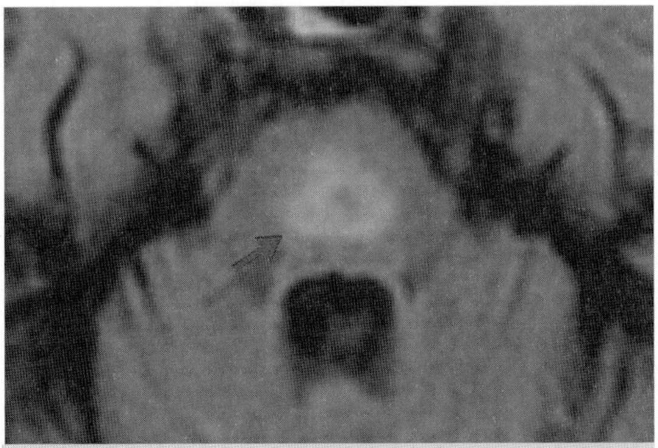

A Central pontine myelinolysis (arrow).

Aphasia	Aphasia = higher-order inability to speak (language deficit). Dysarthria = motor inability to speak (movement deficit).	
Broca's	Nonfluent aphasia with intact comprehension. Broca's area—inferior frontal gyrus of frontal lobe.	**Broca's Broken Boca** (boca = mouth in Spanish).
Wernicke's	Fluent aphasia with impaired comprehension. Wernicke's area—superior temporal gyrus of temporal lobe.	Wernicke's is Wordy but makes no sense. Wernicke's = "What?"
Global	Nonfluent aphasia with impaired comprehension. Both Broca's and Wernicke's areas affected.	
Conduction	Poor repetition but fluent speech, intact comprehension. Can be caused by damage to arcuate fasciculus.	Can't repeat phrases such as, "No ifs, ands, or buts."

Cerebral arteries—cortical distribution

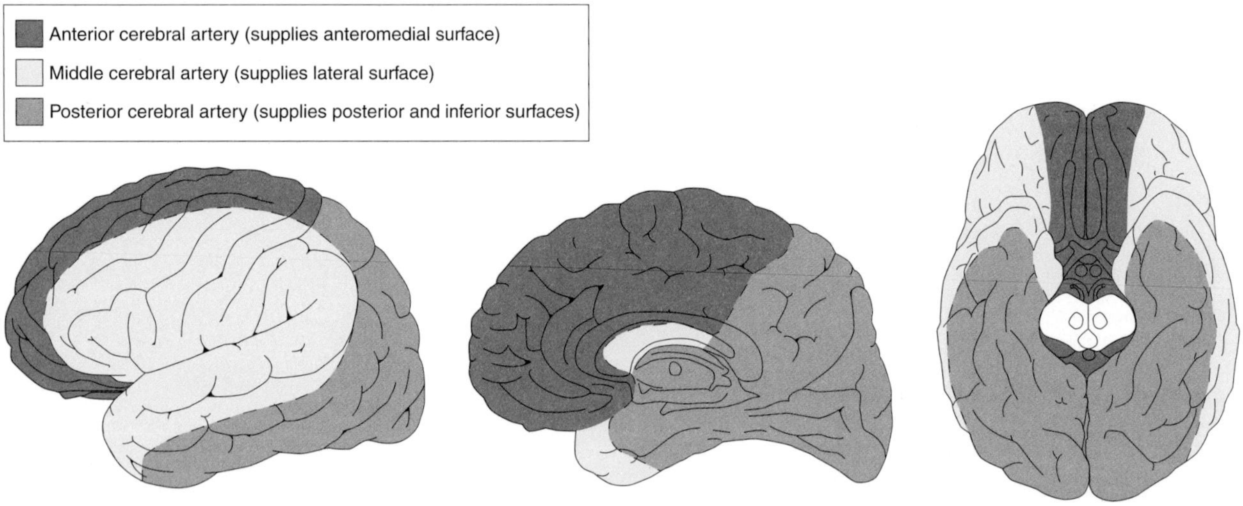
Anterior cerebral artery (supplies anteromedial surface)
Middle cerebral artery (supplies lateral surface)
Posterior cerebral artery (supplies posterior and inferior surfaces)

Watershed zones	Between anterior cerebral/middle cerebral, posterior cerebral/middle cerebral arteries. Damage in severe hypotension → upper leg/upper arm weakness, defects in higher-order visual processing.

Regulation of cerebral perfusion

Brain perfusion relies on tight autoregulation. Cerebral perfusion is primarily driven by P_{CO_2} (P_{O_2} also modulates perfusion in severe hypoxia).

Therapeutic hyperventilation (↓ P_{CO_2}) helps ↓ ICP in cases of acute cerebral edema (stroke, trauma) via decreasing cerebral perfusion.

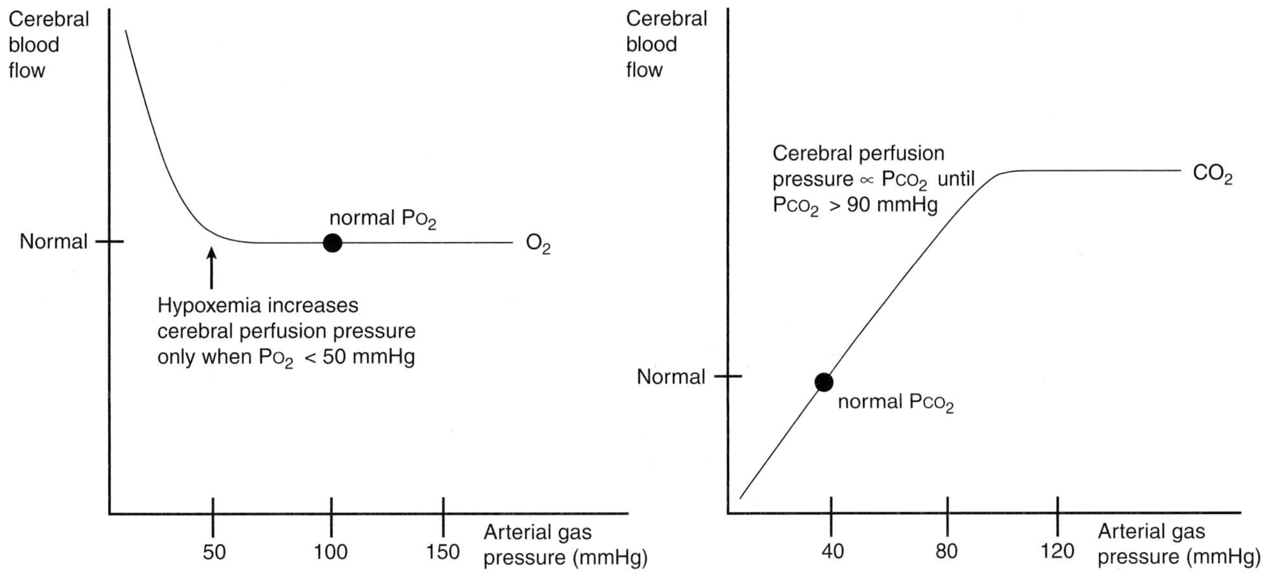

Effects of strokes

ARTERY	AREA OF LESION	SYMPTOMS	NOTES
Anterior circulation			
MCA	Motor cortex—upper limb and face.	Contralateral paralysis—upper limb and face.	
	Sensory cortex—upper limb and face.	Contralateral loss of sensation—upper limb and face.	
	Temporal lobe (Wernicke's area); frontal lobe (Broca's area).	Aphasia if in dominant (usually left) hemisphere. Hemineglect if lesion affects nondominant (usually right) side.	
ACA	Motor cortex—lower limb.	Contralateral paralysis—lower limb.	
	Sensory cortex—lower limb.	Contralateral loss of sensation—lower limb.	
Lateral striate artery	Striatum, internal capsule.	Contralateral hemiparesis/hemiplegia.	Common location of lacunar infarcts, 2° to unmanaged hypertension.
Posterior circulation			
ASA	Lateral corticospinal tract.	Contralateral hemiparesis—lower limbs.	Stroke commonly bilateral. **Medial medullary syndrome**—caused by infarct of paramedian branches of ASA and vertebral arteries.
	Medial lemniscus.	↓ contralateral proprioception.	
	Caudal medulla—hypoglossal nerve.	Ipsilateral hypoglossal dysfunction (tongue deviates ipsilaterally).	
PICA	Lateral medulla—vestibular nuclei, lateral spinothalamic tract, spinal trigeminal nucleus, nucleus ambiguus, sympathetic fibers, inferior cerebellar peduncle.	Vomiting, vertigo, nystagmus; ↓ pain and temperature sensation to limbs/face; **dysphagia**, **hoarseness**, ↓ gag reflex; ipsilateral Horner's syndrome; ataxia, dysmetria.	**Lateral medullary (Wallenberg's) syndrome.** Nucleus ambiguus effects are specific to PICA lesions. "Don't **pick a** (**PICA**) **horse** (hoarseness) that **can't eat** (dysphagia)."
AICA	Lateral pons—cranial nerve nuclei; vestibular nuclei, facial nucleus, spinal trigeminal nucleus, cochlear nuclei, sympathetic fibers.	Vomiting, vertigo, nystagmus. **Paralysis** of face, ↓ lacrimation, salivation, ↓ taste from anterior ⅔ of tongue, ↓ corneal reflex. Face—↓ pain and temperature sensation. Ipsilateral ↓ hearing. Ipsilateral Horner's syndrome.	Lateral pontine syndrome. Facial nucleus effects are specific to AICA lesions. "**Facial droop** means AICA's **pooped**."
	Middle and inferior cerebellar peduncles.	Ataxia, dysmetria.	
PCA	Occipital cortex, visual cortex.	Contralateral hemianopia with macular sparing.	
Communicating arteries			
AComm	Common site of saccular (berry) aneurysm → impingement on cranial nerves.	Visual field defects.	Lesions are typically aneurysms, not strokes.
PComm	Common site of saccular (berry) aneurysm.	CN III palsy—eye is "down and out" with ptosis and pupil dilation.	Lesions are typically aneurysms, not strokes.

Aneurysms	In general, an abnormal dilation of artery due to weakening of vessel wall.
Berry aneurysm	Occurs at the bifurcations in the circle of Willis A. Most common site is bifurcation of the anterior communicating artery. Rupture (most common complication) leads to subarachnoid hemorrhage ("worst headache of life") or hemorrhagic stroke. Can also cause bitemporal hemianopia via compression of optic chiasm. Associated with ADPKD, Ehlers-Danlos syndrome, and Marfan's syndrome. Other risk factors: advanced age, hypertension, smoking, race (higher risk in blacks).
Charcot-Bouchard microaneurysm	Associated with chronic hypertension; affects small vessels (e.g., in basal ganglia, thalamus).

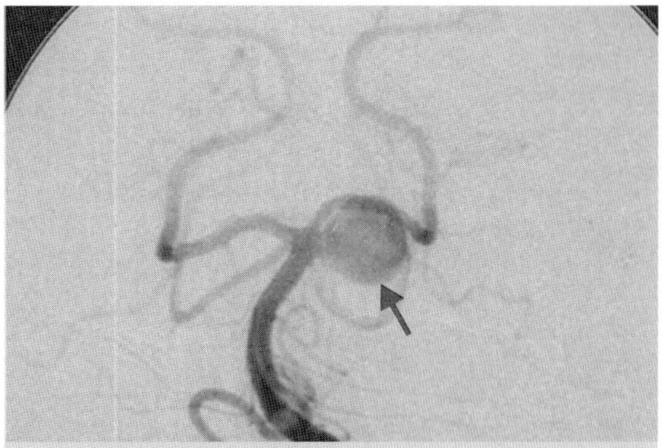

A Berry aneurysm (arrow).

Intracranial hemorrhage

Epidural hematoma

Rupture of middle meningeal artery (branch of maxillary artery), often 2° to fracture of temporal bone. Lucid interval. Rapid expansion under systemic arterial pressure → transtentorial herniation, CN III palsy.

CT shows biconvex (lentiform), hyperdense blood collection A not crossing suture lines. Can cross falx, tentorium.

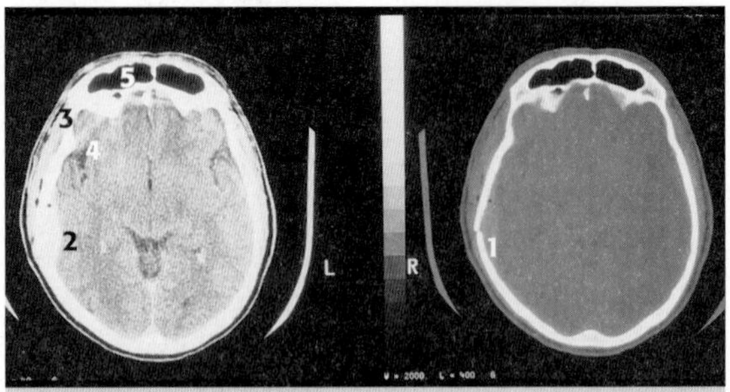

A **Epidural hematoma.** 1–fracture; 2–epidural hematoma; 3–temporalis muscle; 4–Sylvian fissure; 5–frontal sinus.

Subdural hematoma

Rupture of bridging veins. Slow venous bleeding (less pressure = hematoma develops over time). Seen in elderly individuals, alcoholics, blunt trauma, shaken baby (predisposing factors: brain atrophy, shaking, whiplash).

Crescent-shaped hemorrhage that crosses suture lines B. Midline shift. Cannot cross falx, tentorium.

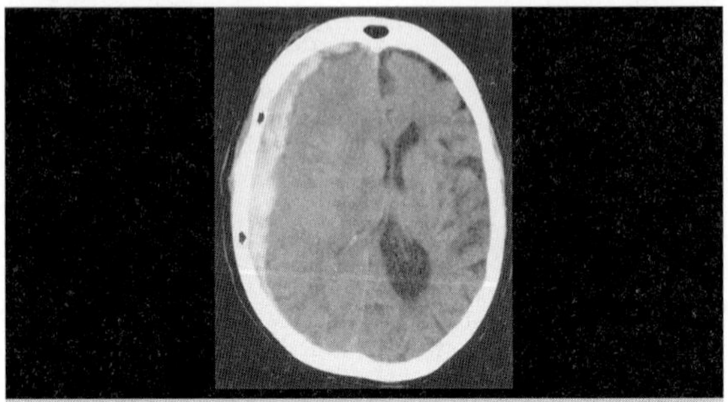

B **Subdural hematoma.** Note crescent-shaped hemorrhage that crosses suture lines.

Subarachnoid hemorrhage

Rupture of an aneurysm (such as a berry [saccular] aneurysm, as seen in Marfan's, Ehlers-Danlos, ADPKD) or an AVM. Rapid time course. Patients complain of "worst headache of my life (WHOML)." Bloody or yellow (xanthochromic) spinal tap. 2–3 days afterward, risk of vasospasm due to blood breakdown (not visible on CT, treat with nimodipine) and rebleed (visible on CT) C.

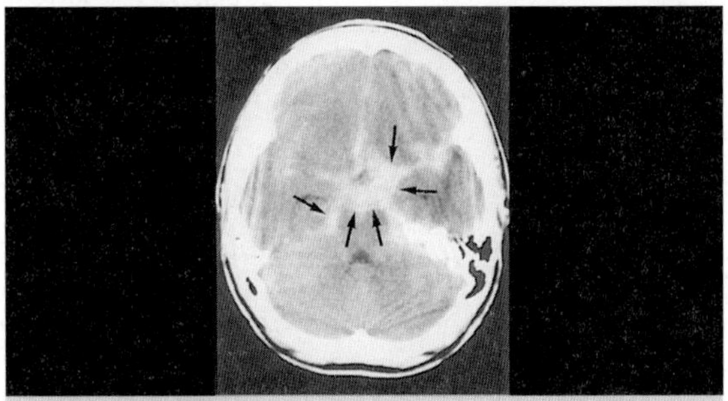

C **Subarachnoid hemorrhage.** Arrows show characteristic blood in cisterns.

Intraparenchymal (hypertensive) hemorrhage

Most commonly caused by systemic hypertension D. Also seen with amyloid angiopathy, vasculitis, and neoplasm. Typically occurs in basal ganglia and internal capsule (Charcot-Bouchard aneurysm of lenticulostriate vessels), but can be lobar.

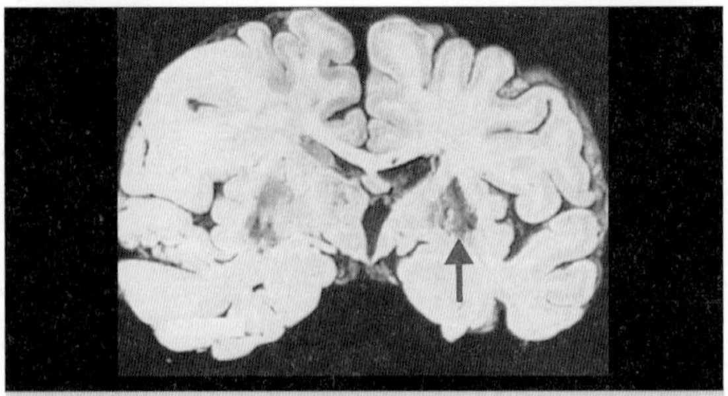

D **Hypertensive hemorrhage.**

Ischemic brain disease/stroke	Irreversible damage begins after 5 minutes of hypoxia. Most vulnerable—hippocampus, neocortex, cerebellum, watershed areas. Irreversible neuronal injury—red neurons (12–48 hours), necrosis + neutrophils (24–72 hours), macrophages (3–5 days), reactive gliosis + vascular proliferation (1–2 weeks), glial scar (> 2 weeks). Stroke imaging: bright on diffusion-weighted MRI in 3–30 minutes and remains bright for 10 days, dark on noncontrast CT in ~ 24 hours. Bright areas on noncontrast CT indicate hemorrhage (tPA contraindicated).
Atherosclerosis	Thrombi lead to ischemic stroke with subsequent necrosis. Form cystic cavity with reactive gliosis.
Hemorrhagic stroke	Intracerebral bleeding, often due to hypertension, anticoagulation, and cancer (abnormal vessels can bleed). May be 2° to ischemic stroke followed by reperfusion (↑ vessel fragility).
Ischemic stroke	Atherosclerotic emboli block large vessels; etiologies include atrial fibrillation, carotid dissection, patent foramen ovale, endocarditis. Lacunar strokes block small vessels, may be 2° to hypertension. Treatment: tPA within 4.5 hours (so long as patient presents within 3 hours of onset and there is no major risk of hemorrhage).
Transient ischemic attack (TIA)	Brief, reversible episode of focal neurologic dysfunction typically lasting < 1 hour **without** acute infarction (⊖ MRI); deficits due to focal ischemia.

Dural venous sinuses Large venous channels that run through the dura. Drain blood from cerebral veins and receive CSF from arachnoid granulations. Empty into internal jugular vein.

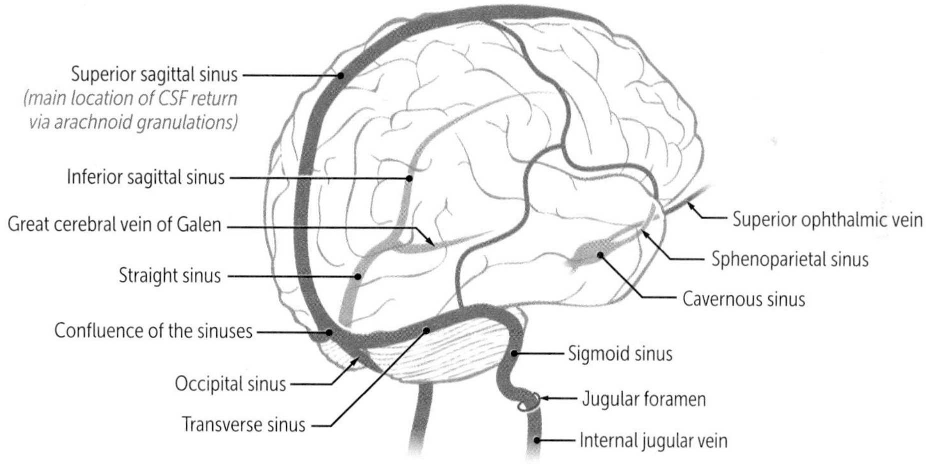
Superior sagittal sinus
(main location of CSF return via arachnoid granulations)
Inferior sagittal sinus
Great cerebral vein of Galen
Straight sinus
Confluence of the sinuses
Occipital sinus
Transverse sinus
Superior ophthalmic vein
Sphenoparietal sinus
Cavernous sinus
Sigmoid sinus
Jugular foramen
Internal jugular vein

Ventricular system

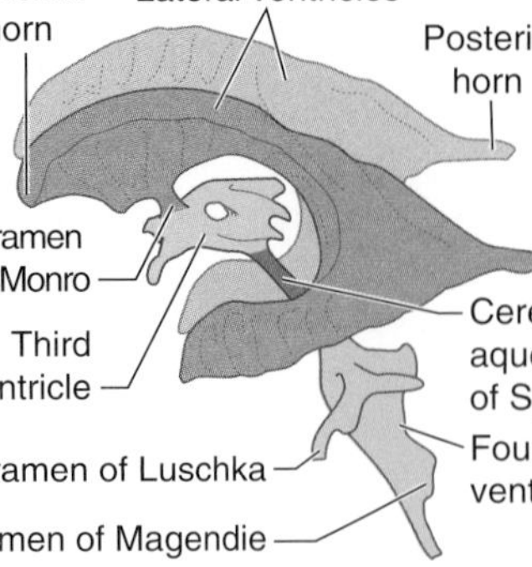
Anterior horn
Lateral ventricles
Posterior horn
Foramen of Monro
Third ventricle
Cerebral aqueduct of Sylvius
Foramen of Luschka
Fourth ventricle
Foramen of Magendie

Lateral ventricle → 3rd ventricle via right and left intraventricular foramina of Monro.
3rd ventricle → 4th ventricle via cerebral aqueduct (of Sylvius).
4th ventricle → subarachnoid space via:
- Foramina of **L**uschka = **L**ateral.
- Foramen of **M**agendie = **M**edial.

CSF is made by ependymal cells of choroid plexus; it is reabsorbed by arachnoid granulations and then drains into dural venous sinuses.

Hydrocephalus

Communicating (nonobstructive)		
Communicating hydrocephalus	↓ CSF absorption by arachnoid granulations, which can lead to ↑ intracranial pressure, papilledema, and herniation (e.g., arachnoid scarring post-meningitis).	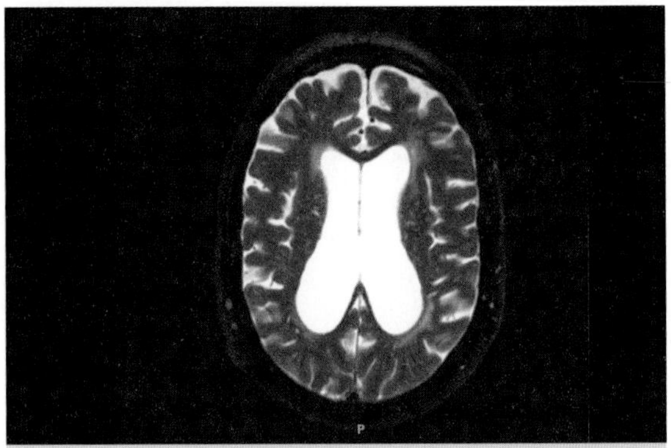 A **Normal pressure hydrocephalus.** Lateral ventricle enlargement in absence of, or out of proportion to, sulcal enlargement (marker for brain atrophy).
Normal pressure hydrocephalus	Results in ↑ subarachnoid space volume but no increase in CSF pressure. Expansion of ventricles distorts the fibers of the corona radiata and leads to the clinical triad of **urinary incontinence**, **ataxia**, and **cognitive dysfunction** (sometimes reversible) A. "**Wet**, **wobbly**, and **wacky**."	
Hydrocephalus ex vacuo	Appearance of ↑ CSF in atrophy (e.g., Alzheimer's disease, advanced HIV, Pick's disease). Intracranial pressure is normal; triad is not seen.	Apparent increase in CSF observed on imaging is actually result of decreased neural tissue due to neuronal atrophy.
Noncommuncating (obstructive)		
Noncommunicating hydrocephalus	Caused by a structural blockage of CSF circulation within the ventricular system (e.g., stenosis of the aqueduct of Sylvius).	

Spinal nerves	There are 31 spinal nerves in total: 8 cervical, 12 thoracic, 5 lumbar, 5 sacral, 1 coccygeal. Nerves C1–C7 exit above the corresponding vertebra. All other nerves exit below (e.g., C3 exits above the 3rd cervical vertebra; L2 exits below the 2nd lumbar vertebra).	**31**, just like **31** flavors of Baskin-Robbins ice cream! Vertebral disc herniation: nucleus pulposus (soft central disc) herniates through anulus fibrosus (outer ring); usually occurs posterolaterally at L4–L5 or L5–S1.
Spinal cord–lower extent	In adults, spinal cord extends to lower border of L1–L2 vertebrae. Subarachnoid space (which contains the CSF) extends to lower border of S2 vertebra. Lumbar puncture is usually performed between L3–L4 or L4–L5 (level of cauda equina).	Goal of lumbar puncture is to obtain sample of CSF without damaging spinal cord. To **keep** the cord **alive,** keep the spinal needle between **L3** and **L5.**

Spinal cord and associated tracts

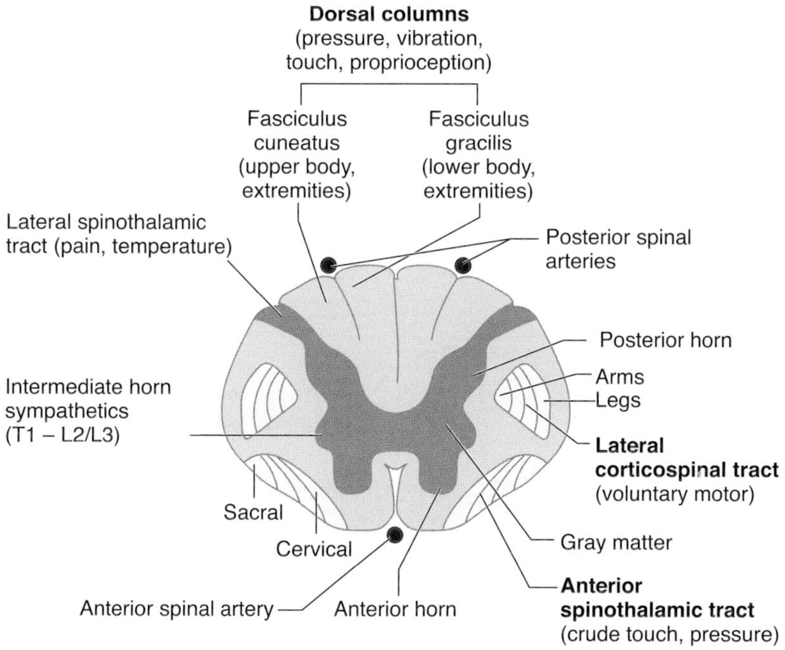

Legs are Lateral in Lateral corticospinal, spinothalamic tracts.

Dorsal column is organized as you are, with hands at sides. Arms outside, legs inside.

Spinal tract anatomy and functions

Remember, ascending tracts synapse and then cross.

TRACT AND FUNCTION	1ST-ORDER NEURON	SYNAPSE 1	2ND-ORDER NEURON	SYNAPSE 2	3RD-ORDER NEURON
Dorsal column Medial lemniscal pathway Ascending pressure, vibration, fine touch, and proprioception	Sensory nerve ending → cell body in dorsal root ganglion → enters spinal cord, ascends ipsilaterally in dorsal column	Ipsilateral nucleus cuneatus or gracilis (medulla)	Decussates in medulla → ascends contralaterally in medial lemniscus	VPL (thalamus)	Sensory cortex
Spinothalamic tract Lateral: pain, temperature Anterior: crude touch, pressure	Sensory nerve ending (Aδ and C fibers) (cell body in dorsal root ganglion) → enters spinal cord	Ipsilateral gray matter (spinal cord)	Decussates at anterior white commissure → ascends contralaterally	VPL (thalamus)	Sensory cortex
Lateral corticospinal tract Descending voluntary movement of contralateral limbs	UMN: cell body in 1° motor cortex → descends ipsilaterally (through internal capsule) until decussating at caudal medulla (pyramidal decussation) → descends contralaterally	Cell body of anterior horn (spinal cord)	LMN: leaves spinal cord	NMJ	

Motor neuron signs

SIGN	UMN LESION	LMN LESION	COMMENTS
Weakness	+	+	**Lower** MN = everything **lower**ed (less muscle mass, ↓ muscle tone, ↓ reflexes, downgoing toes). **Up**per MN = everything **up** (tone, DTRs, toes). Fasciculation = muscle twitching. Positive Babinski is normal in infants.
Atrophy	–	+	
Fasciculations	–	+	
Reflexes	↑	↓	
Tone	↑	↓	
Babinski	+	–	
Spastic paralysis	+	–	
Flaccid paralysis	–	+	
Clasp knife spasticity	+	–	

Spinal cord lesions

AREA AFFECTED	DISEASE	CHARACTERISTICS
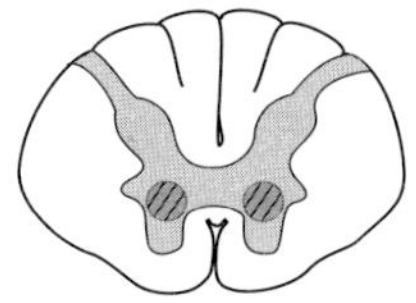	Poliomyelitis and Werdnig-Hoffman disease	LMN lesions only, due to destruction of anterior horns; flaccid paralysis.
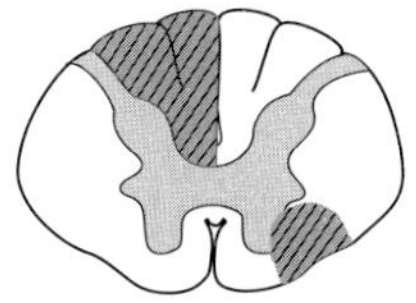	Multiple sclerosis	Mostly white matter of cervical region; random and asymmetric lesions, due to demyelination; scanning speech, intention tremor, nystagmus.
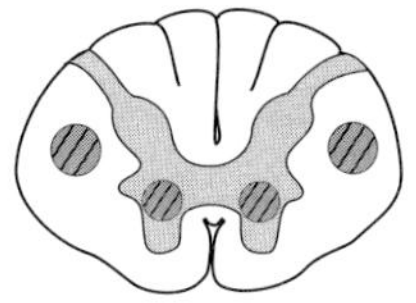	Amyotrophic lateral sclerosis (ALS)	Combined UMN and LMN deficits with no sensory, cognitive, or oculomotor deficits; both UMN and LMN signs. Can be caused by defect in superoxide dismutase 1. Commonly presents as fasciculations with eventual atrophy; progressive and fatal. Riluzole treatment modestly ↑ survival by ↓ presynaptic glutamate release. Commonly known as Lou Gehrig's disease. Stephen Hawking is a well-known patient who highlights the lack of cognitive deficit.
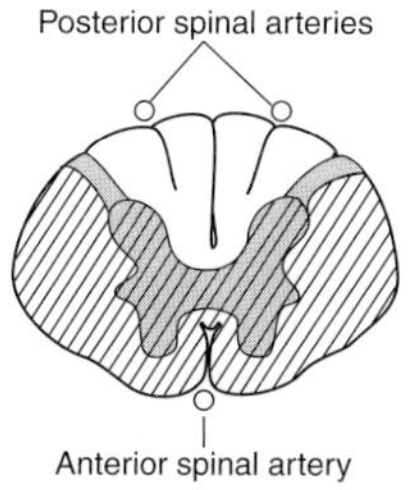	Complete occlusion of anterior spinal artery	Spares dorsal columns and Lissauer's tract; upper thoracic ASA territory is a watershed area, as artery of Adamkiewicz supplies ASA below ~T8.
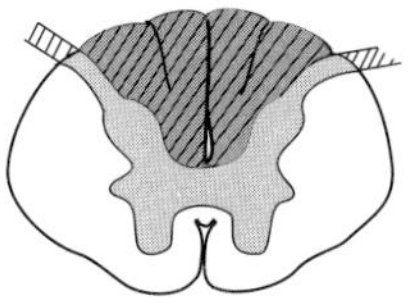	Tabes dorsalis	Caused by 3° syphilis. Results from degeneration (demyelination) of dorsal columns and roots → impaired sensation and proprioception and progressive sensory ataxia (inability to sense or feel the legs). Associated with Charcot's joints, shooting pain, Argyll Robertson pupils (small bilateral pupils that further constrict to accommodation but not to light). Exam will demonstrate absence of DTRs and positive Romberg.
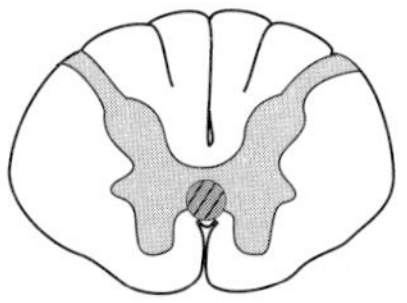	Syringomyelia	Syrinx expands and damages anterior white commissure of spinothalamic tract (2nd-order neurons) → bilateral loss of pain and temperature sensation (usually C8–T1); seen with Chiari I malformation; can expand and affect other tracts.
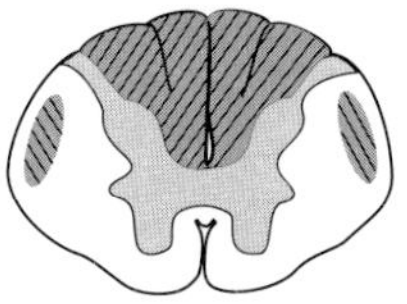	Vitamin B_{12} or vitamin E deficiency	Subacute combined degeneration—demyelination of dorsal columns, lateral corticospinal tracts, and spinocerebellar tracts; ataxic gait, paresthesia, impaired position and vibration sense.

Poliomyelitis	Caused by poliovirus (fecal-oral transmission). Replicates in the oropharynx and small intestine before spreading via the bloodstream to the CNS. Infection causes destruction of cells in anterior horn of spinal cord (LMN death).
SYMPTOMS	LMN lesion signs—weakness, hypotonia, flaccid paralysis, atrophy, fasciculations, hyporeflexia, and muscle atrophy. Signs of infection—malaise, headache, fever, nausea, etc.
FINDINGS	CSF with ↑ WBCs with slight elevation of protein (with no change in CSF glucose). Virus recovered from stool or throat.

Werdnig-Hoffman disease

Congenital degeneration of anterior horns of spinal cord → LMN lesion. "Floppy baby" with marked hypotonia and tongue fasciculations. Infantile type has median age of death of 7 months. Autosomal-recessive inheritance.

Friedreich's ataxia

Autosomal-recessive trinucleotide repeat disorder (GAA) in gene that encodes frataxin. Leads to impairment in mitochondrial functioning. **Staggering** gait, frequent **falling**, nystagmus, dysarthria, pes cavus, hammer toes, hypertrophic cardiomyopathy (cause of death). Presents in childhood with kyphoscoliosis.

Friedreich is Fratastic (**frataxin**): he's your favorite **frat** brother, always stumbling, **staggering**, and **falling**.

Brown-Séquard syndrome

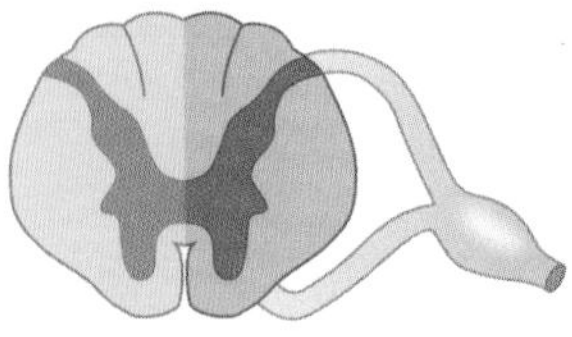
Lesion

Hemisection of spinal cord. Findings:

- Ipsilateral UMN signs below the level of the lesion (due to corticospinal tract damage)
- Ipsilateral loss of tactile, vibration, proprioception sense below the level of the lesion (due to dorsal column damage)
- Contralateral pain and temperature loss below the level of the lesion (due to spinothalamic tract damage)
- Ipsilateral loss of all sensation at the level of the lesion
- Ipsilateral LMN signs (e.g., flaccid paralysis) at the level of the lesion

If lesion occurs above T1, patient may present with Horner's syndrome due to damage of sympathetic ganglion.

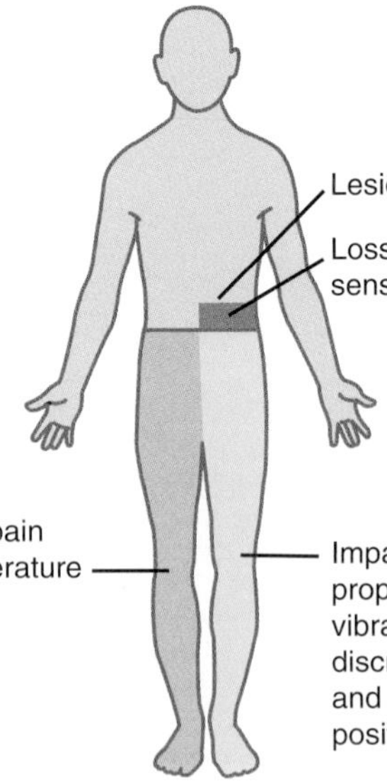
Lesion
Loss of all sensation
Impaired pain and temperature sensation
Impaired proprioception, vibration, 2-point discrimination, and joint and position sensation

Horner's syndrome

Sympathectomy of face:
- Ptosis (slight drooping of eyelid: superior tarsal muscle)
- Anhidrosis (absence of sweating) and flushing (rubor) of affected side of face
- Miosis (pupil constriction)

Associated with lesion of spinal cord above T1 (e.g., Pancoast tumor, Brown-Séquard syndrome [cord hemisection], late-stage syringomyelia).

PAM is **horny** (Horner's).
Ptosis, anhidrosis, and **miosis** (rhyming).

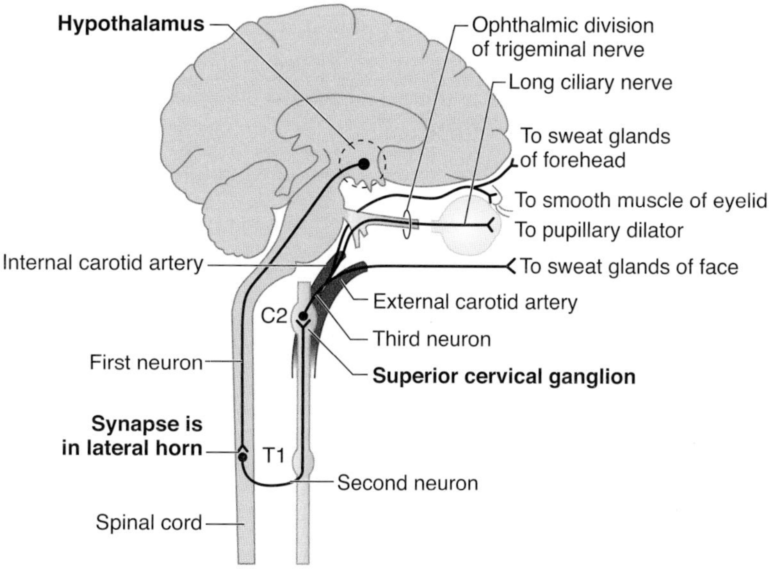

The 3-neuron oculosympathetic pathway projects from the hypothalamus to the intermediolateral column of the spinal cord, then to the superior cervical (sympathetic) ganglion, and finally to the pupil, the smooth muscle of the eyelids, and the sweat glands of the forehead and face. Interruption of any of these pathways results in Horner's syndrome.

Landmark dermatomes

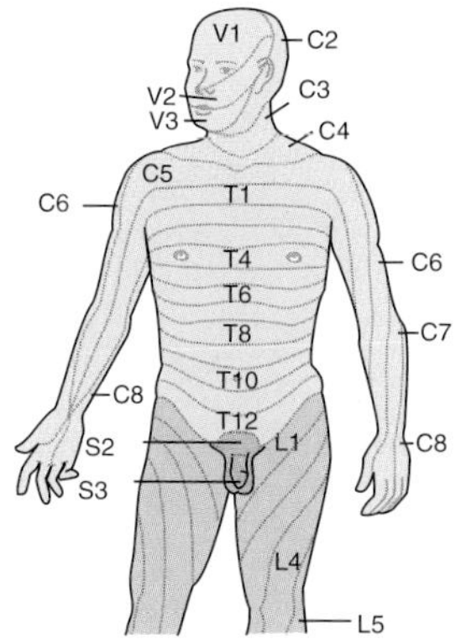

C2—posterior half of a skull "cap."
C3—high turtleneck shirt.
C4—low-collar shirt.
T4—at the nipple.
T7—at the xiphoid process.
T10—at the umbilicus (important for early appendicitis pain referral).
L1—at the inguinal ligament.
L4—includes the kneecaps.
S2, S3, S4—erection and sensation of penile and anal zones.

Diaphragm and gallbladder pain referred to the right shoulder via the phrenic nerve.

T4 at the **teat pore**.

T10 at the belly **butten**.

L1 is **IL** (**I**nguinal **L**igament).
Down on **ALL** 4's (**L4**).
"**S2, 3, 4** keep the penis off the **floor**."

Clinical reflexes

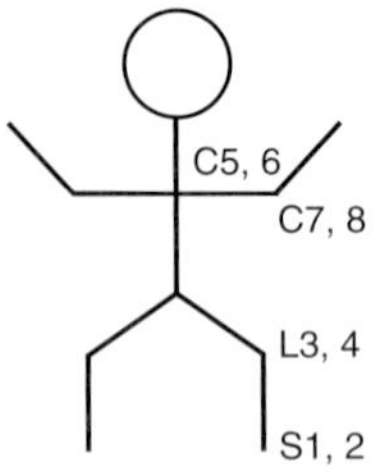

Biceps = C5 nerve root.
Triceps = C7 nerve root.
Patella = L4 nerve root.
Achilles = S1 nerve root.
Babinski—dorsiflexion of the big toe and fanning of other toes; sign of UMN lesion, but normal reflex in 1st year of life.

Reflexes count up in order:
S1, 2
L3, 4
C5, 6
C7, 8

Primitive reflexes

CNS reflexes that are present in a healthy infant, but are absent in a neurologically intact adult.
Normally disappear within 1st year of life. These "primitive" reflexes are inhibited by a mature/developing frontal lobe. They may reemerge in adults following frontal lobe lesions → loss of inhibition of these reflexes.

Moro reflex	"Hang on for life" reflex—abduct/extend limbs when startled, and then draw together
Rooting reflex	Movement of head toward one side if cheek or mouth is stroked (nipple seeking)
Sucking reflex	Sucking response when roof of mouth is touched
Palmar reflex	Curling of fingers if palm is stroked
Plantar reflex	Dorsiflexion of large toe and fanning of other toes with plantar stimulation Babinski sign—presence of this reflex in an adult, which may signify a UMN lesion
Galant reflex	Stroking along one side of the spine while newborn is in ventral suspension (face down) causes lateral flexion of lower body toward stimulated side

---

Brain stem—ventral view

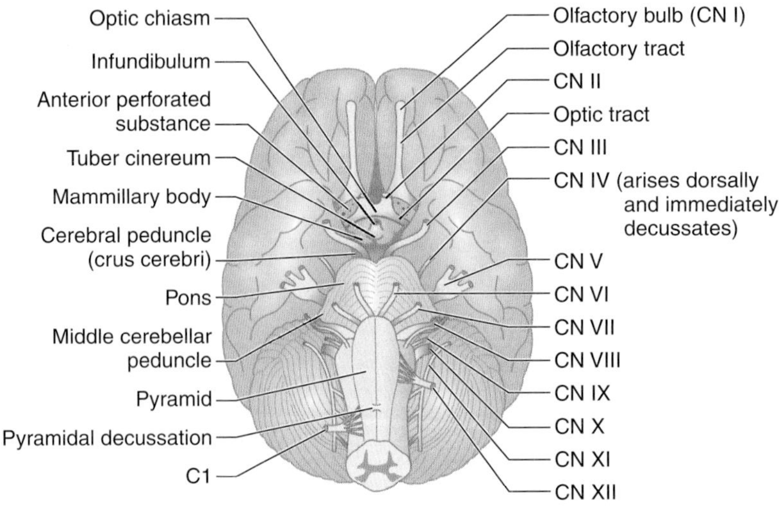

CNs that lie medially at brain stem: **III, VI, XII**. 3(×2) = 6(×2) = 12 (Motor = Medial).

Brain stem–dorsal view (cerebellum removed)

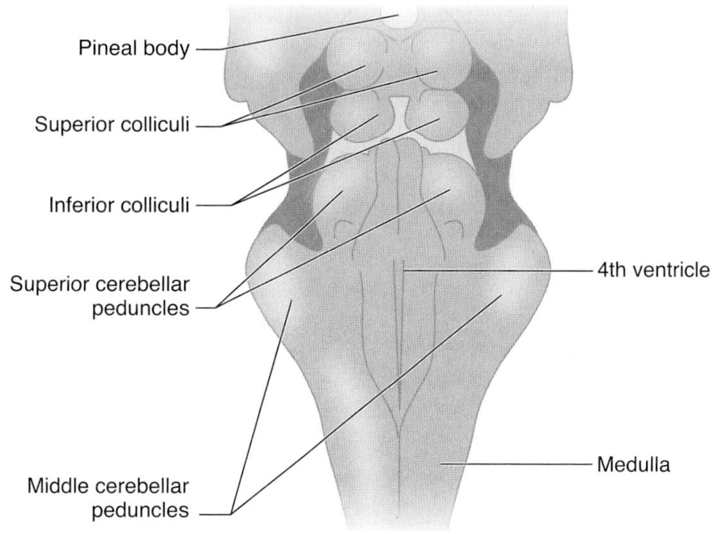
Pineal body
Superior colliculi
Inferior colliculi
Superior cerebellar peduncles
Middle cerebellar peduncles
4th ventricle
Medulla

Pineal gland—melatonin secretion, circadian rhythms.

Superior colliculi—conjugate vertical gaze center.

Inferior colliculi—auditory.

Parinaud syndrome—paralysis of conjugate vertical gaze due to lesion in superior colliculi (e.g., pinealoma).

Your eyes are **above** your ears, and the superior colliculus (visual) is **above** the inferior colliculus (auditory).

Cranial nerves

NERVE	CN	FUNCTION	TYPE	MNEMONIC
Olfactory	I	Smell (only CN without thalamic relay to cortex)	Sensory	Some
Optic	II	Sight	Sensory	Say
Oculomotor	III	Eye movement (SR, IR, MR, IO), pupillary constriction (sphincter pupillae: Edinger-Westphal nucleus, muscarinic receptors), accommodation, eyelid opening (levator palpebrae)	Motor	Marry
Trochlear	IV	Eye movement (SO)	Motor	Money
Trigeminal	V	Mastication, facial sensation (ophthalmic, maxillary, mandibular divisions), somatosensation from anterior 2/3 of tongue	Both	But
Abducens	VI	Eye movement (LR)	Motor	My
Facial	VII	Facial movement, taste from anterior 2/3 of tongue, lacrimation, salivation (submandibular and sublingual glands), eyelid closing (orbicularis oculi), stapedius muscle in ear (note: nerve courses through the parotid gland, but does not innervate it)	Both	Brother
Vestibulocochlear	VIII	Hearing, balance	Sensory	Says
Glossopharyngeal	IX	Taste and somatosensation from posterior 1/3 of tongue, swallowing, salivation (parotid gland), monitoring carotid body and sinus chemo- and baroreceptors, and stylopharyngeus (elevates pharynx, larynx)	Both	Big
Vagus	X	Taste from epiglottic region, swallowing, palate elevation, midline uvula, talking, coughing, thoracoabdominal viscera, monitoring aortic arch chemo- and baroreceptors	Both	Brains
Accessory	XI	Head turning, shoulder shrugging (SCM, trapezius)	Motor	Matter
Hypoglossal	XII	Tongue movement	Motor	Most

Cranial nerve nuclei

Located in tegmentum portion of brain stem (between dorsal and ventral portions):
- Midbrain—nuclei of CN III, IV
- Pons—nuclei of CN V, VI, VII, VIII
- Medulla—nuclei of CN IX, X, XII
- Spinal cord—nucleus of CN XI

Lateral nuclei = sensory (aLar plate).
—Sulcus limitans—
Medial nuclei = Motor (basal plate).

Cranial nerve reflexes

REFLEX	AFFERENT	EFFERENT
Corneal	V_1 ophthalmic (nasociliary branch)	VII (temporal branch: orbicularis oculi)
Lacrimation	V_1 (loss of reflex does not preclude emotional tears)	VII
Jaw jerk	V_3 (sensory—muscle spindle from masseter)	V_3 (motor—masseter)
Pupillary	II	III
Gag	IX	X

Vagal nuclei		
Nucleus Solitarius	Visceral Sensory information (e.g., taste, baroreceptors, gut distention).	VII, IX, X.
Nucleus aMbiguus	Motor innervation of pharynx, larynx, and upper esophagus (e.g., swallowing, palate elevation).	IX, X.
Dorsal motor nucleus	Sends autonomic (parasympathetic) fibers to heart, lungs, and upper GI.	X.

Cranial nerve and vessel pathways	Cribriform plate (CN I). Middle cranial fossa (CN II–VI)—through sphenoid bone: ▪ Optic canal (CN II, ophthalmic artery, central retinal vein) ▪ Superior orbital fissure (CN III, IV, V_1, VI, ophthalmic vein, sympathetic fibers) ▪ Foramen Rotundum (CN V_2) ▪ Foramen Ovale (CN V_3) ▪ Foramen spinosum (middle meningeal artery) Posterior cranial fossa (CN VII–XII)—through temporal or occipital bone: ▪ Internal auditory meatus (CN VII, VIII) ▪ Jugular foramen (CN IX, X, XI, jugular vein) ▪ Hypoglossal canal (CN XII) ▪ Foramen magnum (spinal roots of CN XI, brain stem, vertebral arteries)	Divisions of CN V exit owing to Standing Room Only.

Cavernous sinus

A collection of venous sinuses on either side of the pituitary. Blood from eye and superficial cortex → cavernous sinus → internal jugular vein.

CN III, IV, V_1, V_2, and VI and postganglionic sympathetic fibers en route to the orbit all pass through the cavernous sinus. Cavernous portion of internal carotid artery is also here.

The nerves that control extraocular muscles (plus V_1 and V_2) pass through the cavernous sinus.

Cavernous sinus syndrome (e.g., due to mass effect, fistula, thrombosis)—ophthalmoplegia and ↓ corneal and maxillary sensation with normal vision.

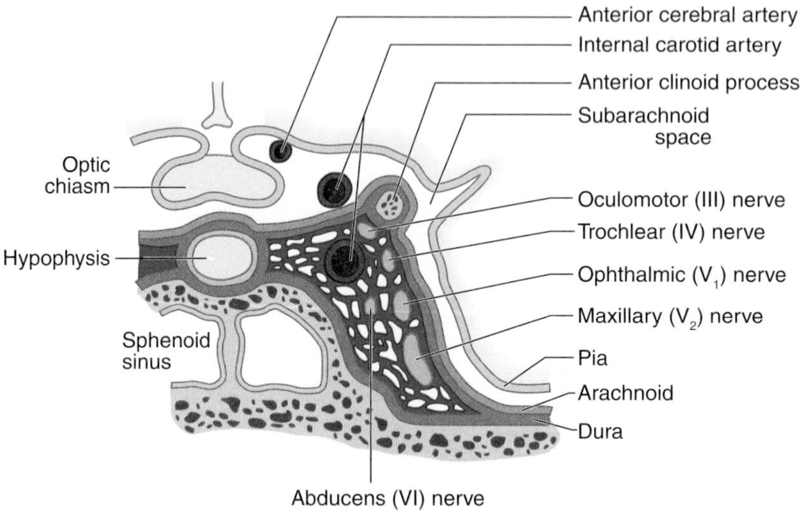

Common cranial nerve lesions

CN V motor lesion	Jaw deviates **toward** side of lesion due to unopposed force from the opposite pterygoid muscle.
CN X lesion	Uvula deviates **away** from side of lesion. Weak side collapses and uvula points away.
CN XI lesion	Weakness turning head to contralateral side of lesion (SCM). Shoulder droop on side of lesion (trapezius). The left SCM contracts to help turn the head to the right.
CN XII lesion (LMN)	Tongue deviates **toward** side of lesion ("lick your wounds") due to weakened tongue muscles on the affected side.

Hearing loss

	RINNE TEST	WEBER TEST
Conductive	Abnormal (bone > air)	Localizes to affected ear
Sensorineural	Normal (air > bone)	Localizes to unaffected ear

Noise-induced	Damage to stereociliated cells in organ of Corti; loss of high-frequency hearing 1st; sudden extremely loud noises can produce hearing loss due to tympanic membrane rupture.

Facial lesions

UMN lesion	Lesion of motor cortex or connection between cortex and facial nucleus. Contralateral paralysis of lower face; forehead spared due to bilateral UMN innervation.
LMN lesion	Ipsilateral paralysis of upper **and** lower face.
Facial nerve palsy	Complete destruction of the facial nucleus itself or its branchial efferent fibers (facial nerve proper). Peripheral ipsilateral facial paralysis with inability to close eye on involved side. Can occur idiopathically; gradual recovery in most cases. Seen as a complication in AIDS, Lyme disease, herpes simplex and (less common) herpes zoster, sarcoidosis, tumors, and diabetes. Called Bell's palsy when idiopathic.

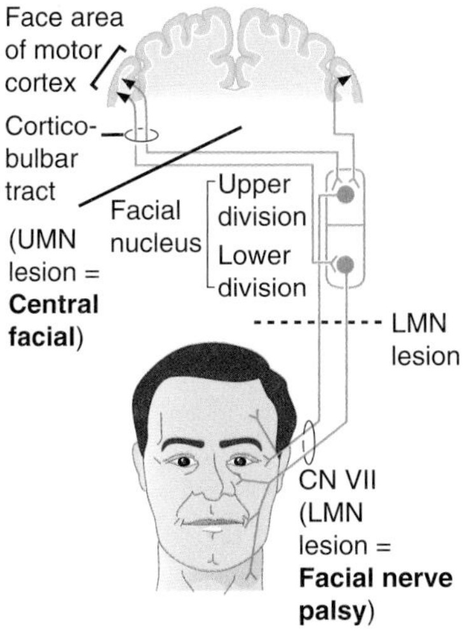
Face area of motor cortex
Cortico-bulbar tract
(UMN lesion = **Central facial**)
Facial nucleus
Upper division
Lower division
LMN lesion
CN VII (LMN lesion = **Facial nerve palsy**)

Mastication muscles

3 muscles close jaw: **M**asseter, te**M**poralis, **M**edial pterygoid. 1 opens: lateral pterygoid. All are innervated by the trigeminal nerve (V_3).

M's **M**unch.
Lateral **L**owers (when speaking of pterygoids with respect to jaw motion).
"It takes more muscle to keep your mouth shut."

Eye and retina

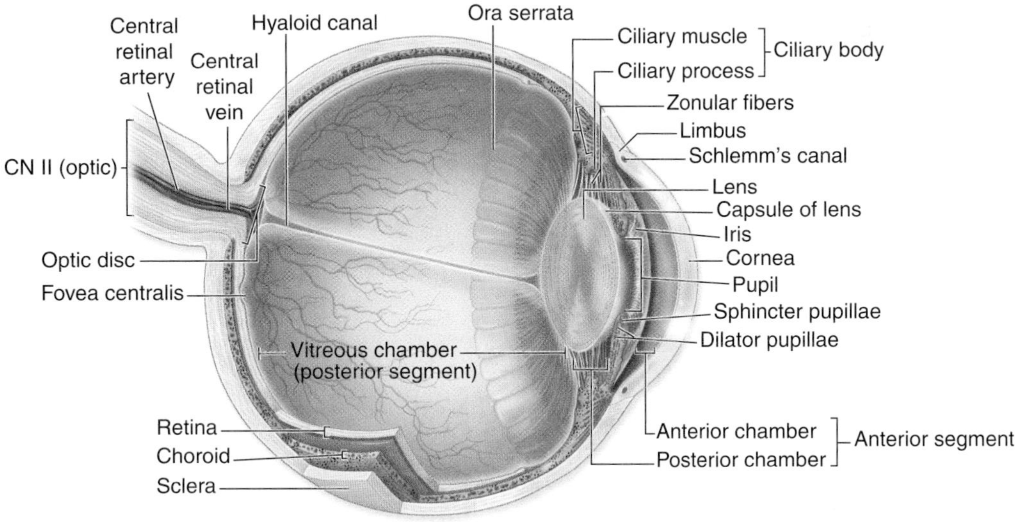
Central retinal artery
Hyaloid canal
Central retinal vein
Ora serrata
Ciliary muscle
Ciliary process
Ciliary body
Zonular fibers
Limbus
Schlemm's canal
CN II (optic)
Lens
Capsule of lens
Iris
Cornea
Optic disc
Pupil
Fovea centralis
Sphincter pupillae
Dilator pupillae
Vitreous chamber (posterior segment)
Retina
Choroid
Sclera
Anterior chamber
Posterior chamber
Anterior segment

(Reproduced, with permission, from Mescher AL. *Junqueira's Basic Histology: Text & Atlas,* 12th ed. New York: McGraw-Hill, 2010: Fig. 23-1.)

Common eye conditions

Refractive errors	Impaired vision that improves with glasses. Hyperopia: eye too short for refractive power of cornea and lens → light focused behind retina. Myopia: eye too long for refractive power of cornea and lens → light focused in front of retina. Astigmatism: abnormal curvature of cornea resulting in different refractive power at different axes. Accommodation: focusing on near objects → ciliary muscles tighten → zonular fibers relax → lens becomes more convex. Occurs with convergence and miosis. Presbyopia: ↓ change in focusing ability during accommodation due to sclerosis and decreased elasticity.
Uveitis	Inflammation of uveal coat (consists of iris, ciliary body, and choroid). Often associated with systemic inflammatory disorders (e.g., sarcoid, rheumatoid arthritis, juvenile idiopathic arthritis, TB, HLA-B27–associated conditions).
Retinitis	Retinal edema and necrosis leading to scar. Often viral (CMV, HSV, HZV). Associated with immunosuppression.
Central retinal artery occlusion	Acute, painless monocular vision loss. Retina whitening with cherry-red spot.

Aqueous humor pathway

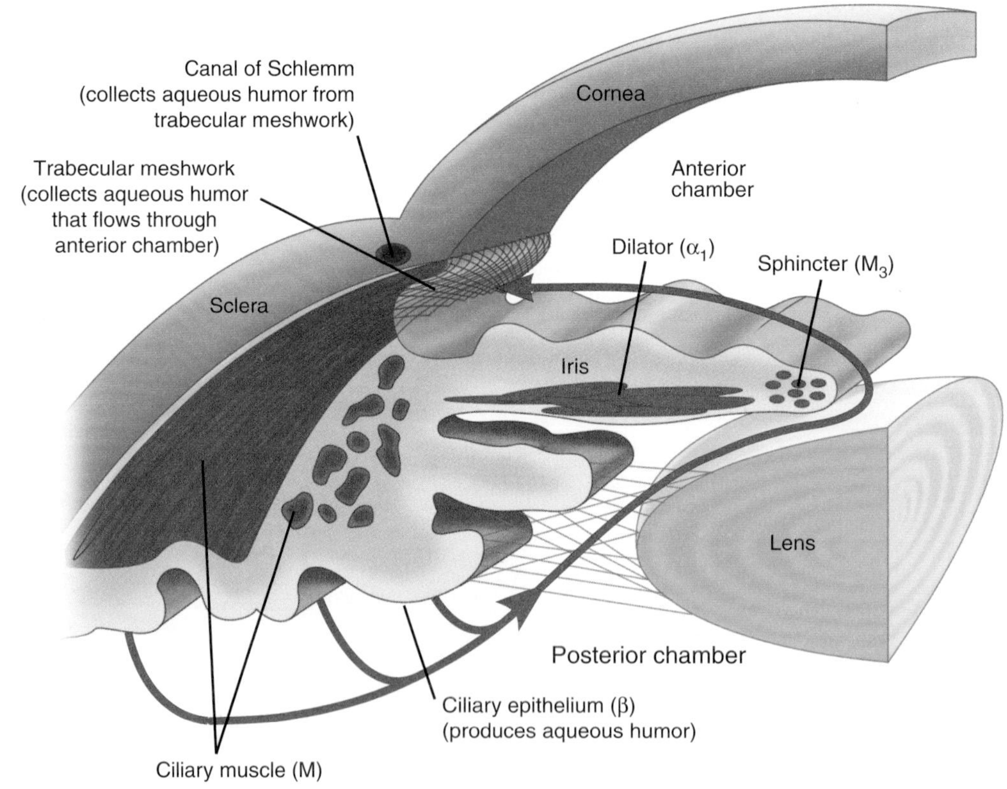
Canal of Schlemm (collects aqueous humor from trabecular meshwork)
Cornea
Trabecular meshwork (collects aqueous humor that flows through anterior chamber)
Anterior chamber
Dilator (α_1)
Sphincter (M_3)
Sclera
Iris
Lens
Posterior chamber
Ciliary epithelium (β) (produces aqueous humor)
Ciliary muscle (M)

(Adapted, with permission, from Riordan-Eva P, Whitcher JP. *Vaughan & Asbury's General Ophthalmology,* 17th ed. New York: McGraw-Hill, 2008.)

Glaucoma	Optic neuropathy, usually with ↑ intraocular pressure (IOP).
Open/wide angle	Characterized by peripheral then central vision loss usually with ↑ IOP; optic disc atrophy with cupping; associated with ↑ age, African-American race, family history, ↑ IOP. Painless, more common in U.S. Primary cause unclear. Secondary causes include uveitis, trauma, corticosteroids, and vasoproliferative retinopathy that can block or ↓ outflow at the trabecular meshwork.
Closed/narrow angle	Enlargement or forward movement of lens against central iris leads to obstruction of normal aqueous flow through pupil → fluid builds up behind iris, pushing peripheral iris against cornea and impeding flow through the trabecular meshwork. Chronic closure: Often asymptomatic with damage to optic nerve and peripheral vision. Acute closure: True ophthalmic emergency. ↑ IOP pushes iris forward → angle closes abruptly. Very painful, sudden vision loss, halos around lights, rock-hard eye, frontal headache. Do not give epinephrine because of its mydriatic effect.
Cataract	Painless, often bilateral, opacification of lens → ↓ in vision. Risk factors: age, smoking, EtOH, excessive sunlight, prolonged corticosteroid use, classic galactosemia, galactokinase deficiency, diabetes (sorbitol), trauma, infection.
Papilledema	Optic disc swelling (usually bilateral) due to ↑ intracranial pressure (e.g., 2° to mass effect). Enlarged blind spot and elevated optic disc with blurred margins seen on fundoscopic exam.

Extraocular muscles and nerves

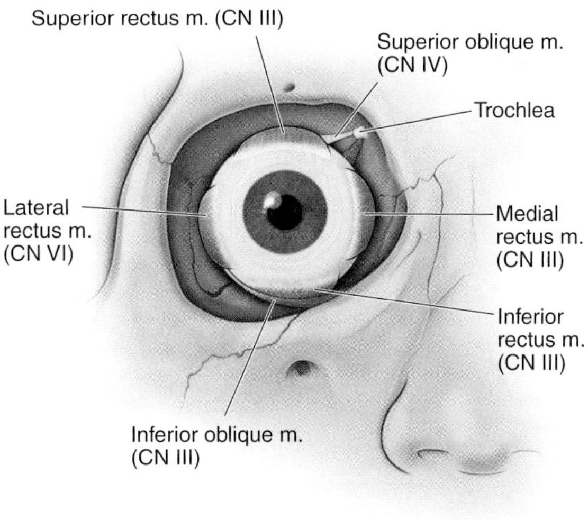
Superior rectus m. (CN III)
Superior oblique m. (CN IV)
Trochlea
Lateral rectus m. (CN VI)
Medial rectus m. (CN III)
Inferior rectus m. (CN III)
Inferior oblique m. (CN III)

(Reproduced, with permission, from Morton D et al. *The Big Picture: Gross Anatomy.* New York: McGraw-Hill, 2011: Fig. 18-3C.)

CN III damage—eye looks down and out; ptosis, pupillary dilation, loss of accommodation.
CN IV damage—eye moves upward, particularly with contralateral gaze and ipsilateral head tilt (problems going down stairs).
CN VI damage—medially directed eye that cannot abduct.

CN **VI** innervates the **L**ateral **R**ectus.
CN **IV** innervates the **S**uperior **O**blique.
CN **III** innervates the **R**est.
The "chemical formula" $LR_6SO_4R_3$.
The superior oblique abducts, intorts, and depresses while adducted.

Testing extraocular muscles

To test the function of each muscle, have the patient look in the following directions (e.g., to test SO, have patient depress eye from adducted position):

IOU: to test Inferior Oblique, have patient look Up.
Obliques move the eye in the Opposite direction.

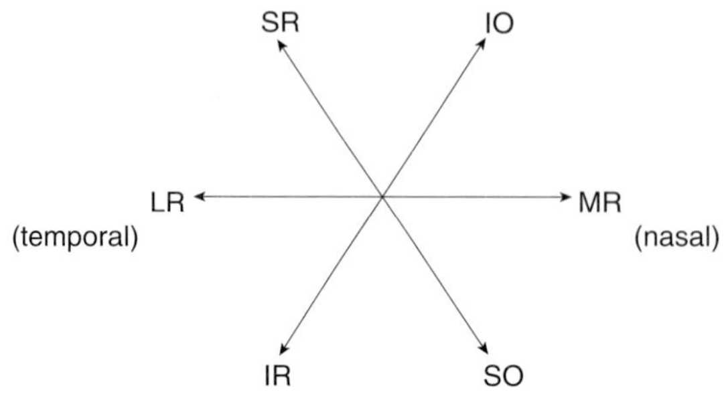

SR
IO
LR
(temporal)
MR
(nasal)
IR
SO

Pupillary control

Miosis (constriction, parasympathetic):
- 1st neuron: Edinger-Westphal nucleus to ciliary ganglion via CN III
- 2nd neuron: short ciliary nerves to pupillary sphincter muscles

Mydriasis (dilation, sympathetic)
- 1st neuron: hypothalamus to ciliospinal center of Budge (C8–T2)
- 2nd neuron: exit at T1 to superior cervical ganglion (travels along cervical sympathetic chain near lung apex, subclavian vessels)
- 3rd neuron: plexus along internal carotid, through cavernous sinus; enters orbit as long ciliary nerve to pupillary dilator muscles

---

Pupillary light reflex

Light in either retina sends a signal via CN II to pretectal nuclei (dashed lines) in midbrain that activate **bilateral** Edinger-Westphal nuclei; pupils contract bilaterally (consensual reflex).
Result: illumination of 1 eye results in **bilateral** pupillary constriction.
Marcus Gunn pupil—afferent pupillary defect (e.g., due to optic nerve damage or retinal detachment). ↓ bilateral pupillary constriction when light is shone in affected eye relative to unaffected eye. Tested with the "swinging flashlight test."

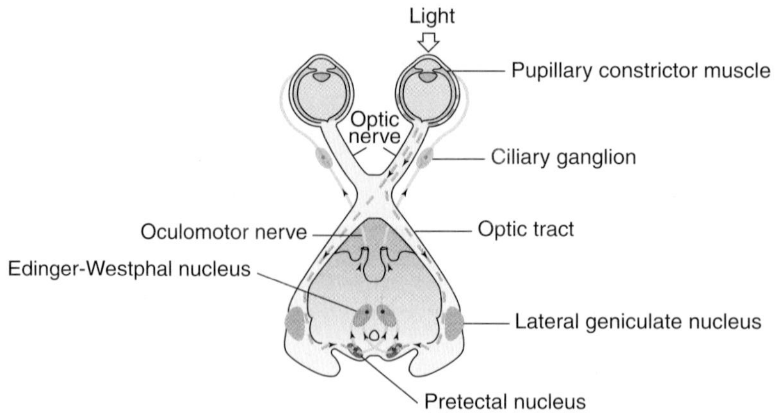

Light
Pupillary constrictor muscle
Optic nerve
Ciliary ganglion
Oculomotor nerve
Optic tract
Edinger-Westphal nucleus
Lateral geniculate nucleus
Pretectal nucleus

(Adapted, with permission, from Simon RP et al. *Clinical Neurology,* 7th ed. New York: McGraw-Hill, 2009: Fig. 4-12.)

Cranial nerve III

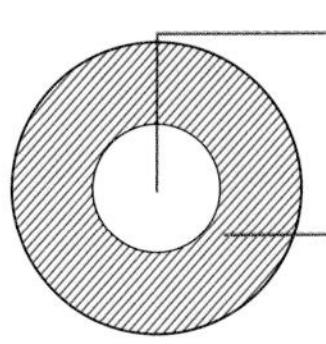

CN III has both motor (central) and parasympathetic (peripheral) components.

Motor output to ocular muscles—affected primarily by vascular disease (e.g., diabetes: glucose → sorbitol) due to ↓ diffusion of oxygen and nutrients to the interior fibers from compromised vasculature that resides on outside of nerve. Signs: ptosis, "down and out" gaze.

Parasympathetic output—fibers on the periphery are 1st affected by compression (e.g., posterior communicating artery aneurysm, uncal herniation). Signs: diminished or absent pupillary light reflex, "blown pupil."

Retinal detachment

Separation of neurosensory layer of retina (photoreceptor layer with rods and cones) from outermost pigmented epithelium (normally shields excess light, supports retina) → degeneration of photoreceptors → vision loss. May be 2° to retinal breaks, diabetic traction, inflammatory effusions.

Breaks more common in patients with high myopia and are often preceded by posterior vitreous detachment (flashes and floaters) and eventual monocular loss of vision like a "curtain drawn down." Surgical emergency.

Age-related macular degeneration

Degeneration of macula (central area of retina). Causes distortion (metamorphopsia) and eventual loss of central vision (scotomas).

- Dry (nonexudative, > 80%)—deposition of yellowish extracellular material beneath retinal pigment epithelium ("drusen") with gradual ↓ in vision. Prevent progression with multivitamin and antioxidant supplements.
- Wet (exudative, 10–15%)—rapid loss of vision due to bleeding secondary to choroidal neovascularization. Treat with anti-vascular endothelial growth factor injections (anti-VEGF) or laser.

Visual field defects

1. Right anopia
2. Bitemporal hemianopia
3. Left homonymous hemianopia
4. Left upper quadrantic anopia (right temporal lesion, MCA)
5. Left lower quadrantic anopia (right parietal lesion, MCA)
6. Left hemianopia with macular sparing (PCA infarct), macula → bilateral projection to occiput
7. Central scotoma (macular degeneration)

Meyer's loop—inferior retina; loops around inferior horn of lateral ventricle.

Dorsal optic radiation—superior retina; takes shortest path via internal capsule.

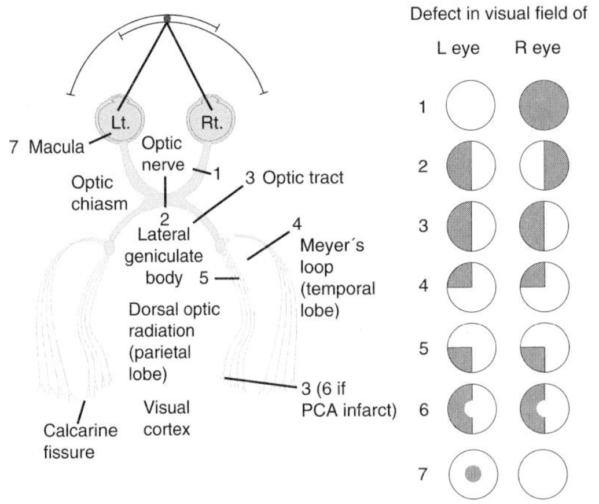

Note: When an image hits 1° visual cortex, it is upside down and left-right reversed.

Internuclear ophthalmoplegia (MLF syndrome)

Medial longitudinal fasciculus (MLF): pair of tracts that allows for crosstalk between CN VI and CN III nuclei. Coordinates both eyes to move in same horizontal direction. Highly myelinated (must communicate quickly so eyes move at same time). Lesions seen in patients with demyelination (e.g., multiple sclerosis).

Lesion in MLF = INO: lack of communication such that when CN VI nucleus activates ipsilateral lateral rectus, contralateral CN III nucleus does not stimulate medial rectus to fire. Abducting eye gets nystagmus (CN VI overfires to stimulate CN III). Convergence normal.

MLF in MS.

When looking left, the left nucleus of CN VI fires, which contracts the left lateral rectus and stimulates the contralateral (right) nucleus of CN III via the right MLF to contract the right medial rectus.

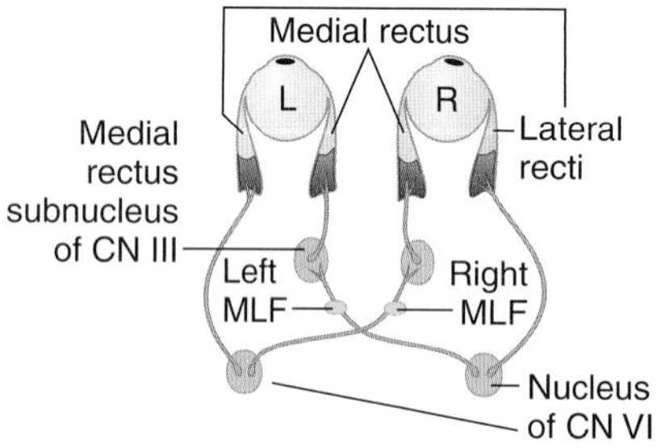

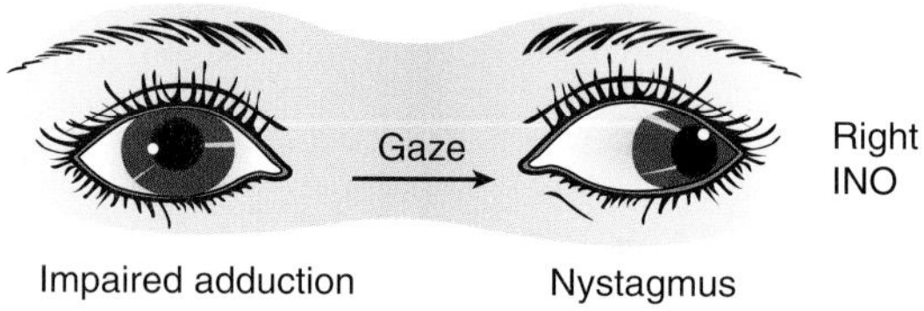

▸ NEUROLOGY—PATHOLOGY

Dementia A ↓ in cognitive ability, memory, or function with intact consciousness.

DISEASE	DESCRIPTION	HISTOLOGIC/GROSS FINDINGS
Alzheimer's disease 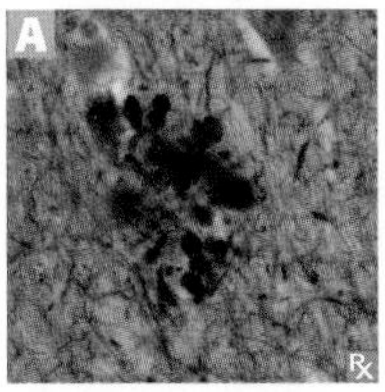	Most common cause in elderly. Down syndrome patients have an ↑ risk of developing Alzheimer's. Familial form (10%) associated with the following altered proteins (respective chromosomes in parentheses): ▪ Early onset: APP (21), presenilin-1 (14), presenilin-2 (1) ▪ Late onset: ApoE4 (19) ApoE2 (19) is protective.	Widespread cortical atrophy ↓ ACh Senile plaques A: extracellular β-amyloid core; may cause amyloid angiopathy → intracranial hemorrhage; Aβ (amyloid-β) synthesized by cleaving amyloid precursor protein Neurofibrillary tangles: intracellular, abnormally phosphorylated tau protein = insoluble cytoskeletal elements; tangles correlate with degree of dementia
Pick's disease (frontotemporal dementia)	Dementia, aphasia, parkinsonian aspects; change in personality. Spares parietal lobe and posterior ⅔ of superior temporal gyrus.	Pick bodies: spherical tau protein aggregates Frontotemporal atrophy
Lewy body dementia	Parkinsonism with dementia and hallucinations.	α-synuclein defect
Creutzfeldt-Jakob disease (CJD)	Rapidly progressive (weeks to months) dementia with myoclonus ("startle myoclonus").	Spongiform cortex Prions (PrP^c → PrP^{sc} sheet [β-pleated sheet resistant to proteases])
Other causes	Multi-infarct (2nd most common cause of dementia in elderly); syphilis; HIV; vitamins B_1, B_3, or B_{12} deficiency; Wilson's disease; and NPH.	

Multiple sclerosis	Autoimmune inflammation and demyelination of CNS (brain and spinal cord). Patients can present with optic neuritis (sudden loss of vision), MLF syndrome (internuclear ophthalmoplegia), hemiparesis, hemisensory symptoms, or bladder/bowel incontinence. Relapsing and remitting course. Most often affects women in their 20s and 30s; more common in whites.	Charcot's classic triad of MS is a **SIN**: ▪ **S**canning speech ▪ **I**ntention tremor (also **I**ncontinence and **I**nternuclear ophthalmoplegia) ▪ **N**ystagmus
FINDINGS	↑ protein (IgG) in CSF. Oligoclonal bands are diagnostic. MRI is gold standard. Periventricular plaques A (areas of oligodendrocyte loss and reactive gliosis) with destruction of axons.	
TREATMENT	β-interferon, immunosuppression, natalizumab. Symptomatic treatment for neurogenic bladder (catheterization, muscarinic antagonists), spasticity (baclofen, GABA receptor agonist), pain (opioids).	

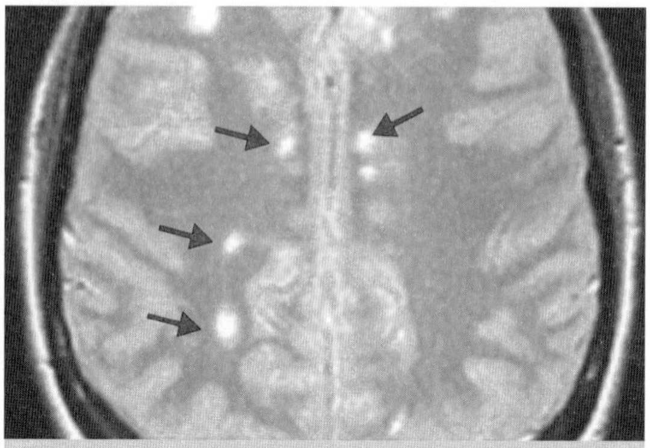

A **Multiple sclerosis.** T2-weighted MRI shows typical plaques (arrows).

Acute inflammatory demyelinating polyradiculopathy	Most common variant of Guillain-Barré syndrome. Autoimmune condition that destroys Schwann cells → inflammation and demyelination of peripheral nerves and motor fibers. Results in symmetric ascending muscle weakness/paralysis beginning in lower extremities. Facial paralysis in 50% of cases. Autonomic function may be severely affected (e.g., cardiac irregularities, hypertension, or hypotension). Almost all patients survive; the majority recover completely after weeks to months. Findings: ↑ CSF protein with normal cell count (albuminocytologic dissociation). ↑ protein → papilledema.	Associated with infections (*Campylobacter jejuni* and CMV) → autoimmune attack of peripheral myelin due to molecular mimicry, inoculations, and stress, but no definitive link to pathogens. Respiratory support is critical until recovery. Additional treatment: plasmapheresis, IV immune globulins.

Other demyelinating and dysmyelinating diseases

Progressive multifocal leukoencephalopathy (PML)	Demyelination of CNS due to destruction of oligodendrocytes. Associated with JC virus. Seen in 2–4% of AIDS patients (reactivation of latent viral infection). Rapidly progressive, usually fatal.
Acute disseminated (postinfectious) encephalomyelitis	Multifocal perivenular inflammation and demyelination after infection (commonly measles or VZV) or certain vaccinations (e.g., rabies, smallpox).
Metachromatic leukodystrophy	Autosomal-recessive lysosomal storage disease, most commonly due to arylsulfatase A deficiency. Buildup of sulfatides leads to impaired production of myelin sheath.
Charcot-Marie-Tooth disease	Also known as hereditary motor and sensory neuropathy (HMSN). Group of progressive hereditary nerve disorders related to the defective production of proteins involved in the structure and function of peripheral nerves or the myelin sheath.
Krabbe's disease	Autosomal-recessive lysosomal storage disease due to deficiency of galactocerebrosidase. Buildup of galactocerebroside destroys myelin sheath.

Seizures

Characterized by synchronized, high-frequency neuronal firing. Variety of forms.

Partial (focal) seizures	Affect 1 area of the brain. Most commonly originate in medial temporal lobe. Often preceded by seizure aura; can secondarily generalize. Types: ▪ **Simple partial** (consciousness intact)—motor, sensory, autonomic, psychic ▪ **Complex partial** (impaired consciousness)	**Epilepsy**—a disorder of recurrent seizures (febrile seizures are not epilepsy). **Status epilepticus**—continuous seizure for > 30 min or recurrent seizures without regaining consciousness between seizures for > 30 min. Medical emergency. Causes of seizures by age: ▪ Children—genetic, infection (febrile), trauma, congenital, metabolic ▪ Adults—tumors, trauma, stroke, infection ▪ Elderly—stroke, tumor, trauma, metabolic, infection
Generalized seizures	Diffuse. Types: ▪ **Absence** (petit mal)—3 Hz, no postictal confusion, blank stare ▪ **Myoclonic**—quick, repetitive jerks ▪ **Tonic-clonic** (grand mal)—alternating stiffening and movement ▪ **Tonic**—stiffening ▪ **Atonic**—"drop" seizures (falls to floor); commonly mistaken for fainting	

Differentiating headaches Pain due to irritation of structures such as the dura, cranial nerves, or extracranial structures.

CLASSIFICATION	LOCALIZATION	DURATION	DESCRIPTION	TREATMENT
Cluster[a]	Unilateral	15 min–3 hr; repetitive	Repetitive brief headaches. Excruciating periorbital pain with lacrimation and rhinorrhea. May induce Horner's syndrome. More common in males.	Inhaled oxygen, sumatriptan
Tension	Bilateral	> 30 min (typically 4–6 hr); constant	Steady pain. No photophobia or phonophobia. No aura.	
Migraine	Unilateral	4–72 hr	Pulsating pain with nausea, photophobia, or phonophobia. May have "aura." Due to irritation of CN V, meninges, or blood vessels (release of substance P, CGRP, vasoactive peptides).	Abortive therapies (e.g., triptans) and prophylactic (propranolol, topiramate)

Other causes of headache include subarachnoid hemorrhage ("worst headache of life"), meningitis, hydrocephalus, neoplasia, and arteritis.

[a] Cluster headaches can be differentiated from trigeminal neuralgia (TN) based on duration. TN produces repetitive shooting pain in the distribution of CN V that lasts (typically) for < 1 minute. The pain from cluster headaches lasts considerably longer (> 15 minutes).

Vertigo	Sensation of spinning while actually stationary. Subtype of "dizziness," but distinct from "lightheadedness."
Peripheral vertigo	More common. Inner ear etiology (e.g., semicircular canal debris, vestibular nerve infection, Ménière's disease). Positional testing → delayed horizontal nystagmus.
Central vertigo	Brain stem or cerebellar lesion (e.g., stroke affecting vestibular nuclei or posterior fossa tumor). Findings: directional change of nystagmus, skew deviation, diplopia, dysmetria. Positional testing → immediate nystagmus in any direction; may change directions.

Neurocutaneous disorders

Sturge-Weber syndrome	Congenital disorder with port-wine stains (aka nevus flammeus), typically in V_1 ophthalmic distribution; ipsilateral leptomeningeal angiomas, pheochromocytomas. Can cause glaucoma, seizures, hemiparesis, and mental retardation. Occurs sporadically.
Tuberous sclerosis	**HAMARTOMAS**: **H**amartomas in CNS and skin; **A**denoma sebaceum (cutaneous angiofibromas); **M**itral regurgitation; **A**sh-leaf spots; cardiac **R**habdomyoma; (**T**uberous sclerosis); autosomal d**O**minant; **M**ental retardation; renal **A**ngiomyolipoma; **S**eizures.
Neurofibromatosis type I (von Recklinghausen's disease)	Café-au-lait spots, Lisch nodules (pigmented iris hamartomas), neurofibromas in skin, optic gliomas, pheochromocytomas. Autosomal dominant, 100% penetrant, variable expression. Mutated *NF1* gene on chromosome 17.
von Hippel–Lindau disease	Cavernous hemangiomas in skin, mucosa, organs; bilateral renal cell carcinoma, hemangioblastoma in retina, brain stem, cerebellum; pheochromocytomas. Autosomal dominant; mutated tumor suppressor *VHL* gene on chromosome 3.

Adult primary brain tumors

Glioblastoma multiforme (grade IV astrocytoma)	Most common 1° brain tumor. Malignant with < 1-year life expectancy. Found in cerebral hemispheres. Can cross corpus callosum ("butterfly glioma") A. Stain astrocytes for GFAP. "Pseudopalisading" pleomorphic tumor cells—border central areas of necrosis and hemorrhage.	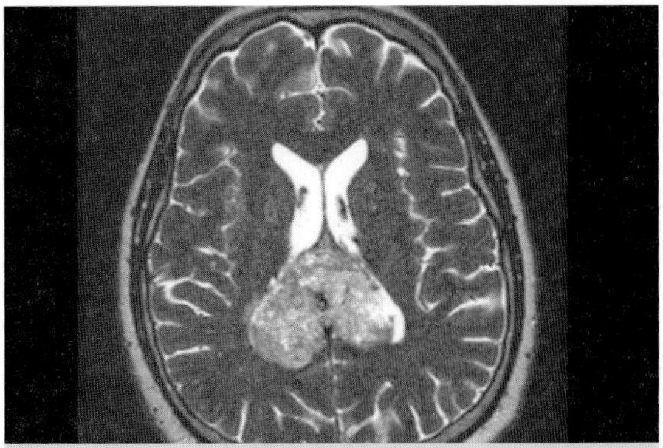 A **Glioblastoma multiforme.** T2-weighted MRI shows a lobulated mass near the corpus callosum that enhances with contrast and crosses the midline in an adult with positional headaches.
Meningioma	2nd most common 1° brain tumor. Most often occurs in convexities of hemispheres (near surfaces of brain) and parasagittal region. Arise from arachnoid cells, are extra-axial (external to brain parenchyma), and may have a dural attachment ("tail"). Typically benign and resectable. Often asymptomatic; may present with seizures or focal signs.	Spindle cells concentrically arranged in a whorled pattern; psammoma bodies (laminated calcifications).
Schwannoma	3rd most common 1° brain tumor. Schwann cell origin; often localized to CN VIII → acoustic schwannoma (aka acoustic neuroma). Resectable or treated with stereotactic radiosurgery. Usually found at cerebellopontine angle; S-100 positive.	Bilateral acoustic schwannoma found in neurofibromatosis type 2.
Oligodendroglioma	Relatively rare, slow growing. Most often in frontal lobes. Chicken-wire capillary pattern. Oligodendrocytes = "fried egg" cells—round nuclei with clear cytoplasm B. Often calcified in oligodendroglioma.	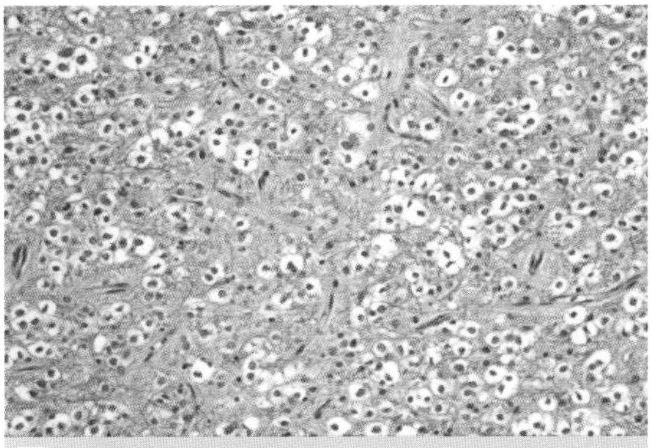 B **Oligodendroglioma.** Infiltrating tumor cells with perinuclear halos and prominent delicate vasculature.
Pituitary adenoma	Most commonly prolactinoma. Bitemporal hemianopia (due to pressure on optic chiasm) and hyper- or hypopituitarism are sequelae.	

Childhood primary brain tumors

Pilocytic (low-grade) astrocytoma	Usually well circumscribed. In children, most often found in posterior fossa (e.g., cerebellum). May be supratentorial. GFAP positive. Benign; good prognosis.	Rosenthal fibers—eosinophilic, corkscrew fibers. Cystic + solid (gross).
Medulloblastoma	Highly malignant cerebellar tumor. A form of primitive neuroectodermal tumor. Can compress 4th ventricle, causing hydrocephalus. Can send "drop metastases" to spinal cord.	Homer-Wright rosettes. Solid (gross), small blue cells (histology). Radiosensitive.
Ependymoma	Ependymal cell tumors most commonly found in 4th ventricle. Can cause hydrocephalus. Poor prognosis.	Characteristic perivascular pseudorosettes. Rod-shaped blepharoplasts (basal ciliary bodies) found near nucleus.
Hemangioblastoma	Most often cerebellar; associated with von Hippel–Lindau syndrome when found with retinal angiomas. Can produce EPO → 2° polycythemia.	Foamy cells and high vascularity are characteristic.
Craniopharyngioma	Benign childhood tumor, confused with pituitary adenoma (can also cause bitemporal hemianopia). Most common childhood supratentorial tumor.	Derived from remnants of Rathke's pouch. Calcification is common (tooth enamel–like).

Herniation syndromes

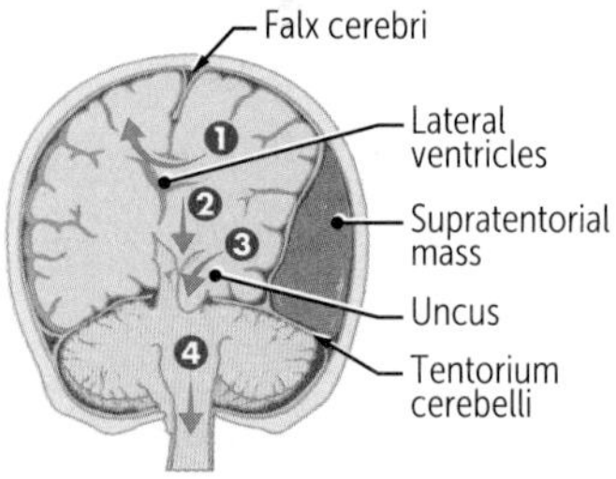
Falx cerebri
Lateral ventricles
Supratentorial mass
Uncus
Tentorium cerebelli
❶
❷
❸
❹

❶ Cingulate (subfalcine) herniation under falx cerebri	Can compress anterior cerebral artery.
❷ Downward transtentorial (central) herniation	
❸ Uncal herniation	Uncus = medial temporal lobe.
❹ Cerebellar tonsillar herniation into the foramen magnum	Coma and death result when these herniations compress the brain stem.

▶ NEUROLOGY–PHARMACOLOGY

Glaucoma drugs ↓ intraocular pressure via ↓ amount of aqueous humor (inhibit synthesis/secretion or increase drainage).

DRUG	MECHANISM	SIDE EFFECTS
α-agonists		
Epinephrine	↓ aqueous humor synthesis via vasoconstriction	Mydriasis; do not use in closed-angle glaucoma
Brimonidine (α_2)	↓ aqueous humor synthesis	Blurry vision, ocular hyperemia, foreign body sensation, ocular allergic reactions, ocular pruritus
β-blockers		
Timolol, betaxolol, carteolol	↓ aqueous humor synthesis	No pupillary or vision changes
Diuretics		
Acetazolamide	↓ aqueous humor synthesis via inhibition of carbonic anhydrase	No pupillary or vision changes
Cholinomimetics		
Direct (pilocarpine, carbachol) **Indirect (physostigmine, echothiophate)**	↑ outflow of aqueous humor via contraction of ciliary muscle and opening of trabecular meshwork Use pilocarpine in emergencies—very effective at opening meshwork into canal of Schlemm	Miosis and cyclospasm (contraction of ciliary muscle)
Prostaglandin		
Latanoprost ($PGF_{2\alpha}$)	↑ outflow of aqueous humor	Darkens color of iris (browning)

Opioid analgesics Morphine, fentanyl, codeine, heroin, methadone, meperidine, dextromethorphan, diphenoxylate.

MECHANISM	Act as agonists at opioid receptors (mu = morphine, delta = enkephalin, kappa = dynorphin) to modulate synaptic transmission—open K^+ channels, close Ca^{2+} channels → ↓ synaptic transmission. Inhibit release of ACh, NE, 5-HT, glutamate, substance P.
CLINICAL USE	Pain, cough suppression (dextromethorphan), diarrhea (loperamide and diphenoxylate), acute pulmonary edema, maintenance programs for addicts (methadone).
TOXICITY	Addiction, respiratory depression, constipation, miosis (pinpoint pupils), additive CNS depression with other drugs. Tolerance does not develop to miosis and constipation. Toxicity treated with naloxone or naltrexone (opioid receptor antagonist).

Butorphanol

MECHANISM	Mu-opioid receptor **partial** agonist and kappa-opioid receptor agonist; produces analgesia.
CLINICAL USE	Severe pain (migraine, labor, etc.). Causes less respiratory depression than full opioid agonists.
TOXICITY	Can cause opioid withdrawal symptoms if patient is also taking full opioid agonist (competition for opioid receptors). Overdose not easily reversed with naloxone.

Tramadol

MECHANISM	Very weak opioid agonist; also inhibits serotonin and NE reuptake (works on multiple neurotransmitters—"**tram it all**" in with **tramadol**).
CLINICAL USE	Chronic pain.
TOXICITY	Similar to opioids. Decreases seizure threshold.

Epilepsy drugs

	PARTIAL (FOCAL)		GENERALIZED				
	SIMPLE	COMPLEX	TONIC-CLONIC	ABSENCE	STATUS EPILEPTICUS	MECHANISM	NOTES
Phenytoin	✓	✓	1st line		1st line for prophylaxis	↑ Na^+ channel inactivation	Fosphenytoin for parenteral use
Carbamazepine	1st line	1st line	1st line			↑ Na^+ channel inactivation	1st line for trigeminal neuralgia
Lamotrigine	✓	✓	✓			Blocks voltage-gated Na^+ channels	
Gabapentin	✓	✓	✓			Designed as GABA analog, but primarily inhibits high-voltage-activated Ca^{2+} channels	Also used for peripheral neuropathy, postherpetic neuralgia, migraine prophylaxis, bipolar disorder
Topiramate	✓	✓	✓			Blocks Na^+ channels, ↑ GABA action	Also used for migraine prevention
Phenobarbital	✓	✓	✓			↑ $GABA_A$ action	1st line in children
Valproic acid	✓	✓	1st line	✓		↑ Na^+ channel inactivation, ↑ GABA concentration	Also used for myoclonic seizures
Ethosuximide				1st line		Blocks thalamic T-type Ca^{2+} channels	
Benzodiazepines (diazepam or lorazepam)					1st line for acute	↑ $GABA_A$ action	Also used for seizures of eclampsia (1st line is $MgSO_4$)
Tiagabine	✓	✓				Inhibits GABA reuptake	
Vigabatrin	✓	✓				Irreversibly inhibits GABA transaminase → ↑ GABA	
Levetiracetam	✓	✓	✓			Unknown; may modulate GABA and glutamate release	

Epilepsy drug toxicities

Benzodiazepines	Sedation, tolerance, dependence.	Stevens-Johnson syndrome—prodrome of malaise and fever followed by rapid onset of erythematous/purpuric macules (oral, ocular, genital). Skin lesions progress to epidermal necrosis and sloughing.
Carbamazepine	Diplopia, ataxia, blood dyscrasias (agranulocytosis, aplastic anemia), liver toxicity, teratogenesis, induction of cytochrome P-450, SIADH, Stevens-Johnson syndrome.	
Ethosuximide	GI distress, fatigue, headache, urticaria, Stevens-Johnson syndrome.	EFGH—Ethosuximide, Fatigue, GI, Headache.
Phenobarbital	Sedation, tolerance, dependence, induction of cytochrome P-450.	
Phenytoin	Nystagmus, diplopia, ataxia, sedation, gingival hyperplasia, hirsutism, megaloblastic anemia, teratogenesis (fetal hydantoin syndrome), SLE-like syndrome, induction of cytochrome P-450, lymphadenopathy, Stevens-Johnson syndrome, osteopenia.	
Valproic acid	GI distress, rare but fatal hepatotoxicity (measure LFTs), neural tube defects in fetus (spina bifida), tremor, weight gain. Contraindicated in pregnancy.	
Lamotrigine	Stevens-Johnson syndrome.	
Gabapentin	Sedation, ataxia.	
Topiramate	Sedation, mental dulling, kidney stones, weight loss.	

Phenytoin

MECHANISM	Use-dependent blockade of Na^+ channels; inhibition of glutamate release from excitatory presynaptic neuron.
CLINICAL USE	Tonic-clonic seizures. Also a class IB antiarrhythmic.
TOXICITY	Nystagmus, ataxia, diplopia, sedation, SLE-like syndrome, induction of cytochrome P-450. Chronic use produces gingival hyperplasia in children, peripheral neuropathy, hirsutism, megaloblastic anemia (↓ folate absorption). Teratogenic (fetal hydantoin syndrome).

Barbiturates	Phenobarbital, pentobarbital, thiopental, secobarbital.
MECHANISM	Facilitate $GABA_A$ action by ↑ **duration** of Cl^- channel opening, thus ↓ neuron firing (barbi**durates** ↑ **duration**). Contraindicated in porphyria.
CLINICAL USE	Sedative for anxiety, seizures, insomnia, induction of anesthesia (thiopental).
TOXICITY	Respiratory and cardiovascular depression (can be fatal); CNS depression (can be exacerbated by EtOH use); dependence; drug interactions (induces P-450). Overdose treatment is supportive (assist respiration and maintain BP).

Benzodiazepines	Diazepam, lorazepam, triazolam, temazepam, oxazepam, midazolam, chlordiazepoxide, alprazolam.	
MECHANISM	Facilitate $GABA_A$ action by ↑ **frequency** of Cl^- channel opening. ↓ REM sleep. Most have long half-lives and active metabolites (exceptions: triazolam, oxazepam, and midazolam are short acting → higher addictive potential).	**Fre**nzodiazepines ↑ **fre**quency. Benzos, barbs, and EtOH all bind the $GABA_A$ receptor, which is a ligand-gated chloride channel.
CLINICAL USE	Anxiety, spasticity, status epilepticus (lorazepam and diazepam), detoxification (especially alcohol withdrawal–DTs), night terrors, sleepwalking, general anesthetic (amnesia, muscle relaxation), hypnotic (insomnia).	
TOXICITY	Dependence, additive CNS depression effects with alcohol. Less risk of respiratory depression and coma than with barbiturates. Treat overdose with flumazenil (competitive antagonist at GABA benzodiazepine receptor).	

Nonbenzodiazepine hypnotics	Zolpidem (Ambien), zaleplon, eszopiclone.
MECHANISM	Act via the BZ1 subtype of the GABA receptor. Effects reversed by flumazenil.
CLINICAL USE	Insomnia.
TOXICITY	Ataxia, headaches, confusion. Short duration because of rapid metabolism by liver enzymes. Unlike older sedative-hypnotics, cause only modest day-after psychomotor depression and few amnestic effects. Lower dependence risk than benzodiazepines.

Anesthetics—general principles

CNS drugs must be lipid soluble (cross the blood-brain barrier) or be actively transported.
Drugs with ↓ solubility in blood = rapid induction and recovery times.

Drugs with ↑ solubility in lipids = ↑ potency = $\frac{1}{MAC}$

MAC = minimal alveolar concentration at which 50% of the population is anesthetized. Varies with age.
Examples: N_2O has ↓ blood and lipid solubility, and thus fast induction and low potency. Halothane, in contrast, has ↑ lipid and blood solubility, and thus high potency and slow induction.

Inhaled anesthetics	Halothane, enflurane, isoflurane, sevoflurane, methoxyflurane, nitrous oxide.
MECHANISM	Mechanism unknown.
EFFECTS	Myocardial depression, respiratory depression, nausea/emesis, ↑ cerebral blood flow (↓ cerebral metabolic demand).
TOXICITY	Hepatotoxicity (halothane), nephrotoxicity (methoxyflurane), proconvulsant (enflurane), malignant hyperthermia (all but nitrous oxide; rare, life-threatening, inherited susceptibility), expansion of trapped gas in a body cavity (nitrous oxide).

Intravenous anesthetics

Barbiturates	Thiopental—high potency, high lipid solubility, rapid entry into brain. Used for induction of anesthesia and short surgical procedures. Effect terminated by rapid redistribution into tissue (i.e., skeletal muscle) and fat. ↓ cerebral blood flow.	B. B. King on OPIOIDS PROPOses FOOLishly.
Benzodiazepines	Midazolam most common drug used for endoscopy; used adjunctively with gaseous anesthetics and narcotics. May cause severe postoperative respiratory depression, ↓ BP (treat overdose with flumazenil), and amnesia.	
Arylcyclohexylamines (Ketamine)	PCP analogs that act as dissociative anesthetics. Block NMDA receptors. Cardiovascular stimulants. Cause disorientation, hallucination, and bad dreams. ↑ cerebral blood flow.	
Opioids	Morphine, fentanyl used with other CNS depressants during general anesthesia.	
Propofol	Used for sedation in ICU, rapid anesthesia induction, and short procedures. Less postoperative nausea than thiopental. Potentiates $GABA_A$.	Not recommended for home use by pop stars.

Local anesthetics

Esters—procaine, cocaine, tetracaine.
Amides—lIdocaIne, mepIvacaIne, bupIvacaIne (amIdes have 2 I's in name).

MECHANISM	Block Na^+ channels by binding to specific receptors on inner portion of channel. Preferentially bind to activated Na^+ channels, so most effective in rapidly firing neurons. 3° amine local anesthetics penetrate membrane in uncharged form, then bind to ion channels as charged form.
PRINCIPLE	Can be given with vasoconstrictors (usually epinephrine) to enhance local action—↓ bleeding, ↑ anesthesia by ↓ systemic concentration. In infected (acidic) tissue, alkaline anesthetics are charged and cannot penetrate membrane effectively → need more anesthetic. Order of nerve blockade: small-diameter fibers > large diameter. Myelinated fibers > unmyelinated fibers. Overall, size factor predominates over myelination such that small myelinated fibers > small unmyelinated fibers > large myelinated fibers > large unmyelinated fibers. Order of loss: (1) pain, (2) temperature, (3) touch, (4) pressure.
CLINICAL USE	Minor surgical procedures, spinal anesthesia. If allergic to esters, give amides.
TOXICITY	CNS excitation, severe cardiovascular toxicity (bupivacaine), hypertension, hypotension, and arrhythmias (cocaine).

Neuromuscular blocking drugs	Used for muscle paralysis in surgery or mechanical ventilation. Selective for motor (vs. autonomic) nicotinic receptor.
Depolarizing	Succinylcholine—strong ACh receptor agonist; produces sustained depolarization and prevents muscle contraction. Reversal of blockade: ▪ Phase I (prolonged depolarization)—no antidote. Block potentiated by cholinesterase inhibitors. ▪ Phase II (repolarized but blocked; ACh receptors are available, but desensitized)—antidote consists of cholinesterase inhibitors (e.g., neostigmine). Complications include hypercalcemia, hyperkalemia, and malignant hyperthermia.
Nondepolarizing	Tubocurarine, atracurium, mivacurium, pancuronium, vecuronium, rocuronium. Competitive antagonists—compete with ACh for receptors. Reversal of blockade—neostigmine, edrophonium, and other cholinesterase inhibitors.

Dantrolene

MECHANISM	Prevents the release of Ca^{2+} from the sarcoplasmic reticulum of skeletal muscle.
CLINICAL USE	Used in the treatment of **malignant hyperthermia**, a rare but life-threatening side effect of inhalation anesthetics (except N_2O) and succinylcholine. Also used to treat neuroleptic malignant syndrome (a toxicity of antipsychotic drugs).

Parkinson's disease drugs

Parkinsonism is due to loss of dopaminergic neurons and excess cholinergic activity.

STRATEGY	AGENTS	
Dopamine agonists	**B**romocriptine (ergot), pramipexole, ropinirole (non-ergot); non-ergots are preferred	BALSA: Bromocriptine Amantadine Levodopa (with carbidopa) Selegiline (and COMT inhibitors) Antimuscarinics For essential or familial tremors, use a β-blocker (e.g., propranolol).
↑ dopamine	**A**mantadine (may ↑ dopamine release); also used as an antiviral against influenza A and rubella; toxicity = ataxia L-dopa/carbidopa (converted to dopamine in CNS)	
Prevent dopamine breakdown	**S**elegiline (selective MAO type B inhibitor); entacapone, tolcapone (COMT inhibitors—prevent L-dopa degradation, thereby increasing dopamine availability)	
Curb excess cholinergic activity	**Benz**tropine (**A**ntimuscarinic; improves tremor and rigidity but has little effect on bradykinesia)	**Park** your Mercedes-**Benz**.

L-dopa (levodopa)/carbidopa

MECHANISM	↑ level of dopamine in brain. Unlike dopamine, L-dopa can cross blood-brain barrier and is converted by dopa decarboxylase in the CNS to dopamine. Carbidopa, a peripheral decarboxylase inhibitor, is given with L-dopa to ↑ the bioavailability of L-dopa in the brain and to limit peripheral side effects.
CLINICAL USE	Parkinson's disease.
TOXICITY	Arrhythmias from increased peripheral formation of catecholamines. Long-term use can lead to dyskinesia following administration, akinesia between doses.

Selegiline

MECHANISM	Selectively inhibits MAO-B, which preferentially metabolizes dopamine over NE and 5-HT, thereby increasing the availability of dopamine.
CLINICAL USE	Adjunctive agent to L-dopa in treatment of Parkinson's disease.
TOXICITY	May enhance adverse effects of L-dopa.

Alzheimer's drugs

Memantine

MECHANISM	NMDA receptor antagonist; helps prevent excitotoxicity (mediated by Ca^{2+}).
TOXICITY	Dizziness, confusion, hallucinations.

Donepezil, galantamine, rivastigmine

MECHANISM	Acetylcholinesterase inhibitors.
TOXICITY	Nausea, dizziness, insomnia.

Huntington's drugs

Neurotransmitter changes in Huntington's disease: ↓ GABA, ↓ ACh, ↑ dopamine.

Treatments:
- Tetrabenazine and reserpine—inhibit VMAT; limit dopamine vesicle packaging and release.
- Haloperidol—dopamine receptor antagonist.

Sumatriptan

MECHANISM	$5\text{-HT}_{1B/1D}$ agonist. Inhibits trigeminal nerve activation; prevents vasoactive peptide release; induces vasoconstriction. Half-life < 2 hours.	A **SUM**o wrestler **TRIP**s **AN**d falls on your **head**.
CLINICAL USE	Acute migraine, cluster **head**ache attacks.	
TOXICITY	Coronary vasospasm (contraindicated in patients with CAD or Prinzmetal's angina), mild tingling.	

HIGH-YIELD PRINCIPLES IN

Psychiatry

"A Freudian slip is when you say one thing but mean your mother."

—Anonymous

"Men will always be mad, and those who think they can cure them are the maddest of all."

—Voltaire

"Anyone who goes to a psychiatrist ought to have his head examined."

—Samuel Goldwyn

▶ PSYCHIATRY–PSYCHOLOGY

Classical conditioning	Learning in which a natural response (salivation) is elicited by a conditioned, or learned, stimulus (bell) that previously was presented in conjunction with an unconditioned stimulus (food).	Pavlov's classical experiments with dogs—ringing the bell provoked salivation.

Operant conditioning	Learning in which a particular action is elicited because it produces a reward.
Positive reinforcement	Desired reward produces action (mouse presses button to get food).
Negative reinforcement	Target behavior (response) is followed by removal of aversive stimulus (mouse presses button to turn off continuous loud noise).
Punishment	Repeated application of aversive stimulus extinguishes unwanted behavior.
Extinction	Discontinuation of reinforcement (positive or negative) eventually eliminates behavior.

Transference and countertransference	
Transference	Patient projects feelings about formative or other important persons onto physician (e.g., psychiatrist is seen as parent).
Countertransference	Doctor projects feelings about formative or other important persons onto patient.

Ego defenses Unconscious mental processes used to resolve conflict and prevent undesirable feelings (e.g., anxiety, depression).

IMMATURE DEFENSES	DESCRIPTION	EXAMPLE
Acting out	Unacceptable feelings and thoughts are expressed through actions.	Tantrums.
Dissociation	Temporary, drastic change in personality, memory, consciousness, or motor behavior to avoid emotional stress.	Extreme forms can result in dissociative identity disorder (multiple personality disorder).
Denial	Avoidance of awareness of some painful reality.	A common reaction in newly diagnosed AIDS and cancer patients.
Displacement	Process whereby avoided ideas and feelings are transferred to some neutral person or object (vs. projection).	Mother yells at her child, because her husband yelled at her.
Fixation	Partially remaining at a more childish level of development (vs. regression).	Men fixating on sports games.
Identification	Modeling behavior after another person who is more powerful (though not necessarily admired).	Abused child identifies himself/herself with an abuser.
Isolation (of affect)	Separation of feelings from ideas and events.	Describing murder in graphic detail with no emotional response.
Projection	An unacceptable internal impulse is attributed to an external source (vs. displacement).	A man who wants another woman thinks his wife is cheating on him.

Ego defenses *(continued)*

IMMATURE DEFENSES	DESCRIPTION	EXAMPLE
Rationalization	Proclaiming logical reasons for actions actually performed for other reasons, usually to avoid self-blame.	After getting fired, claiming that the job was not important anyway.
Reaction formation	Process whereby a warded-off idea or feeling is replaced by an (unconsciously derived) emphasis on its opposite (vs. sublimation).	A patient with libidinous thoughts enters a monastery.
Regression	Turning back the maturational clock and going back to earlier modes of dealing with the world (vs. fixation).	Seen in children under stress such as illness, punishment, or birth of a new sibling (e.g., bedwetting in a previously toilet-trained child when hospitalized).
Repression	Involuntary withholding of an idea or feeling from conscious awareness (vs. suppression).	Not remembering a conflictual or traumatic experience; pressing bad thoughts into the unconscious.
Splitting	Belief that people are either all good or all bad at different times due to intolerance of ambiguity. Seen in borderline personality disorder.	A patient says that all the nurses are cold and insensitive but that the doctors are warm and friendly.
MATURE DEFENSES		
Altruism	Guilty feelings alleviated by unsolicited generosity toward others.	Mafia boss makes large donation to charity.
Humor	Appreciating the amusing nature of an anxiety-provoking or adverse situation.	Nervous medical student jokes about the boards.
Sublimation	Process whereby one replaces an unacceptable wish with a course of action that is similar to the wish but does not conflict with one's value system (vs. reaction formation).	Teenager's aggression toward his father is redirected to perform well in sports.
Suppression	Voluntary withholding of an idea or feeling from conscious awareness (vs. repression).	Choosing not to think about the USMLE until the week of the exam.
	Mature adults wear a **SASH**: **S**ublimation, **A**ltruism, **S**uppression, **H**umor.	

▸ PSYCHIATRY—PATHOLOGY

Infant deprivation effects	Long-term deprivation of affection results in: ▪ ↓ muscle tone ▪ Poor language skills ▪ Poor socialization skills ▪ Lack of basic trust ▪ Anaclitic depression (infant withdrawn/unresponsive) ▪ Weight loss ▪ Physical illness	The 4 **W**'s: **W**eak, **W**ordless, **W**anting (socially), **W**ary. Deprivation for > 6 months can lead to irreversible changes. Severe deprivation can result in infant death.

Child abuse

	Physical abuse	Sexual abuse
EVIDENCE	Healed fractures on x-ray, burns (e.g., cigarette, scalding), subdural hematomas, multiple bruises, retinal hemorrhage or detachment	Genital, anal, or oral trauma; STIs; UTIs
ABUSER	Usually male caregiver	Known to victim, usually male
EPIDEMIOLOGY	~3000 deaths/yr in U.S., 80% < 3 yr of age	Peak incidence 9–12 years of age

Child neglect	Failure to provide a child with adequate food, shelter, supervision, education, and/or affection. Most common form of child maltreatment. Evidence: poor hygiene, malnutrition, withdrawal, impaired social/emotional development, failure to thrive. As with child abuse, child neglect must be reported to local child protective services.

Childhood and early-onset disorders

Attention-deficit hyperactivity disorder (ADHD)	Onset before age 7. Limited attention span and poor impulse control. Characterized by hyperactivity, impulsivity, and inattention in multiple settings (school, home, places of worship, etc.). Normal intelligence, but commonly coexists with difficulties in school. Continues into adulthood in as many as 50% of individuals. Associated with ↓ frontal lobe volumes. Treatment: methylphenidate, amphetamines, atomoxetine, behavioral interventions (reinforcement, reward).
Conduct disorder	Repetitive and pervasive behavior violating the basic rights of others (e.g., physical aggression, destruction of property, theft). After 18 years of age, many of these patients will meet criteria for diagnosis of antisocial personality disorder.
Oppositional defiant disorder	Enduring pattern of hostile, defiant behavior toward authority figures in the absence of serious violations of social norms.
Tourette's syndrome	Onset before age 18. Characterized by sudden, rapid, recurrent, nonrhythmic, stereotyped motor and vocal tics that persist for **> 1 year.** Lifetime prevalence of 0.1–1.0% in the general population. Coprolalia (involuntary obscene speech) found in only 10–20% of patients. Associated with OCD. Treatment: antipsychotics and behavioral therapy.
Separation anxiety disorder	Common onset at 7–9 years of age. Overwhelming fear of separation from home or loss of attachment figure. May lead to factitious physical complaints to avoid going to or staying at school. Treatment: SSRIs and relaxation techniques/behavioral interventions.

Pervasive developmental disorders	Characterized by difficulties with language and failure to acquire or early loss of social skills.
Autistic disorder	Severe language impairment and poor social interactions. Greater focus on objects than on people. Characterized by repetitive behavior and usually below-normal intelligence. Rarely accompanied by unusual abilities (savants). More common in boys. Treatment: behavioral and supportive therapy to improve communication and social skills. Medication when appropriate (i.e., disruptive/harmful behavior).
Asperger's disorder	Milder form of autism. Characterized by all-absorbing interests, repetitive behavior, and problems with social relationships. Children are of normal intelligence and lack verbal or cognitive deficits. No language impairment.
Rett's disorder	X-linked disorder seen almost exclusively in girls (affected males die in utero or shortly after birth). Symptoms usually become apparent around ages 1–4, including regression characterized by loss of development, loss of verbal abilities, mental retardation, ataxia, and stereotyped hand-wringing.
Childhood disintegrative disorder	Common age of onset is 3–4 years. Marked regression in multiple areas of functioning after at least 2 years of apparently normal development. Significant loss of expressive or receptive language skills, social skills or adaptive behavior, bowel or bladder control, play, or motor skills. More common in boys.

Neurotransmitter changes with disease

DISORDER	NEUROTRANSMITTER CHANGES
Anxiety	↑ NE, ↓ GABA, ↓ serotonin (5-HT)
Depression	↓ NE, ↓ serotonin (5-HT), ↓ dopamine
Alzheimer's dementia	↓ ACh
Huntington's disease	↓ GABA, ↓ ACh, ↑ dopamine
Schizophrenia	↑ dopamine
Parkinson's disease	↓ dopamine, ↑ serotonin (5-HT), ↑ ACh

Understanding these changes can help guide pharmacologic treatment choice.

Orientation

Patient's ability to know who he or she is, where he or she is, and the date and time.

Common causes of loss of orientation: alcohol, drugs, fluid/electrolyte imbalance, head trauma, hypoglycemia, nutritional deficiencies.

Order of loss: 1st—time; 2nd—place; last—person.

Often abbreviated in the medical chart as "alert and oriented × 3" (AO×3).

Amnesias

Retrograde amnesia	Inability to remember things that occurred before a CNS insult.
Anterograde amnesia	Inability to remember things that occurred after a CNS insult (no new memory).
Korsakoff's amnesia	Classic anterograde amnesia caused by thiamine deficiency and the associated destruction of mammillary bodies. May also include some retrograde amnesia. Seen in alcoholics, and associated with confabulations.
Dissociative amnesia	Inability to recall important personal information, usually subsequent to severe trauma or stress.

Cognitive disorder	Significant change in cognition (memory, attention, language, judgment) from previous level of functioning. Associated with abnormalities in CNS, a general medical condition, medications, or substance use. Includes delirium and dementia.	
Delirium	"Waxing and waning" level of consciousness with acute onset; rapid ↓ in attention span and level of arousal. Characterized by disorganized thinking, hallucinations (often visual), illusions, misperceptions, disturbance in sleep-wake cycle, cognitive dysfunction. Usually secondary to other illness (e.g., CNS disease, infection, trauma, substance abuse/withdrawal). Most common presentation of altered mental status in inpatient setting. Abnormal EEG. Treatment: ▪ Identify and address underlying cause. ▪ Optimize brain condition (O_2, hydration, pain, etc.) ▪ Antipsychotics (mainly haloperidol).	Del**irium** = changes in senso**rium**. Check for drugs with anticholinergic effects. Often reversible. **T-A-DA** approach (**T**olerate, **A**nticipate, **D**on't **A**gitate) helpful for management.
Dementia	Gradual ↓ in intellectual ability or "cognition" without affecting level of consciousness. Characterized by memory deficits, aphasia, apraxia, agnosia, loss of abstract thought, behavioral/personality changes, impaired judgment. A patient with dementia can develop delirium (e.g., an Alzheimer's patient who develops pneumonia is at increased risk for delirium). Caused by Alzheimer's disease, cerebral vascular infarcts, HIV, Pick's disease, chronic substance abuse (due to neurotoxicity of drugs), Creutzfeldt–Jakob disease, NPH, and many other disorders. ↑ incidence with age. EEG usually normal.	"De**mem**tia" is characterized by **mem**ory loss. Usually irreversible. In elderly patients, depression may present like dementia (pseudodementia).
Psychotic disorder	A distorted perception of reality (psychosis) characterized by delusions, hallucinations, and/or disorganized thinking. Psychosis can occur in patients with medical illness, psychiatric illness, or both.	

Signs of psychosis

Hallucinations	Perceptions in the absence of external stimuli (e.g., seeing a light that is not actually present).
Delusions	False beliefs about oneself or others that persist despite the facts (e.g., thinking the CIA is spying on you).
Disorganized speech	Words and ideas are strung together based on sounds, puns, or "loose associations."

Hallucination types

Visual	More commonly a feature of medical illness (e.g., drug intoxication) than psychiatric illness.
Auditory	More commonly a feature of psychiatric illness (e.g., schizophrenia) than medical illness.
Olfactory	Often occur as an aura of psychomotor epilepsy and in brain tumors.
Gustatory	Rare.
Tactile	Common in alcohol withdrawal (e.g., formication—the sensation of bugs crawling on one's skin). Also seen in cocaine abusers ("cocaine crawlies").
HypnaGOgic	Occurs while GOing to sleep.
HypnoPOMPic	Occurs while waking from sleep ("POMPous upon awakening").

Schizophrenia

Chronic mental disorder with periods of psychosis, disturbed behavior and thought, and decline in functioning that lasts > 6 **months**. Associated with ↑ dopaminergic activity, ↓ dendritic branching.

Diagnosis requires 2 or more of the following (first 4 in this list are "positive symptoms"):
- Delusions
- Hallucinations—often auditory
- Disorganized speech (loose associations)
- Disorganized or catatonic behavior
- "Negative symptoms"—flat affect, social withdrawal, lack of motivation, lack of speech or thought

Brief psychotic disorder—**< 1 month**, usually stress related.

Schizophreniform disorder—**1–6 months**.

Schizoaffective disorder—**at least 2 weeks** of stable mood with psychotic symptoms, plus a major depressive, manic, or mixed (both) episode. 2 subtypes: bipolar or depressive.

5 subtypes:
- Paranoid (delusions)
- Disorganized (with regard to speech, behavior, and affect)
- Catatonic (automatisms)
- Undifferentiated (elements of all types)
- Residual

Genetics and environment contribute to the etiology of schizophrenia.

Frequent cannabis use is associated with psychosis/schizophrenia in teens.

Lifetime prevalence—1.5% (males = females, blacks = whites). Presents earlier in men (late teens to early 20s vs. late 20s to early 30s in women). Patients are at ↑ risk for suicide.

Delusional disorder

Fixed, persistent, nonbizarre belief system **lasting > 1 month**. Functioning otherwise not impaired. Example: a woman who genuinely believes she is married to a celebrity when, in fact, she is not.

Shared psychotic disorder (folie à deux)—development of delusions in a person in a close relationship with someone with delusional disorder. Often resolves upon separation.

Dissociative disorders

Dissociative identity disorder	Formerly known as multiple personality disorder. Presence of 2 or more distinct identities or personality states. More common in women. Associated with history of sexual abuse.
Depersonalization disorder	Persistent feelings of detachment or estrangement from one's own body, a social situation, or the environment.
Dissociative fugue	Abrupt change in geographic location with inability to recall the past, confusion about personal identity, or assumption of a new identity. Associated with traumatic circumstances (e.g., natural disasters, wartime, trauma). Leads to significant distress or impairment. Not the result of substance abuse or general medical condition.

Mood disorder

Characterized by an abnormal range of moods or internal emotional states and loss of control over them. Severity of moods causes distress and impairment in social and occupational functioning. Includes major depressive disorder, bipolar disorder, dysthymic disorder, and cyclothymic disorder. Psychotic features (delusions or hallucinations) may be present.

Manic episode

Distinct period of abnormally and persistently elevated, expansive, or irritable mood and abnormally and persistently increased activity or energy **lasting at least 1 week**. Often disturbing to patient.

Diagnosis requires hospitalization or at least 3 of the following (manics **DIG FAST**):

- Distractibility
- Irresponsibility—seeks pleasure without regard to consequences (hedonistic)
- Grandiosity—inflated self-esteem
- Flight of ideas—racing thoughts
- ↑ in goal-directed Activity/psychomotor Agitation
- ↓ need for Sleep
- Talkativeness or pressured speech

Hypomanic episode

Like manic episode except mood disturbance is not severe enough to cause marked impairment in social and/or occupational functioning or to necessitate hospitalization. No psychotic features.

Bipolar disorder

Defined by the presence of at least 1 manic (bipolar I) or hypomanic (bipolar II) episode. Depressive symptoms always occur eventually. Patient's mood and functioning usually return to normal between episodes. Use of antidepressants can lead to ↑ mania. High suicide risk. Treatment: mood stabilizers (e.g., lithium, valproic acid, carbamazepine), atypical antipsychotics.

Cyclothymic disorder—dysthymia and hypomania; milder form of bipolar disorder **lasting at least 2 years**.

Major depressive disorder	Self-limited disorder, with major depressive episodes usually **lasting 6–12 months**. Episodes characterized by **at least 5** of the following 9 symptoms for **2 or more weeks** (symptoms must include patient-reported depressed mood or anhedonia and occur more frequently as the disorder progresses): Characterized by: ▪ Sleep disturbance ▪ Loss of Interest (anhedonia) ▪ Guilt or feelings of worthlessness ▪ Loss of Energy ▪ Loss of Concentration ▪ Appetite/weight changes ▪ Psychomotor retardation or agitation ▪ Suicidal ideations ▪ Depressed mood **Dysthymia**—milder form of depression **lasting at least 2 years**. **Seasonal affective disorder**—symptoms associated with winter season; improves in response to full-spectrum bright-light exposure.	SIG E CAPS. Commonly used mnemonic for depression screening. Historically used by physicians in prescription writing. **SIG** is short for *signatura* (Latin for "directions"). Depressed patients were directed to take Energy CAPSules. Lifetime prevalence of major depressive episode: 5–12% male, 10–25% female.
Atypical depression	Differs from classical forms of depression. Characterized by mood reactivity (being able to experience improved mood in response to positive events), "reversed" vegetative symptoms (hypersomnia and weight gain), leaden paralysis (heavy feeling in arms and legs), and long-standing interpersonal rejection sensitivity. Most common subtype of depression. Treatment: MAO inhibitors, SSRIs.	

Postpartum mood disturbances

Maternal (postpartum) "blues"	50–85% incidence rate. Characterized by depressed affect, tearfulness, and fatigue starting 2–3 days after delivery. **Usually resolves within 10–14 days**. Treatment: supportive. Follow-up to assess for possible postpartum depression.
Postpartum depression	10–15% incidence rate. Characterized by depressed affect, anxiety, and poor concentration starting within 4 weeks after delivery. **Lasts 2 weeks to a year or more**. Treatment: antidepressants, psychotherapy.
Postpartum psychosis	0.1–0.2% incidence rate. Characterized by delusions, hallucinations, confusion, unusual behavior, and possible homicidal/suicidal ideations or attempts. Usually **lasts days to 4–6 weeks**. Treatment: antipsychotics, antidepressants, possible inpatient hospitalization.

Electroconvulsive therapy

Treatment option for major depressive disorder refractory to other treatment and for pregnant women with major depressive disorder. Also considered when immediate response is necessary (acute suicidality), in depression with psychotic features, and for catatonia. Produces a painless seizure in an anesthetized patient. Major adverse effects are disorientation and temporary anterograde/retrograde amnesia usually fully resolving in 6 months.

Risk factors for suicide completion

Sex (male), Age (teenager or elderly), Depression, Previous attempt, Ethanol or drug use, loss of Rational thinking, Sickness (medical illness, 3 or more prescription medications), Organized plan, No spouse (divorced, widowed, or single, especially if childless), Social support lacking.

Women try more often; men succeed more often.

SAD PERSONS are more likely to complete suicide.

Anxiety disorder

Inappropriate experience of fear/worry and its physical manifestations (anxiety) when the source of the fear/worry is either not real or insufficient to account for the severity of the symptoms. Symptoms interfere with daily functioning. Lifetime prevalence of 30% in women and 19% in men. Includes panic disorder, phobias, OCD, PTSD, and generalized anxiety disorder.

Panic disorder

Defined by the presence of recurrent periods of intense fear and discomfort peaking in 10 minutes with at least 4 of the following: Palpitations, Paresthesias, Abdominal distress, Nausea, Intense fear of dying or losing control, lIght-headedness, Chest pain, Chills, Choking, disConnectedness, Sweating, Shaking, Shortness of breath. Strong genetic component. Treatment: cognitive behavioral therapy (CBT), SSRIs, venlafaxine, benzodiazepines (risk of tolerance, physical dependence).

PANICS.

Described in context of occurrence (e.g., panic disorder with agoraphobia).

Associated with persistent fear of having another attack.

Symptoms are the systemic manifestations of fear.

Specific phobia

Fear that is excessive or unreasonable and interferes with normal function. Cued by presence or anticipation of a specific object or situation. Person recognizes fear is excessive. Can treat with systematic desensitization.

Social phobia (social anxiety disorder)—exaggerated fear of embarrassment in social situations (e.g., public speaking, using public restrooms). Treatment: SSRIs.

Obsessive-compulsive disorder

Recurring intrusive thoughts, feelings, or sensations (obsessions) that cause severe distress; relieved in part by the performance of repetitive actions (compulsions). Ego dystonic: behavior inconsistent with one's own beliefs and attitudes (vs. obsessive-compulsive personality disorder). Associated with Tourette's disorder. Treatment: SSRIs, clomipramine.

Post-traumatic stress disorder	Persistent reexperiencing of a previous traumatic event (e.g., war, rape, robbery, serious accident, fire). May involve nightmares or flashbacks, intense fear, helplessness, or horror. Leads to avoidance of stimuli associated with the trauma and persistently ↑ arousal. **Disturbance lasts > 1 month,** with onset of symptoms beginning anytime after event, and causes significant distress and/or impaired functioning. Treatment: psychotherapy, SSRIs. **Acute stress disorder—lasts between 2 days and 1 month**.
Generalized anxiety disorder	Pattern of uncontrollable anxiety for **at least 6 months** that is unrelated to a specific person, situation, or event. Associated with sleep disturbance, fatigue, GI disturbance, and difficulty concentrating. Treatment: SSRIs, SNRIs. **Adjustment disorder**—emotional symptoms (anxiety, depression) causing impairment following an identifiable psychosocial stressor (e.g., divorce, illness) and **lasting < 6 months** (> 6 months in presence of chronic stressor).
Malingering	Patient consciously fakes or claims to have a disorder in order to attain a specific 2° gain (e.g., avoiding work, obtaining drugs). Poor compliance with treatment or follow-up of diagnostic tests. Complaints cease after gain (vs. factitious disorder).
Factitious disorder	Patient consciously creates physical and/or psychological symptoms in order to assume "sick role" and to get medical attention (1° gain).
Munchausen's syndrome	**Chronic** factitious disorder with predominantly physical signs and symptoms. Characterized by a history of multiple hospital admissions and willingness to receive invasive procedures.
Munchausen's syndrome by proxy	When illness in a child or elderly patient is caused by the caregiver. Motivation is to assume a sick role by proxy. Form of child/elder abuse.
Somatoform disorders	Category of disorders characterized by physical symptoms with no identifiable physical cause. Both illness production and motivation are unconscious drives. Symptoms not intentionally produced or feigned. More common in women.
Somatization disorder	Variety of complaints in multiple organ systems (at least 4 pain, 2 GI, 1 sexual, 1 pseudoneurologic) over a period of years, developing before age 30 years
Conversion	Sudden loss of sensory or motor function (e.g., paralysis, blindness, mutism), often following an acute stressor; patient is aware of but sometimes indifferent toward symptoms ("la belle indifférence"); more common in females, adolescents, and young adults
Hypochondriasis	Preoccupation with and fear of having a serious illness despite medical evaluation and reassurance
Body dysmorphic disorder	Preoccupation with minor or imagined defect in appearance, leading to significant emotional distress or impaired functioning; patients often repeatedly seek cosmetic surgery
Pain disorder	Prolonged pain with no physical findings; pain is the predominant focus of clinical presentation and psychological factors play an important role in severity, exacerbation, or maintenance of the pain

Personality

Personality trait	An enduring, repetitive pattern of perceiving, relating to, and thinking about the environment and oneself.
Personality disorder	Inflexible, maladaptive, and rigidly pervasive pattern of behavior causing subjective distress and/or impaired functioning; person is usually not aware of problem. Usually presents by early adulthood.

Cluster A personality disorders	Odd or eccentric; inability to develop meaningful social relationships. No psychosis; genetic association with schizophrenia.	"**W**eird" (**A**ccusatory, **A**loof, **A**wkward).
Paranoid	Pervasive distrust and suspiciousness; projection is the major defense mechanism.	
Schizoid	Voluntary social withdrawal, limited emotional expression, content with social isolation (vs. avoidant).	Schizoid = distant.
Schizotypal	Eccentric appearance, odd beliefs or magical thinking, interpersonal awkwardness.	Schizotypal = magical thinking.

Cluster B personality disorders	Dramatic, emotional, or erratic; genetic association with mood disorders and substance abuse.	"**W**ild" (**B**ad to the **B**one).
Antisocial	Disregard for and violation of rights of others, criminality; males > females; conduct disorder if < 18 years.	Antisocial = sociopath.
Borderline	Unstable mood and interpersonal relationships, impulsiveness, self-mutilation, boredom, sense of emptiness; females > males; splitting is a major defense mechanism.	
Histrionic	Excessive emotionality and excitability, attention seeking, sexually provocative, overly concerned with appearance.	
Narcissistic	Grandiosity, sense of entitlement; lacks empathy and requires excessive admiration; often demands the "best" and reacts to criticism with rage.	

Cluster C personality disorders	Anxious or fearful; genetic association with anxiety disorders.	"**Worried**" (**C**owardly, **C**ompulsive, **C**lingy).
Avoidant	Hypersensitive to rejection, socially inhibited, timid, feelings of inadequacy, desires relationships with others (vs. schizoid).	
Obsessive-compulsive	Preoccupation with order, perfectionism, and control; ego-syntonic: behavior consistent with one's own beliefs and attitudes (vs. OCD).	
Dependent	Submissive and clinging, excessive need to be taken care of, low self-confidence.	

Keeping "schizo-" straight

Schizoid	<	**Schizotypal**	<	**Schizophrenic**	<	**Schizoaffective**
		(schizoid + odd thinking)		(greater odd thinking than schizotypal)		(schizophrenic psychotic symptoms + bipolar or depressive mood disorder)

Schizophrenia time course:
- **< 1 mo**—brief psychotic disorder, usually stress related
- **1–6 mo**—schizophreniform disorder
- **> 6 mo**—schizophrenia

Eating disorders	
Anorexia nervosa	Excessive dieting +/– purging; intense fear of gaining weight, body image distortion, and ↑ exercise, leading to body weight < 85% of ideal body weight. Associated with ↓ bone density. Severe weight loss, metatarsal stress fractures, amenorrhea, anemia, and electrolyte disturbances. Seen primarily in adolescent girls. Commonly coexists with depression.
Bulimia nervosa	Binge eating +/– purging; often followed by self-induced vomiting or use of laxatives, diuretics, or emetics. Body weight often maintained within normal range. Associated with parotitis, enamel erosion, electrolyte disturbances, alkalosis, dorsal hand calluses from induced vomiting (Russell's sign). Seen predominantly in adolescent girls.

Gender identity disorder

Strong, persistent cross-gender identification. Characterized by persistent discomfort with one's sex, causing significant distress and/or impaired functioning.

Trans**sex**ualism—desire to live as the opposite **sex**, often through surgery or hormone treatment.

Trans**vest**ism—paraphilia; wearing clothes (e.g., **vest**) of the opposite sex (cross-dressing).

Substance dependence

Maladaptive pattern of substance use defined as 3 or more of the following signs in 1 year:
- Tolerance—need more to achieve same effect
- Withdrawal
- Substance taken in larger amounts, or over longer time, than desired
- Persistent desire or unsuccessful attempts to cut down
- Significant energy spent obtaining, using, or recovering from substance
- Important social, occupational, or recreational activities reduced because of substance use
- Continued use in spite of knowing the problems that it causes

Substance abuse

Maladaptive pattern leading to clinically significant impairment or distress.
- Recurrent use resulting in failure to fulfill major obligations at work, school, or home
- Recurrent use in physically hazardous situations
- Recurrent substance-related legal problems
- Continued use in spite of persistent problems caused by use

Stages of change in overcoming substance addiction

1. **Precontemplation**—not yet acknowledging that there is a problem
2. **Contemplation**—acknowledging that there is a problem, but not yet ready or willing to make a change
3. **Preparation/determination**—getting ready to change behavior
4. **Action/willpower**—changing behaviors
5. **Maintenance**—maintaining the behavior change
6. **Relapse**—returning to old behaviors and abandoning new changes

Psychoactive drug intoxication and withdrawal

DRUG	INTOXICATION	WITHDRAWAL
Depressants		
	Nonspecific: mood elevation, ↓ anxiety, sedation, behavioral disinhibition, respiratory depression.	Nonspecific: anxiety, tremor, seizures, insomnia.
Alcohol	Emotional lability, slurred speech, ataxia, coma, blackouts. Serum γ-glutamyltransferase (GGT)—sensitive indicator of alcohol use. Lab AST value is twice ALT value.	Mild alcohol withdrawal: symptoms similar to other depressants. Severe alcohol withdrawal can cause autonomic hyperactivity and DTs. Treatment for DTs: benzodiazepines.
Opioids (e.g., morphine, heroin, methadone)	Euphoria, respiratory and CNS depression, ↓ gag reflex, pupillary constriction (pinpoint pupils), seizures (overdose). Treatment: naloxone, naltrexone.	Sweating, dilated pupils, piloerection ("cold turkey"), fever, rhinorrhea, yawning, nausea, stomach cramps, diarrhea ("flu-like" symptoms). Treatment: long-term support, methadone, buprenorphine.
Barbiturates	Low safety margin, marked respiratory depression. Treatment: symptom management (assist respiration, ↑ BP).	Delirium, life-threatening cardiovascular collapse.
Benzodiazepines	Greater safety margin. Ataxia, minor respiratory depression. Treatment: flumazenil (competitive benzodiazepine antagonist).	Sleep disturbance, depression, rebound anxiety, seizure (severe).

Psychoactive drug intoxication and withdrawal *(continued)*

DRUG	INTOXICATION	WITHDRAWAL
Stimulants		
	Nonspecific: mood elevation, psychomotor agitation, insomnia, cardiac arrhythmias, tachycardia, anxiety.	Nonspecific: post-use "crash," including depression, lethargy, weight gain, headache.
Amphetamines	Euphoria, grandiosity, pupillary dilation, prolonged wakefulness and attention, hypertension, tachycardia, anorexia, paranoia, fever. Severe: cardiac arrest, seizure.	Anhedonia, increased appetite, hypersomnolence, existential crisis.
Cocaine	Impaired judgment, pupillary dilation, hallucinations (including tactile), paranoid ideations, angina, sudden cardiac death. Treatment: benzodiazepines.	Hypersomnolence, malaise, severe psychological craving, depression/suicidality.
Caffeine	Restlessness, ↑ diuresis, muscle twitching.	Lack of concentration, headache.
Nicotine	Restlessness.	Irritability, anxiety, craving. Treatment: nicotine patch, gum, or lozenges; bupropion/varenicline.
Hallucinogens		
PCP	Belligerence, impulsiveness, fever, psychomotor agitation, analgesia, vertical and horizontal nystagmus, tachycardia, homicidality, psychosis, delirium, seizures. Treatment: benzodiazepines, rapid-acting antipsychotic.	Depression, anxiety, irritability, restlessness, anergia, disturbances of thought and sleep.
LSD	Perceptual distortion (visual, auditory), depersonalization, anxiety, paranoia, psychosis, possible flashbacks.	
Marijuana (cannabinoid)	Euphoria, anxiety, paranoid delusions, perception of slowed time, impaired judgment, social withdrawal, ↑ appetite, dry mouth, conjunctival injection, hallucinations. Prescription form is dronabinol (tetrahydrocannabinol isomer): used as antiemetic (chemotherapy) and appetite stimulant (in AIDS).	Irritability, depression, insomnia, nausea, anorexia. Most symptoms peak in 48 hours and last for 5–7 days. Generally detectable in urine for 4–10 days.

Heroin addiction

Users at ↑ risk for hepatitis, abscesses, overdose, hemorrhoids, AIDS, and right-sided endocarditis. Look for track marks (needle sticks in veins).

Methadone—long-acting oral opiate; used for heroin detoxification or long-term maintenance.

Naloxone + buprenorphine—Partial agonist; long acting with fewer withdrawal symptoms than methadone. Naloxone is not active when taken orally, so withdrawal symptoms occur only if injected (lower abuse potential).

Alcoholism	Physiologic tolerance and dependence with symptoms of withdrawal (tremor, tachycardia, hypertension, malaise, nausea, DTs) when intake is interrupted. Complications: alcoholic cirrhosis, hepatitis, pancreatitis, peripheral neuropathy, testicular atrophy. Treatment: disulfiram (to condition the patient to abstain from alcohol use), supportive care. Alcoholics Anonymous and other peer support groups are helpful in sustaining abstinence.
Wernicke-Korsakoff syndrome	Caused by thiamine deficiency. Triad of confusion, ophthalmoplegia, and ataxia (**Wernicke's encephalopathy**). May progress to irreversible memory loss, confabulation, personality change (**Korsakoff's psychosis**). Associated with periventricular hemorrhage/necrosis of mammillary bodies. Treatment: IV vitamin B_1 (thiamine).
Mallory-Weiss syndrome	Longitudinal lacerations at the gastroesophageal junction caused by excessive vomiting. Often presents with hematemesis. Associated with pain (vs. esophageal varices).

Delirium tremens (DTs)	Life-threatening alcohol withdrawal syndrome that peaks 2–5 days after last drink. Symptoms in order of appearance: autonomic system hyperactivity (tachycardia, tremors, anxiety, seizures), psychotic symptoms (hallucinations, delusions), confusion. Treatment: benzodiazepines.

▸ PSYCHIATRY–PHARMACOLOGY

Treatment for selected psychiatric conditions

PSYCHIATRIC CONDITION	PREFERRED DRUGS
Alcohol withdrawal	Benzodiazepines
Anxiety	SSRIs, SNRIs, buspirone
ADHD	Methylphenidate, amphetamines
Bipolar disorder	"Mood stabilizers" (e.g., lithium, valproic acid, carbamazepine), atypical antipsychotics
Bulimia	SSRIs
Depression	SSRIs, SNRIs, TCAs, buspirone, mirtazapine (especially with insomnia)
Obsessive-compulsive disorder	SSRIs, clomipramine
Panic disorder	SSRIs, venlafaxine, benzodiazepines
PTSD	SSRIs
Schizophrenia	Antipsychotics
Social phobias	SSRIs
Tourette's syndrome	Antipsychotics (e.g., haloperidol, risperidone)

CNS stimulants	Methylphenidate, dextroamphetamine, methamphetamine.
MECHANISM	↑ catecholamines at the synaptic cleft, especially NE and dopamine.
CLINICAL USE	ADHD, narcolepsy, appetite control.

Antipsychotics (neuroleptics)

Haloperidol, trifluoperazine, fluphenazine, thioridazine, chlorpromazine (haloperidol + "-azines").

MECHANISM	All typical antipsychotics block dopamine D_2 receptors (↑ [cAMP]).
CLINICAL USE	Schizophrenia (primarily positive symptoms), psychosis, acute mania, Tourette's syndrome.
TOXICITY	Highly lipid soluble and stored in body fat; thus, very slow to be removed from body. Extrapyramidal system (EPS) side effects (e.g., dyskinesias). Endocrine side effects (e.g., dopamine receptor antagonism → hyperprolactinemia → galactorrhea). Side effects arising from blocking muscarinic (dry mouth, constipation), α_1 (hypotension), and histamine (sedation) receptors.
OTHER TOXICITIES	**Neuroleptic malignant syndrome (NMS)**—rigidity, myoglobinuria, autonomic instability, hyperpyrexia. Treatment: dantrolene, D_2 agonists (e.g., bromocriptine). **Tardive dyskinesia**—stereotypic oral-facial movements as a result of long-term antipsychotic use. Often irreversible.

High potency: Trifluoperazine, Fluphenazine, Haloperidol (**T**ry to **Fly High**)—neurologic side effects (extrapyramidal symptoms).

Low potency: Chlorpromazine, Thioridazine (**C**heating **T**hieves are **low**)—non-neurologic side effects (anticholinergic, antihistamine, and α_1-blockade effects).

Chlorpromazine—Corneal deposits; Thioridazine—reTinal deposits; haloperidol—NMS, tardive dyskinesia.

Evolution of EPS side effects:
- 4 hr acute dystonia (muscle spasm, stiffness, oculogyric crisis)
- 4 day akathisia (restlessness)
- 4 wk bradykinesia (parkinsonism)
- 4 mo tardive dyskinesia

For NMS, think **FEVER:**
Fever
Encephalopathy
Vitals unstable
Elevated enzymes
Rigidity of muscles

Atypical antipsychotics

Olanzapine, **clo**zapine, **quet**iapine, **risper**idone, **a**ripiprazole, **z**iprasidone.

It's **atypical** for **o**ld **clo**sets to **quiet**ly **risper** from **A** to **Z**.

MECHANISM	Not completely understood. Varied effects on 5-HT_2, dopamine, and α- and H_1-receptors.	
CLINICAL USE	Schizophrenia—both positive and negative symptoms. Also used for bipolar disorder, OCD, anxiety disorder, depression, mania, Tourette's syndrome.	
TOXICITY	Fewer extrapyramidal and anticholinergic side effects than traditional antipsychotics. Olanzapine/clozapine may cause significant weight gain. Clozapine may cause agranulocytosis (requires weekly WBC monitoring) and seizure. Ziprasidone may prolong the QT interval.	Must watch **clozapine clozely**!

Lithium

MECHANISM	Not established; possibly related to inhibition of phosphoinositol cascade.	**LMNOP**: **L**ithium side effects— **M**ovement (tremor) **N**ephrogenic diabetes insipidus Hyp**O**thyroidism **P**regnancy problems
CLINICAL USE	Mood stabilizer for bipolar disorder; blocks relapse and acute manic events. Also SIADH.	
TOXICITY	Tremor, sedation, edema, heart block, hypothyroidism, polyuria (ADH antagonist causing nephrogenic diabetes insipidus), teratogenesis. Fetal cardiac defects include Ebstein anomaly and malformation of the great vessels. Narrow therapeutic window requires close monitoring of serum levels. Almost exclusively excreted by the kidneys; most is reabsorbed at the proximal convoluted tubules following Na^+ reabsorption.	

Buspirone

MECHANISM	Stimulates $5\text{-}HT_{1A}$ receptors.	I'm always anxious if the **bus** will be **on** time, so I take **buspirone**.
CLINICAL USE	Generalized anxiety disorder. Does not cause sedation, addiction, or tolerance. Takes 1–2 weeks to take effect. Does not interact with alcohol (vs. barbiturates, benzodiazepines).	

Antidepressants

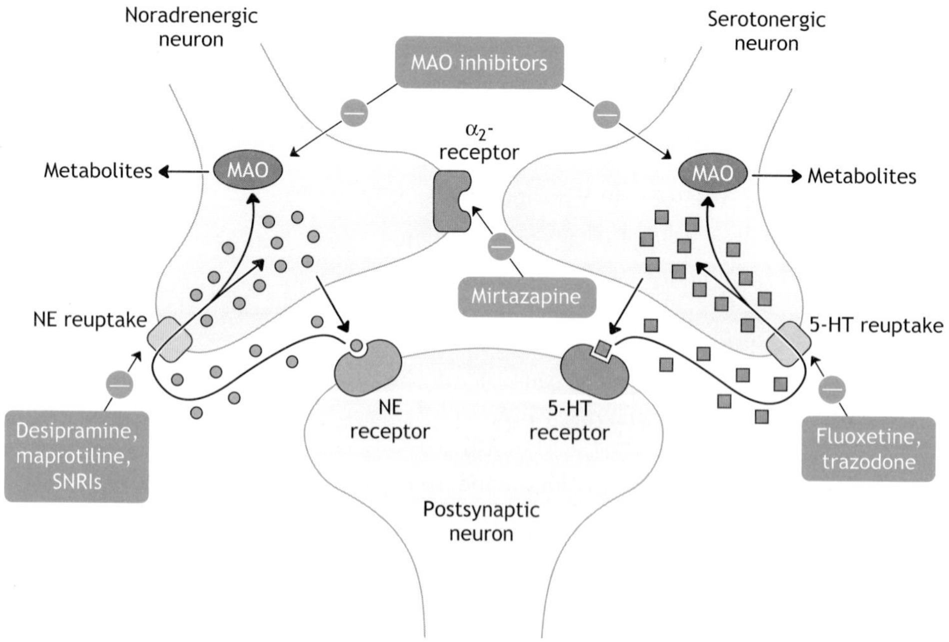

(Adapted, with permission, from Katzung BG, Trevor AJ. *USMLE Road Map: Pharmacology*, 2nd ed. New York: McGraw-Hill, 2006: Fig. 5-7.)

SSRIs	Fluoxetine, paroxetine, sertraline, citalopram.	Flashbacks paralyze senior citizens.
MECHANISM	Serotonin-specific reuptake inhibitors.	It normally takes 4–8 weeks for antidepressants to have an effect.
CLINICAL USE	Depression, generalized anxiety disorder, panic disorder, OCD, bulimia, social phobias, PTSD.	
TOXICITY	Fewer than TCAs. GI distress, sexual dysfunction (anorgasmia and ↓ libido). **Serotonin syndrome** with any drug that ↑ serotonin (e.g., MAO inhibitors, SNRIs, TCAs)—hyperthermia, confusion, myoclonus, cardiovascular collapse, flushing, diarrhea, seizures. Treatment: cyproheptadine (5-HT_2 receptor antagonist).	

SNRIs	Venlafaxine, duloxetine.
MECHANISM	Inhibit serotonin and NE reuptake.
CLINICAL USE	Depression. Venlafaxine is also used in generalized anxiety and panic disorders; duloxetine is also indicated for diabetic peripheral neuropathy. Duloxetine has greater effect on NE.
TOXICITY	↑ BP most common; also stimulant effects, sedation, nausea.

Tricyclic antidepressants	Amitriptyline, nortriptyline, imipramine, desipramine, clomipramine, doxepin, amoxapine (all TCAs end in -iptyline or -ipramine except doxepin and amoxapine).
MECHANISM	Block reuptake of NE and serotonin.
CLINICAL USE	Major depression, bedwetting (imipramine), OCD (clomipramine), fibromyalgia.
TOXICITY	Sedation, α_1-blocking effects including postural hypotension, and atropine-like (anticholinergic) side effects (tachycardia, urinary retention, dry mouth). 3° TCAs (amitriptyline) have more anticholinergic effects than 2° TCAs (nortriptyline) have. Desipramine is less sedating and has higher seizure threshold. Tri-C's: Convulsions, Coma, Cardiotoxicity (arrhythmias); also respiratory depression, hyperpyrexia. Confusion and hallucinations in elderly due to anticholinergic side effects (use nortriptyline). Treatment: $NaHCO_3$ for cardiovascular toxicity.

Monoamine oxidase (MAO) inhibitors	Tranylcypromine, Phenelzine, Isocarboxazid, Selegiline (selective MAO-B inhibitor). (MAO Takes Pride In Shanghai).
MECHANISM	Nonselective MAO inhibition ↑ levels of amine neurotransmitters (NE, serotonin, dopamine).
CLINICAL USE	Atypical depression, anxiety, hypochondriasis.
TOXICITY	Hypertensive crisis (most notably with ingestion of tyramine, which is found in many foods such as wine and cheese); CNS stimulation. Contraindicated with SSRIs, TCAs, St. John's Wort, meperidine, and dextromethorphan (to prevent serotonin syndrome).

Atypical antidepressants

Bupropion	Also used for smoking cessation. ↑ NE and dopamine via unknown mechanism. Toxicity: stimulant effects (tachycardia, insomnia), headache, seizure in bulimic patients. No sexual side effects.	
Mirtazapine	α_2-antagonist (↑ release of NE and serotonin) and potent 5-HT_2 and 5-HT_3 receptor antagonist. Toxicity: sedation (which may be desirable in depressed patients with insomnia), ↑ appetite, weight gain (which may be desirable in elderly or anorexic patients), dry mouth.	
Maprotiline	Blocks NE reuptake. Toxicity: sedation, orthostatic hypotension.	
Trazodone	Primarily inhibits serotonin reuptake. Used primarily for insomnia, as high doses are needed for antidepressant effects. Toxicity: sedation, nausea, priapism, postural hypotension.	Called trazo**bone** due to male-specific side effects.

HIGH-YIELD SYSTEMS

Renal

"But I know all about love already. I know precious little still about kidneys."

—Aldous Huxley, *Antic Hay*

"This too shall pass. Just like a kidney stone."

—Hunter Madsen

"I drink too much. The last time I gave a urine sample it had an olive in it."

—Rodney Dangerfield

▸ RENAL–EMBRYOLOGY

Kidney embryology

Pronephros—week 4; then degenerates
Mesonephros—functions as interim kidney for 1st trimester; later contributes to male genital system
Metanephros—permanent; first appears in 5th week of gestation; nephrogenesis continues through 32–36 weeks of gestation

- Ureteric bud—derived from caudal end of mesonephros; gives rise to ureter, pelvises, calyces, and collecting ducts; fully canalized by 10th week
- Metanephric mesenchyme—ureteric bud interacts with this tissue; interaction induces differentiation and formation of glomerulus through to distal convoluted tubule
- Aberrant interaction between these 2 tissues may result in several congenital malformations of the kidney

Ureteropelvic junction—last to canalize → most common site of obstruction (hydronephrosis) in fetus.

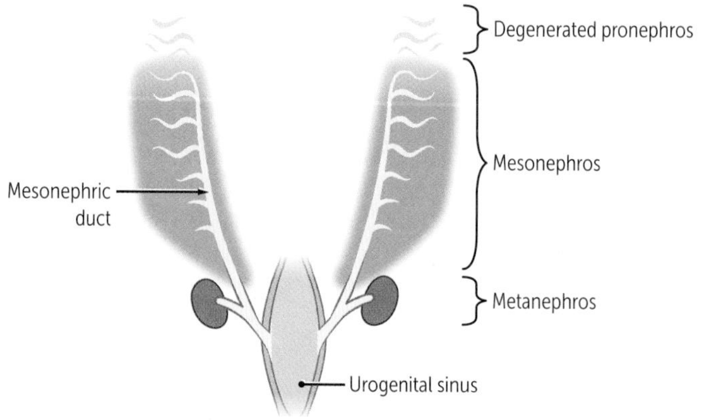

Potter's syndrome

Oligohydramnios → compression of fetus → limb deformities, facial deformities, and pulmonary hypoplasia (cause of death).

Babies who can't "Pee" in utero develop Potter's. Causes include ARPKD, posterior urethral valves, bilateral renal agenesis.

Horseshoe kidney

Inferior poles of both kidneys fuse. As they ascend from pelvis during fetal development, horseshoe kidneys get trapped under inferior mesenteric artery and remain low in the abdomen. Kidney functions normally. Associated with Turner syndrome.

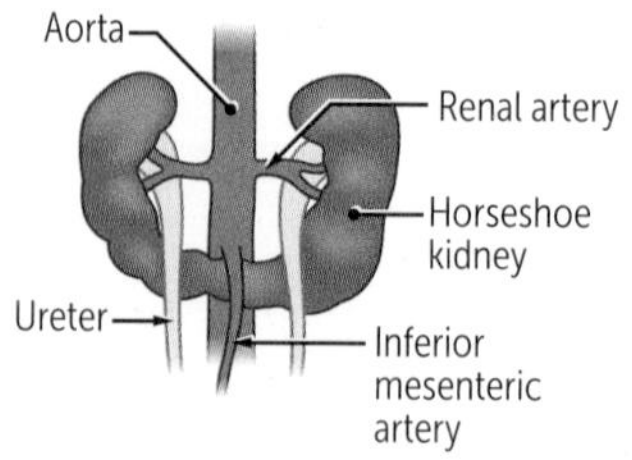

Multicystic dysplastic kidney

Due to abnormal interaction between ureteric bud and metanephric mesenchyme. This leads to a nonfunctional kidney consisting of cysts and connective tissue. If unilateral (most common), generally asymptomatic with compensatory hypertrophy of contralateral kidney. Often diagnosed prenatally via ultrasound.

▸ RENAL–ANATOMY

Kidney anatomy and glomerular structure

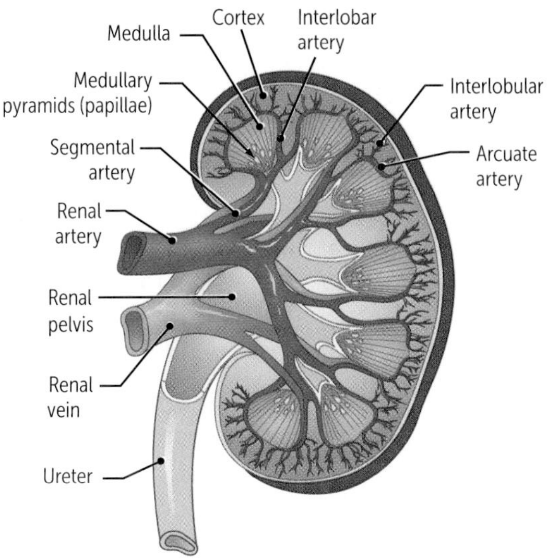

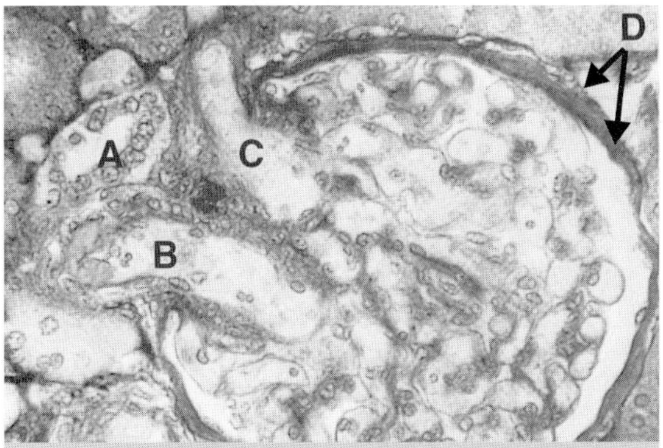

A **Normal glomerulus.** Showing (A) macula densa and distal convoluted tubule, (B) afferent arteriole, (C) efferent arteriole, and (D) Bowman's capsule.

The left kidney is taken during living donor transplantation because it has a longer renal vein.

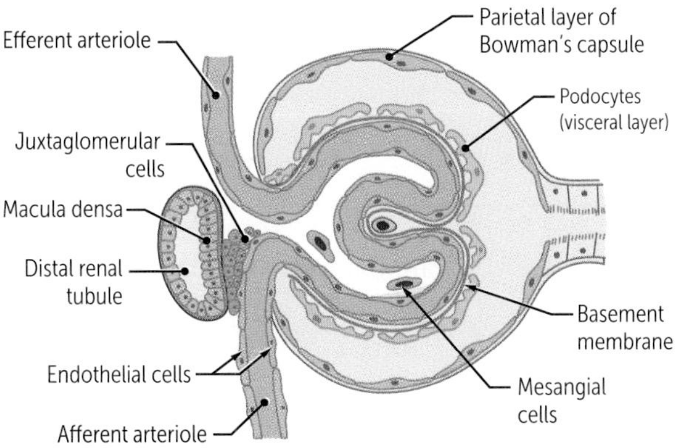

Ureters: course

Ureters pass **under** uterine artery and **under** ductus deferens (retroperitoneal).

"Water (ureters) **under** the bridge (uterine artery, vas deferens)."

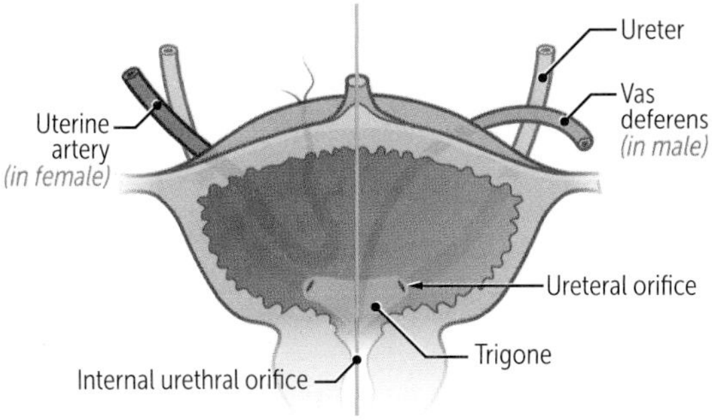

▸ RENAL–PHYSIOLOGY

Fluid compartments

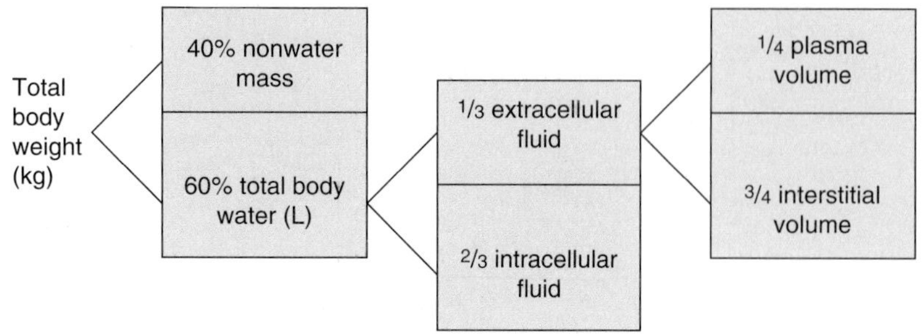

HIKIN': **HI**gh **K** **IN**tracellular.
60–40–20 rule (% of body weight):
- 60% total body water
- 40% ICF
- 20% ECF

Plasma volume measured by radiolabeled albumin.
Extracellular volume measured by inulin.
Osmolarity = 290 mOsm/L.

Glomerular filtration barrier

Responsible for filtration of plasma according to size and net charge.
Composed of:
- Fenestrated capillary endothelium (size barrier)
- Fused basement membrane with heparan sulfate (negative charge barrier)
- Epithelial layer consisting of podocyte foot processes

The charge barrier is lost in nephrotic syndrome, resulting in albuminuria, hypoproteinemia, generalized edema, and hyperlipidemia.

Renal clearance

$C_x = U_xV/P_x$ = volume of plasma from which the substance is completely cleared per unit time.
$C_x <$ GFR: net tubular reabsorption of X.
$C_x >$ GFR: net tubular secretion of X.
$C_x =$ GFR: no net secretion or reabsorption.

Be familiar with calculations.
C_x = clearance of X. Units are mL/min.
U_x = urine concentration of X.
P_x = plasma concentration of X.
V = urine flow rate.

Glomerular filtration rate (GFR)

Inulin clearance can be used to calculate GFR because it is freely filtered and is neither reabsorbed nor secreted.

$GFR = U_{inulin} \times V/P_{inulin} = C_{inulin}$
$= K_f[(P_{GC} - P_{BS}) - (\pi_{GC} - \pi_{BS})]$.

(GC = glomerular capillary; BS = Bowman's space.) π_{BS} normally equals zero.

Normal GFR ≈ 100 mL/min.
Creatinine clearance is an approximate measure of GFR. Slightly overestimates GFR because creatinine is moderately secreted by the renal tubules.
Incremental reductions in GFR define the stages of chronic kidney disease.

Effective renal plasma flow

ERPF can be estimated using PAH clearance because it is both filtered and actively secreted in the proximal tubule. All PAH entering the kidney is excreted.
$ERPF = U_{PAH} \times V/P_{PAH} = C_{PAH}$.
RBF = RPF/(1 – Hct).
ERPF underestimates true RPF by ~10%.

Filtration

Filtration fraction (FF) = GFR/RPF.
Normal FF = 20%.
Filtered load = GFR × plasma concentration.

GFR can be estimated with creatinine clearance.
RPF is best estimated with PAH clearance.

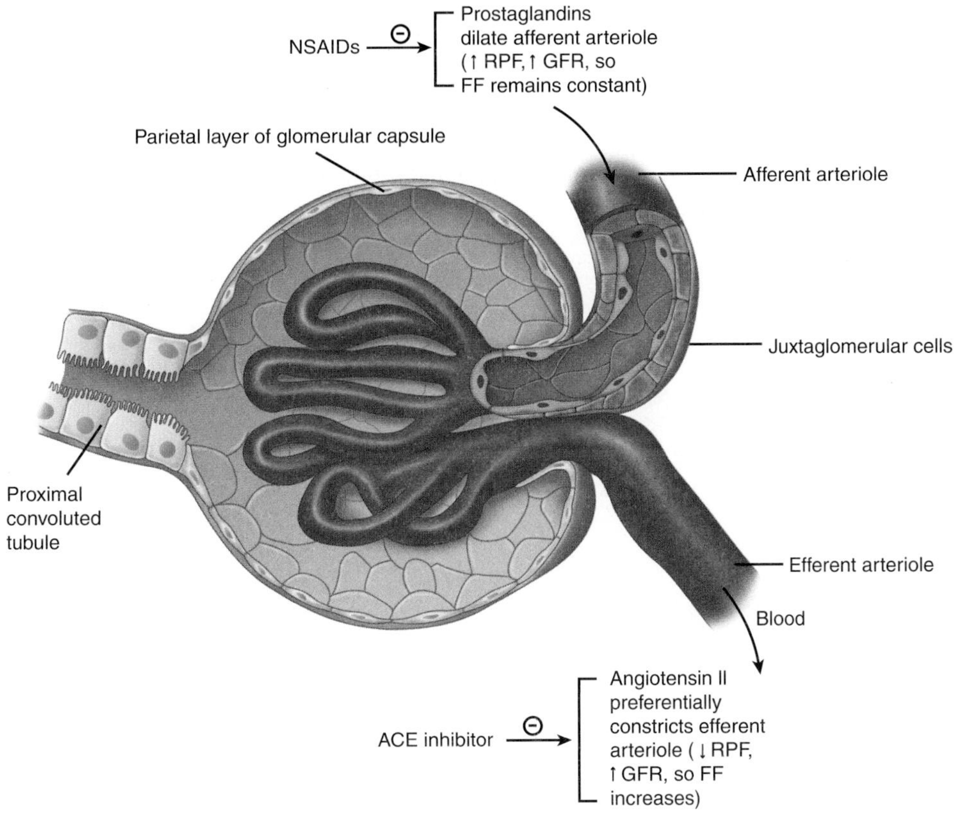
NSAIDs
⊖
Prostaglandins dilate afferent arteriole (↑ RPF, ↑ GFR, so FF remains constant)
Parietal layer of glomerular capsule
Afferent arteriole
Juxtaglomerular cells
Proximal convoluted tubule
Efferent arteriole
Blood
ACE inhibitor
⊖
Angiotensin II preferentially constricts efferent arteriole (↓ RPF, ↑ GFR, so FF increases)

Changes in glomerular dynamics

Effect	RPF	GFR	FF (GFR/RPF)
Afferent arteriole constriction	↓	↓	NC
Efferent arteriole constriction	↓	↑	↑
↑ plasma protein concentration	NC	↓	↓
↓ plasma protein concentration	NC	↑	↑
Constriction of ureter	NC	↓	↓

Calculation of reabsorption and secretion rate

Filtered load = GFR × P_x.
Excretion rate = V × U_x.
Reabsorption = filtered – excreted.
Secretion = excreted – filtered.

Glucose clearance	Glucose at a normal plasma level is completely reabsorbed in proximal tubule by Na^+/glucose cotransport. At plasma glucose of ~160 mg/dL, glucosuria begins (threshold). At 350 mg/dL, all transporters are fully saturated (T_m).	Glucosuria is an important clinical clue to diabetes mellitus. Normal pregnancy reduces reabsorption of glucose and amino acids in the proximal tubule, leading to glucosuria and aminoaciduria.
Amino acid clearance	Sodium-dependent transporters in proximal tubule reabsorb amino acids. Hartnup's disease—deficiency of neutral amino acid (tryptophan) transporter; results in pellagra.	

Nephron physiology

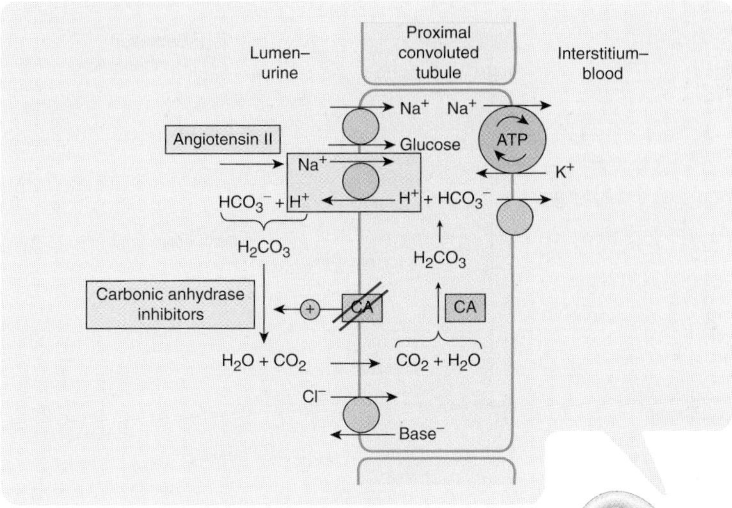

Early proximal tubule—contains brush border. Reabsorbs all of the glucose and amino acids and most of the bicarbonate, sodium, chloride, phosphate, and water. Isotonic absorption. Generates and secretes ammonia, which acts as a buffer for secreted H^+.

PTH—inhibits Na^+/phosphate cotransport → phosphate excretion.

AT II—stimulates Na^+/H^+ exchange → ↑ Na^+, H_2O, and HCO_3^- reabsorption (permitting contraction alkalosis).

65–80% Na^+ reabsorbed.

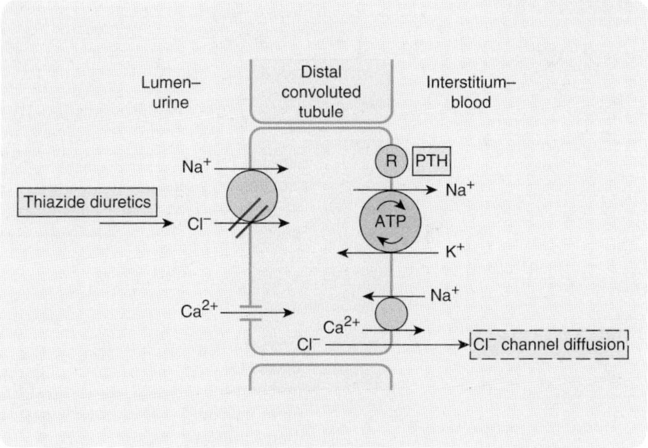

Early distal convoluted tubule—actively reabsorbs Na^+, Cl^-. Makes urine hypotonic.

PTH—↑ Ca^{2+}/Na^+ exchange → Ca^{2+} reabsorption.

5–10% Na^+ reabsorbed.

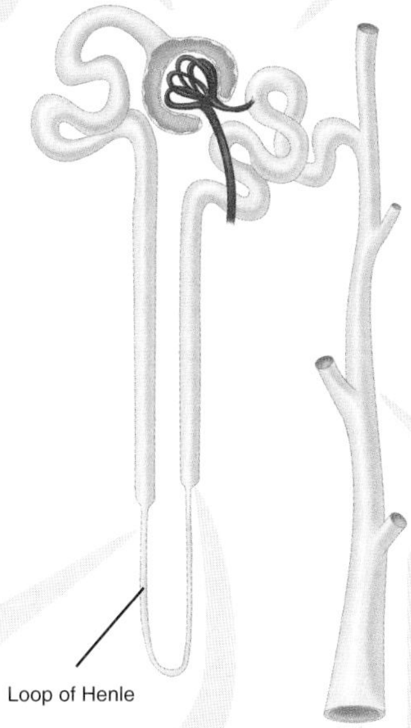

Thin descending loop of Henle—passively reabsorbs water via medullary hypertonicity (impermeable to sodium). Concentrating segment. Makes urine hypertonic.

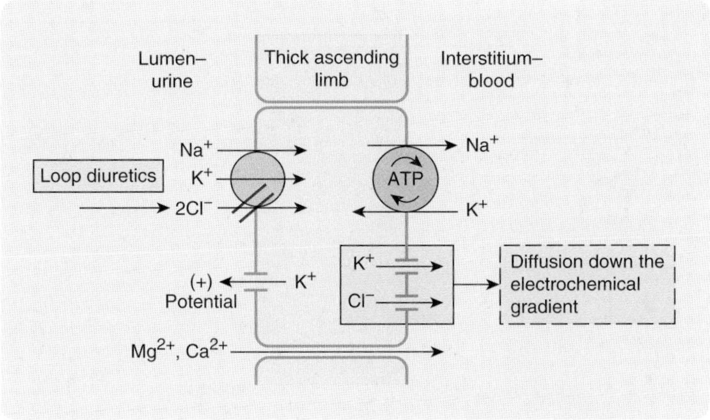

Thick ascending loop of Henle—actively reabsorbs Na^+, K^+, and Cl^-. Indirectly induces the paracellular reabsorption of Mg^{2+} and Ca^{2+} through (+) lumen potential generated by K^+ backleak. Impermeable to H_2O. Makes urine less concentrated as it ascends.

10–20% Na^+ reabsorbed.

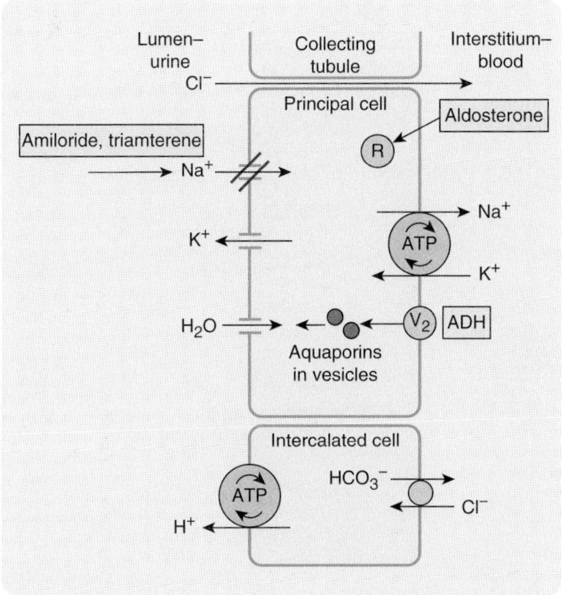

Collecting tubules—reabsorb Na^+ in exchange for secreting K^+ and H^+ (regulated by aldosterone).

Aldosterone—acts on mineralocorticoid receptor → insertion of Na^+ channel on luminal side.

ADH—acts at V_2 receptor → insertion of aquaporin H_2O channels on luminal side.

3–5% Na^+ reabsorbed.

Relative concentrations along proximal tubule

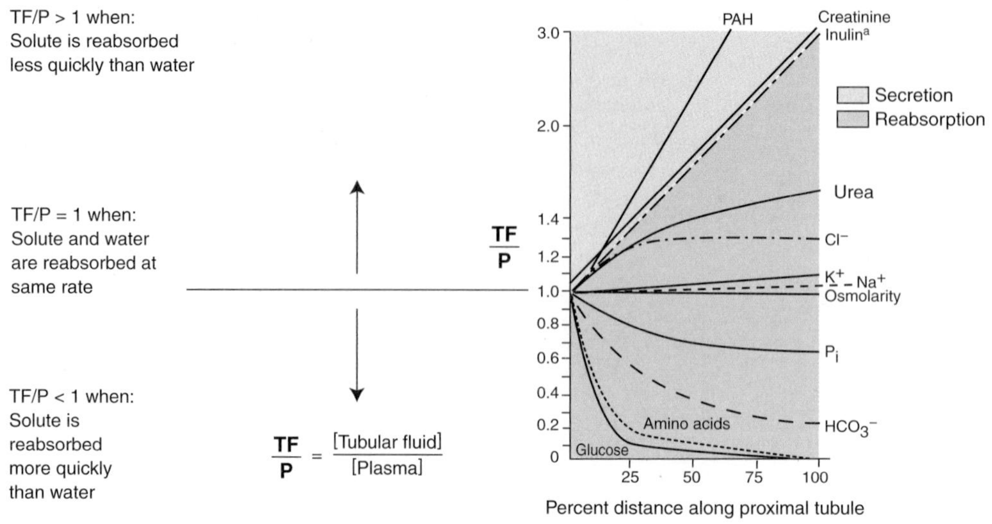
TF/P > 1 when:
Solute is reabsorbed less quickly than water
TF/P = 1 when:
Solute and water are reabsorbed at same rate
TF/P < 1 when:
Solute is reabsorbed more quickly than water
TF/P = [Tubular fluid]/[Plasma]
TF/P
3.0
2.0
1.4
1.2
1.0
0.8
0.6
0.4
0.2
0
25
50
75
100
Percent distance along proximal tubule
PAH
Creatinine
Inulin[a]
Secretion
Reabsorption
Urea
Cl⁻
K⁺ Na⁺
Osmolarity
Pi
Amino acids
Glucose
HCO3⁻

[a]Neither secreted nor reabsorbed; concentration increases as water is reabsorbed.

(Adapted, with permission, from Ganong WF. *Review of Medical Physiology,* 22nd ed. New York: McGraw-Hill, 2005.)

Tubular inulin ↑ in concentration (but not amount) along the proximal tubule as a result of water reabsorption.

Cl^- reabsorption occurs at a slower rate than Na^+ in the proximal ⅓ of the proximal tubule and then matches the rate of Na^+ reabsorption more distally. Thus, its relative concentration ↑ before it plateaus.

Renin-angiotensin-aldosterone system

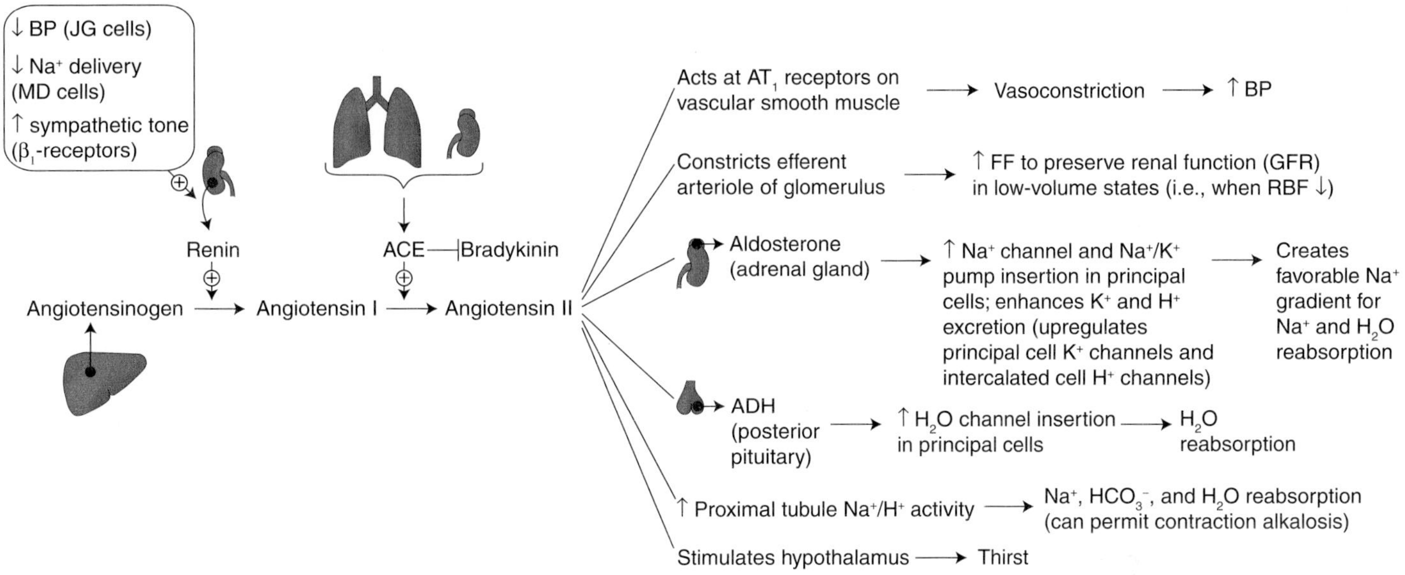

AT II	Affects baroreceptor function; limits reflex bradycardia, which would normally accompany its pressor effects. Helps maintain blood volume and blood pressure.
ANP	Released from atria in response to ↑ volume; may act as a "check" on renin-angiotensin-aldosterone system; relaxes vascular smooth muscle via cGMP, causing ↑ GFR, ↓ renin.
ADH	Primarily regulates osmolarity but also responds to low blood volume, which takes precedence over osmolarity.
Aldosterone	Primarily regulates blood volume; in low-volume states, both ADH and aldosterone act to protect blood volume.

Juxtaglomerular apparatus

Consists of JG cells (modified smooth muscle of afferent arteriole) and the macula densa (NaCl sensor, part of the distal convoluted tubule). JG cells secrete renin in response to ↓ renal blood pressure, ↓ NaCl delivery to distal tubule, and ↑ sympathetic tone (β_1).

JGA defends glomerular filtration rate via renin-angiotensin-aldosterone system.

β-blockers can decrease BP by inhibiting β_1-receptors of the JGA, causing ↓ renin release.

Juxta = close by.

Kidney endocrine functions

Erythropoietin	Released by interstitial cells in the peritubular capillary bed in response to hypoxia.	
1,25-$(OH)_2$ vitamin D	Proximal tubule cells convert 25-OH vitamin D to 1,25-$(OH)_2$ vitamin D (active form).	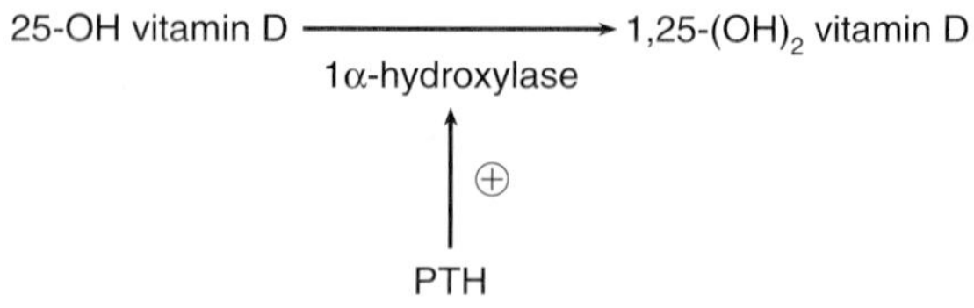
Renin	Secreted by JG cells in response to ↓ renal arterial pressure and ↑ renal sympathetic discharge (β_1 effect).	
Prostaglandins	Paracrine secretion vasodilates the afferent arterioles to ↑ GFR.	NSAIDs can cause acute renal failure by inhibiting the renal production of prostaglandins, which keep the afferent arterioles vasodilated to maintain GFR.

25-OH vitamin D → 1,25-(OH)2 vitamin D
1α-hydroxylase
⊕
PTH

Hormones acting on kidney

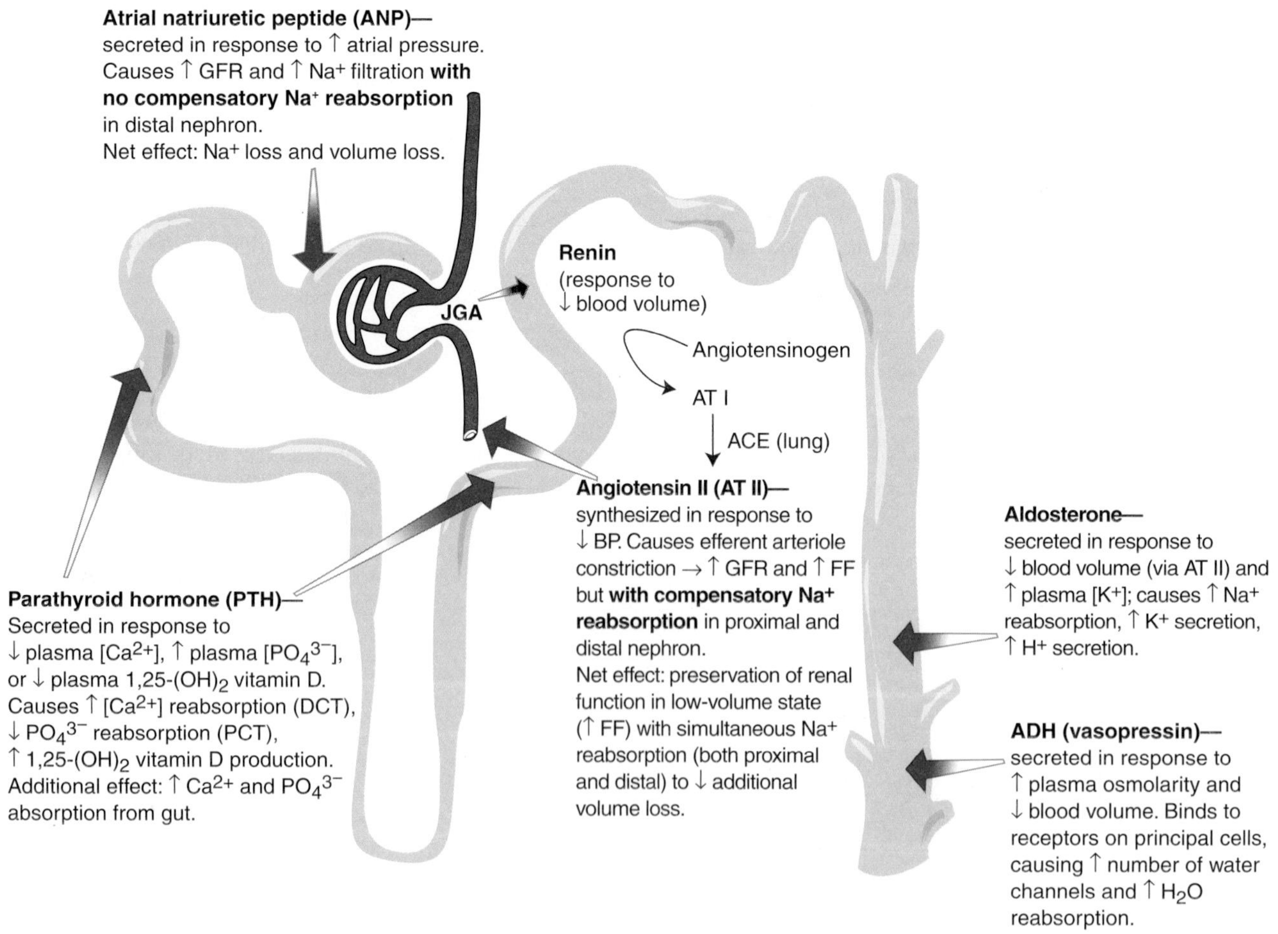

Atrial natriuretic peptide (ANP)—secreted in response to ↑ atrial pressure. Causes ↑ GFR and ↑ Na+ filtration **with no compensatory Na+ reabsorption** in distal nephron. Net effect: Na+ loss and volume loss.
JGA
Renin (response to ↓ blood volume)
Angiotensinogen
AT I
ACE (lung)
Angiotensin II (AT II)—synthesized in response to ↓ BP. Causes efferent arteriole constriction → ↑ GFR and ↑ FF but **with compensatory Na+ reabsorption** in proximal and distal nephron. Net effect: preservation of renal function in low-volume state (↑ FF) with simultaneous Na+ reabsorption (both proximal and distal) to ↓ additional volume loss.
Parathyroid hormone (PTH)—Secreted in response to ↓ plasma [Ca2+], ↑ plasma [PO43−], or ↓ plasma 1,25-(OH)2 vitamin D. Causes ↑ [Ca2+] reabsorption (DCT), ↓ PO43− reabsorption (PCT), ↑ 1,25-(OH)2 vitamin D production. Additional effect: ↑ Ca2+ and PO43− absorption from gut.
Aldosterone—secreted in response to ↓ blood volume (via AT II) and ↑ plasma [K+]; causes ↑ Na+ reabsorption, ↑ K+ secretion, ↑ H+ secretion.
ADH (vasopressin)—secreted in response to ↑ plasma osmolarity and ↓ blood volume. Binds to receptors on principal cells, causing ↑ number of water channels and ↑ H2O reabsorption.

Potassium shifts

SHIFTS K^+ OUT OF CELL (CAUSING HYPERKALEMIA)	SHIFTS K^+ INTO CELL (CAUSING HYPOKALEMIA)
Digitalis	
Hyper**O**smolarity	Hypo-osmolarity
Insulin deficiency	Insulin (↑ Na^+/K^+ ATPase)
Lysis of cells	
Acidosis	Alkalosis
β-adrenergic antagonist	β-adrenergic agonist (↑ Na^+/K^+ ATPase)
Patient with hyperkalemia? **DO Insulin LAβ** work.	**Insulin** shifts K^+ **into** cells

Electrolyte disturbances

Electrolyte	Low serum concentration	High serum concentration
Na^+	Nausea and malaise, stupor, coma	Irritability, stupor, coma
K^+	U waves on ECG, flattened T waves, arrhythmias, muscle weakness	Wide QRS and peaked T waves on ECG, arrhythmias, muscle weakness
Ca^{2+}	Tetany, seizures	**Stones** (renal), **bones** (pain), **groans** (abdominal pain), **psychiatric overtones** (anxiety, altered mental status), but not necessarily calciuria
Mg^{2+}	Tetany, arrhythmias	↓ DTRs, lethargy, bradycardia, hypotension, cardiac arrest, hypocalcemia
PO_4^{3-}	Bone loss, osteomalacia	Renal stones, metastatic calcifications, hypocalcemia

Acid-base physiology

	pH	P_{CO_2}	$[HCO_3^-]$	COMPENSATORY RESPONSE
Metabolic acidosis	↓	↓	**↓**	Hyperventilation (immediate)
Metabolic alkalosis	↑	↑	**↑**	Hypoventilation (immediate)
Respiratory acidosis	↓	**↑**	↑	↑ renal $[HCO_3^-]$ reabsorption (delayed)
Respiratory alkalosis	↑	**↓**	↓	↓ renal $[HCO_3^-]$ reabsorption (delayed)

Key: **↑ ↓** = 1° disturbance; ↓ ↑ = compensatory response.

Henderson-Hasselbalch equation: $pH = 6.1 + \log \frac{[HCO_3^-]}{0.03\ P_{CO_2}}$

The predicted respiratory compensation for a simple metabolic acidosis can be calculated using Winter's formula. If the measured P_{CO_2} differs significantly from the predicted P_{CO_2}, then a mixed acid-base disorder is likely present:

$$P_{CO_2} = 1.5\ (HCO_3^-) + 8 \pm 2$$

Acidosis/alkalosis

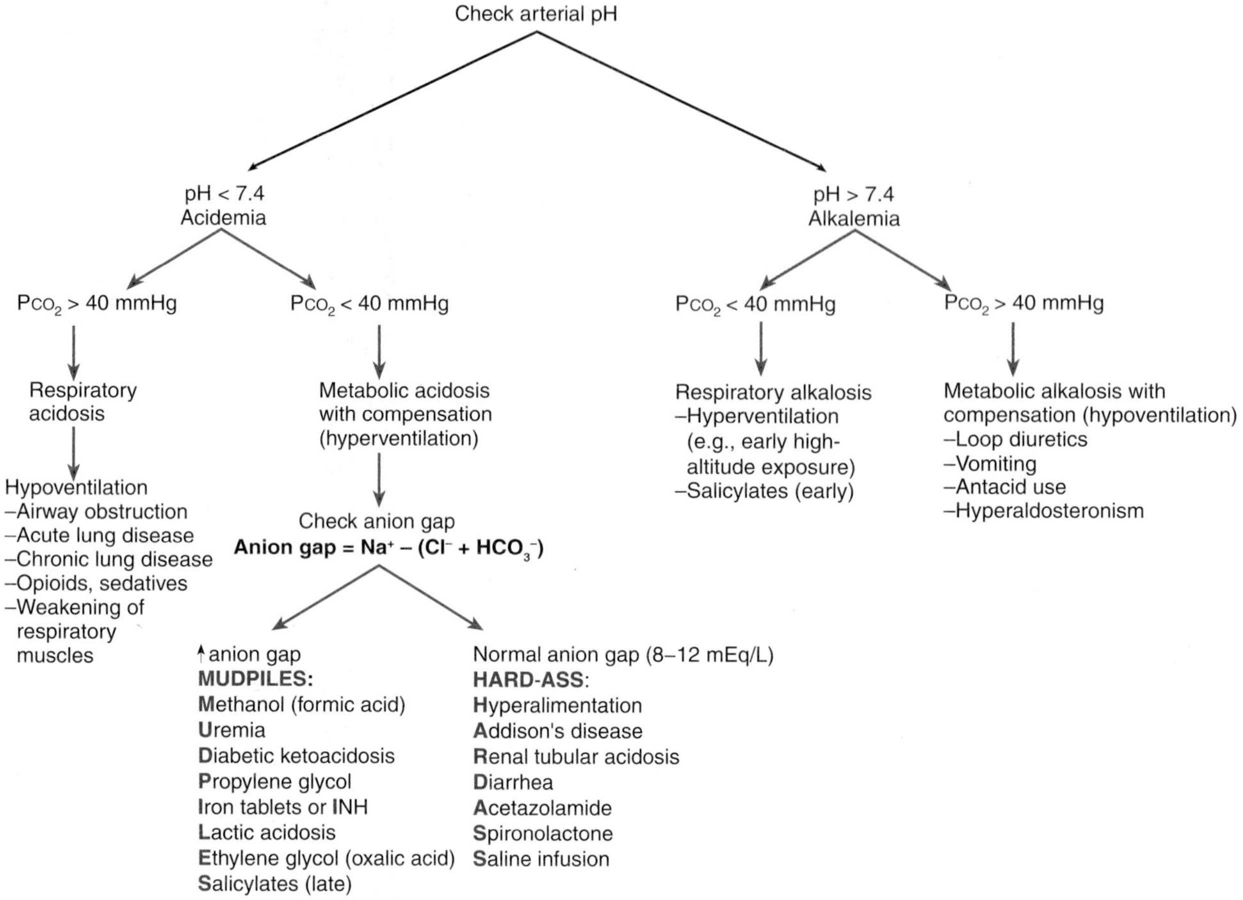

Renal tubular acidosis (RTA)

Type 1 ("distal")	Defect in collecting tubule's ability to excrete H^+. Untreated patients have urine pH > 5.5. Associated with hypokalemia. ↑ risk for calcium phosphate kidney stones as a result of ↑ urine pH and bone resorption.
Type 2 ("proximal")	Defect in proximal tubule HCO_3^- reabsorption. May be seen with Fanconi's syndrome. Untreated patients typically have urine pH < 5.5. Associated with hypokalemia. ↑ risk for hypophosphatemic rickets.
Type 4 ("hyperkalemic")	Hypoaldosteronism or lack of collecting tubule response to aldosterone. The resulting hyperkalemia impairs ammoniagenesis in the proximal tubule, leading to ↓ buffering capacity and ↓ urine pH.

▸ RENAL–PATHOLOGY

Casts in urine	Presence of casts indicates that hematuria/pyuria is of renal (vs. bladder) origin.	
RBC casts	Glomerulonephritis, ischemia, or malignant hypertension.	Bladder cancer, kidney stones → hematuria, no casts.
WBC casts	Tubulointerstitial inflammation, acute pyelonephritis, transplant rejection.	Acute cystitis → pyuria, no casts.
Fatty casts ("oval fat bodies")	Nephrotic syndrome.	
Granular ("muddy brown") casts	Acute tubular necrosis.	
Waxy casts	Advanced renal disease/chronic renal failure.	
Hyaline casts	Nonspecific, can be a normal finding.	

Nomenclature of glomerular disorders

TYPE	CHARACTERISTICS	EXAMPLE
Focal	< 50% of glomeruli are involved	Focal segmental glomerulosclerosis
Diffuse	> 50% of glomeruli are involved	Diffuse proliferative glomerulonephritis
Proliferative	Hypercellular glomeruli	Mesangial proliferative
Membranous	Thickening of glomerular basement membrane	Membranous nephropathy
1° glomerular disease	Involves only glomeruli, thus a primary disease of the kidney	Minimal change disease
2° glomerular disease	Involves glomeruli and other organs, thus a disease of another organ system, or a systemic disease that has impact on the kidney	SLE, diabetic nephropathy

Glomerular diseases

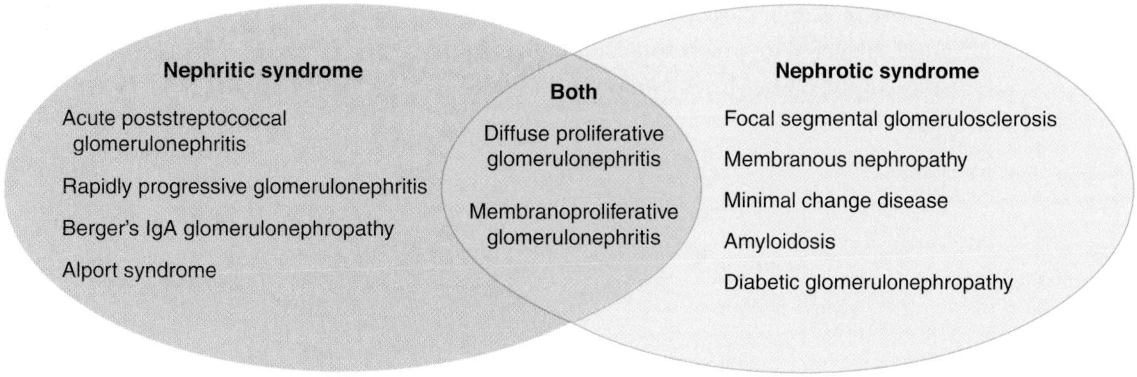
Nephritic syndrome
Acute poststreptococcal glomerulonephritis
Rapidly progressive glomerulonephritis
Berger's IgA glomerulonephropathy
Alport syndrome
Both
Diffuse proliferative glomerulonephritis
Membranoproliferative glomerulonephritis
Nephrotic syndrome
Focal segmental glomerulosclerosis
Membranous nephropathy
Minimal change disease
Amyloidosis
Diabetic glomerulonephropathy

Nephrotic syndrome

NephrOtic syndrome presents with massive prOteinuria (> 3.5g/day, frothy urine), hyperlipidemia, fatty casts, edema. Associated with thromboembolism (hypercoagulable state due to AT III loss in urine) and ↑ risk of infection (loss of immunoglobulins).

Focal segmental glomerulosclerosis

LM—segmental sclerosis and hyalinosis A.

EM—effacement of foot process similar to minimal change disease.

Most common cause of nephrotic syndrome in adults.

Associated with HIV infection, heroin abuse, massive obesity, interferon treatment, and chronic kidney disease due to congenital absence or surgical removal.

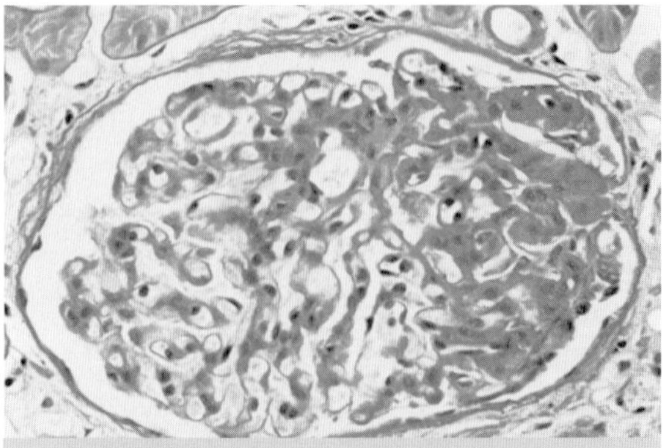

A Focal segmental glomerulosclerosis.

Membranous nephropathy

LM—diffuse capillary and GBM thickening B.

EM—"spike and dome" appearance with subepithelial deposits.

IF—granular. SLE's nephrotic presentation.

Second most common cause of primary nephrotic syndrome in adults. Can be idiopathic or caused by drugs, infections, SLE, solid tumors.

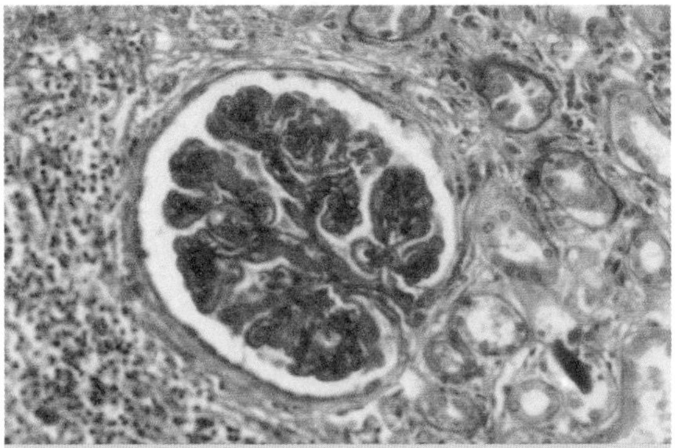

B Membranous nephropathy.

Minimal change disease (lipoid nephrosis)

LM—normal glomeruli.

EM—foot process effacement C.

Selective loss of albumin, not globulins, caused by GBM polyanion loss.

May be triggered by a recent infection or an immune stimulus. Most common in children. Responds to corticosteroids.

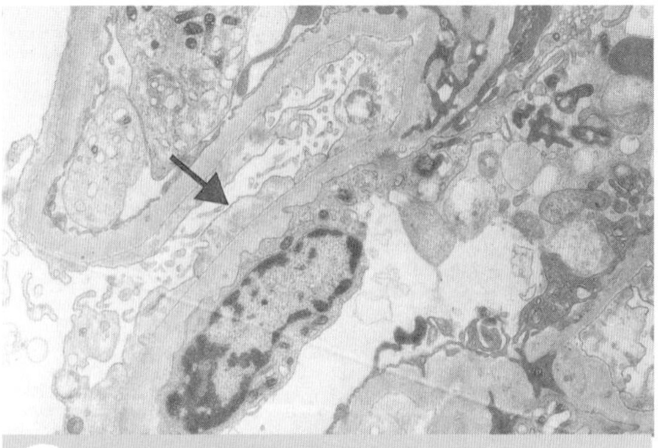

C **Minimal change disease (lipoid nephrosis).** Note effacement of foot processes on EM (red arrow).

Amyloidosis

LM—Congo red stain shows apple-green birefringence under polarized light.

Associated with chronic conditions (e.g., multiple myeloma, TB, RA).

Nephrotic syndrome *(continued)*

Membrano-proliferative glomerulonephritis (MPGN)	Type I—subendothelial IC deposits with granular IF; "tram-track" appearance due to GBM splitting caused by mesangial ingrowth D. Type II—intramembranous IC deposits; "dense deposits." Can also present as nephritic syndrome. Type I is associated with HBV, HCV. Type II is associated with C3 nephritic factor.	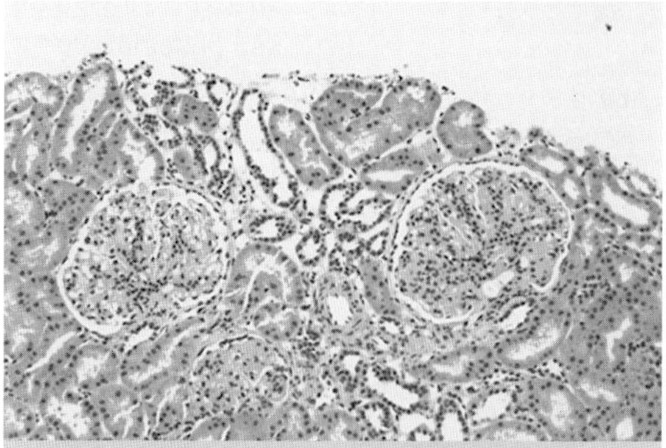 D Membranoproliferative glomerulonephritis.
Diabetic glomerulo-nephropathy	Nonenzymatic glycosylation (NEG) of GBM → ↑ permeability, thickening. NEG of efferent arterioles → ↑ GFR → mesangial expansion. LM—mesangial expansion, GBM thickening, eosinophilic nodular glomerulosclerosis (Kimmelstiel-Wilson lesion) E.	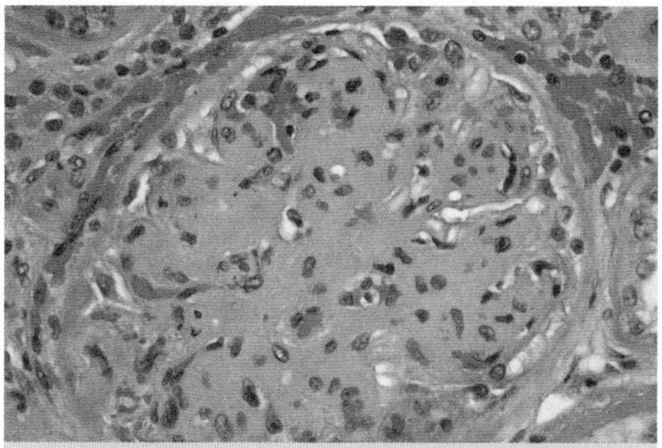 E Diabetic glomerulosclerosis.

Nephritic syndrome	Nephr**I**tic syndrome = an **I**nflammatory process. When it involves glomeruli, it leads to hematuria and RBC casts in urine. Associated with azotemia, oliguria, hypertension (due to salt retention), and proteinuria (< 3.5 g/day).	
Acute poststreptococcal glomerulonephritis	LM—glomeruli enlarged and hypercellular, neutrophils, "lumpy-bumpy" appearance. EM—subepithelial immune complex (IC) humps. IF—granular appearance due to IgG, IgM, and C3 deposition along GBM and mesangium.	Most frequently seen in children. Peripheral and periorbital edema, dark urine, and hypertension. Resolves spontaneously.
Rapidly progressive (crescentic) glomerulonephritis (RPGN) 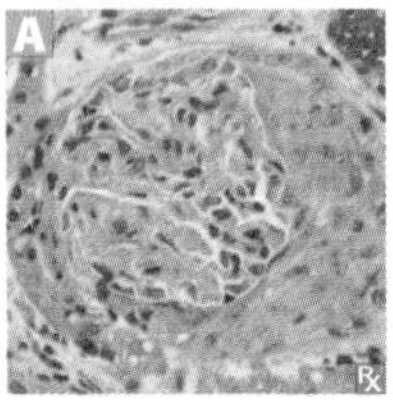	LM and IF—crescent-moon shape A. Crescents consist of fibrin and plasma proteins (e.g., C3b) with glomerular parietal cells, monocytes, and macrophages. Several disease processes may result in this pattern, including: ▪ **Goodpasture's syndrome**—type II hypersensitivity; antibodies to GBM and alveolar basement membrane → linear IF ▪ Granulomatosis with polyangiitis (Wegener's) ▪ Microscopic polyangiitis	Poor prognosis. Rapidly deteriorating renal function (days to weeks). Hematuria/hemoptysis. c-ANCA. p-ANCA.
Diffuse proliferative glomerulonephritis (DPGN)	Due to SLE or MPGN. LM—"wire looping" of capillaries. EM—subendothelial and sometimes intramembranous IgG-based ICs often with C3 deposition. IF—granular.	Most common cause of death in SLE. SLE and MPGN can present as nephrotic syndrome and nephritic syndrome concurrently.
Berger's disease (IgA nephropathy)	Related to Henoch-Schönlein purpura. LM—mesangial proliferation. EM—mesangial IC deposits. IF—IgA-based IC deposits in mesangium.	Often presents/flares with a URI or acute gastroenteritis.
Alport syndrome	Mutation in type IV collagen → split basement membrane. X-linked.	Glomerulonephritis, deafness, and, less commonly, eye problems.

LM = light microscopy; EM = electron microscopy; IF = immunofluorescence.

Kidney stones

Can lead to severe complications, such as hydronephrosis and pyelonephritis. Treat and prevent by encouraging fluid intake.

CONTENT	FREQUENCY	PRECIPITATES AT	X-RAY	NOTES
Calcium	80%	↑ pH (calcium phosphate) ↓ pH (calcium oxalate)	Radiopaque	Calcium oxalate, calcium phosphate, or both. Conditions that cause hypercalcemia (cancer, ↑ PTH) can → hypercalciuria and stones. Oxalate crystals can result from ethylene glycol (antifreeze) or vitamin C abuse. Treatments for recurrent stones include thiazides and citrate. Most common kidney stone presentation: calcium oxalate stone in a patient with hypercalciuria and normocalcemia.
Ammonium magnesium phosphate ("struvite") 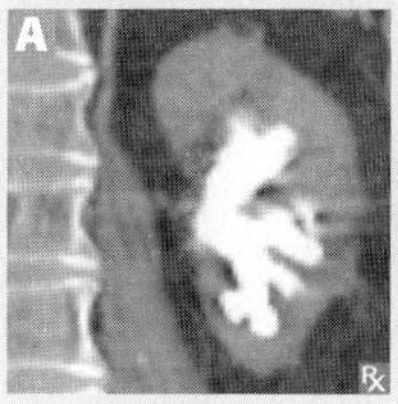	15%	↑ pH	Radiopaque	Caused by infection with urease-positive bugs (*Proteus mirabilis, Staphylococcus, Klebsiella*) that hydrolyze urea to ammonia → urine alkalinization. Can form staghorn calculi A that can be a nidus for UTIs.
Uric acid	5%	↓ pH	RadiolUcent	Visible on CT and ultrasound but not x-ray. Strong association with hyperuricemia (e.g., gout). Often seen in diseases with ↑ cell turnover, such as leukemia. Treat with alkalinization of urine.
Cystine	1%	↓ pH	Radiopaque	Most often 2° to cystinuria. Hexagonal crystals. Treat with alkalinization of urine.

Hydronephrosis

Back-up of urine into the kidney. Can be caused by urinary tract obstruction or vesicoureteral reflux. Causes dilation of renal pelvis and calyces proximal to obstruction. May result in parenchymal thinning in chronic, severe cases.

Renal cell carcinoma	Originates from proximal tubule cells → polygonal clear cells A filled with accumulated lipids and carbohydrates. Most common in men 50–70 years of age. ↑ incidence with smoking and obesity. Manifests clinically with hematuria, palpable mass B, 2° polycythemia, flank pain, fever, and weight loss. Invades renal vein then IVC and spreads hematogenously; metastasizes to lung and bone.	Most common renal malignancy. Associated with gene deletion on chromosome 3 (deletion may be sporadic or inherited as von Hippel-Lindau syndrome). Associated with paraneoplastic syndromes (ectopic EPO, ACTH, PTHrP). "Silent" cancer because in retroperitoneum, commonly presents as a metastatic neoplasm. Treatment: resection if localized disease. Resistant to conventional chemotherapy and radiation therapy.

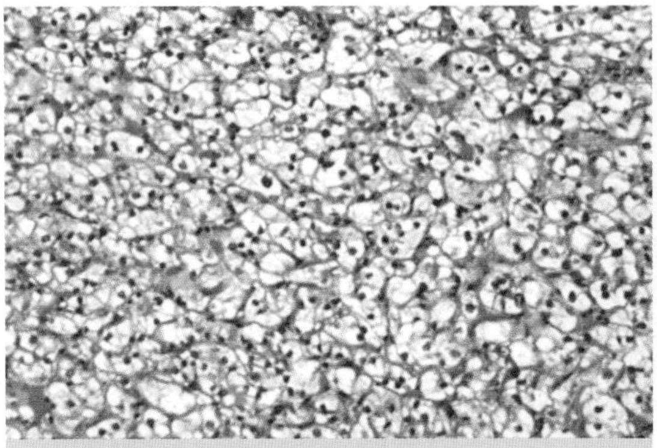

A Renal cell carcinoma (histology).

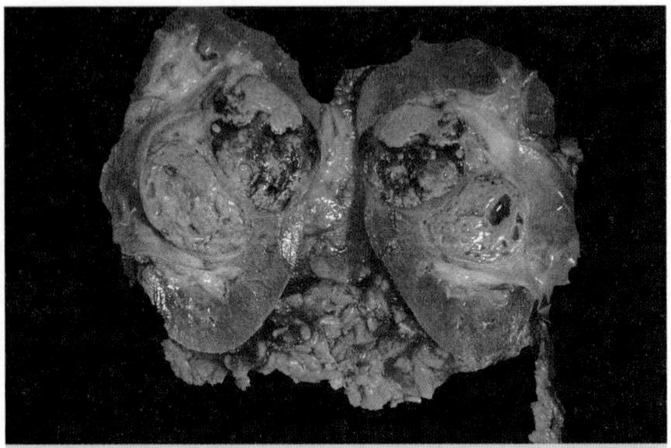

B Renal cell carcinoma (gross).

Wilms' tumor (nephroblastoma)	Most common renal malignancy of early childhood (ages 2–4). Contains embryonic glomerular structures. Presents with huge, palpable flank mass and/or hematuria.	Deletion of tumor suppressor gene *WT1* on chromosome 11. May be part of Beckwith-Wiedemann syndrome or **WAGR** complex: **W**ilms' tumor, **A**niridia, **G**enitourinary malformation, and mental **R**etardation.
Transitional cell carcinoma	Most common tumor of urinary tract system (can occur in renal calyces, renal pelvis, ureters, and bladder) A. Painless hematuria (no casts) suggests bladder cancer. Associated with problems in your **P**ee **SAC**: **P**henacetin, **S**moking, **A**niline dyes, and **C**yclophosphamide.	

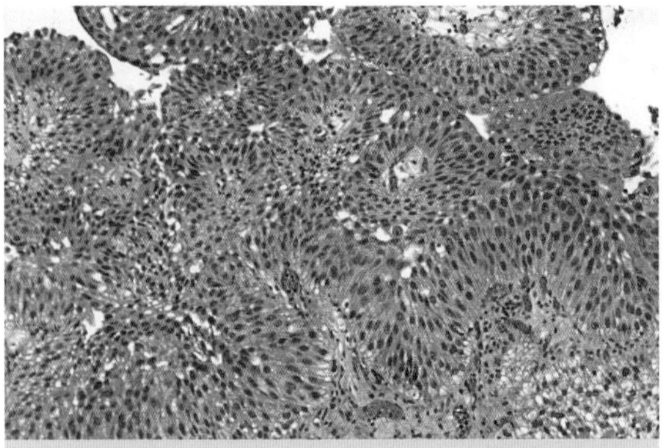

A **Transitional cell carcinoma.** Papillary growth lined by transitional epithelium with mild nuclear atypia and pleomorphism.

Pyelonephritis

Acute	Affects cortex with relative sparing of glomeruli/vessels A. Presents with fever, costovertebral angle tenderness, nausea, and vomiting. White cell casts in urine are classic.	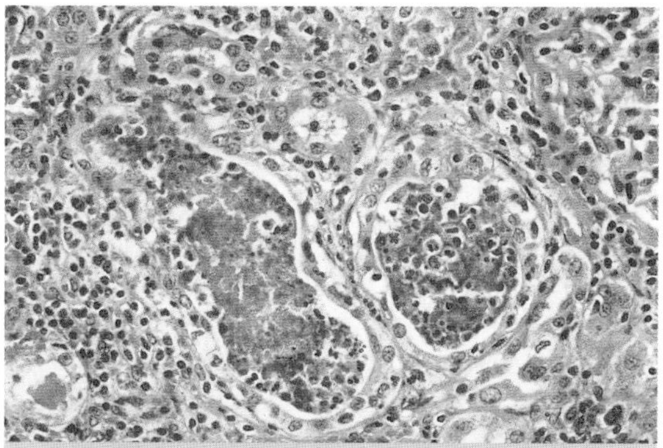 A **Acute pyelonephritis.** Neutrophilic infiltration into renal interstitium.
Chronic	The result of recurrent episodes of acute pyelonephritis. Typically requires predisposition to infection such as vesicoureteral reflux or chronically obstructing kidney stones. Coarse, asymmetric corticomedullary scarring, blunted calyx B. Tubules can contain eosinophilic casts (thyroidization of kidney).	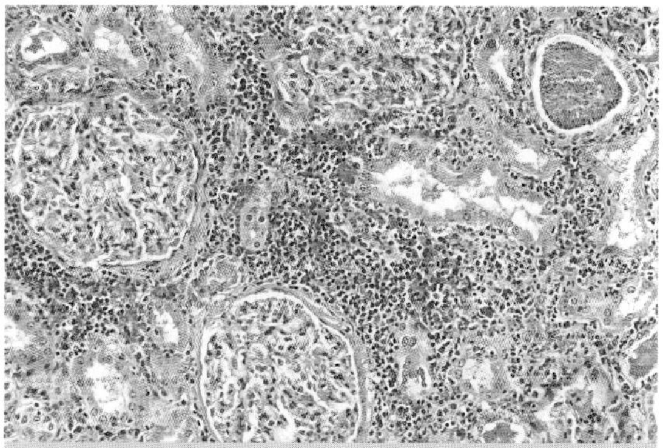 B **Chronic pyelonephritis.** Lymphocytic invasion with fibrosis.

Drug-induced interstitial nephritis (tubulointerstitial nephritis)	Acute interstitial renal inflammation. Pyuria (classically eosinophils) and azotemia occurring after administration of drugs that act as haptens, inducing hypersensitivity. Nephritis typically occurs 1–2 weeks after certain drugs (e.g., diuretics, penicillin derivatives, sulfonamides, rifampin), but can occur months after starting NSAIDs.	Associated with fever, rash, hematuria, and costovertebral angle tenderness, but can be asymptomatic.
Diffuse cortical necrosis	Acute generalized cortical infarction of both kidneys. Likely due to a combination of vasospasm and DIC.	Associated with obstetric catastrophes (e.g., abruptio placentae) and septic shock.

Acute tubular necrosis

Most common cause of intrinsic renal failure. Self-reversible in some cases, but can be fatal if left untreated. Death most often occurs during initial oliguric phase.

3 stages:

1. Inciting event
2. Maintenance phase—oliguric; lasts 1–3 weeks; risk of hyperkalemia
3. Recovery phase—polyuric; BUN and serum creatinine fall; risk of hypokalemia

Associated with renal ischemia (e.g., shock, sepsis), crush injury (myoglobinuria), drugs, toxins.

Key finding: granular ("muddy brown") casts.

Renal papillary necrosis

Sloughing of renal papillae → gross hematuria and proteinuria. May be triggered by a recent infection or immune stimulus. Associated with:

- Diabetes mellitus
- Acute pyelonephritis
- Chronic phenacetin use (acetaminophen is phenacetin derivative)
- Sickle cell anemia and trait

Acute renal failure (acute kidney injury)

In normal nephron, BUN is reabsorbed (for countercurrent multiplication), but creatinine is not. Acute renal failure is defined as an abrupt decline in renal function with ↑ creatinine and ↑ BUN over a period of several days.

Prerenal azotemia

As a result of ↓ RBF (e.g., hypotension) → ↓ GFR. Na^+/H_2O and urea retained by kidney in an attempt to conserve volume, so BUN/creatinine ratio ↑.

Intrinsic renal failure

Generally due to acute tubular necrosis or ischemia/toxins; less commonly due to acute glomerulonephritis (e.g., RPGN). Patchy necrosis leads to debris obstructing tubule and fluid backflow across necrotic tubule → ↓ GFR. Urine has epithelial/granular casts. BUN reabsorption is impaired → ↓ BUN/creatinine ratio.

Postrenal azotemia

Due to outflow obstruction (stones, BPH, neoplasia, congenital anomalies). Develops only with bilateral obstruction.

Variable	Prerenal	Intrinsic Renal	Postrenal
Urine osmolality (mOsm/kg)	> 500	< 350	< 350
Urine Na (mEq/L)	< 20	> 40	> 40
Fe_{Na}	< 1%	> 2%	> 2%
Serum BUN/Cr	> 20	< 15	> 15

Consequences of renal failure	Inability to make urine and excrete nitrogenous wastes.
	Consequences:
	▪ Na^+/H_2O retention (CHF, pulmonary edema, hypertension)
	▪ Hyperkalemia
	▪ Metabolic acidosis
	▪ Uremia—clinical syndrome marked by ↑ BUN and ↑ creatinine
	  ▪ Nausea and anorexia
	  ▪ Pericarditis
	  ▪ Asterixis
	  ▪ Encephalopathy
	  ▪ Platelet dysfunction
	▪ Anemia (failure of erythropoietin production)
	▪ Renal osteodystrophy (see below)
	▪ Dyslipidemia (especially ↑ triglycerides)
	▪ Growth retardation and developmental delay (in children)
		2 forms of renal failure—acute (e.g., ATN) and chronic (e.g., hypertension and diabetes).

Renal osteodystrophy	Failure of vitamin D hydroxylation, hypocalcemia, and hyperphosphatemia → 2° hyperparathyroidism. Hyperphosphatemia also independently ↓ serum Ca^{2+} by causing tissue calcifications, whereas ↓ 1,25-$(OH)_2$ vitamin D → ↓ intestinal Ca^{2+} absorption. Causes subperiosteal thinning of bones.	

Renal cysts

ADPKD	Formerly adult polycystic kidney disease. Multiple, large, bilateral cysts A that ultimately destroy the kidney parenchyma. Presents with flank pain, hematuria, hypertension, urinary infection, progressive renal failure. Autosomal-Dominant mutation in *PKD1* or *PKD2*. Death from complications of chronic kidney disease or hypertension (caused by ↑ renin production). Associated with berry aneurysms, mitral valve prolapse, benign hepatic cysts.	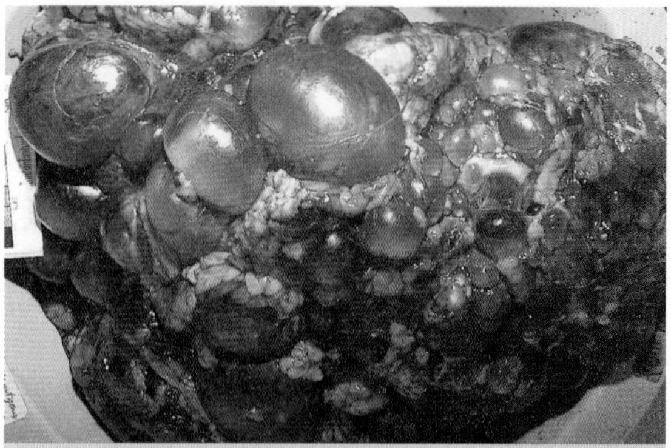 A **ADPKD.** Distended kidney with multiple fluid-filled cysts.
ARPKD	Formerly infantile polycystic kidney disease. Infantile presentation in parenchyma. Autosomal Recessive. Associated with congenital hepatic fibrosis. Significant renal failure in utero can lead to Potter's syndrome. Concerns beyond neonatal period include hypertension, portal hypertension, and progressive renal insufficiency.	
Medullary cystic disease	Inherited disease causing tubulointerstitial fibrosis and progressive renal insufficiency with inability to concentrate urine. Medullary cysts usually not visualized; shrunken kidneys on ultrasound. Poor prognosis.	

▶ RENAL–PHARMACOLOGY

Diuretics: site of action

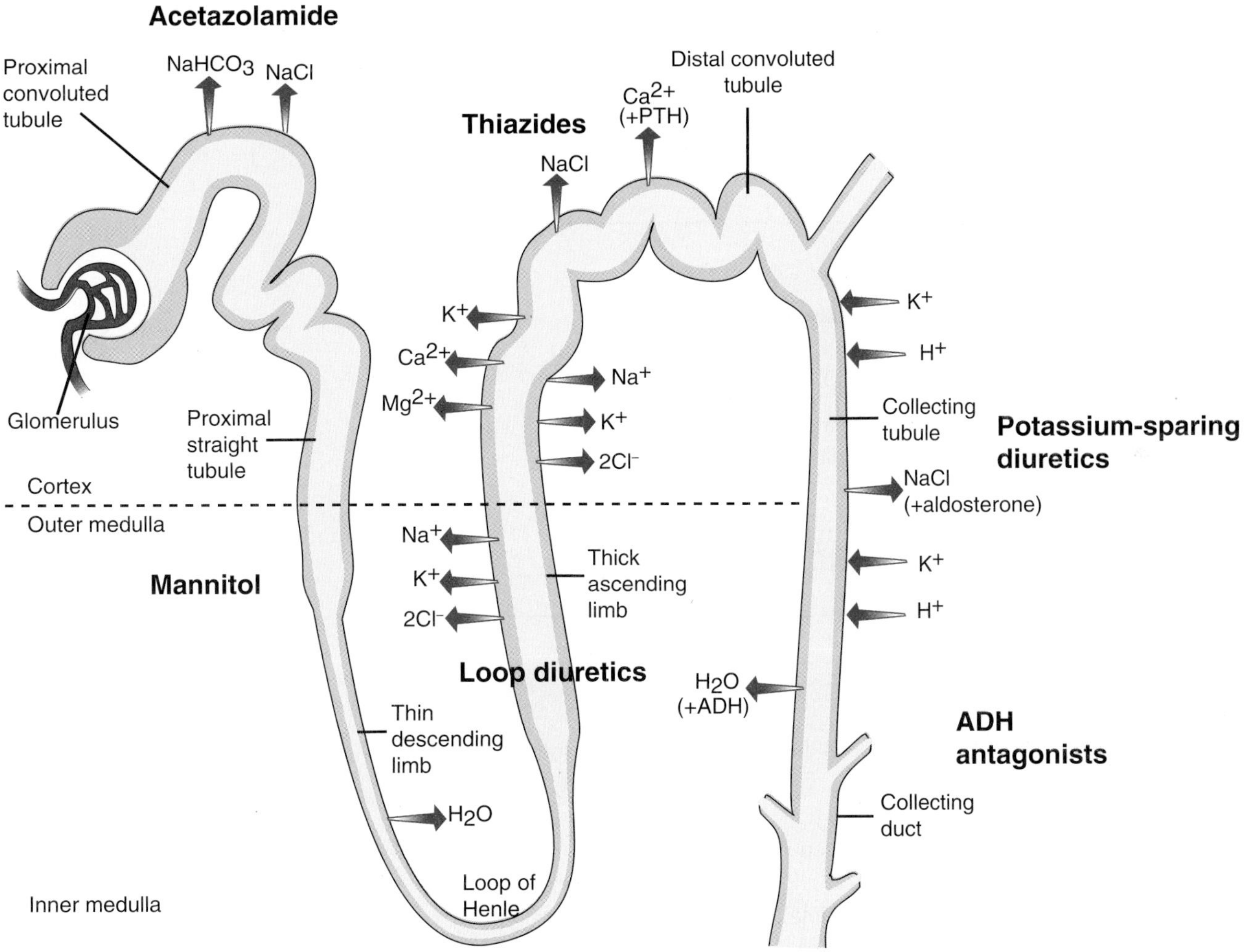

(Adapted, with permission, from Katzung BG. *Basic and Clinical Pharmacology,* 7th ed. Stamford, CT: Appleton & Lange, 1997: 243.)

Mannitol

MECHANISM	Osmotic diuretic, ↑ tubular fluid osmolarity, producing ↑ urine flow, ↓ intracranial/intraocular pressure.
CLINICAL USE	Drug overdose, elevated intracranial/intraocular pressure.
TOXICITY	Pulmonary edema, dehydration. Contraindicated in anuria, CHF.

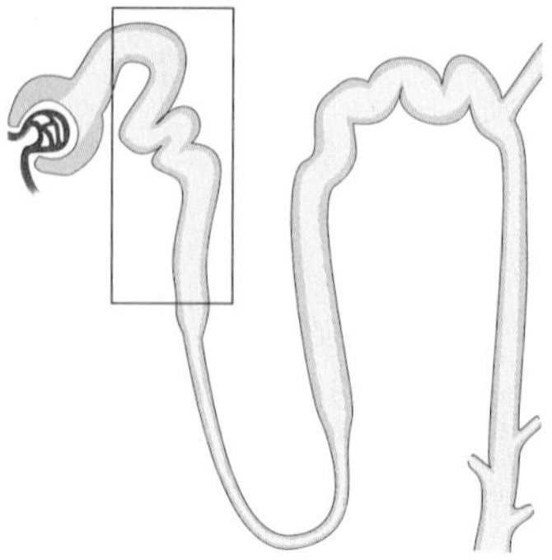

Acetazolamide

MECHANISM	Carbonic anhydrase inhibitor. Causes self-limited $NaHCO_3$ diuresis and reduction in total-body HCO_3^- stores.	
CLINICAL USE	Glaucoma, urinary alkalinization, metabolic alkalosis, altitude sickness, pseudotumor cerebri.	
TOXICITY	Hyperchloremic metabolic acidosis, paresthesias, NH_3 toxicity, sulfa allergy.	"**ACID**"azolamide causes **ACID**osis.

Loop diuretics

Furosemide

MECHANISM	Sulfonamide loop diuretic. Inhibits cotransport system (Na^+, K^+, 2 Cl^-) of thick ascending limb of loop of Henle. Abolishes hypertonicity of medulla, preventing concentration of urine. Stimulates PGE release (vasodilatory effect on afferent arteriole); inhibited by NSAIDs. ↑ Ca^{2+} excretion. **L**oops **L**ose calcium.	
CLINICAL USE	Edematous states (CHF, cirrhosis, nephrotic syndrome, pulmonary edema), hypertension, hypercalcemia.	
TOXICITY	**O**totoxicity, **H**ypokalemia, **D**ehydration, **A**llergy (sulfa), **N**ephritis (interstitial), **G**out.	**OH DANG**!

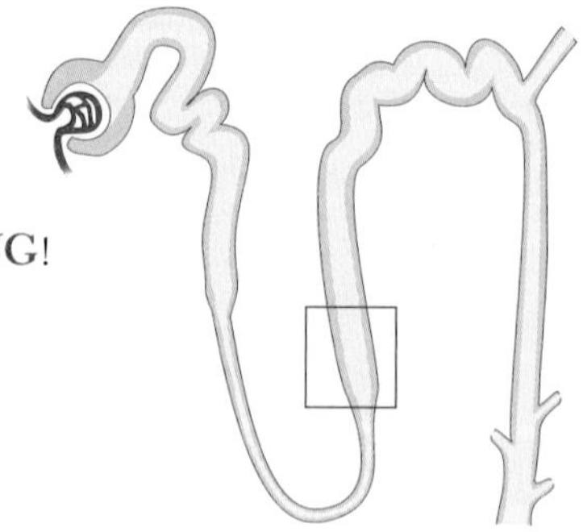

Ethacrynic acid

MECHANISM	Phenoxyacetic acid derivative (not a sulfonamide). Essentially same action as furosemide.
CLINICAL USE	Diuresis in patients allergic to sulfa drugs.
TOXICITY	Similar to furosemide; can cause hyperuricemia; never use to treat gout.

Hydrochlorothiazide

MECHANISM	Thiazide diuretic. Inhibits NaCl reabsorption in early distal tubule, reducing diluting capacity of the nephron. ↓ Ca^{2+} excretion.	
CLINICAL USE	Hypertension, CHF, idiopathic hypercalciuria, nephrogenic diabetes insipidus.	
TOXICITY	Hypokalemic metabolic alkalosis, hyponatremia, hyper**G**lycemia, hyper**L**ipidemia, hyper**U**ricemia, and hyper**C**alcemia. Sulfa allergy.	Hyper**GLUC**.

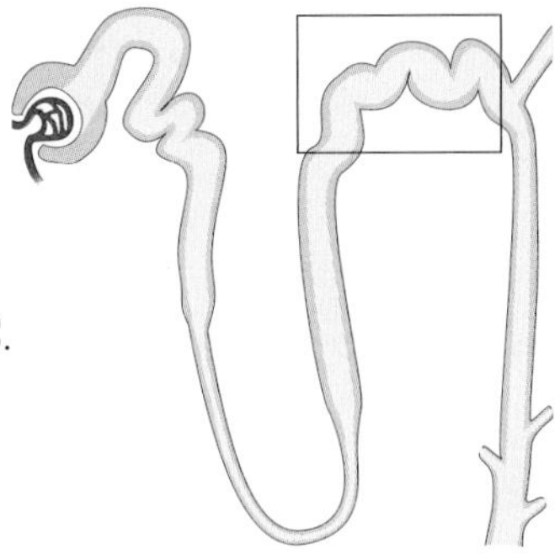

K^+-sparing diuretics

Spironolactone and eplerenone; **T**riamterene, and **A**miloride. — The K^+ **STA**ys.

MECHANISM	Spironolactone and eplerenone are competitive aldosterone receptor antagonists in the cortical collecting tubule. Triamterene and amiloride act at the same part of the tubule by blocking Na^+ channels in the CCT.
CLINICAL USE	Hyperaldosteronism, K^+ depletion, CHF.
TOXICITY	Hyperkalemia (can lead to arrhythmias), endocrine effects with spironolactone (e.g., gynecomastia, antiandrogen effects).

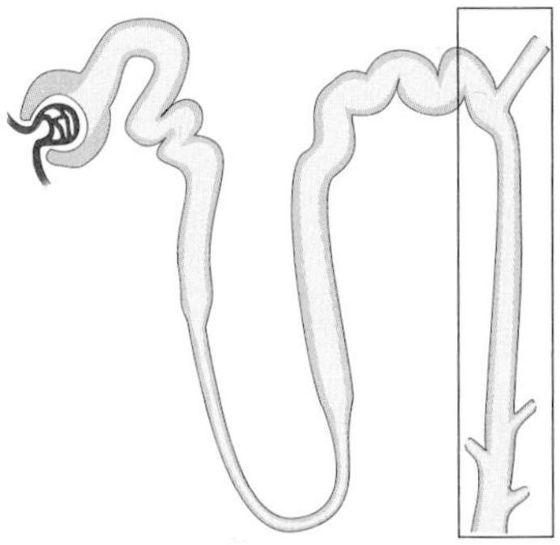

Diuretics: electrolyte changes

Urine NaCl	↑ (all diuretics). Serum NaCl may ↓ as a result.
Urine K^+	↑ (all except K^+-sparing diuretics). Serum K^+ may ↓ as a result.
Blood pH	↓ (**acidemia**): carbonic anhydrase inhibitors— ↓ HCO_3^- reabsorption. K^+ sparing—aldosterone blockade prevents K^+ secretion and H^+ secretion. Additionally, hyperkalemia leads to K^+ entering all cells (via H^+/K^+ exchanger) in exchange for H^+ exiting cells. ↑ (**alkalemia**): loop diuretics and thiazides cause alkalemia through several mechanisms: ▪ Volume contraction → ↑ AT II → ↑ Na^+/H^+ exchange in proximal tubule → ↑ HCO_3^- reabsorption ("contraction alkalosis") ▪ K^+ loss leads to K^+ exiting all cells (via H^+/K^+ exchanger) in exchange for H^+ entering cells ▪ In low K^+ state, H^+ (rather than K^+) is exchanged for Na^+ in cortical collecting tubule, leading to alkalosis and "paradoxical aciduria"
Urine Ca^{2+}	↑ with loop diuretics: ↓ paracellular Ca^{2+} reabsorption → hypocalcemia. ↓ with **thiazides**: Enhanced paracellular Ca^{2+} reabsorption in proximal tubule and loop of Henle.

ACE inhibitors	Captopril, enalapril, lisinopril.	
MECHANISM	Inhibit angiotensin-converting enzyme (ACE) → ↓ angiotensin II → ↓ GFR by preventing constriction of efferent arterioles. Levels of renin ↑ as a result of loss of feedback inhibition. Inhibition of ACE also prevents inactivation of bradykinin, a potent vasodilator.	Angiotensin II receptor blockers (-sartans) have effects similar to ACE inhibitors but do not ↑ bradykinin → no cough or angioedema.
CLINICAL USE	Hypertension, CHF, proteinuria, diabetic renal disease. Prevent unfavorable heart remodeling as a result of chronic hypertension.	
TOXICITY	**C**ough, **A**ngioedema, **T**eratogen (fetal renal malformations), **C**reatinine increase (↓ GFR), **H**yperkalemia, and **H**ypotension. Avoid in bilateral renal artery stenosis, because ACE inhibitors will further ↓ GFR → renal failure.	Captopril's **CATCHH**.

HIGH-YIELD SYSTEMS

Reproductive

"Artificial insemination is when the farmer does it to the cow instead of the bull."

—Student essay

"Whoever called it necking was a poor judge of anatomy."

—Groucho Marx

"See, the problem is that God gives men a brain and a penis, and only enough blood to run one at a time."

—Robin Williams

▸ REPRODUCTIVE–EMBRYOLOGY

Important genes of embryogenesis

Sonic hedgehog gene	Produced at base of limbs in zone of polarizing activity. Involved in patterning along anterior-posterior axis. Involved in CNS development; mutation can cause holoprosencephaly.
***Wnt-7* gene**	Produced at apical ectodermal ridge (thickened ectoderm at distal end of each developing limb). Necessary for proper organization along dorsal-ventral axis.
***FGF* gene**	Produced at apical ectodermal ridge. Stimulates mitosis of underlying mesoderm, providing for lengthening of limbs.
Homeobox (Hox) genes	Involved in segmental organization of embryo in a craniocaudal direction. Hox mutations → appendages in wrong locations.

Early fetal development

DAY 0	Fertilization by sperm forming zygote, initiating embryogenesis.
WITHIN WEEK 1	hCG secretion begins after implantation of blastocyst.
WITHIN WEEK 2	Bilaminar disc (epiblast, hypoblast). 2 weeks = 2 layers.
WITHIN WEEK 3	Trilaminar disc. 3 weeks = 3 layers. Gastrulation. Primitive streak, notochord, mesoderm and its organization, and neural plate begin to form.
WEEKS 3–8 (EMBRYONIC PERIOD)	Neural tube formed by neuroectoderm and closes by week 4. Organogenesis. Extremely susceptible to teratogens.
WEEK 4	Heart begins to beat. Upper and lower limb buds begin to form. 4 weeks = 4 limbs.
WEEK 8 (START OF FETAL PERIOD)	Fetal movement, fetus looks like a baby.
WEEK 10	Genitalia have male/female characteristics.

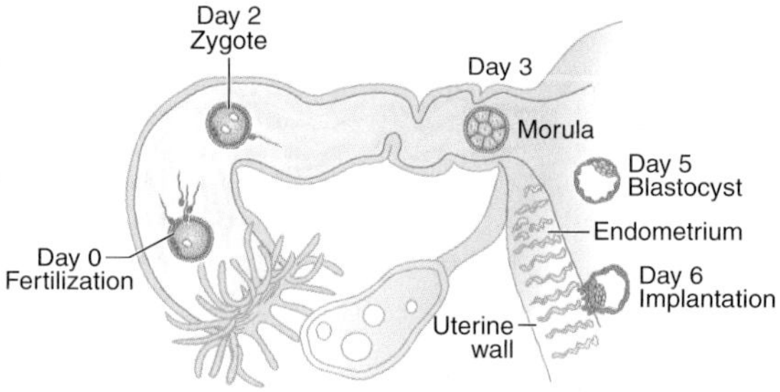

Gastrulation

Process that forms the trilaminar embryonic disc. Establishes the ectoderm, mesoderm, and endoderm germ layers. Starts with the epiblast invaginating to form the primitive streak.

Embryologic derivatives

Ectoderm		
Surface ectoderm	Adenohypophysis (from Rathke's pouch); lens of eye; epithelial linings of oral cavity, sensory organs of ear, and olfactory epithelium; epidermis; anal canal below the pectinate line; parotid, sweat, and mammary glands.	Craniopharyngioma—benign Rathke's pouch tumor with cholesterol crystals, calcifications.
Neuroectoderm	Brain (neurohypophysis, CNS neurons, oligodendrocytes, astrocytes, ependymal cells, pineal gland), retina and optic nerve, spinal cord.	Neuroectoderm—think CNS.
Neural crest	PNS (dorsal root ganglia, cranial nerves, celiac ganglion, Schwann cells, ANS), melanocytes, chromaffin cells of adrenal medulla, parafollicular (C) cells of thyroid, Schwann cells, pia and arachnoid, bones of the skull, odontoblasts, aorticopulmonary septum.	Neural crest—think PNS and non-neural structures nearby.
Mesoderm	Muscle, bone, connective tissue, serous linings of body cavities (e.g., peritoneum), spleen (derived from foregut mesentery), cardiovascular structures, lymphatics, blood, wall of gut tube, wall of bladder, urethra, vagina, kidneys, adrenal cortex, dermis, testes, ovaries. Notochord induces ectoderm to form neuroectoderm (neural plate). Its only postnatal derivative is the nucleus pulposus of the intervertebral disc.	Mesodermal defects = **VACTERL**: **V**ertebral defects **A**nal atresia **C**ardiac defects **T**racheo-**E**sophageal fistula **R**enal defects **L**imb defects (bone and muscle)
Endoderm	Gut tube epithelium (including anal canal above the pectinate line) and luminal epithelial derivatives (e.g., lungs, liver, gallbladder, pancreas, eustachian tube, thymus, parathyroid, thyroid follicular cells).	

Types of errors in organ morphogenesis

Agenesis	Absent organ due to absent primordial tissue.
Aplasia	Absent organ despite present primordial tissue.
Deformation	Extrinsic disruption; occurs after the embryonic period.
Hypoplasia	Incomplete organ development; primordial tissue present.
Malformation	Intrinsic disruption; occurs during the embryonic period (weeks 3–8).

Teratogens

Most susceptible in 3rd–8th weeks (embryonic period—organogenesis) of pregnancy. Before week 3: all-or-none effects. After week 8: growth and function affected.

TERATOGEN	EFFECTS ON FETUS	NOTES
Medications		
ACE inhibitors	Renal damage	
Alkylating agents	Absence of digits, multiple anomalies	
Aminoglycosides	CN VIII toxicity	**A mean guy** hit the baby in the ear.
Carbamazepine	Neural tube defects, craniofacial defects, fingernail hypoplasia, developmental delay, IUGR	
Diethylstilbestrol (DES)	Vaginal clear cell adenocarcinoma, congenital Müllerian anomalies	
Folate antagonists	Neural tube defects	
Lithium	Ebstein's anomaly (atrialized right ventricle)	
Phenytoin	Fetal hydantoin syndrome: microcephaly, dysmorphic craniofacial features, hypoplastic nails and distal phalanges, cardiac defects, IUGR, mental retardation	
Tetracyclines	Discolored teeth	
Thalidomide	Limb defects ("flipper" limbs)	**Limb** defects with "tha-**limb**-domide."
Valproate	Inhibition of maternal folate absorption → neural tube defects	
Warfarin	Bone deformities, fetal hemorrhage, abortion, ophthalmologic abnormalities	Do not wage **warfare** on the baby; keep it **heppy** with **heparin** (does not cross placenta).
Substance abuse		
Alcohol	Leading cause of birth defects and mental retardation; fetal alcohol syndrome	
Cocaine	Abnormal fetal development and fetal addiction; placental abruption	
Smoking (nicotine, CO)	Preterm labor, placental problems, IUGR, ADHD	
Other		
Iodide (lack or excess)	Congenital goiter or hypothyroidism (cretinism)	
Maternal diabetes	Caudal regression syndrome (anal atresia to sirenomelia), congenital heart defects, neural tube defects	
Vitamin A (excess)	Extremely high risk for spontaneous abortions and birth defects (cleft palate, cardiac abnormalities)	
X-rays	Microcephaly, mental retardation	

Fetal infections and certain antibiotics can also cause congenital malformations (see the Microbiology chapter).

Fetal alcohol syndrome Leading cause of congenital malformations in the United States. Newborns of mothers who consumed significant amounts of alcohol during pregnancy have an ↑ incidence of congenital abnormalities, including mental retardation, pre- and postnatal developmental retardation, microcephaly, holoprosencephaly, facial abnormalities, limb dislocation, and heart and lung fistulas.

Twinning Dizygotic twins arise from 2 eggs that are separately fertilized by 2 different sperm (always 2 zygotes), and will have 2 separate amniotic sacs and 2 separate placentas (chorions). Monozygotic twins arise from 1 fertilized egg (1 egg + 1 sperm) that splits into 2 zygotes in early pregnancy. The degree of separation between monozygotic twins depends on when the fertilized egg splits into 2 zygotes. The timing of this separation determines the number of chorions and the number of amnions.

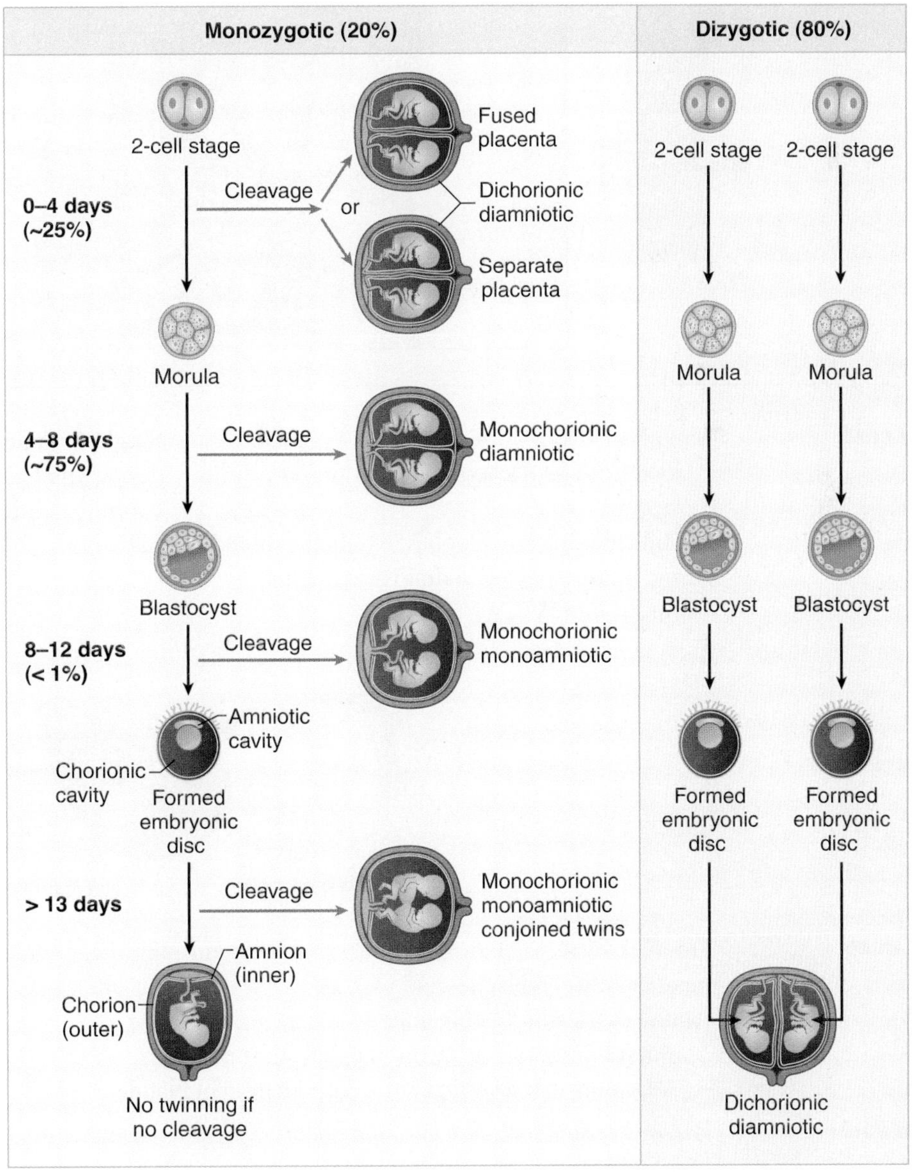

(Adapted, with permission, from Cunningham FG et al. *Williams Obstetrics*, 23rd ed. New York: McGraw-Hill, 2009: Fig. 39-2.)

Placental development	1° site of nutrient and gas exchange between mother and fetus.	
Fetal component		
Cytotrophoblast	Inner layer of chorionic villi.	Cytotrophoblast makes Cells.
Syncytiotrophoblast	Outer layer of chorionic villi; secretes hCG (structurally similar to LH; stimulates corpus luteum to secrete progesterone during first trimester).	
Maternal component		
Decidua basalis	Derived from the endometrium. Maternal blood in lacunae.	

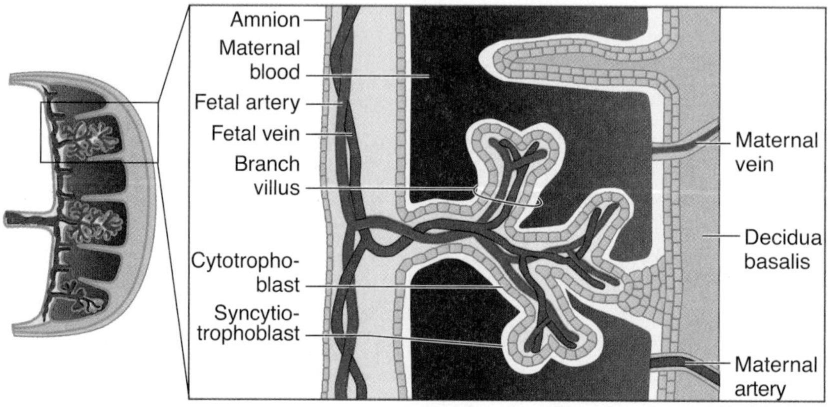

Umbilical cord	Umbilical arteries (2)—return deoxygenated blood from fetal internal iliac arteries to placenta. Umbilical vein (1)—supplies oxygenated blood from placenta to fetus; drains via ductus venosus into IVC.	Single umbilical artery is associated with congenital and chromosomal anomalies. Umbilical arteries and veins are derived from allantois.

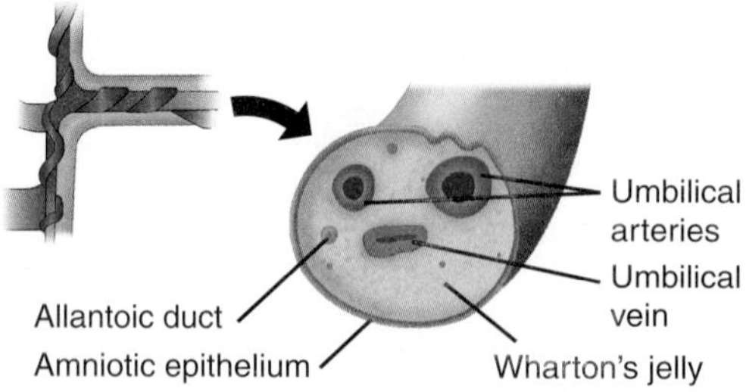

Urachal duct

3rd week—yolk sac forms allantois, which extends into urogenital sinus. Allantois becomes urachus, a duct between bladder and yolk sac.

Failure of urachus to obliterate:

- **Patent urachus**—urine discharge from umbilicus.
- **Vesicourachal diverticulum**—outpouching of bladder.

Vitelline duct

7th week—obliteration of vitelline duct (omphalo-mesenteric duct), which connects yolk sac to midgut lumen.

Failure of vitelline duct to close:

- **Vitelline fistula** → meconium discharge from umbilicus.
- **Meckel's diverticulum**—partial closure, with patent portion attached to ileum. May have ectopic gastric mucosa → melena, periumbilical pain, and ulcer.

Aortic arch derivatives	Develop into the arterial system.	
1st	Part of **max**illary artery (branch of external carotid).	1st arch is **max**imal.
2nd	Stapedial artery and hyoid artery.	Second = Stapedial.
3rd	Common Carotid artery and proximal part of internal Carotid artery.	C is 3rd letter of alphabet.
4th	On left, aortic arch; on right, proximal part of right subclavian artery.	4th arch (4 limbs) = systemic.
6th	Proximal part of pulmonary arteries and (on left only) ductus arteriosus.	6th arch = pulmonary and the pulmonary-to-systemic shunt (ductus arteriosus).

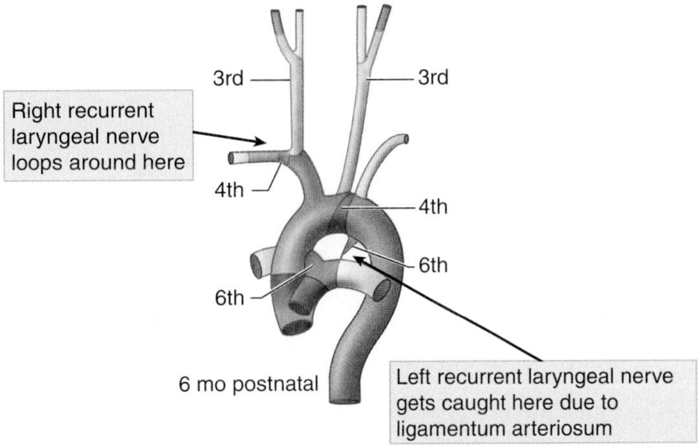

3rd
3rd
Right recurrent laryngeal nerve loops around here
4th
4th
6th
6th
6 mo postnatal
Left recurrent laryngeal nerve gets caught here due to ligamentum arteriosum

Branchial apparatus	Also called pharyngeal apparatus. Composed of branchial clefts, arches, and pouches. Branchial clefts—derived from ectoderm. Also called branchial grooves. Branchial arches—derived from mesoderm (muscles, arteries) and neural crest (bones, cartilage). Branchial pouches—derived from endoderm.	CAP covers outside from inside: Clefts = ectoderm Arches = mesoderm Pouches = endoderm

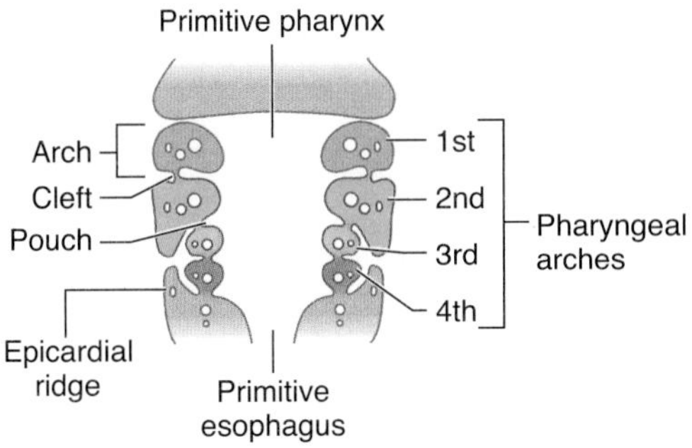

Primitive pharynx
Arch
Cleft
Pouch
1st
2nd
3rd
4th
Pharyngeal arches
Epicardial ridge
Primitive esophagus

Branchial cleft derivatives	1st cleft develops into external auditory meatus. 2nd through 4th clefts form temporary cervical sinuses, which are obliterated by proliferation of 2nd arch mesenchyme. Persistent cervical sinus → branchial cleft cyst within lateral neck.

Branchial arch derivatives

ARCH	CARTILAGE	MUSCLES	NERVES[a]	ABNORMALITIES/COMMENTS
1st arch	Meckel's cartilage: **M**andible, **M**alleus, incus, spheno-**M**andibular ligament	Muscles of **M**astication (temporalis, **M**asseter, lateral and **M**edial pterygoids), **M**ylohyoid, anterior belly of digastric, tensor tympani, tensor veli palatini	CN V_2 and V_3 **chew**	Treacher Collins syndrome: 1st-arch neural crest fails to migrate → mandibular hypoplasia, facial abnormalities
2nd arch	Reichert's cartilage: **S**tapes, **S**tyloid process, lesser horn of hyoid, **S**tylohyoid ligament	Muscles of facial expression, **S**tapedius, **S**tylohyoid, posterior belly of digastric	CN VII (facial expression) **smile**	
3rd arch	Cartilage: greater horn of hyoid	Stylopharyngeus (think of stylo**pharyngeus** innervated by glosso**pharyngeal** nerve)	CN IX (**stylo**-pharyngeus) **swallow styl**ishly	Congenital pharyngo-cutaneous fistula: persistence of cleft and pouch → fistula between tonsillar area, cleft in lateral neck
4th–6th arches	Cartilages: thyroid, cricoid, arytenoids, corniculate, cuneiform	4th arch: most pharyngeal constrictors; cricothyroid, levator veli palatini 6th arch: all intrinsic muscles of larynx except cricothyroid	4th arch: CN X (superior laryngeal branch) **simply swallow** 6th arch: CN X (recurrent laryngeal branch) **speak**	Arches 3 and 4 form posterior ⅓ of tongue; arch 5 makes no major developmental contributions

[a]These are the only CNs with both motor and sensory components (except V_2, which is sensory only).

When at the restaurant of the golden **arches**, children tend to first **chew** (1), then **smile** (2), then **swallow styl**ishly (3) or **simply swallow** (4), and then **speak** (6).

Branchial pouch derivatives

1st pouch	Develops into middle ear cavity, eustachian tube, mastoid air cells.	1st pouch contributes to endoderm-lined structures of ear.	**Ear, tonsils, bottom-to-top**: 1 (**ear**), 2 (**tonsils**), 3 dorsal (**bottom** for inferior parathyroids), 3 ventral (**to** = thymus), 4 (**top** = superior parathyroids).
2nd pouch	Develops into epithelial lining of palatine tonsil.		
3rd pouch	Dorsal wings—develops into **inferior** parathyroids. Ventral wings—develops into thymus.	3rd pouch contributes to 3 structures (thymus, left and right inferior parathyroids). 3rd-pouch structures end up **below** 4th-pouch structures.	
4th pouch	Dorsal wings—develops into **superior** parathyroids.		
DiGeorge syndrome	Aberrant development of 3rd and 4th pouches → T-cell deficiency (thymic aplasia) and hypocalcemia (failure of parathyroid development).		
MEN 2A	Mutation of germline *RET* (neural crest cells): ▪ Adrenal medulla (pheochromocytoma). ▪ Parathyroid (tumor): 3rd/4th pharyngeal pouch. ▪ Parafollicular cells (medullary thyroid cancer): derived from neural crest cells; associated with the 4th/5th pharyngeal pouches.		

Cleft lip and cleft palate

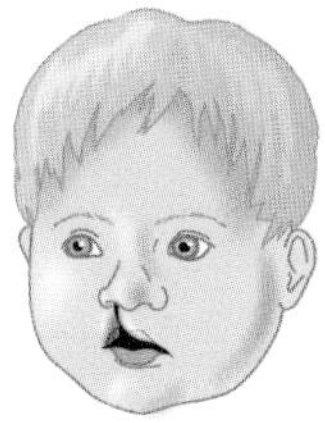

Cleft lip

Cleft lip—failure of fusion of the maxillary and medial nasal processes (formation of 1° palate).

Cleft palate—failure of fusion of the lateral palatine processes, the nasal septum, and/or the median palatine process (formation of 2° palate).

Cleft lip and cleft palate have two distinct etiologies, but often occur together.

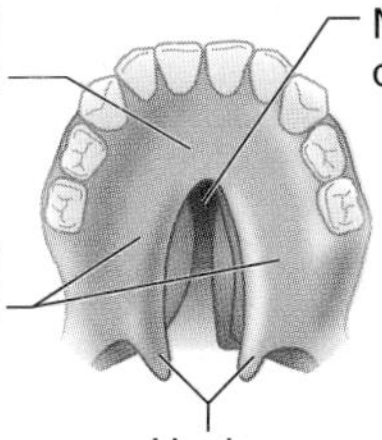
Roof of mouth
Nasal cavity
Palatine shelves (2° palate)
Uvula

Cleft palate (partial)

Genital embryology

Female	Default development. Mesonephric duct degenerates and paramesonephric duct develops.
Male	*SRY* gene on Y chromosome—produces testis-determining factor (testes development). Sertoli cells secrete Müllerian inhibitory factor (MIF) that suppresses development of paramesonephric ducts. Leydig cells secrete androgens that stimulate the development of mesonephric ducts.
Paramesonephric (Müllerian) duct	Develops into female internal structures—fallopian tubes, uterus, and upper portion of vagina (lower portion from urogenital sinus). Müllerian duct abnormalities result in anatomical defects that may present as primary amenorrhea in females with fully developed secondary sexual characteristics (indicator of functional ovaries).
Mesonephric (Wolffian) duct	Develops into male internal structures (except prostate)—**S**eminal vesicles, **E**pididymis, **E**jaculatory duct, and **D**uctus deferens (**SEED**).

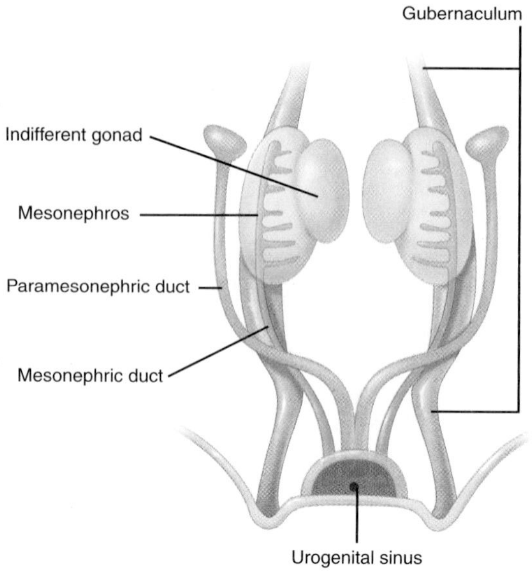
Gubernaculum
Indifferent gonad
Mesonephros
Paramesonephric duct
Mesonephric duct
Urogenital sinus

Bicornuate uterus	Results from incomplete fusion of the paramesonephric ducts. Can lead to urinary tract abnormalities and miscarriages.

SRY gene

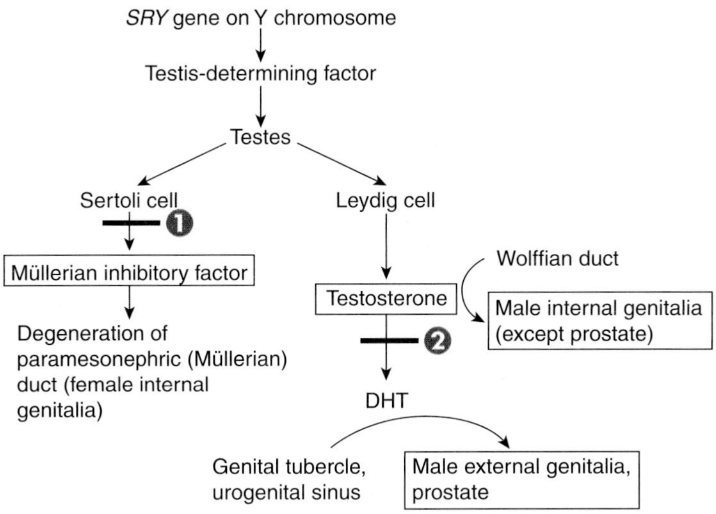

SRY gene on Y chromosome
Testis-determining factor
Testes
Sertoli cell
Leydig cell
❶
Müllerian inhibitory factor
Degeneration of paramesonephric (Müllerian) duct (female internal genitalia)
Wolffian duct
Testosterone
Male internal genitalia (except prostate)
❷
DHT
Genital tubercle, urogenital sinus
Male external genitalia, prostate

❶ No Sertoli cells or lack of Müllerian inhibitory factor: develop both male and female internal genitalia and male external genitalia

❷ 5α-reductase deficiency: male internal genitalia, ambiguous external genitalia until puberty

Male/female genital homologues

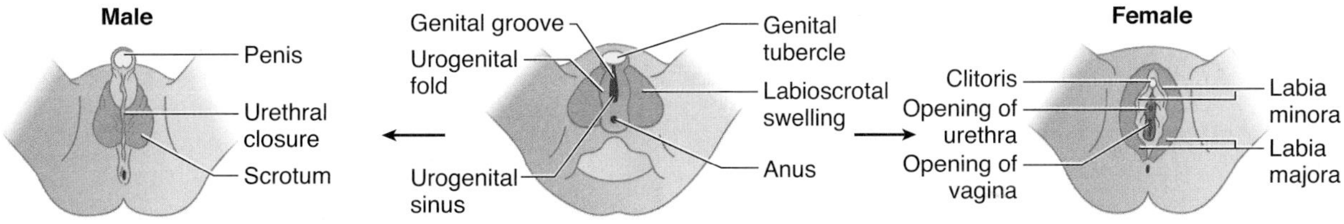

Male
Penis
Urethral closure
Scrotum
Genital groove
Urogenital fold
Urogenital sinus
Genital tubercle
Labioscrotal swelling
Anus
Female
Clitoris
Opening of urethra
Opening of vagina
Labia minora
Labia majora

Male (← Dihydrotestosterone)		Female (Estrogen →)
Glans penis	Genital tubercle	Glans clitoris
Corpus cavernosum and spongiosum	Genital tubercle	Vestibular bulbs
Bulbourethral glands (of Cowper)	Urogenital sinus	Greater vestibular glands (of Bartholin)
Prostate gland	Urogenital sinus	Urethral and paraurethral glands (of Skene)
Ventral shaft of penis (penile urethra)	Urogenital folds	Labia minora
Scrotum	Labioscrotal swelling	Labia majora

(Adapted, with permission, from Strong B et al. *Human Sexuality: Diversity in Contemporary America,* 5th ed. New York: McGraw-Hill, 2005: Fig. 3.1)

Congenital penile abnormalities

Hypospadias 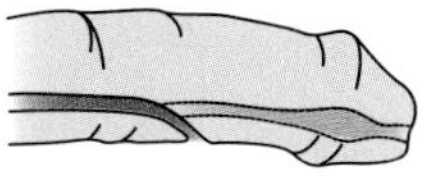	Abnormal opening of penile urethra on **inferior** (ventral) side of penis due to failure of urethral folds to close.	Hypospadias is more common than epispadias. Fix hypospadias to prevent UTIs. **Hypo** is **below**.
Epispadias 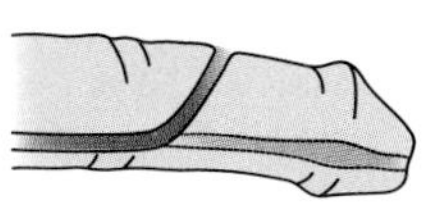	Abnormal opening of penile urethra on superior (dorsal) side of penis due to faulty positioning of genital tubercle.	Exstrophy of the bladder is associated with **E**pispadias. When you have **E**pispadias, you hit your **E**ye when you p**EE**.

Descent of testes and ovaries

	MALE REMNANT	FEMALE REMNANT
Gubernaculum (band of fibrous tissue)	Anchors testes within scrotum.	Ovarian ligament + round ligament of uterus.
Processus vaginalis (evagination of peritoneum)	Forms tunica vaginalis.	Obliterated.

▶ REPRODUCTIVE–ANATOMY

Gonadal drainage

Venous drainage	Left ovary/testis → left gonadal vein → left renal vein → IVC. Right ovary/testis → right gonadal vein → IVC.	Just as the left adrenal vein drains to the left renal vein before the IVC. Because the left spermatic vein enters the left renal vein at a 90° angle, flow is less continuous on the left than on the right. → left venous pressure > right venous pressure → varicocele more common on the left.
Lymphatic drainage	Ovaries/testes → para-aortic lymph nodes. Distal $^{1}/_{3}$ of vagina/vulva/scrotum → superficial inguinal nodes. Proximal $^{2}/_{3}$ of vagina/uterus → obturator, external iliac and hypogastric nodes.	

Female reproductive anatomy

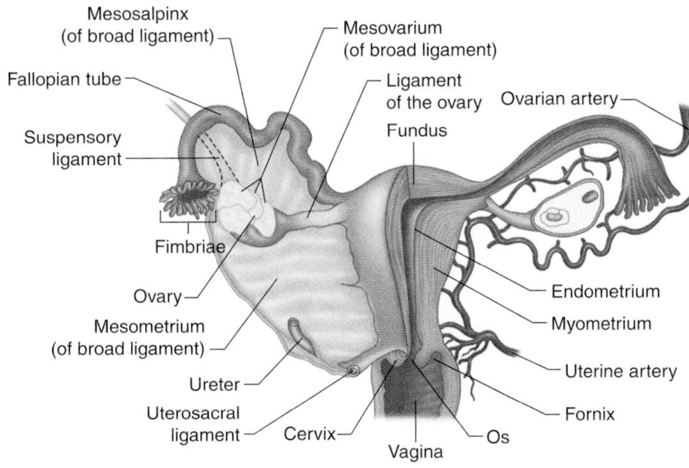

Posterior view

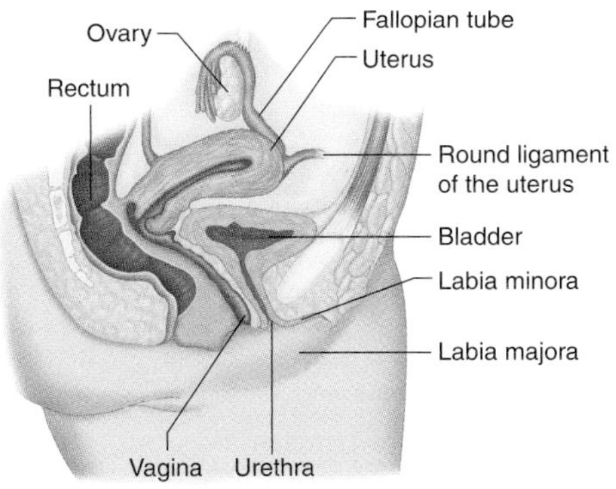

Sagittal view

LIGAMENT	CONNECTS	STRUCTURES CONTAINED	NOTES
Suspensory ligament of the ovaries	Ovaries to lateral pelvic wall	Ovarian vessels	Ureter at risk of injury during ligation of ovarian vessels in oophorectomy. Suspensory ligament suspends ovary to pelvic wall.
Cardinal ligament (not labeled)	Cervix to side wall of pelvis	Uterine vessels	Ureter at risk of injury during ligation of uterine vessels in hysterectomy.
Round ligament of the uterus	Uterine fundus to labia majora	Artery of Sampson	Derivative of gubernaculum. Travels through **round** inguinal canal.
Broad ligament	Uterus, fallopian tubes, and ovaries to pelvic side wall	Ovaries, fallopian tubes, and round ligaments of uterus	Mesosalpinx, mesometrium, and mesovarium are the components of the broad ligament.
Ligament of the ovary	Medial pole of ovary to lateral uterus	None	Ligament of the ovary **L**atches ovary to **L**ateral uterus; is a derivative of the gubernaculum.

Female reproductive epithelial histology

TISSUE	HISTOLOGY
Vagina	Stratified squamous epithelium, nonkeratinized
Ectocervix	Stratified squamous epithelium
Endocervix	Simple columnar epithelium
Uterus	Simple columnar epithelium, pseudostratified tubular glands
Fallopian tube	Simple columnar epithelium, ciliated
Ovary	Simple cuboidal epithelium

Male reproductive anatomy

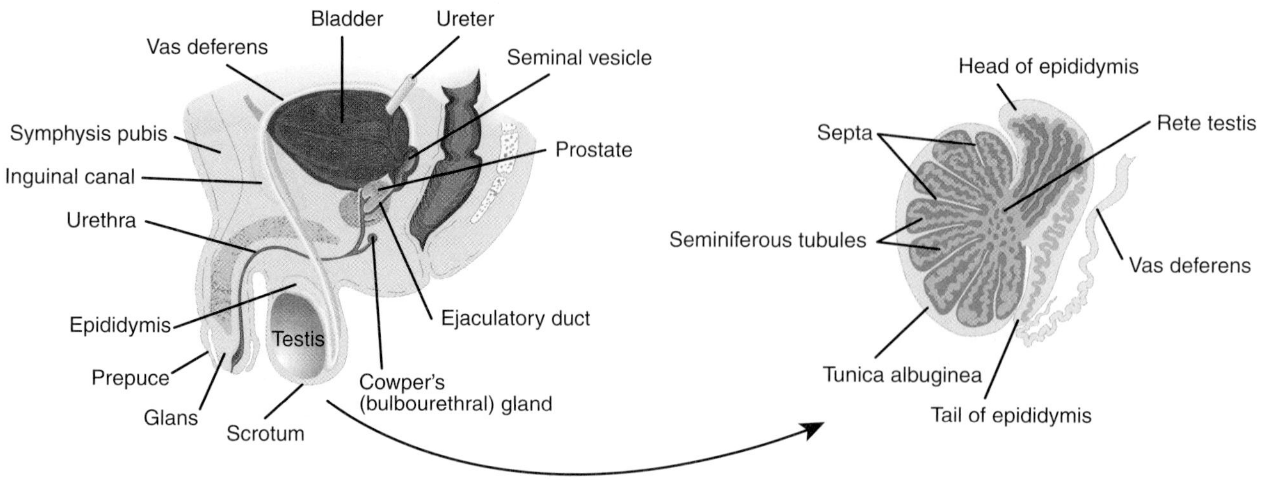

Pathway of sperm during ejaculation—
SEVEN UP:
Seminiferous tubules
Epididymis
Vas deferens
Ejaculatory ducts
(**N**othing)
Urethra
Penis

Autonomic innervation of the male sexual response

Erection—Parasympathetic nervous system (pelvic nerve):
- NO → ↑ cGMP → smooth muscle relaxation → vasodilation → proerectile.
- NE → ↑ $[Ca^{2+}]_{in}$ → smooth muscle contraction → vasoconstriction → antierectile.

Emission—Sympathetic nervous system (hypogastric nerve).

Ejaculation—visceral and somatic nerves (pudendal nerve).

Point and **S**hoot.

Sildenafil and vardenafil inhibit cGMP breakdown.

Seminiferous tubules

CELL	FUNCTION	LOCATION/NOTES
Spermatogonia (germ cells)	Maintain germ pool and produce 1° spermatocytes	Line seminiferous tubules A
Sertoli cells (non–germ cells)	Secrete inhibin → inhibit FSH Secrete androgen-binding protein (ABP) → maintain local levels of testosterone Tight junctions between adjacent Sertoli cells form blood-testis barrier → isolate gametes from autoimmune attack Support and nourish developing spermatozoa Regulate spermatogenesis Produce anti-müllerian hormone Temperature sensitive; ↓ sperm production and ↓ inhibin with ↑ temperature	Line seminiferous tubules Sertoli cells Support Sperm Synthesis ↑ temperature seen in varicocele, cryptorchidism
Leydig cells (endocrine cells)	Secrete testosterone; testosterone production unaffected by temperature	Interstitium

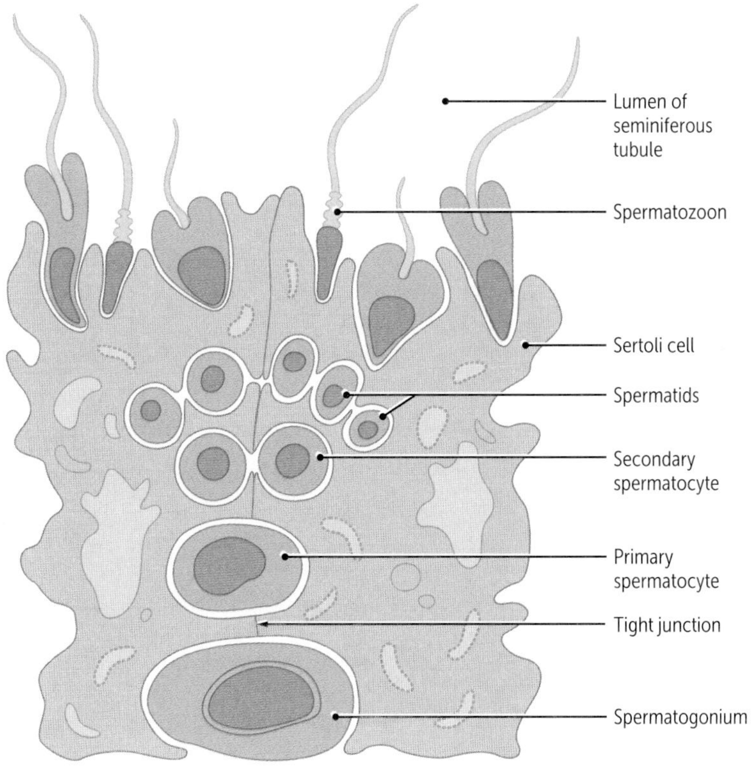
Lumen of seminiferous tubule
Spermatozoon
Sertoli cell
Spermatids
Secondary spermatocyte
Primary spermatocyte
Tight junction
Spermatogonium

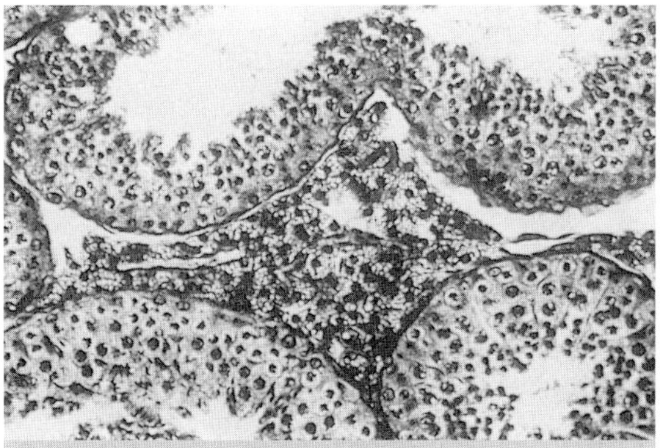

A **Seminiferous tubules.**

▸ REPRODUCTIVE–PHYSIOLOGY

Spermatogenesis

Spermatogenesis begins at puberty with spermatogonia. Full development takes 2 months. Occurs in seminiferous tubules. Produces spermatids that undergo spermiogenesis (loss of cytoplasmic contents, gain of acrosomal cap) to form mature spermatozoon.

"**Gonium**" is **going** to be a sperm; "Zoon" is "Zooming" to egg.

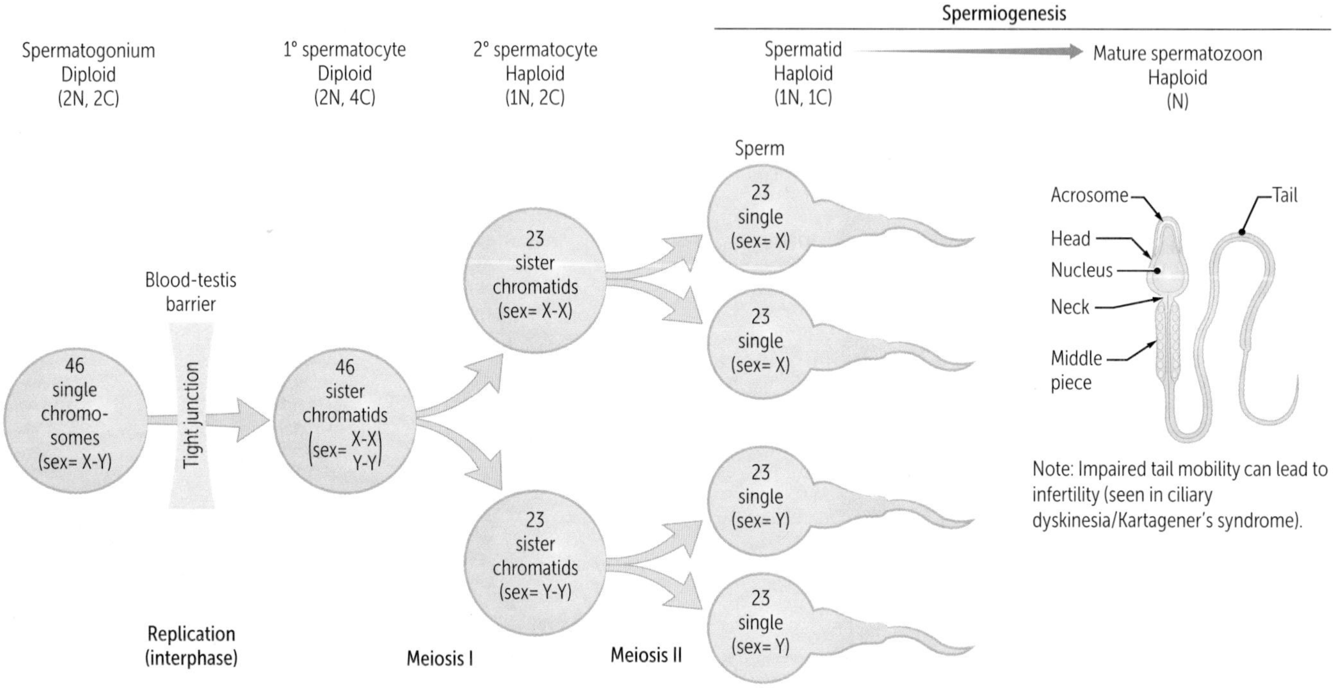
Spermiogenesis
Spermatogonium Diploid (2N, 2C)
1° spermatocyte Diploid (2N, 4C)
2° spermatocyte Haploid (1N, 2C)
Spermatid Haploid (1N, 1C)
Mature spermatozoon Haploid (N)
Sperm
46 single chromo-somes (sex= X-Y)
Blood-testis barrier
Tight junction
46 sister chromatids (sex= X-X Y-Y)
23 sister chromatids (sex= X-X)
23 sister chromatids (sex= Y-Y)
23 single (sex= X)
23 single (sex= X)
23 single (sex= Y)
23 single (sex= Y)
Replication (interphase)
Meiosis I
Meiosis II
Acrosome
Head
Nucleus
Neck
Middle piece
Tail
Note: Impaired tail mobility can lead to infertility (seen in ciliary dyskinesia/Kartagener's syndrome).

Regulation of spermatogenesis

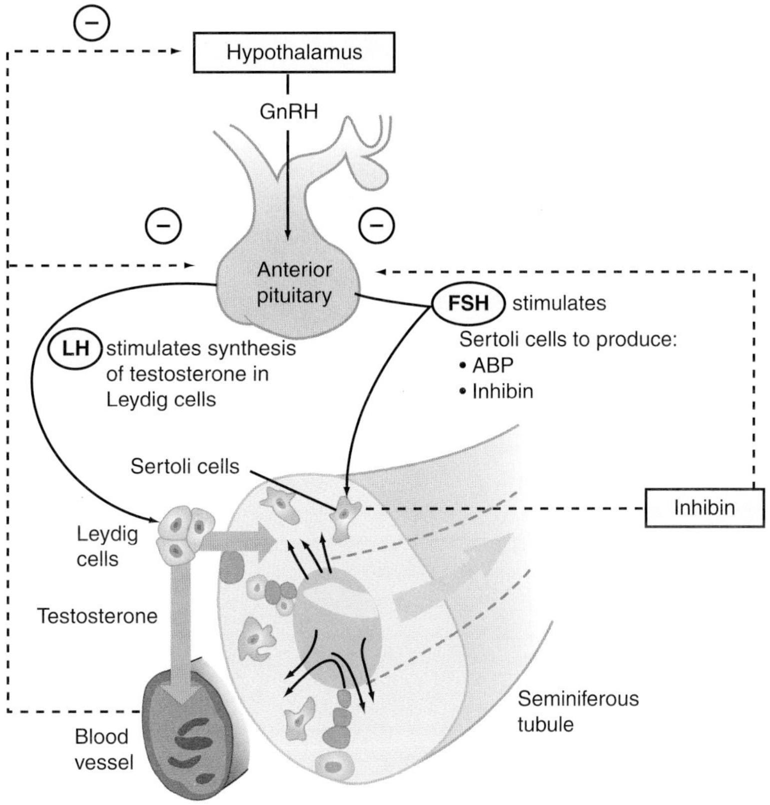

Androgens	Testosterone, dihydrotestosterone (DHT), androstenedione.	
SOURCE	DHT and testosterone (testis), **A**n**D**rostenedione (**AD**renal)	Potency: DHT > testosterone > androstenedione.

FUNCTION	Testosterone:
	▪ Differentiation of epididymis, vas deferens, seminal vesicles (internal genitalia, except prostate)
	▪ Growth spurt
	  ▪ Penis
	  ▪ Seminal vesicles
	  ▪ Sperm
	  ▪ Muscle
	  ▪ RBCs
	▪ Deepening of voice
	▪ Closing of epiphyseal plates (via estrogen converted from testosterone)
	▪ Libido
	DHT:
	▪ Early—differentiation of penis, scrotum, prostate
	▪ Late—prostate growth, balding, sebaceous gland activity
		Testosterone is converted to DHT by the enzyme 5α-reductase, which is inhibited by finasteride.
		Testosterone and androstenedione are converted to estrogen in adipose tissue and Leydig cells by the enzyme aromatase. Aromatase is the key enzyme in the conversion of androgens to estrogen.
		Exogenous testosterone → inhibition of hypothalamic–pituitary–gonadal axis → ↓ intratesticular testosterone → ↓ testicular size → azoospermia.

Estrogen

SOURCE	Ovary (17β-estradiol), placenta (estriol), adipose tissue (estrone via aromatization)	Potency: estradiol > estrone > estriol
FUNCTION	Development of genitalia and breast, female fat distribution Growth of follicle, endometrial proliferation, ↑ myometrial excitability Upregulation of estrogen, LH, and progesterone receptors; feedback inhibition of FSH and LH, then LH surge; stimulation of prolactin secretion (but blocks its action at breast) ↑ transport proteins, SHBG; ↑ HDL; ↓ LDL	Pregnancy: ▪ 50-fold ↑ in estradiol and estrone ▪ 1000-fold ↑ in estriol (indicator of fetal well-being) Estrogen receptors expressed in the cytoplasm; translocate to the nucleus when bound by ligand

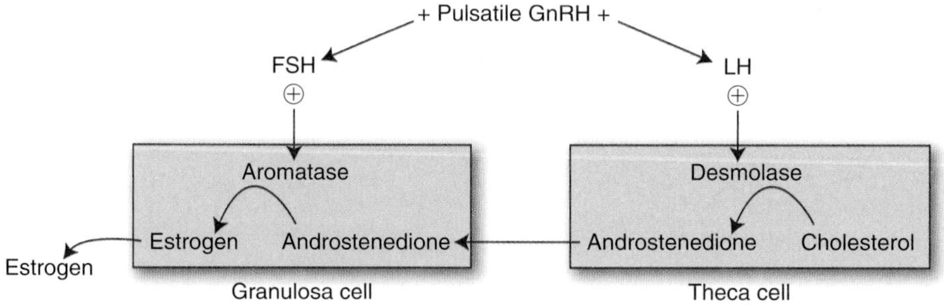
+ Pulsatile GnRH +
FSH
LH
Aromatase
Desmolase
Estrogen
Androstenedione
Androstenedione
Cholesterol
Estrogen
Granulosa cell
Theca cell

Progesterone

SOURCE	Corpus luteum, placenta, adrenal cortex, testes	Elevation of progesterone is indicative of ovulation. **Progest**erone is **pro-gest**ation.
FUNCTION	Stimulation of endometrial glandular secretions and spiral artery development Maintenance of pregnancy ↓ myometrial excitability Production of thick cervical mucus, which inhibits sperm entry into the uterus ↑ body temperature Inhibition of gonadotropins (LH, FSH) Uterine smooth muscle relaxation (preventing contractions) ↓ estrogen receptor expressivity	

Tanner stages of sexual development

I. Childhood
II. Pubic hair appears (pubarche); breast bud forms (thelarche)
III. Pubic hair darkens and becomes curly; penis size/length ↑; breast enlarges
IV. Penis width ↑, darker scrotal skin, development of glans; raised areolae
V. Adult; areolae are no longer raised

Menstrual cycle

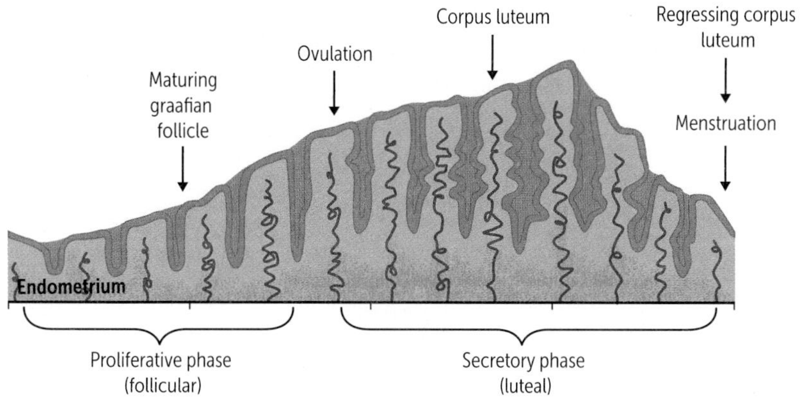

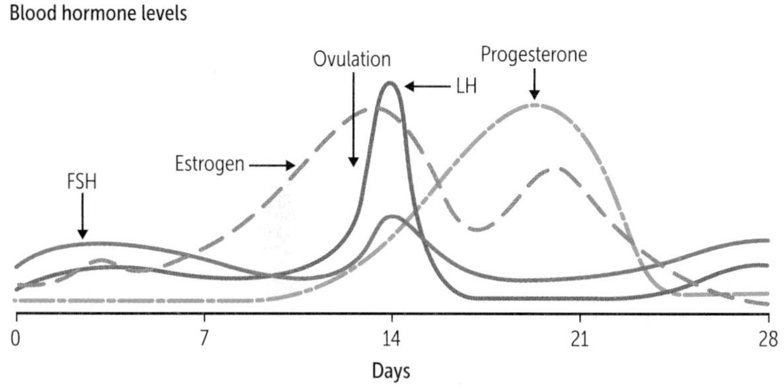

Follicular phase can vary in length. Luteal phase is usually a constant 14 days. Ovulation day + 14 days = menstruation.
Follicular growth is fastest during 2nd week of proliferative phase.
Estrogen stimulates endometrial proliferation.
Progesterone maintains endometrium to support implan tation.
↓ progesterone → ↓ fertility.
Oligomenorrhea: > 35-day cycle.
Polymenorrhea: < 21-day cycle.
Metrorrhagia: frequent but irregular menstruation.
Menometrorrhagia: heavy, irregular menstruation at irregular intervals.

↑ estrogen
↓
LH surge
↓
Ovulation
↓
Progesterone (from corpus luteum)
↓
Progesterone levels fall
↓
Menstruation (via apoptosis of endometrial cells)

Ovulation

↑ estrogen, ↑ GnRH receptors on anterior pituitary. Estrogen surge then stimulates LH release, causing ovulation (rupture of follicle).
↑ temperature (progesterone induced).

Mittelschmerz—blood from ruptured follicle or follicular enlargement causes peritoneal irritation that can mimic appendicitis.

Oogenesis

1° oocytes begin meiosis I during fetal life and complete meiosis I just prior to ovulation.

Meiosis I is arrested in prOphase I for years until Ovulation (1° oocytes).

Meiosis II is arrested in **met**aphase II until fertilization (2° oocytes). An egg **met** a sperm.

If fertilization does not occur within 1 day, the 2° oocyte degenerates.

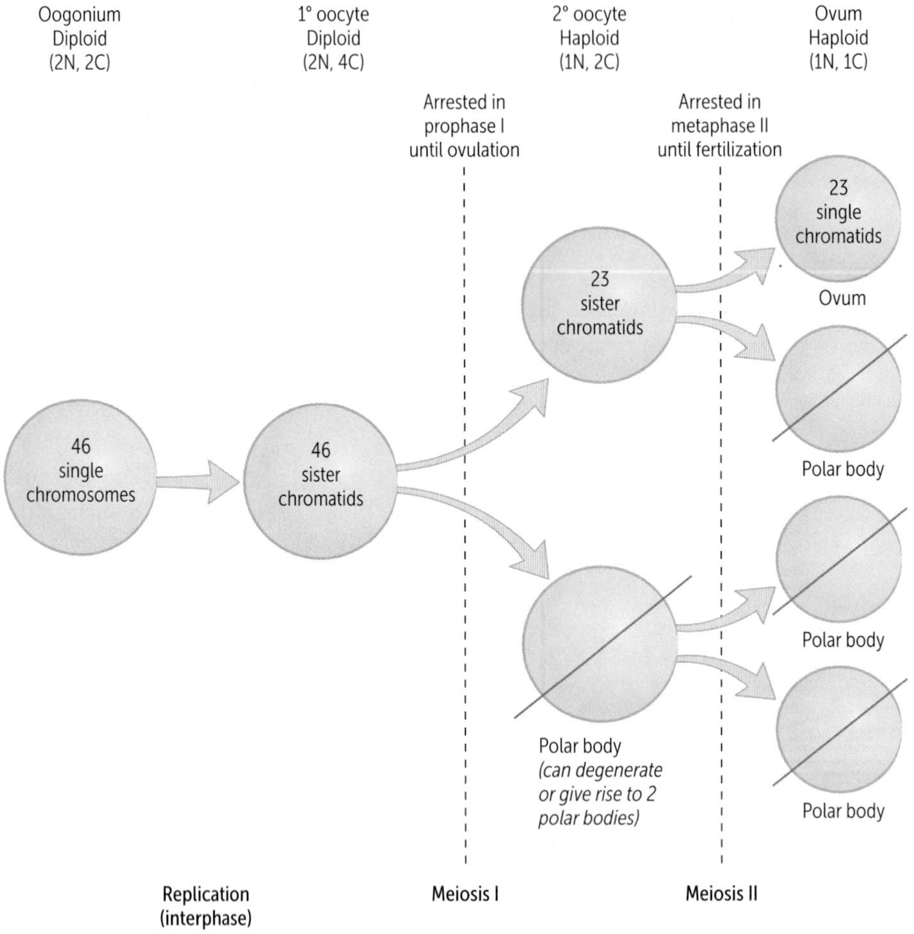
Oogonium
Diploid
(2N, 2C)
1° oocyte
Diploid
(2N, 4C)
2° oocyte
Haploid
(1N, 2C)
Ovum
Haploid
(1N, 1C)
Arrested in prophase I until ovulation
Arrested in metaphase II until fertilization
46 single chromosomes
46 sister chromatids
23 sister chromatids
23 single chromatids
Ovum
Polar body
Polar body
Polar body
Polar body
(can degenerate or give rise to 2 polar bodies)
Replication
(interphase)
Meiosis I
Meiosis II

Pregnancy

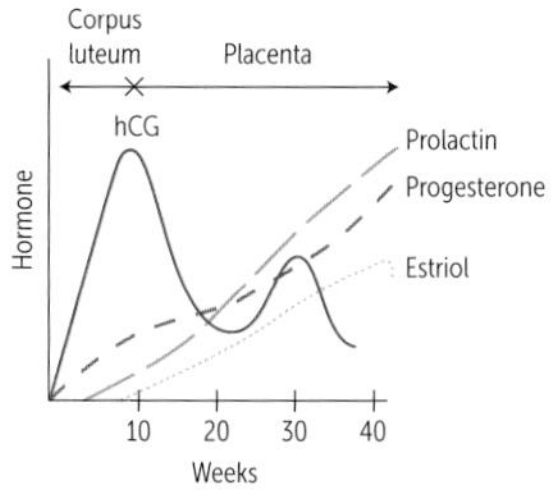

Fertilization most commonly occurs in upper end of fallopian tube (the ampulla). Occurs within 1 day of ovulation.

Implantation within the wall of the uterus occurs 6 days after fertilization. Trophoblasts secrete hCG, which is detectable in blood 1 week after conception and on home test in urine 2 weeks after conception.

Lactation

After labor, the ↓ in progesterone disinhibits lactation. Suckling is required to maintain milk production, since ↑ nerve stimulation ↑ oxytocin and prolactin.
Prolactin—induces and maintains lactation and ↓ reproductive function.
Oxytocin—appears to help with milk letdown and may be involved with uterine contractions (function not yet entirely known).

hCG

SOURCE	Syncytiotrophoblast of placenta.
FUNCTION	Maintains the corpus luteum (and thus progesterone) for the 1st trimester by acting like LH (otherwise no luteal cell stimulation, and abortion results). In the 2nd and 3rd trimesters, the placenta synthesizes its own estriol and progesterone and the corpus luteum degenerates. Used to detect pregnancy because it appears early in the urine (see above). Elevated hCG in pathologic states (e.g., hydatidiform moles, choriocarcinoma).

Menopause

↓ estrogen production due to age-linked decline in number of ovarian follicles. Average age at onset is 51 years (earlier in smokers).

Usually preceded by 4–5 years of abnormal menstrual cycles. Source of estrogen (estrone) after menopause becomes peripheral conversion of androgens. ↑ androgens cause hirsutism.

↑↑ FSH is the best test to confirm menopause (loss of negative feedback for FSH due to ↓ estrogen).

Hormonal changes: ↓ estrogen, ↑↑ FSH, ↑ LH (no surge), ↑ GnRH.
Menopause causes **HHAVOC**: **H**irsutism, **H**ot flashes, **A**trophy of the **V**agina, **O**steoporosis, **C**oronary artery disease.
Menopause before age 40 can indicate premature ovarian failure.

▸ REPRODUCTIVE–PATHOLOGY

Sex chromosome disorders

Klinefelter's syndrome [male] (XXY), 1:850 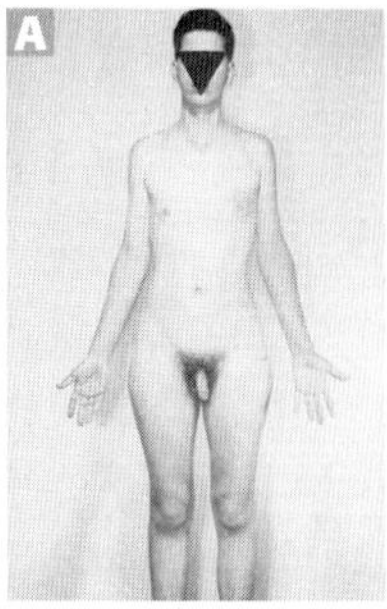	Testicular atrophy, eunuchoid body shape, tall, long extremities, gynecomastia, female hair distribution A. May present with developmental delay. Presence of inactivated X chromosome (Barr body). Common cause of hypogonadism seen in infertility work-up.	Dysgenesis of seminiferous tubules → ↓ inhibin → ↑ FSH. Abnormal Leydig cell function → ↓ testosterone → ↑ LH → ↑ estrogen.
Turner syndrome [female] (XO) 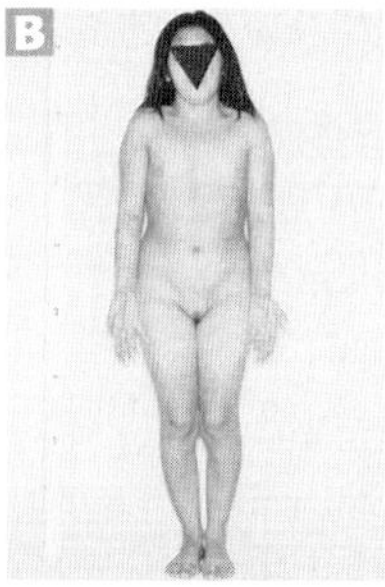	Short stature (if left untreated, < 5 feet), ovarian dysgenesis (streak ovary with infertility), shield chest, bicuspid aortic valve, defects in lymphatics → webbing of neck (cystic hygroma) and lymphedema in feet and hands, preductal coarctation of the aorta, horseshoe kidney, dysgerminoma B. Most common cause of 1° amenorrhea. No Barr body.	"Hugs and kisses" (**XO**) from Tina **Turner**. Menopause before menarche. ↓ estrogen leads to ↑ LH and FSH.
Double Y males [male] (XYY), 1:1000	Phenotypically normal, very tall, severe acne, antisocial behavior (seen in 1–2% of XYY males). Normal fertility. Small percentage diagnosed with autism spectrum disorders.	

Diagnosing disorders of sex hormones

Testosterone	LH	Diagnosis
↑	↑	Defective androgen receptor
↑	↓	Testosterone-secreting tumor, exogenous steroids
↓	↑	1° hypogonadism
↓	↓	Hypogonadotropic hypogonadism

Pseudo-hermaphroditism

Disagreement between the phenotypic (external genitalia) and gonadal (testes vs. ovaries) sex.

Female pseudo-hermaphrodite (XX)	Ovaries present, but external genitalia are virilized or ambiguous. Due to excessive and inappropriate exposure to androgenic steroids during early gestation (e.g., congenital adrenal hyperplasia or exogenous administration of androgens during pregnancy).
Male pseudo-hermaphrodite (XY)	Testes present, but external genitalia are female or ambiguous. Most common form is androgen insensitivity syndrome (testicular feminization).

True hermaphroditism (46,XX or 47,XXY)

Both ovary and testicular tissue present (ovotestis); ambiguous genitalia. Very rare.

Androgen insensitivity syndrome (46,XY)

Defect in androgen receptor resulting in normal-appearing female; female external genitalia with rudimentary vagina; uterus and fallopian tubes generally absent; presents with scant sexual hair; develops testes (often found in labia majora; surgically removed to prevent malignancy). ↑ testosterone, estrogen, LH (vs. sex chromosome disorders).

5α-reductase deficiency

Autosomal recessive; sex limited to genetic males. Inability to convert testosterone to DHT. Ambiguous genitalia until puberty, when ↑ testosterone causes masculinization/↑ growth of external genitalia. Testosterone/estrogen levels are normal; LH is normal or ↑. Internal genitalia are normal.

Kallmann syndrome

Defective migration of GnRH cells and formation of olfactory bulb; ↓ synthesis of GnRH in the hypothalamus; anosmia; lack of secondary sexual characteristics; ↓ GnRH, FSH, LH, testosterone, and sperm count.

Hydatidiform mole

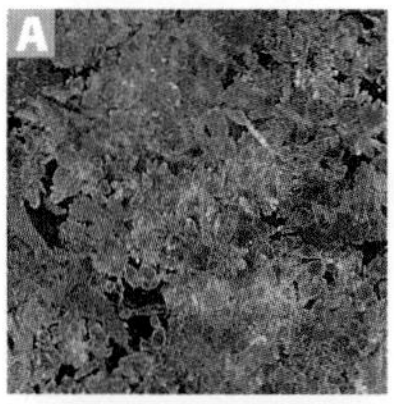

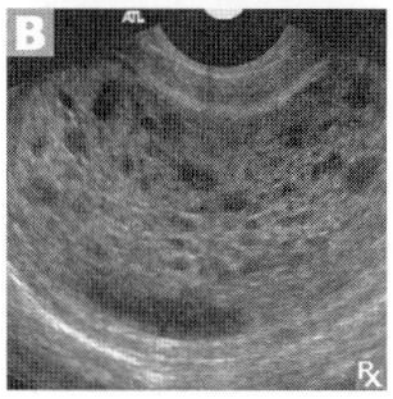

Cystic swelling of chorionic villi and proliferation of chorionic epithelium (trophoblast) that presents with abnormal vaginal bleeding. Most common precursor of choriocarcinoma. ↑ β-hCG. "Honeycombed uterus" or "cluster of grapes" appearance A, abnormally enlarged uterus. Complete moles classically have "snowstorm" appearance with no fetus during 1st sonogram B. Moles can lead to uterine rupture. Treatment: dilation and curettage and methotrexate. Monitor β-hCG.

	Complete mole	Partial mole
KARYOTYPE	46,XX; 46,XY	69,XXX; 69,XXY; 69,XYY
hCG	↑↑↑↑	↑
UTERINE SIZE	↑	—
CONVERT TO CHORIOCARCINOMA	2%	Rare
FETAL PARTS	No	Yes (**partial** = fetal **parts**)
COMPONENTS	2 sperm + empty egg	2 sperm + 1 egg
RISK OF COMPLICATIONS	15–20% malignant trophoblastic disease	Low risk of malignancy (< 5%)

Pregnancy-induced hypertension (preeclampsia-eclampsia)	**Preeclampsia**—hypertension, proteinuria, and edema. **Eclampsia**—preeclampsia + seizures. Preeclampsia occurs in 7% of pregnant women from 20 weeks' gestation to 6 weeks postpartum (before 20 weeks suggests molar pregnancy). ↑ incidence in patients with preexisting hypertension, diabetes, chronic renal disease, and autoimmune disorders. Caused by placental ischemia due to impaired vasodilation of spiral arteries, resulting in ↑ vascular tone. Can be associated with **HELLP** syndrome (**H**emolysis, **E**levated **L**iver enzymes, **L**ow **P**latelets). Mortality as a result of cerebral hemorrhage and ARDS.
CLINICAL FEATURES	Headache, blurred vision, abdominal pain, edema of face and extremities, altered mentation, hyperreflexia; lab findings may include thrombocytopenia, hyperuricemia.
TREATMENT	Delivery of fetus as soon as viable. Otherwise bed rest, monitoring, and treatment of hypertension. Treatment: IV magnesium sulfate to prevent and treat seizures of eclampsia.

Pregnancy complications

Abruptio placentae

Premature detachment of placenta from implantation site. May be associated with DIC. ↑ risk with smoking, hypertension, cocaine use.

Painful bleeding in 3rd trimester. **Abrupt** detachment. Life threatening for both fetus and mother.

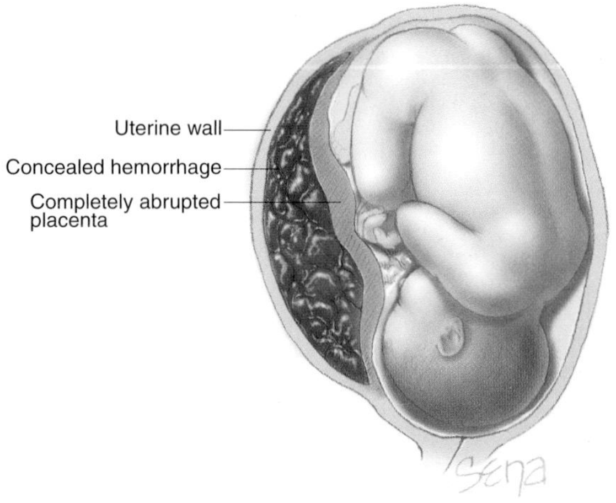
Uterine wall
Concealed hemorrhage
Completely abrupted placenta
Sena

(Reproduced, with permission, from Cunningham FG et al. *Williams Obstetrics*, 23rd ed. New York: McGraw-Hill, 2010, Fig. 35-4.)

Placenta accreta

Defective decidual layer allows placenta to attach to myometrium. No separation of placenta after birth. ↑ risk with prior C-section, inflammation, and placenta previa.

Massive bleeding after delivery.

Accreta = "encased in" = encased in myometrium.

Pregnancy complications *(continued)*

Placenta previa	Attachment of placenta to lower uterine segment. Lies near or extends over internal cervical os. ↑ risk with multiparity and prior C-section. Painless bleeding in any trimester.	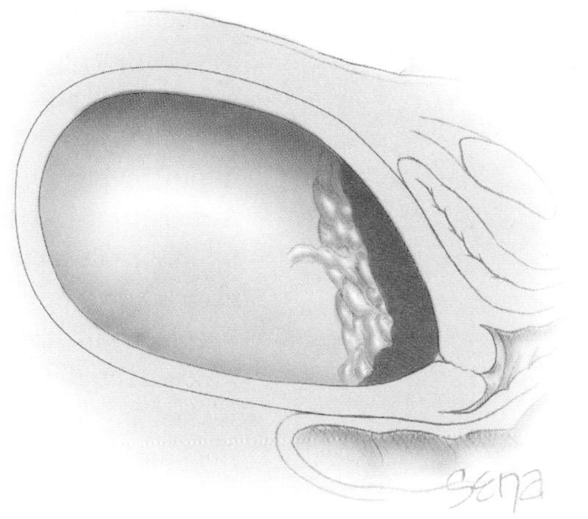 (Reproduced, with permission, from Cunningham FG et al. *Williams Obstetrics*, 23rd ed. New York: McGraw-Hill, 2010, Fig. 35-11.)
Retained placental tissue	May cause postpartum hemorrage, ↑ risk of infection.	
Ectopic pregnancy	Most often in fallopian tubes. Suspect with history of amenorrhea, lower-than-expected ↑ hCG based on dates, and sudden lower abdominal pain; confirm with ultrasound. Often clinically mistaken for appendicitis. Endometrial biopsy shows decidualized endometrium but no chorionic villi (develop only in intra-uterine pregnancy).	Pain with or without bleeding. Risk factors: ▪ History of infertility ▪ Salpingitis (PID) ▪ Ruptured appendix ▪ Prior tubal surgery

Amniotic fluid abnormalities

Polyhydramnios	> 1.5–2 L of amniotic fluid; associated with esophageal/duodenal atresia, causing inability to swallow amniotic fluid, and with anencephaly.
Oligohydramnios	< 0.5 L of amniotic fluid; associated with placental insufficiency, bilateral renal agenesis, or posterior urethral valves (in males) and resultant inability to excrete urine. Can give rise to Potter's syndrome.

Cervical pathology

Dysplasia and carcinoma in situ	Disordered epithelial growth; begins at basal layer of squamo-columnar junction and extends outward. Classified as CIN 1, CIN 2, or CIN 3 (severe dysplasia or carcinoma in situ), depending on extent of dysplasia. Associated with HPV 16 (E6 gene product inhibits *p53* suppressor gene), and HPV 18 (E7 gene product inhibits *RB* suppressor gene). Vaccine available. May progress slowly to invasive carcinoma if left untreated. Risk factors: multiple sexual partners (#1), smoking, early sexual intercourse, HIV infection.	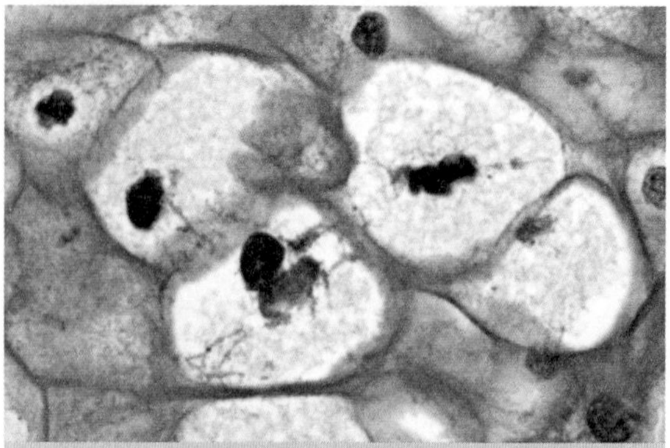 A **Koilocytes in cervical condyloma.** Note the wrinkled, "raisinoid" nuclei, some of which have clearing or a perinuclear halo.
Invasive carcinoma	Often squamous cell carcinoma. Pap smear can catch cervical dysplasia (koilocytes A) before it progresses to invasive carcinoma. Lateral invasion can block ureters, causing renal failure.	

Endometritis

Inflammation of the endometrium associated with retained products of conception following delivery (vaginal/C-section)/miscarriage/abortion or foreign body such as an IUD. Retained material in uterus promotes infection by bacterial flora from vagina or intestinal tract.
Treatment: gentamycin + clindamycin with or without ampicillin.

Endometriosis

Non-neoplastic endometrial glands/stroma in abnormal locations outside the uterus. Characterized by cyclic bleeding (menstrual type) from ectopic endometrial tissue, resulting in blood-filled "chocolate cysts." In ovary or on peritoneum. Manifests clinically as severe menstrual-related pain. Often results in painful intercourse and infertility. Can be due to retrograde menstrual flow. Treatment: oral contraceptives, NSAIDs, leuprolide, danazol.	Menorrhagia, dysmenorrhea, dyspareunia, infertility; uterus is **normal sized**.
Adenomyosis—endometrium within the myometrium. Treatment: hysterectomy.	Menorrhagia, dysmenorrhea, pelvic pain; uterus is **enlarged**.

Endometrial proliferation

Endometrial hyperplasia	Abnormal endometrial gland proliferation usually caused by excess estrogen stimulation. ↑ risk for endometrial carcinoma. Clinically manifests as postmenopausal vaginal bleeding. Risk factors include anovulatory cycles, hormone replacement therapy, polycystic ovarian syndrome, and granulosa cell tumor.
Endometrial carcinoma	Most common gynecologic malignancy. Peak occurrence at 55–65 years of age. Clinically presents with vaginal bleeding. Typically preceded by endometrial hyperplasia. Risk factors include prolonged use of estrogen without progestins, obesity, diabetes, hypertension, nulliparity, and late menopause. ↑ myometrial invasion → ↓ prognosis.

Myometrial tumors

Leiomyoma (fibroid) 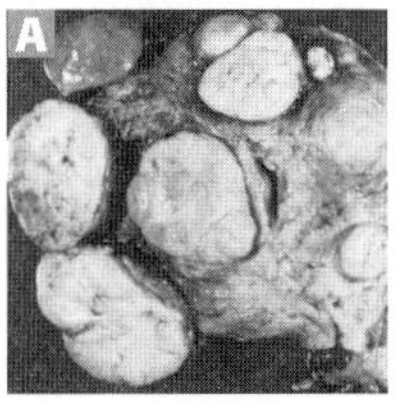	Most common of all tumors in females. Often presents with multiple tumors with well-demarcated borders A. ↑ incidence in blacks. Benign smooth muscle tumor; malignant transformation is rare. Estrogen sensitive—tumor size ↑ with pregnancy and ↓ with menopause. Peak occurrence at 20–40 years of age. May be asymptomatic, cause abnormal uterine bleeding, or result in miscarriage. Severe bleeding may lead to iron deficiency anemia. Does not progress to leiomyosarcoma. Whorled pattern of smooth muscle bundles.
Leiomyosarcoma	Bulky, irregularly shaped tumor with areas of necrosis and hemorrhage, typically arising de novo (not from leiomyoma). ↑ incidence in blacks. Highly aggressive tumor with tendency to recur. May protrude from cervix and bleed. Most commonly seen in middle-aged women.

Gynecologic tumor epidemiology	Incidence—endometrial > ovarian > cervical (data pertain to the United States; cervical cancer is most common worldwide). Worst prognosis—ovarian > cervical > endometrial.

Premature ovarian failure	Premature atresia of ovarian follicles in women of reproductive age. Patients present with signs of menopause after puberty but before age 40.	↓ estrogen, ↑ LH, FSH.

Most common causes of anovulation	Pregnancy, polycystic ovarian syndrome, obesity, HPO axis abnormalities, premature ovarian failure, hyperprolactinemia, thyroid disorders, eating disorders, Cushing's syndrome, adrenal insufficiency.

Polycystic ovarian syndrome	↑ LH production leads to anovulation and therefore no progesterone, hyperandrogenism due to deranged steroid synthesis by theca cells. Enlarged, bilateral cystic ovaries A manifest clinically with amenorrhea, infertility, obesity, and hirsutism. Associated with insulin resistance. ↑ risk of endometrial cancer, secondary to ↑ in estrogens from the aromatization of testosterone in fat cells without progesterone to oppose. Treatment: weight reduction, low-dose OCPs or medroxyprogesterone (↓ LH and androgenesis), spironolactone (treats acne and hirsutism), clomiphene (for women who want to get pregnant), metformin (for patients with features of diabetes or metabolic syndrome).	↑ LH, ↓ FSH, ↑ testosterone, ↑ estrogen (from testosterone aromatization). 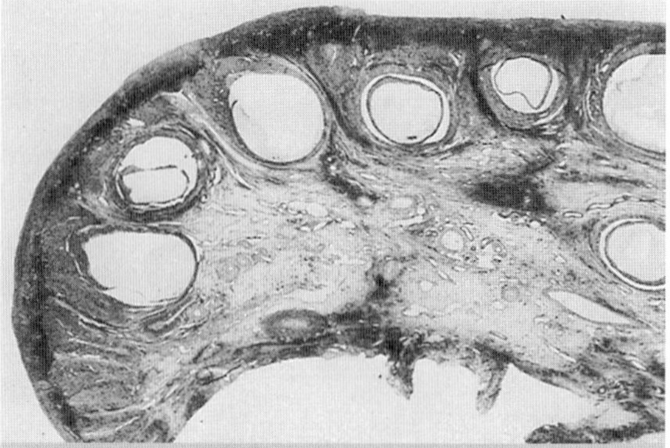 A Polycystic ovary.

Ovarian cysts

Follicular cyst	Distention of unruptured graafian follicle. May be associated with hyperestrinism and endometrial hyperplasia. Most common ovarian mass in young women.
Corpus luteum cyst	Hemorrhage into persistent corpus luteum. Commonly regresses spontaneously.
Theca-lutein cyst	Often bilateral/multiple. Due to gonadotropin stimulation. Associated with choriocarcinoma and moles.
Hemorrhagic cyst	Blood vessel rupture in cyst wall. Cyst grows with ↑ blood retention; usually self-resolves.
Dermoid cyst	Mature teratoma. Cystic growths filled with various types of tissue such as fat, hair, teeth, bits of bone, and cartilage.
Endometrioid cyst	Endometriosis within ovary with cyst formation. Varies with menstrual cycle. When filled with dark, reddish-brown blood it is called a "chocolate cyst."

Ovarian germ cell tumors

Most common in adolescents.

TYPE	CHARACTERISTICS	TUMOR MARKERS
Dysgerminoma	Malignant, equivalent to male seminoma but rarer (1% of germ cell tumors in females vs. 30% in males). Sheets of uniform cells. Associated with Turner syndrome.	hCG, LDH
Choriocarcinoma	Rare but malignant; can develop during or after pregnancy in mother or baby. Malignancy of trophoblastic tissue; chorionic villi are **not** present. ↑ frequency of theca-lutein cysts. Along with moles, comprise spectrum of gestational trophoblastic neoplasia. Early hematogenous spread to lungs.	hCG
Yolk sac (endodermal sinus) tumor	Aggressive malignancy in ovaries (testes in boys) and sacrococcygeal area of young children. Yellow, friable, solid masses. 50% have Schiller-Duval bodies (resemble glomeruli).	AFP
Teratoma	90% of ovarian germ cell tumors. Contain cells from 2 or 3 germ layers A B. Mature teratoma ("dermoid cyst")—most common ovarian germ cell tumor; mostly benign. Immature teratoma—aggressively malignant. Struma ovarii—contains functional thyroid tissue. Can present as hyperthyroidism.	

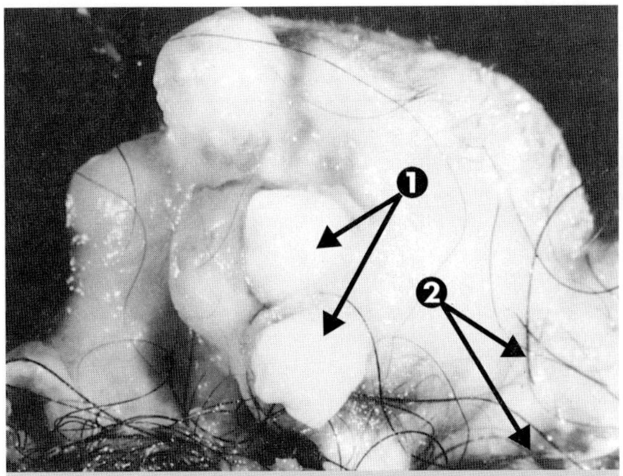

A **Teratoma of the ovary (gross).** Note the teeth (1) and hair (2).

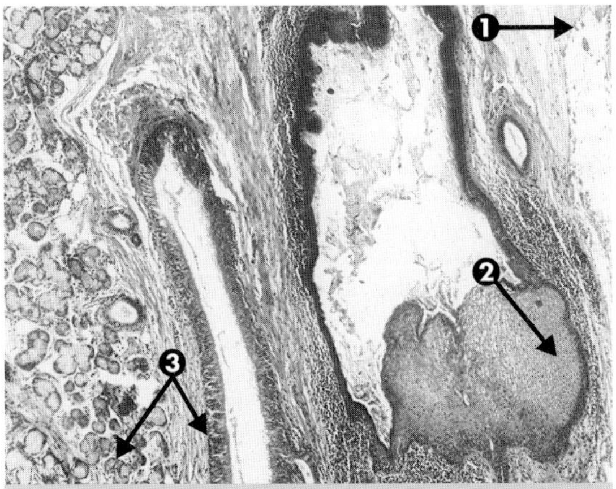

B **Teratoma, histology.** Note the glial tissue (1), stratified squamous epithelium (2), and respiratory epithelium (3).

Ovarian non–germ cell tumors

Serous cystadenoma	45% of ovarian tumors. Frequently bilateral, lined with fallopian tube–like epithelium. Benign.	↑ CA-125 is general ovarian cancer marker. Good for monitoring progression, not for screening.
Serous cystadenocarcinoma	45% of ovarian tumors, malignant and frequently bilateral. Psammoma bodies seen on histology.	Risk factors—*BRCA-1*, *BRCA-2*, HNPCC. Significant genetic predisposition makes family history the most important risk factor.
Mucinous cystadenoma	Multilocular cyst lined by mucus-secreting epithelium A. Benign. Intestine-like tissue.	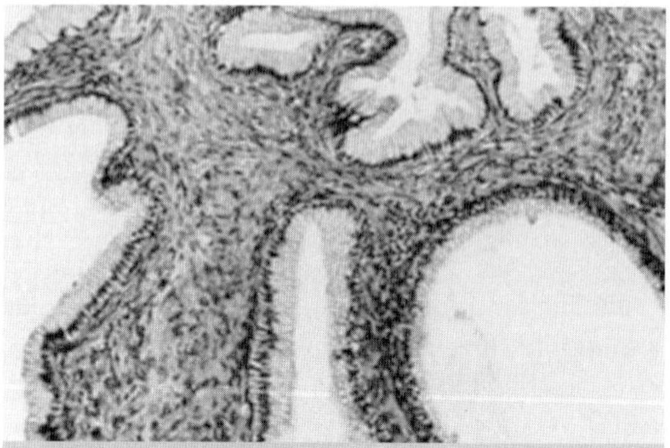 A Mucinous cystadenoma.
Mucinous cystadenocarcinoma	Malignant. Pseudomyxoma peritonei—intraperitoneal accumulation of mucinous material from ovarian or appendiceal tumor.	
Brenner tumor	Benign and unilateral. Looks like bladder. Solid tumor that is pale yellow-tan in color and appears encapsulated. "Coffee bean" nuclei on H&E staining.	
Fibromas	Bundles of spindle-shaped fibroblasts. Meigs' syndrome—triad of ovarian fibroma, ascites, and hydrothorax. Pulling sensation in groin.	
Granulosa cell tumor	Secretes estrogen → precocious puberty (kids). Can cause endometrial hyperplasia or carcinoma in adults. Call-Exner bodies—small follicles filled with eosinophilic secretions. Abnormal uterine bleeding.	
Krukenberg tumor	GI malignancy that metastasizes to ovaries, causing a mucin-secreting signet cell adenocarcinoma.	

Vaginal tumors	Squamous cell carcinoma (SCC)—usually 2° to cervical SCC; 1° vaginal carcinoma rare. Clear cell adenocarcinoma—affects women who had exposure to DES in utero. Sarcoma botryoides (rhabdomyosarcoma variant)—affects girls < 4 years of age; spindle-shaped tumor cells that are desmin positive.

Breast pathology

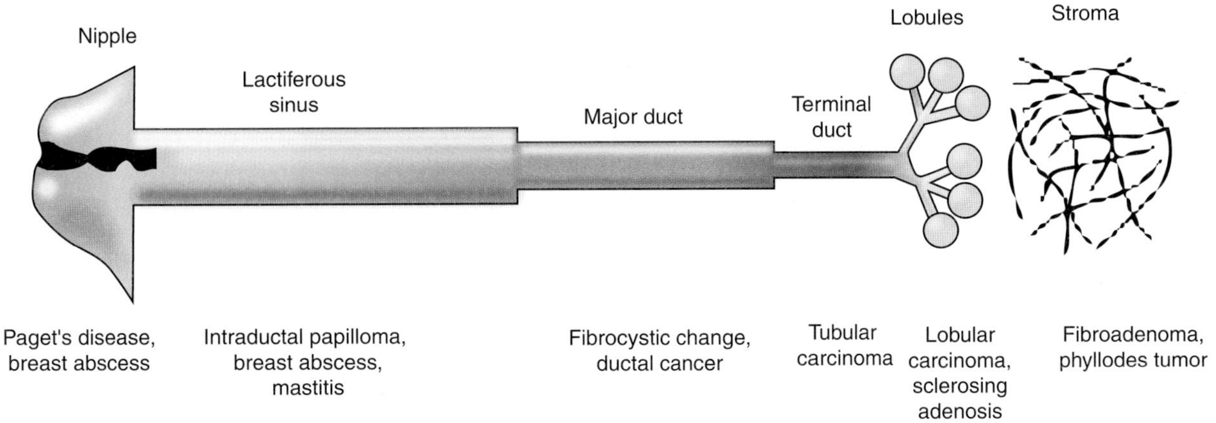
Nipple
Lactiferous sinus
Major duct
Terminal duct
Lobules
Stroma
Paget's disease, breast abscess
Intraductal papilloma, breast abscess, mastitis
Fibrocystic change, ductal cancer
Tubular carcinoma
Lobular carcinoma, sclerosing adenosis
Fibroadenoma, phyllodes tumor

Benign breast tumors

TYPE	CHARACTERISTICS	EPIDEMIOLOGY	NOTES
Fibroadenoma	**Small**, mobile, firm mass with sharp edges.	Most common tumor in those < 35 years of age.	↑ size and tenderness with ↑ estrogen (e.g., pregnancy, menstruation). Not a precursor to breast cancer.
Intraductal papilloma	Small tumor that grows in lactiferous ducts. Typically beneath areola.		Serous or bloody nipple discharge. Slight (1.5–2 ×) ↑ in risk for carcinoma.
Phyllodes tumor	**Large** bulky mass of connective tissue and cysts. "Leaf-like" projections.	Most common in 6th decade.	Some may become malignant.

Malignant breast tumors	Common postmenopause. Usually arise from terminal duct lobular unit. Overexpression of estrogen/progesterone receptors or *c-erbB2* (HER-2, an EGF receptor) is common; affects therapy and prognosis. Axillary lymph node involvement indicating metastasis is the single most important prognostic factor. Most often located in upper-outer quadrant of breast.	Risk factors: ↑ estrogen exposure, ↑ total number of menstrual cycles, older age at 1st live birth, obesity (↑ estrogen exposure as adipose tissue converts androstenedione to estrone), *BRCA1* and *BRCA2* gene mutations.

TYPE	CHARACTERISTICS	NOTES
Noninvasive		
Ductal carcinoma in situ (DCIS)	Fills ductal lumen. Arises from ductal hyperplasia.	Early malignancy without basement membrane penetration.
Comedocarcinoma	Ductal, caseous necrosis A. Subtype of DCIS.	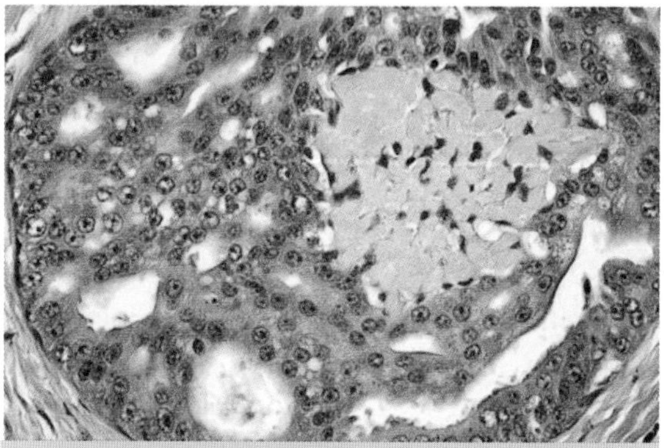 A **Comedocarcinoma.** Note central necrosis surrounded by cancer cells.
Invasive		
Invasive ductal	Firm, fibrous, "rock-hard" mass with sharp margins and small, glandular, duct-like cells. Classic "stellate" morphology.	Worst and most invasive. Most common (76% of all breast cancers).
Invasive lobular	Orderly row of cells ("Indian file").	Often bilateral with multiple lesions in the same location.
Medullary	Fleshy, cellular, lymphocytic infiltrate.	Good prognosis.
Inflammatory	Dermal lymphatic invasion by breast carcinoma. Peau d'orange (breast skin resembles orange peel); neoplastic cells block lymphatic drainage.	50% survival at 5 years.
Paget's disease	Eczematous patches on nipple. Paget cells = large cells in epidermis with clear halo.	Suggests underlying DCIS. Also seen on vulva.

Common breast conditions

Fibrocystic disease	Most common cause of "breast lumps" from age 25 to menopause. Presents with premenstrual breast pain and multiple lesions, often bilateral. Fluctuation in size of mass. Usually does not indicate ↑ risk of carcinoma. Histologic types: ▪ Fibrosis—hyperplasia of breast stroma. ▪ Cystic—fluid filled, blue dome. Ductal dilation. ▪ Sclerosing adenosis—↑ acini and intralobular fibrosis. Associated with calcifications. Often confused with cancer. ▪ Epithelial hyperplasia—↑ in number of epithelial cell layers in terminal duct lobule. ↑ risk of carcinoma with atypical cells. Occurs in women > 30 years of age.
Acute mastitis	Breast abscess; during breast-feeding, ↑ risk of bacterial infection through cracks in the nipple; *S. aureus* is the most common pathogen.
Fat necrosis	A benign, usually painless lump; forms as a result of injury to breast tissue. Up to 50% of patients may not report trauma.
Gynecomastia	Occurs in males. Results from hyperestrogenism (cirrhosis, testicular tumor, puberty, old age), Klinefelter's syndrome, or drugs (estrogen, marijuana, heroin, psychoactive drugs, **S**pironolactone, **D**igitalis, **C**imetidine, **A**lcohol, **K**etoconazole). ("**S**ome **D**rugs **C**reate **A**wkward **K**nockers.")

Prostate pathology

Prostatitis—dysuria, frequency, urgency, low back pain. Acute: bacterial (e.g., *E. coli*); chronic: bacterial or abacterial (most common).

Benign prostatic hyperplasia (BPH)

Common in men > 50 years of age. Hyperplasia (not hypertrophy) of the prostate gland. Characterized by a nodular enlargement of the periurethral (lateral and middle) lobes, which compress the urethra into a vertical slit. Not considered a premalignant lesion.

Often presents with ↑ frequency of urination, nocturia, difficulty starting and stopping the stream of urine, and dysuria. May lead to distention and hypertrophy of the bladder, hydronephrosis, and UTIs. ↑ free prostate-specific antigen (PSA).

Treatment: α_1-antagonists (terazosin, tamsulosin), which cause relaxation of smooth muscle; finasteride.

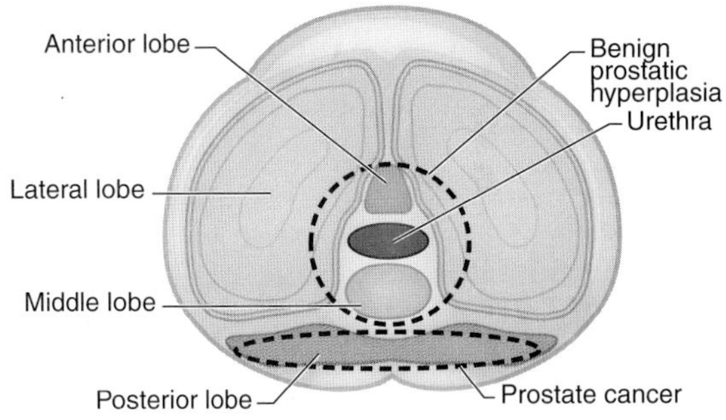
Anterior lobe
Benign prostatic hyperplasia
Urethra
Lateral lobe
Middle lobe
Posterior lobe
Prostate cancer

Prostatic adenocarcinoma

Common in men > 50 years of age. Arises most often from the posterior lobe (peripheral zone) of the prostate gland A and is most frequently diagnosed by ↑ PSA and subsequent needle core biopsies. Prostatic acid phosphatase (PAP) and PSA are useful tumor markers (↑ total PSA, with ↓ fraction of free PSA). Osteoblastic metastases in bone may develop in late stages, as indicated by lower back pain and an ↑ in serum alkaline phosphatase and PSA.

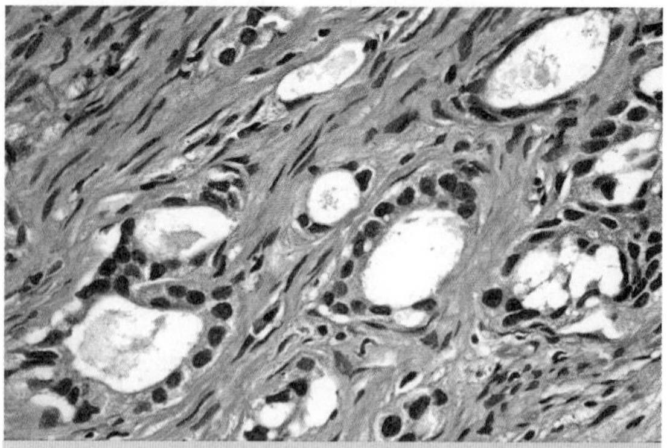

A **Prostatic adenocarcinoma.** Note the small infiltrating glands with prominent nucleoli.

Cryptorchidism

Undescended testis (one or both); impaired spermatogenesis (since sperm develop best at temperatures < 37°C); can have normal testosterone levels (Leydig cells are unaffected by temperature); associated with ↑ risk of germ cell tumors. Prematurity ↑ the risk of cryptorchidism. ↓ inhibin, ↑ FSH, and ↑ LH; testosterone ↓ in bilateral cryptorchidism, normal in unilateral.

Varicocele

Dilated veins in pampiniform plexus as a result of ↑ venous pressure; most common cause of scrotal enlargement in adult males; most often on the left side because of ↑ resistance to flow from left gonadal vein drainage into the left renal vein; can cause infertility because of ↑ temperature; "bag of worms" appearance; diagnosed by ultrasound.

Treatment: varicocelectomy, embolization by interventional radiologist.

Testicular germ cell tumors	~95% of all testicular tumors. Most often malignant. Can present as a mixed germ cell tumor. Differential diagnosis for testicular mass that does not transilluminate: cancer.
Seminoma	Malignant; painless, homogenous testicular enlargement; most common testicular tumor, mostly affecting males age 15–35. Large cells in lobules with watery cytoplasm and a "fried egg" appearance. ↑ placental alkaline phosphatase (PLAP). Radiosensitive. Late metastasis, excellent prognosis.
Yolk sac (endodermal sinus) tumor	Yellow, mucinous. Analogous to ovarian yolk sac tumor. Schiller-Duval bodies resemble primitive glomeruli (↑ AFP).
Choriocarcinoma	Malignant, ↑ hCG. Disordered syncytiotrophoblastic and cytotrophoblastic elements. Hematogenous metastases to lungs. May produce gynecomastia as hCG is an LH analog.
Teratoma	Unlike in females, mature teratoma in adult males is more often malignant. Benign in children. ↑ hCG and/or AFP in 50% of cases.
Embryonal carcinoma	Malignant; painful; worse prognosis than seminoma. Often glandular/papillary morphology. "Pure" embryonal carcinoma is rare; most commonly mixed with other tumor types. May be associated with ↑ hCG and normal AFP levels when pure (↑ AFP when mixed).

Testicular non–germ cell tumors	5% of all testicular tumors. Mostly benign.
Leydig cell	Contains Reinke crystals; usually androgen producing, gynecomastia in men, precocious puberty in boys. Golden brown color.
Sertoli cell	Androblastoma from sex cord stroma.
Testicular lymphoma	Most common testicular cancer in older men. Not a primary cancer, arises from lymphoma metastases to testes. Aggressive.

Tunica vaginalis lesions	Lesions in the serous covering of testis present as testicular masses that can be transilluminated (vs. testicular tumors). Hydrocele—↑ fluid 2° to incomplete fusion of processus vaginalis Spermatocele—dilated epididymal duct

Penile pathology	
Squamous cell carcinoma (SCC)	More common in Asia, Africa, and South America. Commonly associated with HPV, lack of circumcision.
Peyronie's disease	Bent penis due to acquired fibrous tissue formation.
Priapism	Painful sustained erection not associated with sexual stimulation or desire. Associated with trauma, sickle cell disease (sickled RBCs get trapped in vascular channels), medications (anticoagulants, PDE5 inhibitors, antidepressants, α-blockers, cocaine).

▶ REPRODUCTIVE–PHARMACOLOGY

Control of reproductive hormones

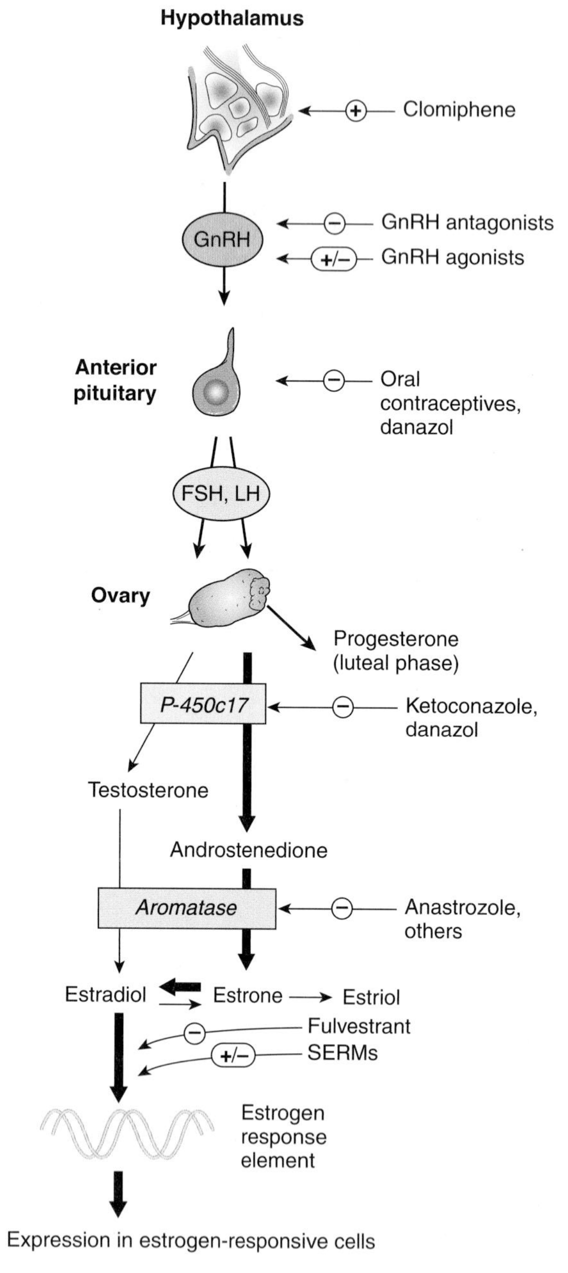

Control of female hormones

(Adapted, with permission, from Katzung BG. *Basic & Clinical Pharmacology, 10th ed.* New York: McGraw-Hill, 2006, Fig. 40-5.)

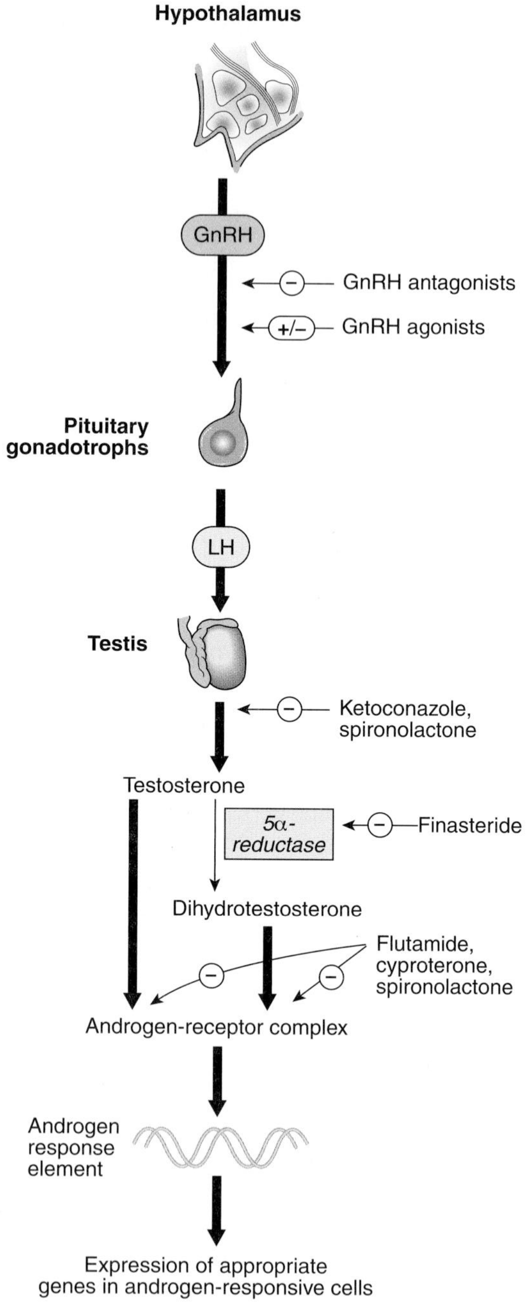

Control of androgen secretion

(Adapted, with permission, from Katzung BG. *Basic & Clinical Pharmacology,* 10th ed. New York: McGraw-Hill, 2006, Fig. 40-6.)

Leuprolide

MECHANISM	GnRH analog with agonist properties when used in pulsatile fashion; antagonist properties when used in continuous fashion (downregulates GnRH receptor in pituitary → ↓ FSH/LH).	**Leu**prolide can be used in **lieu** of GnRH.
CLINICAL USE	Infertility (pulsatile), prostate cancer (continuous—use with flutamide), uterine fibroids (continuous), precocious puberty (continuous).	
TOXICITY	Antiandrogen, nausea, vomiting.	

Testosterone, methyltestosterone

MECHANISM	Agonist at androgen receptors.
CLINICAL USE	Treats hypogonadism and promotes development of 2° sex characteristics; stimulation of anabolism to promote recovery after burn or injury.
TOXICITY	Causes masculinization in females; reduces intratesticular testosterone in males by inhibiting release of LH (via negative feedback), leading to gonadal atrophy. Premature closure of epiphyseal plates. ↑ LDL, ↓ HDL.

Antiandrogens

Testosterone $\xrightarrow{5\alpha\text{-reductase}}$ DHT (more potent).

Finasteride	A 5α-reductase inhibitor (↓ conversion of testosterone to DHT). Useful in BPH. Also promotes hair growth—used to treat male-pattern baldness.	To prevent male-pattern hair loss, give a drug that will encourage female breast growth.
Flutamide	A nonsteroidal competitive inhibitor of androgens at the testosterone receptor. Used in prostate carcinoma.	
Ketoconazole	Inhibits steroid synthesis (inhibits 17,20-desmolase).	Ketoconazole and spironolactone are used in the treatment of polycystic ovarian syndrome to prevent hirsutism. Both have side effects of gynecomastia and amenorrhea.
Spironolactone	Inhibits steroid binding.	

Estrogens (ethinyl estradiol, DES, mestranol)

MECHANISM	Bind estrogen receptors.
CLINICAL USE	Hypogonadism or ovarian failure, menstrual abnormalities, HRT in postmenopausal women; use in men with androgen-dependent prostate cancer.
TOXICITY	↑ risk of endometrial cancer, bleeding in postmenopausal women, clear cell adenocarcinoma of vagina in females exposed to DES in utero, ↑ risk of thrombi. Contraindications—ER-positive breast cancer, history of DVTs.

Selective estrogen receptor modulators—SERMs

Clomiphene	Partial agonist at estrogen receptors in hypothalamus. Prevents normal feedback inhibition and ↑ release of LH and FSH from pituitary, which stimulates ovulation. Used to treat infertility and polycystic ovarian syndrome. May cause hot flashes, ovarian enlargement, multiple simultaneous pregnancies, and visual disturbances.
Tamoxifen	Antagonist on breast tissue; used to treat and prevent recurrence of ER-positive breast cancer.
Raloxifene	Agonist on bone; reduces resorption of bone; used to treat osteoporosis.

Hormone replacement therapy

Used for relief or prevention of menopausal symptoms (e.g., hot flashes, vaginal atrophy) and osteoporosis (↑ estrogen, ↓ osteoclast activity).

Unopposed estrogen replacement therapy (ERT) ↑ the risk of endometrial cancer, so progesterone is added. Possible ↑ CV risk.

Anastrozole/exemestane

Aromatase inhibitors used in postmenopausal women with breast cancer.

Progestins

MECHANISM	Bind progesterone receptors, reduce growth and ↑ vascularization of endometrium.
CLINICAL USE	Used in oral contraceptives and in the treatment of endometrial cancer and abnormal uterine bleeding.

Mifepristone (RU-486)

MECHANISM	Competitive inhibitor of progestins at progesterone receptors.
CLINICAL USE	Termination of pregnancy. Administered with misoprostol (PGE_1).
TOXICITY	Heavy bleeding, GI effects (nausea, vomiting, anorexia), abdominal pain.

Oral contraception (synthetic progestins, estrogen)

Estrogen and progestins inhibit LH/FSH and thus prevent estrogen surge. No estrogen surge → no LH surge → no ovulation.

Progestins cause thickening of the cervical mucus, thereby limiting access of sperm to uterus. Progestins also inhibit endometrial proliferation, thus making endometrium less suitable for the implantation of an embryo.

Contraindications—smokers > 35 years of age (↑ risk of cardiovascular events), patients with history of thromboembolism and stroke or history of estrogen-dependent tumor.

Terbutaline

β_2-agonist that relaxes the uterus; reduces premature uterine contractions.

Tamsulosin

α_1-antagonist used to treat BPH by inhibiting smooth muscle contraction. Selective for $\alpha_{1A,D}$ receptors (found on prostate) vs. vascular α_{1B} receptors.

Sildenafil, vardenafil

MECHANISM	Inhibit phosphodiesterase 5, causing ↑ cGMP, smooth muscle relaxation in the corpus cavernosum, ↑ blood flow, and penile erection.	Sildena**fil** and vardena**fil** **fill** the penis.
CLINICAL USE	Treatment of erectile dysfunction.	
TOXICITY	Headache, flushing, dyspepsia, impaired blue-green color vision. Risk of life-threatening hypotension in patients taking nitrates.	"**H**ot and sweaty," but then **H**eadache, **H**eartburn, **H**ypotension.

Danazol

MECHANISM	Synthetic androgen that acts as partial agonist at androgen receptors.
CLINICAL USE	Endometriosis and hereditary angioedema.
TOXICITY	Weight gain, edema, acne, hirsutism, masculinization, ↓ HDL levels, hepatotoxicity.

NOTES

HIGH-YIELD SYSTEMS

Respiratory

"There's so much pollution in the air now that if it weren't for our lungs, there'd be no place to put it all."

—Robert Orben

"Mars is essentially in the same orbit. Somewhat the same distance from the Sun, which is very important. We have seen pictures where there are canals, we believe, and water. If there is water, that means there is oxygen. If there is oxygen, that means we can breathe."

—Former Vice President Dan Quayle

"None of us is different either as barbarian or as Greek; for we all breathe into the air with mouth and nostrils."

—Antiphon

▸ RESPIRATORY–ANATOMY

Respiratory tree

Conducting zone

Large airways consist of nose, pharynx, trachea, and bronchi. Small airways consist of bronchioles and terminal bronchioles.

Warms, humidifies, and filters air but does not participate in gas exchange → "anatomic dead space."

Extending to end of bronchi:
- Cartilage
- Goblet cells

Extending to end of terminal bronchioles:
- Pseudostratified ciliated columnar cells (beat mucus up and out of lungs)
- Smooth muscle of the airway walls (sparse beyond this point)

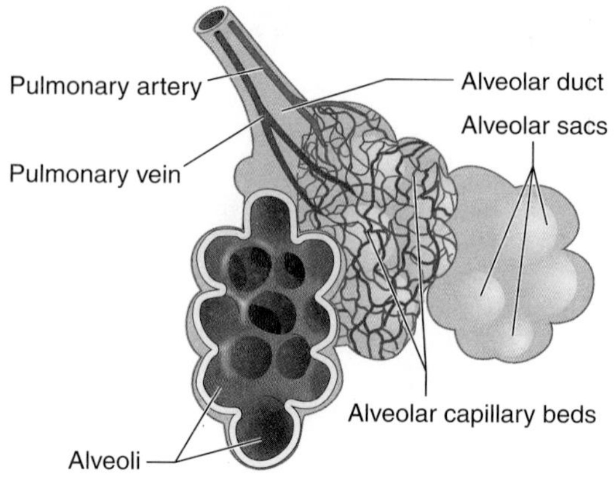

Pulmonary artery
Pulmonary vein
Alveolar duct
Alveolar sacs
Alveolar capillary beds
Alveoli

Respiratory zone

Lung parenchyma; consists of respiratory bronchioles, alveolar ducts, and alveoli. Participates in gas exchange.

Mostly cuboidal cells in respiratory bronchioles, then simple squamous cells up to alveoli. No cilia. Alveolar macrophages clear debris and participate in immune response.

Pneumocytes

Type I cells

97% of alveolar surfaces. Line the alveoli. Squamous; thin for optimal gas diffusion.

Type II cells

Secrete pulmonary surfactant → ↓ alveolar surface tension and prevention of alveolar collapse (atelectasis). Cuboidal and clustered. Also serve as precursors to type I cells and other type II cells. Type II cells proliferate during lung damage.

Clara cells

Nonciliated; columnar with secretory granules. Secrete component of surfactant; degrade toxins; act as reserve cells.

$$\text{Collapsing pressure} = P = \frac{2\ (\text{surface tension})}{\text{radius}}$$

Alveoli have ↑ tendency to collapse on expiration as radius ↓ (law of Laplace).

Pulmonary surfactant is a complex mix of lecithins, the most important of which is dipalmitoylphosphatidylcholine.

Surfactant synthesis begins around week 26 of gestation, but mature levels are not achieved until around week 35.

A lecithin-to-sphingomyelin ratio > 2.0 in amniotic fluid indicates fetal lung maturity.

Lung relations

Right lung has 3 lobes; **L**eft has 2 **L**obes and **L**ingula (homologue of right middle lobe). Right lung is more common site for inhaled foreign body because the right main stem bronchus is wider and more vertical than the left.

Aspirate a peanut:
- While upright—lower portion of right inferior lobe.
- While supine—superior portion of right inferior lobe.

Instead of a middle lobe, the left lung has a space occupied by the heart. The relation of the pulmonary artery to the bronchus at each lung hilus is described by **RALS**—**R**ight **A**nterior; **L**eft **S**uperior.

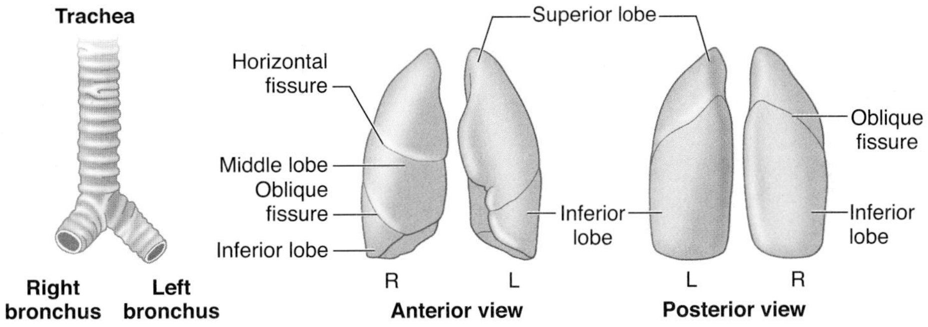

Diaphragm structures

Structures perforating diaphragm:
- At T8: IVC
- At T**10**: esophagus, vagus (2 trunks)
- At T12: aorta (red), thoracic duct (white), azygos vein (blue) ("At **T-1-2** it's the **red**, **white**, and **blue**")

Diaphragm is innervated by **C3, 4,** and **5** (phrenic nerve). Pain from the diaphragm can be referred to the shoulder (C5) and the trapezius ridge (C3, 4).

Number of letters = T level:
T8: vena cava
T10: esophagus
T12: aortic hiatus

I (IVC) **ate** (8) **ten** (10) **eggs** (esophagus) **at** (aorta) **twelve** (12).

C3, 4, 5 keeps the diaphragm **alive**.

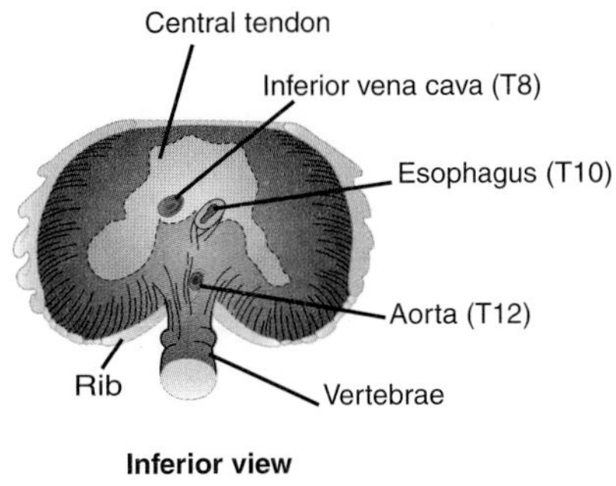

Muscles of respiration

Quiet breathing:
- Inspiration—diaphragm
- Expiration—passive

Exercise:
- InSpiration—external intercostals, Scalene muscles, Sternocleidomastoids
- Expiration—rectus abdominis, internal and external obliques, transversus abdominis, internal intercostals

▸ RESPIRATORY–PHYSIOLOGY

Lung volumes

Inspiratory reserve volume (IRV)	Air that can still be breathed in after normal inspiration
Tidal volume (TV)	Air that moves into lung with each quiet inspiration, typically 500 mL
Expiratory reserve volume (ERV)	Air that can still be breathed out after normal expiration
Residual volume (RV)	Air in lung after maximal expiration; cannot be measured on spirometry
Inspiratory capacity (IC)	IRV + TV
Functional residual capacity (FRC)	RV + ERV (volume in lungs after normal expiration)
Vital capacity (VC)	TV + IRV + ERV Maximum volume of gas that can be expired after a maximal inspiration
Total lung capacity (TLC)	TLC = IRV + TV + ERV + RV Volume of gas present in lungs after a maximal inspiration

Lung volumes (**LITER**):

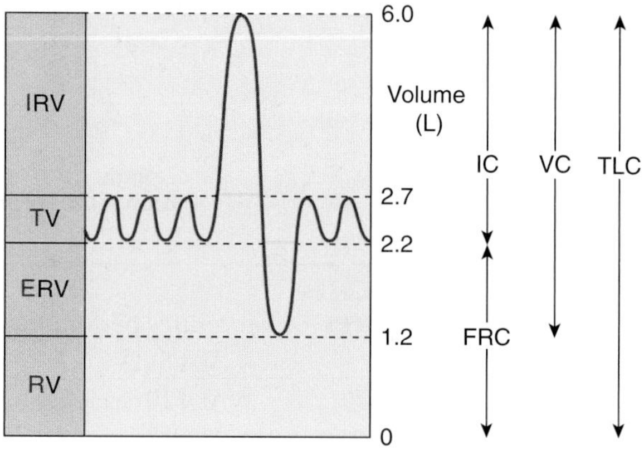

A capacity is a sum of ≥ 2 volumes.

Determination of physiologic dead space

$$V_D = V_T \times \frac{(Pa_{CO_2} - Pe_{CO_2})}{Pa_{CO_2}}$$

V_D = physiologic dead space = anatomic dead space of conducting airways plus functional dead space in alveoli; apex of healthy lung is largest contributor of functional dead space. Volume of inspired air that does not take part in gas exchange.

V_T = tidal volume.

Pa_{CO_2} = arterial P_{CO_2}, Pe_{CO_2} = expired air P_{CO_2}.

Taco, **P**aco, **PE**co, **P**aco (refers to order of variables in equation)

Lung and chest wall	Tendency for lungs to collapse inward and chest wall to spring outward. At FRC, inward pull of lung is balanced by outward pull of chest wall, and system pressure is atmospheric. Elastic properties of both chest wall and lungs determine their combined volume. At FRC, airway and alveolar pressures are 0, and intrapleural pressure is negative (prevents pneumothorax). Compliance—change in lung volume for a given change in pressure; ↓ in pulmonary fibrosis, pneumonia, and pulmonary edema; ↑ in emphysema and normal aging.	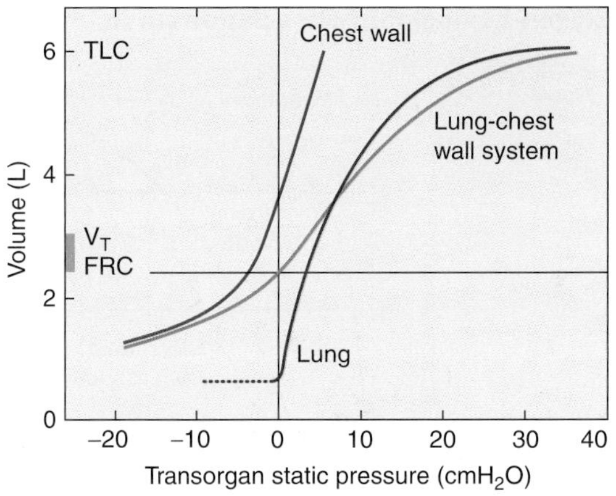

Hemoglobin 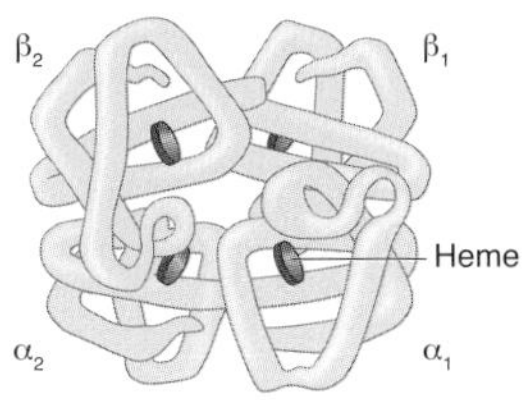	Hemoglobin is composed of 4 polypeptide subunits (2 α and 2 β) and exists in 2 forms: ▪ T (taut) form has low affinity for O_2. ▪ R (relaxed) form has high affinity for O_2 (300×). Hemoglobin exhibits positive cooperativity and negative allostery. ↑ Cl^-, H^+, CO_2, 2,3-BPG, and temperature favor taut form over relaxed form (shifts dissociation curve to right, leading to ↑ O_2 unloading).	Fetal hemoglobin (2 α and 2 γ subunits) has lower affinity for 2,3-BPG than adult hemoglobin and thus has higher affinity for O_2. **T**aut in **T**issues. **R**elaxed in **R**espiratory.

Hemoglobin modifications	Lead to tissue hypoxia from ↓ O_2 saturation and ↓ O_2 content.	
Methemoglobin	Oxidized form of hemoglobin (ferric, Fe^{3+}) that does not bind O_2 as readily, but has ↑ affinity for cyanide. Iron in hemoglobin is normally in a reduced state (ferrous, Fe^{2+}). To treat cyanide poisoning, use nitrites to oxidize hemoglobin to methemoglobin, which binds cyanide, allowing cytochrome oxidase to function. Use thiosulfate to bind this cyanide, forming thiocyanate, which is renally excreted.	**Meth**emoglobinemia can be treated with **meth**ylene blue. Nitrites cause poisoning by oxidizing Fe^{2+} to Fe^{3+}.
Carboxyhemoglobin	Form of hemoglobin bound to CO in place of O_2. Causes ↓ oxygen-binding capacity with a left shift in the oxygen-hemoglobin dissociation curve. ↓ oxygen unloading in tissues.	CO has 200× greater affinity than O_2 for hemoglobin.

Oxygen-hemoglobin dissociation curve

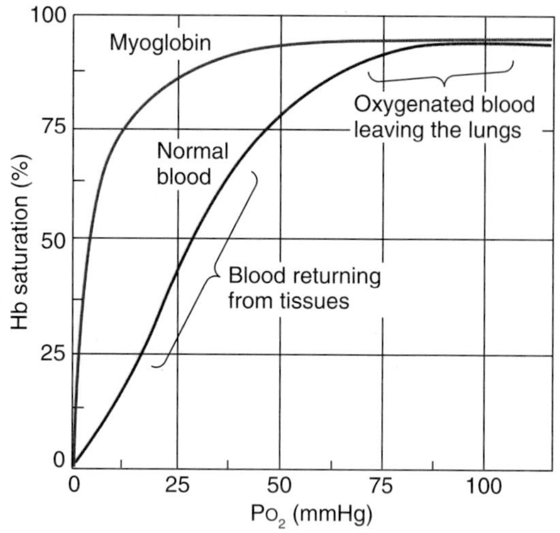

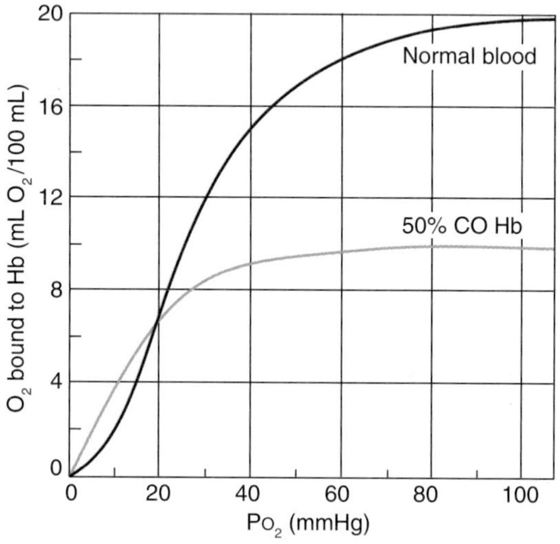

Sigmoidal shape due to positive cooperativity (i.e., tetrameric hemoglobin molecule can bind 4 oxygen molecules and has higher affinity for each subsequent oxygen molecule bound). Myoglobin is monomeric and thus does not show positive cooperativity; curve lacks sigmoidal appearance.

When curve shifts to the right, ↓ affinity of hemoglobin for O_2 (facilitates unloading of O_2 to tissue).

An ↑ in all factors (except pH) causes a shift of the curve to the right.

A ↓ in all factors (except pH) causes a shift of the curve to the left.

Fetal Hb has a higher affinity for oxygen than adult Hb, so its dissociation curve is shifted left.

Right shift—**C-BEAT**:

- **C**O_2
- **B**PG (2,3-BPG)
- **E**xercise
- **A**cid/**A**ltitude
- **T**emperature

Pulmonary circulation

Normally a low-resistance, high-compliance system. P_{O_2} and P_{CO_2} exert opposite effects on pulmonary and systemic circulation. A ↓ in P_{AO_2} causes a hypoxic vasoconstriction that shifts blood away from poorly ventilated regions of lung to well-ventilated regions of lung.

Perfusion limited—O_2 (normal health), CO_2, N_2O. Gas equilibrates early along the length of the capillary. Diffusion can be ↑ only if blood flow ↑.

Diffusion limited—O_2 (emphysema, fibrosis), CO. Gas does not equilibrate by the time blood reaches the end of the capillary.

A consequence of pulmonary hypertension is cor pulmonale and subsequent right ventricular failure (jugular venous distention, edema, hepatomegaly).

Diffusion: $V_{gas} = A/T \times D_k(P_1 - P_2)$ where A = area, T = thickness, and $D_k(P_1 - P_2) \approx$ difference in partial pressures:

- A ↓ in emphysema.
- T ↑ in pulmonary fibrosis.

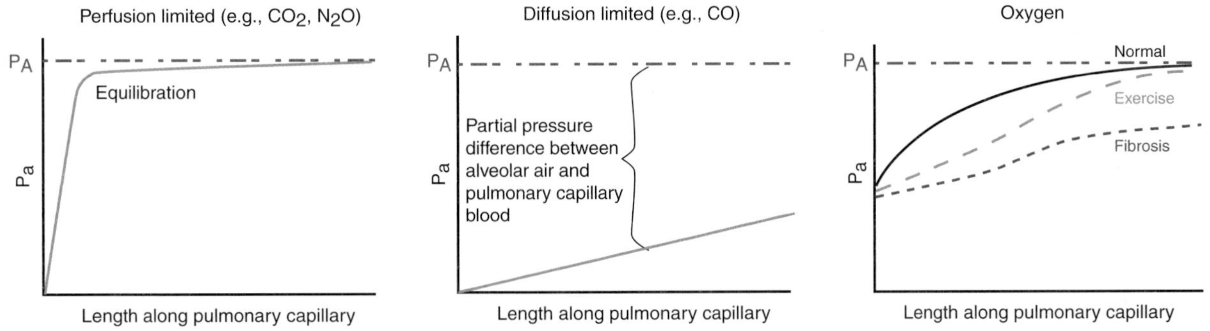

P_a = partial pressure of gas in pulmonary capillary blood
P_A = partial pressure of gas in alveolar air

Pulmonary hypertension

Normal pulmonary artery pressure = 10–14 mmHg; pulmonary hypertension ≥ 25 mmHg or > 35 mmHg during exercise. Results in arteriosclerosis, medial hypertrophy, and intimal fibrosis of pulmonary arteries.

Primary—due to an inactivating mutation in the *BMPR2* gene (normally functions to inhibit vascular smooth muscle proliferation); poor prognosis.

Secondary—due to COPD (destruction of lung parenchyma); mitral stenosis (↑ resistance → ↑ pressure); recurrent thromboemboli (↓ cross-sectional area of pulmonary vascular bed); autoimmune disease (e.g., systemic sclerosis; inflammation → intimal fibrosis → medial hypertrophy); left-to-right shunt (↑ shear stress → endothelial injury); sleep apnea or living at high altitude (hypoxic vasoconstriction).

Course: severe respiratory distress → cyanosis and RVH → death from decompensated cor pulmonale.

Pulmonary vascular resistance

$$PVR = \frac{P_{pulm\ artery} - P_{L\ atrium}}{\text{Cardiac output}}$$

Remember: $\Delta P = Q \times R$, so $R = \Delta P / Q$

$R = 8\eta l / \pi r^4$

$P_{pulm\ artery}$ = pressure in pulmonary artery
$P_{L\ atrium}$ = pulmonary wedge pressure

η = the viscosity of blood; l = vessel length; r = vessel radius

Oxygen content of blood

O_2 content = (O_2 binding capacity × % saturation) + dissolved O_2.
Normally 1 g Hb can bind 1.34 mL O_2; normal Hb amount in blood is 15 g/dL. Cyanosis results when deoxygenated Hb > 5 g/dL.
O_2 binding capacity ≈ 20.1 mL O_2/dL.
O_2 content of arterial blood ↓ as Hb falls, but O_2 saturation and arterial Po_2 do not.
Oxygen delivery to tissues = cardiac output × oxygen content of blood.

Alveolar gas equation

$$PA_{O_2} = PI_{O_2} - \frac{Pa_{CO_2}}{R}$$

Can normally be approximated:
$PA_{O_2} = 150 - Pa_{CO_2} / 0.8$

PA_{O_2} = alveolar Po_2 (mmHg).
PI_{O_2} = Po_2 in inspired air (mmHg).
Pa_{CO_2} = arterial Pco_2 (mmHg).
R = respiratory quotient = CO_2 produced/O_2 consumed.
A-a gradient = $PA_{O_2} - Pa_{O_2}$ = 10–15 mmHg.
↑ A-a gradient may occur in hypoxemia; causes include shunting, V/Q mismatch, fibrosis (impairs diffusion).

Oxygen deprivation

Hypoxemia (↓ Pa_{O_2})	Hypoxia (↓ O_2 delivery to tissue)	Ischemia (loss of blood flow)
Normal A-a gradient ▪ High altitude ▪ Hypoventilation ↑ A-a gradient ▪ V/Q mismatch ▪ Diffusion limitation ▪ Right-to-left shunt	↓ cardiac output Hypoxemia Anemia CO poisoning	Impeded arterial flow Reduced venous drainage

V/Q mismatch

Ideally, ventilation is matched to perfusion (i.e., V/Q = 1) in order for adequate gas exchange to occur.

Lung zones:

- Apex of the lung—V/Q = 3 (wasted ventilation)
- Base of the lung—V/Q = 0.6 (wasted perfusion)

Both ventilation and perfusion are greater at the base of the lung than at the apex of the lung.

With exercise (↑ cardiac output), there is vasodilation of apical capillaries, resulting in a V/Q ratio that approaches 1.

Certain organisms that thrive in high O_2 (e.g., TB) flourish in the apex.

V/Q → 0 = airway obstruction (shunt). In shunt, 100% O_2 does not improve Po_2.

V/Q → ∞ = blood flow obstruction (physiologic dead space). Assuming < 100% dead space, 100% O_2 improves Po_2.

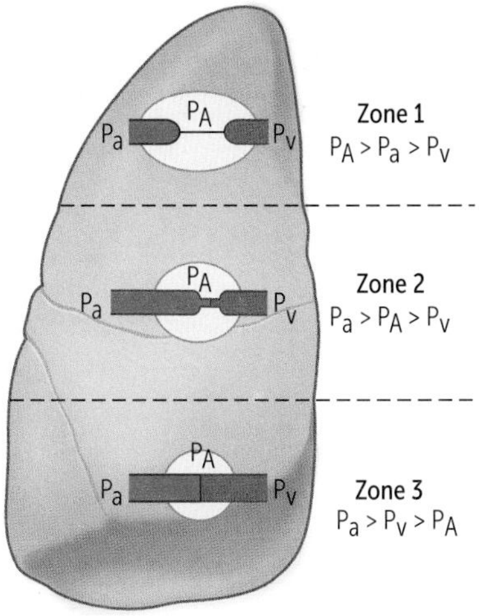

Pa
PA
Pv
Zone 1
PA > Pa > Pv
Zone 2
Pa > PA > Pv
Zone 3
Pa > Pv > PA

CO_2 transport

Carbon dioxide is transported from tissues to the lungs in 3 forms:

- Bicarbonate (90%).
- Carbaminohemoglobin or $HbCO_2$ (5%). CO_2 bound to hemoglobin at N-terminus of globin (not heme). CO_2 binding favors taut form (O_2 unloaded).
- Dissolved CO_2 (5%).

In lungs, oxygenation of Hb promotes dissociation of H^+ from Hb. This shifts equilibrium toward CO_2 formation; therefore, CO_2 is released from RBCs (Haldane effect).

In peripheral tissue, ↑ H^+ from tissue metabolism shifts curve to right, unloading O_2 (Bohr effect).

Majority of blood CO_2 is carried as bicarbonate in the plasma.

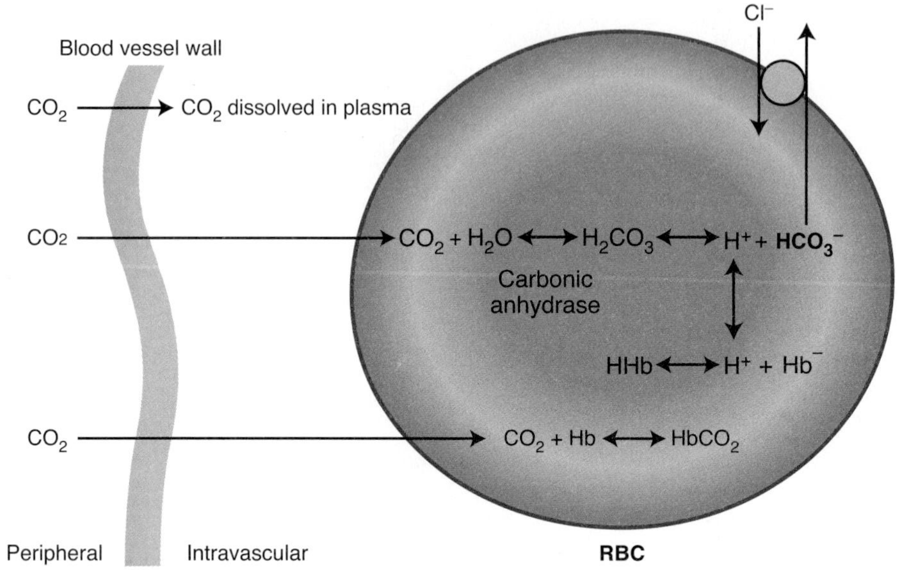

Response to high altitude

Acute ↑ in ventilation, ↓ P_{O_2} and P_{CO_2}
Chronic ↑ in ventilation
↑ erythropoietin → ↑ hematocrit and hemoglobin (chronic hypoxia)
↑ 2,3-BPG (binds to hemoglobin so that hemoglobin releases more O_2)
Cellular changes (↑ mitochondria)
↑ renal excretion of bicarbonate (e.g., can augment by use of acetazolamide) to compensate for the respiratory alkalosis
Chronic hypoxic pulmonary vasoconstriction results in RVH

Response to exercise

↑ CO_2 production
↑ O_2 consumption
↑ ventilation rate to meet O_2 demand
V/Q ratio from apex to base becomes more uniform
↑ pulmonary blood flow due to ↑ cardiac output
↓ pH during strenuous exercise (2° to lactic acidosis)
No change in Pa_{O_2} and Pa_{CO_2}, but ↑ in venous CO_2 content and ↓ in venous O_2 content

▶ RESPIRATORY–PATHOLOGY

Deep venous thrombosis

Predisposed by Virchow's triad:
- Stasis
- Hypercoagulability (e.g., defect in coagulation cascade proteins, most commonly factor V Leiden)
- Endothelial damage (exposed collagen triggers clotting cascade)

Can lead to pulmonary embolus.
Homans' sign—dorsiflexion of foot → calf pain.
Use heparin for prevention and acute management; use warfarin for long-term prevention of DVT recurrence.

Pulmonary emboli

Sudden-onset dyspnea, chest pain, tachypnea. May present as sudden death.
Types: **F**at, **A**ir, **T**hrombus, **B**acteria, **A**mniotic fluid, **T**umor. Fat emboli—associated with long bone fractures and liposuction; classic triad of hypoxemia, neurologic abnormalities, and petechial rash.
Amniotic fluid emboli—can lead to DIC, especially postpartum. A B.

An embolus moves like a **FAT BAT**.
Approximately 95% of pulmonary emboli arise from deep leg veins.
CT pulmonary angiography is the imaging test of choice for a PE.

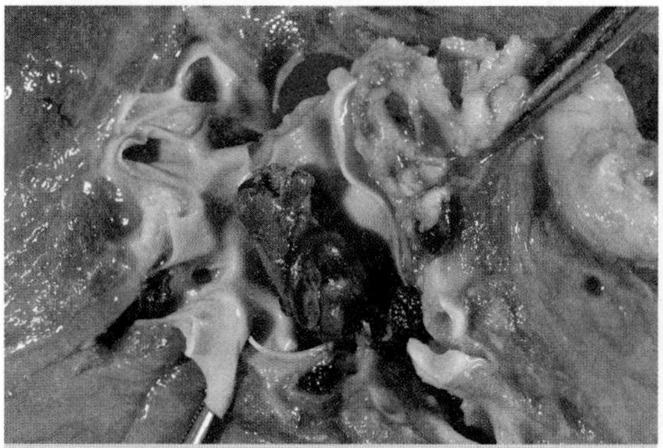

A **Pulmonary embolism.** Note saddle embolus in the pulmonary artery. ℞

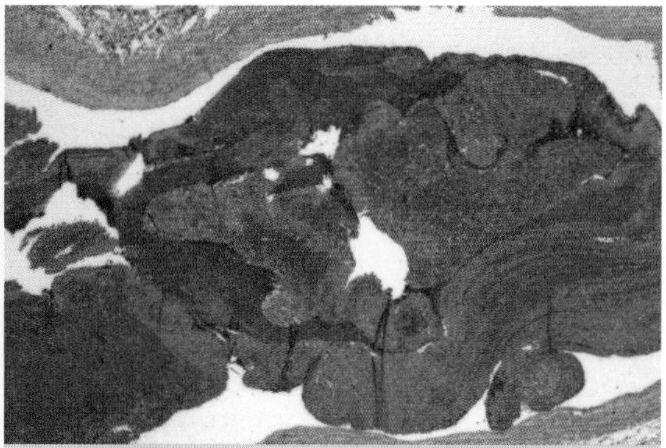

B **Pulmonary thromboembolus.** Lines of Zahn are interdigitating areas of pink (platelets, fibrin) and red (RBCs) found only in thrombi formed before death. Help distinguish pre- and postmortem thrombi. ℞

Obstructive lung diseases

Obstruction of air flow resulting in air trapping in the lungs. Airways close prematurely at high lung volumes, resulting in ↑ RV and ↓ FVC. PFTs: ↓↓ FEV_1, ↓ FVC → ↓ FEV_1/FVC ratio (hallmark), V/Q mismatch.

TYPE	PATHOLOGY	OTHER
Chronic bronchitis ("blue bloater")	A form of COPD along with emphysema. Hypertrophy of mucus-secreting glands in the bronchi → Reid index (thickness of gland layer/total thickness of bronchial wall) > 50%.	Productive cough for > 3 months per year (not necessarily consecutive) for > 2 years. Disease of small airways. Findings: wheezing, crackles, cyanosis (early-onset hypoxemia due to shunting), late-onset dyspnea.
Emphysema ("pink puffer," barrel-shaped chest)	Enlargement of air spaces and ↓ recoil resulting from destruction of alveolar walls A B; ↑ compliance. Two types: ▪ Centriacinar—associated with smoking. ▪ Panacinar—associated with α_1-antitrypsin deficiency.	↑ elastase activity. ↑ lung compliance due to loss of elastic fibers. Exhalation through pursed lips to ↑ airway pressure and prevent airway collapse during respiration.

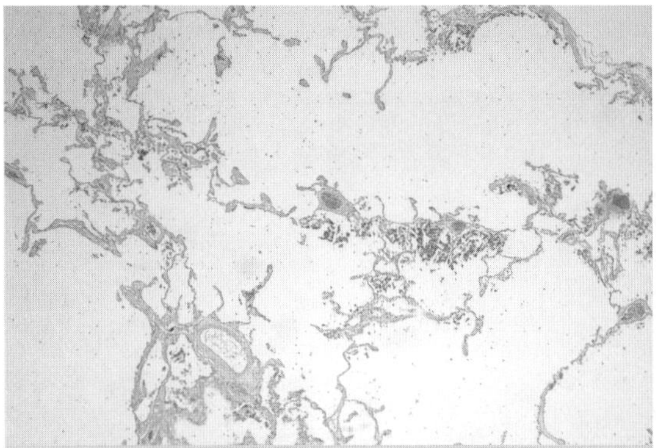

A **Emphysema.** On microscopy, enlarged alveoli are seen separated by thin septa, some of which appear to float in the alveolar spaces. Rx

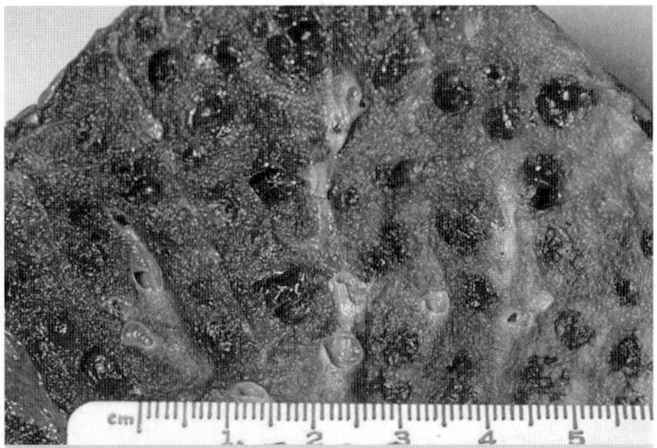

B **Emphysema.** Gross specimen showing multiple cavities linked by heavy black carbon deposits.

TYPE	PATHOLOGY	OTHER
Asthma	Bronchial hyperresponsiveness causes reversible bronchoconstriction. Smooth muscle hypertrophy, Curschmann's spirals (shed epithelium forms mucus plugs), and Charcot-Leyden crystals (formed from breakdown of eosinophils in sputum).	Can be triggered by viral URIs, allergens, and stress. Test with methacholine challenge. Findings: cough, wheezing, tachypnea, dyspnea, hypoxemia, ↓ I/E ratio, pulsus paradoxus, mucus plugging.
Bronchiectasis	Chronic necrotizing infection of bronchi → permanently dilated airways, purulent sputum, recurrent infections, hemoptysis.	Associated with bronchial obstruction, poor ciliary motility (smoking), Kartagener's syndrome, cystic fibrosis, allergic bronchopulmonary aspergillosis.

Restrictive lung disease

Restricted lung expansion causes ↓ lung volumes (↓ FVC and TLC). PFTs—FEV_1/FVC ratio > 80%.

Types:

- Poor breathing mechanics (extrapulmonary, peripheral hypoventilation, normal A-a gradient):
  - Poor muscular effort—polio, myasthenia gravis
  - Poor structural apparatus—scoliosis, morbid obesity
- Interstitial lung diseases (pulmonary, lowered diffusing capacity, ↑ A-a gradient):
  - Acute respiratory distress syndrome (ARDS)
  - Neonatal respiratory distress syndrome (hyaline membrane disease)
  - Pneumoconioses (anthracosis, silicosis, asbestosis)
  - Sarcoidosis: bilateral hilar lymphadenopathy, noncaseating granuloma; ↑ ACE and calcium
  - Idiopathic pulmonary fibrosis (repeated cycles of lung injury and wound healing with ↑ collagen deposition)
  - Goodpasture's syndrome
  - Granulomatosis with polyangiitis (Wegener's)
  - Langerhans cell histiocytosis (eosinophilic granuloma)
  - Hypersensitivity pneumonitis
  - Drug toxicity (bleomycin, busulfan, amiodarone, methotrexate)

Pneumoconioses	Anthracosis, silicosis, and asbestosis → ↑ risk of cor pulmonale and Caplan's syndrome.	
Anthracosis	Associated with coal mines ("coal miner's lung").	Affects upper lobes.
Silicosis	Associated with foundries, sandblasting, and mines. Macrophages respond to silica and release fibrogenic factors, leading to fibrosis. It is thought that silica may disrupt phagolysosomes and impair macrophages, increasing susceptibility to TB. Also increases risk of bronchogenic carcinoma.	Affects upper lobes. "Eggshell" calcification of hilar lymph nodes.
Asbestosis 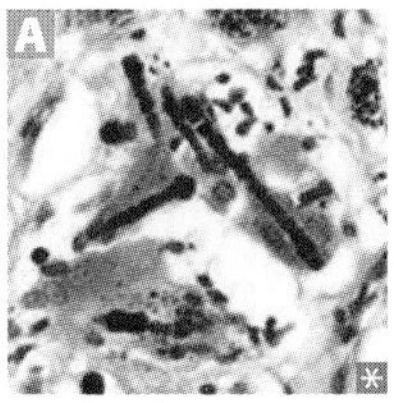	Associated with shipbuilding, roofing, and plumbing. "Ivory white," calcified pleural plaques are pathognomonic of asbestos exposure, but are not precancerous. Associated with an ↑ incidence of bronchogenic carcinoma and mesothelioma.	Affects lower lobes. Asbestos bodies are golden-brown fusiform rods resembling dumbbells A.

Neonatal respiratory distress syndrome

Surfactant deficiency leading to ↑ surface tension, resulting in alveolar collapse. A lecithin:sphingomyelin ratio < 1.5 in amniotic fluid is predictive of neonatal respiratory distress syndrome. Persistently low O_2 tension → risk of PDA. Therapeutic supplemental O_2 can result in retinopathy of prematurity and bronchopulmonary dysplasia.

Risk factors: prematurity, maternal diabetes (due to elevated fetal insulin), cesarean delivery (↓ release of fetal glucocorticoids).

Treatment: maternal steroids before birth; artificial surfactant for infant.

Acute respiratory distress syndrome (ARDS)

May be caused by trauma, sepsis, shock, gastric aspiration, uremia, acute pancreatitis, or amniotic fluid embolism. Diffuse alveolar damage → ↑ alveolar capillary permeability → protein-rich leakage into alveoli. Results in formation of intra-alveolar hyaline membrane A. Initial damage due to release of neutrophilic substances toxic to alveolar wall, activation of coagulation cascade, and oxygen-derived free radicals.

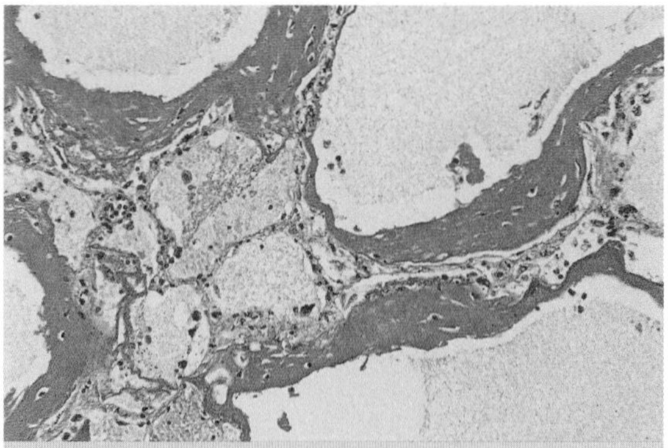

A **Acute respiratory distress syndrome.** Note the alveolar fluid and the hyaline membranes.

Obstructive vs. restrictive lung disease

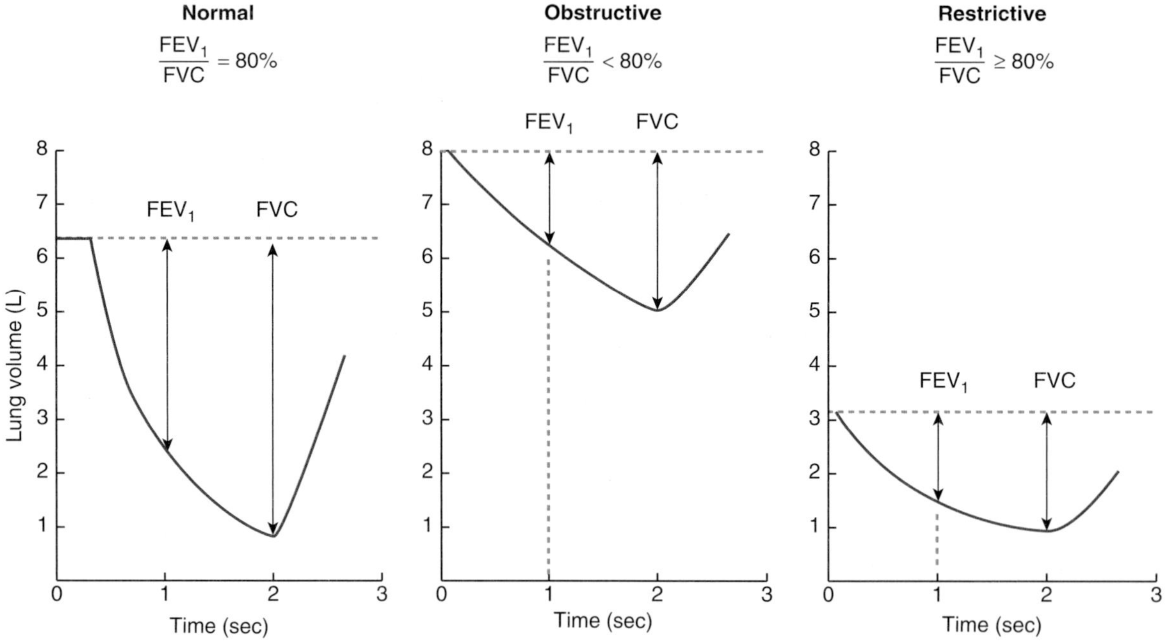

Note: Obstructive lung volumes > normal (↑ TLC, ↑ FRC, ↑ RV); restrictive lung volumes < normal. In both obstructive and restrictive, FEV_1 and FVC are reduced. In obstructive, however, FEV_1 is more dramatically reduced compared to FVC, resulting in a ↓ FEV_1/FVC ratio.

Sleep apnea

Repeated cessation of breathing > 10 seconds during sleep → disrupted sleep → daytime somnolence.

Central sleep apnea—no respiratory effort.

Obstructive sleep apnea—respiratory effort against airway obstruction. Associated with obesity, loud snoring, systemic/pulmonary hypertension, arrhythmias, and possibly sudden death.

Treatment: weight loss, CPAP, surgery.

Hypoxia → ↑ EPO release → ↑ erythropoiesis.

Lung—physical findings

ABNORMALITY	BREATH SOUNDS	PERCUSSION	FREMITUS	TRACHEAL DEVIATION
Pleural effusion	↓	Dull	↓	—
Atelectasis (bronchial obstruction)	↓	Dull	↓	Toward side of lesion
Spontaneous pneumothorax	↓	Hyperresonant	↓	Toward side of lesion
Tension pneumothorax	↓	Hyperresonant	↓	Away from side of lesion
Consolidation (lobar pneumonia, pulmonary edema)	Bronchial breath sounds; late inspiratory crackles	Dull	↑	—

Lung cancer

Lung cancer is the leading cause of cancer death.
Presentation: cough, hemoptysis, bronchial obstruction, wheezing, pneumonic "coin" lesion on x-ray film or noncalcified nodule on CT.
Metastatic cancer is most common cause. Most often from breast, colon, prostate, and bladder cancer.
Sites of metastases—adrenals, brain, bone (pathologic fracture), liver (jaundice, hepatomegaly).

SPHERE of complications:
- **S**uperior vena cava syndrome
- **P**ancoast tumor
- **H**orner's syndrome
- **E**ndocrine (paraneoplastic)
- **R**ecurrent laryngeal symptoms (hoarseness)
- **E**ffusions (pleural or pericardial)

All lung cancer types except **bro**nchioloalveolar and **bro**nchial carcinoid are associated with smoking.

TYPE	LOCATION	CHARACTERISTICS	HISTOLOGY
Adenocarcinoma	Peripheral	Most common lung cancer in nonsmokers and females. Activating mutations in k-*ras* common. Associated with hypertrophic osteoarthropathy (clubbing). Bronchioloalveolar subtype: CXR often shows hazy infiltrates similar to pneumonia; excellent prognosis.	Bronchioloalveolar subtype: grows along alveolar septa → apparent "thickening" of alveolar walls.
Squamous cell carcinoma	Central	Hilar mass arising from bronchus; **C**avitation; **C**igarettes (linked to smoking); hyper**C**alcemia (produces PTHrP).	Keratin pearls and intercellular bridges B.
Small cell (oat cell) carcinoma	Central	Undifferentiated → very aggressive. May produce **A**CTH, **A**DH, or **A**ntibodies against presynaptic calcium channels (Lambert-Eaton syndrome). Amplification of *myc* oncogenes common. Inoperable; treated with chemotherapy.	Neoplasm of neuroendocrine Kulchitsky cells → small dark blue cells A.
Large cell carcinoma	Peripheral	Highly anaplastic undifferentiated tumor; poor prognosis. Less responsive to chemotherapy; removed surgically.	Pleomorphic giant cells.
Bronchial carcinoid tumor	—	Excellent prognosis; metastasis rare. Symptoms usually due to mass effect; occasionally carcinoid syndrome (serotonin secretion → flushing, diarrhea, wheezing).	Nests of neuroendocrine cells; chromogranin positive.

Lung cancer *(continued)*

TYPE	LOCATION	CHARACTERISTICS	HISTOLOGY
Mesothelioma	Pleural	Malignancy of the pleura associated with asbestosis. Results in hemorrhagic pleural effusions and pleural thickening.	Psammoma bodies.

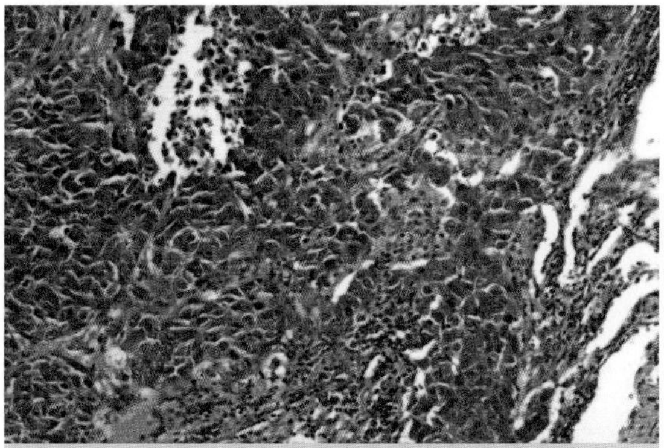

A **Small cell carcinoma.** Sheets of tumor cells with nuclear molding, high mitotic rate, necrosis, and "salt and pepper" neuroendocrine-type chromatin.

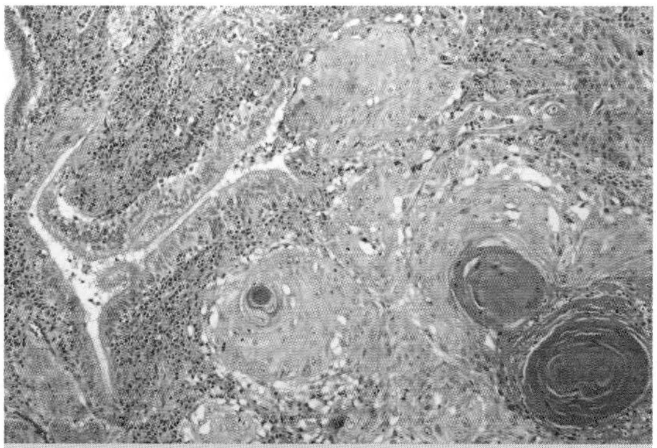

B **Squamous cell carcinoma.** Note sheets of large squamous cells with dysplasia and keratin "pearls."

Pancoast tumor

Carcinoma that occurs in apex of lung may affect cervical sympathetic plexus, causing Horner's syndrome.

Horner's syndrome—ipsilateral ptosis, miosis, anhidrosis.

Superior vena cava syndrome

An obstruction of the SVC that impairs blood drainage from the head ("facial plethora"), neck (jugular venous distention), and upper extremities (edema). Commonly caused by malignancy and thombosis from indwelling catheters. Medical emergency. Can raise intracranial pressure (if obstruction severe) → headaches, dizziness, and ↑ risk of aneurysm/rupture of cranial arteries.

Pneumonia

TYPE	ORGANISM(S)	CHARACTERISTICS
Lobar	*S. pneumoniae* most frequently, *Klebsiella*	Intra-alveolar exudate → consolidation; may involve entire lung A.
Bronchopneumonia	*S. pneumoniae, S. aureus, H. influenzae, Klebsiella*	Acute inflammatory infiltrates from bronchioles into adjacent alveoli; patchy distribution involving ≥ 1 lobe B C.
Interstitial (atypical) pneumonia	Viruses (influenza, RSV, adenoviruses), *Mycoplasma, Legionella, Chlamydia*	Diffuse patchy inflammation localized to interstitial areas at alveolar walls; distribution involving ≥ 1 lobe D. Generally follows a more indolent course.

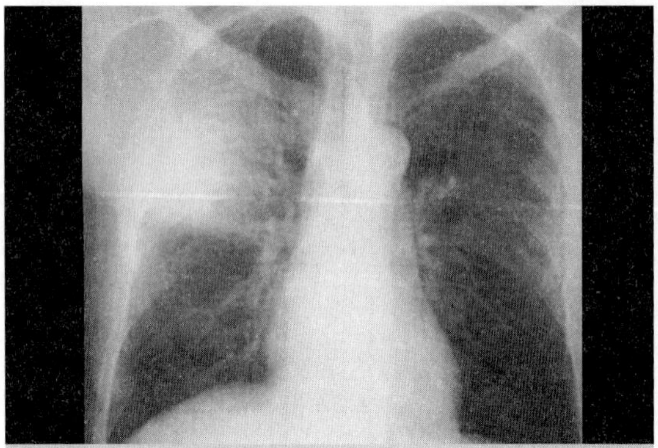

A **Lobar pneumonia.**

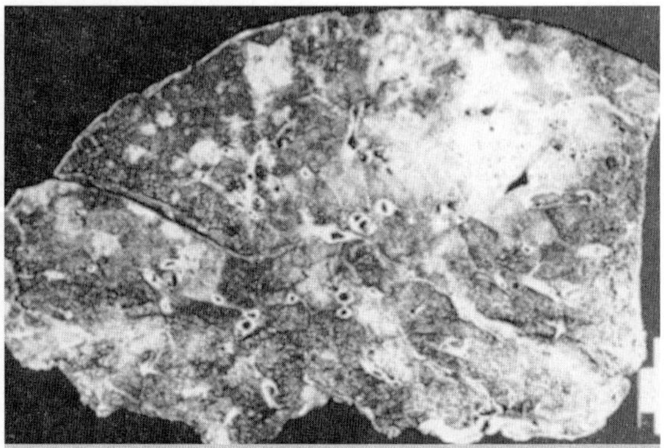

B **Bronchopneumonia.** Gross specimen shows large area of consolidation at the base.

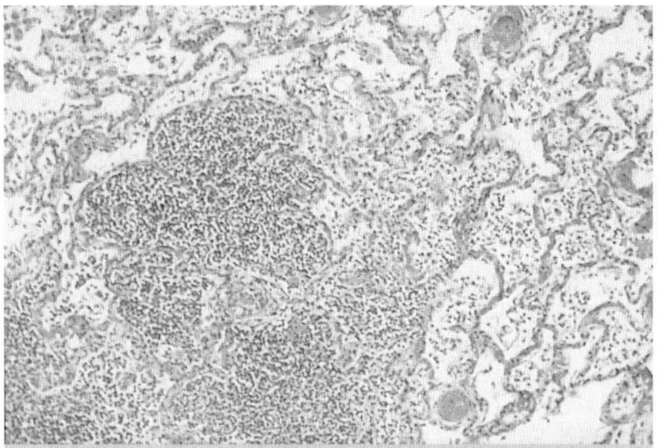

C **Bronchopneumonia.** Note neutrophils in the alveolar spaces.

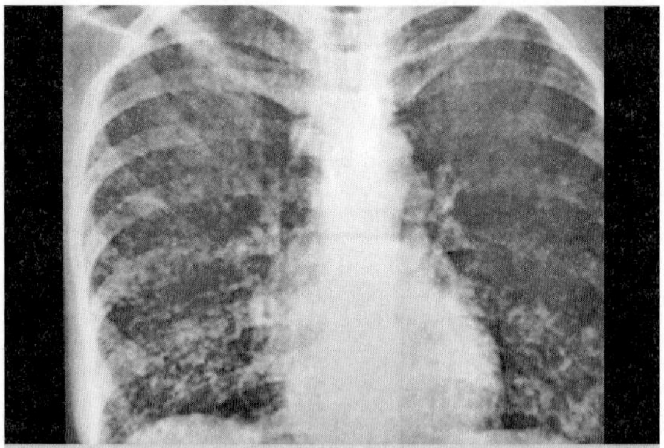

D **Interstitial pneumonia.**

Lung abscess	Localized collection of pus within parenchyma. Caused by: bronchial obstruction (e.g., cancer); aspiration of oropharyngeal contents (especially in patients predisposed to loss of consciousness [e.g., alcoholics or epileptics]).	Air-fluid levels often seen on CXR. Often due to *S. aureus* or anaerobes (*Bacteroides, Fusobacterium, Peptostreptococcus*).
Hypersensitivity pneumonitis	Mixed type III/IV hypersensitivity reaction to environmental antigen → dyspnea, cough, chest tightness, headache. Often seen in farmers and those exposed to birds.	

Pleural effusions

Transudate	↓ protein content. Due to CHF, nephrotic syndrome, or hepatic cirrhosis.
Exudate	↑ protein content, cloudy. Due to malignancy, pneumonia, collagen vascular disease, trauma (occurs in states of ↑ vascular permeability). Must be drained in light of risk of infection.
Lymphatic	Also known as chylothorax. Due to thoracic duct injury from trauma, malignancy. Milky-appearing fluid; ↑ triglycerides.

Pneumothorax

Unilateral chest pain and dyspnea, unilateral chest expansion, ↓ tactile fremitus, hyperresonance, diminished breath sounds.

Spontaneous pneumothorax

Accumulation of air in the pleural space A. Occurs most frequently in tall, thin, young males because of rupture of apical blebs. Trachea deviates toward affected lung.

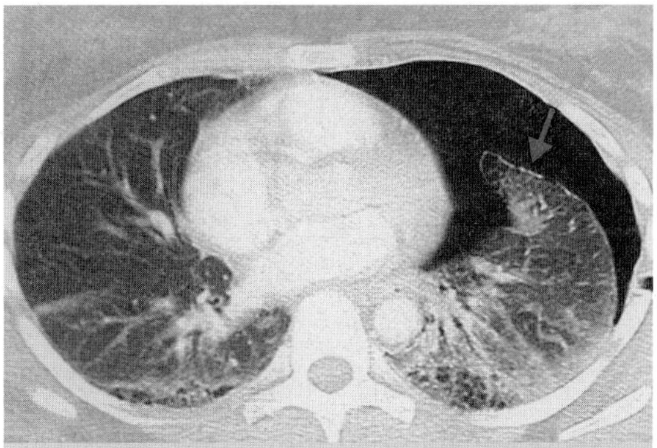

A **Spontaneous pneumothorax.** CT shows collapsed left lung (arrow).

Tension pneumothorax

Usually occurs in setting of trauma or lung infection. Air is capable of entering pleural space but not exiting. Trachea deviates away from affected lung B.

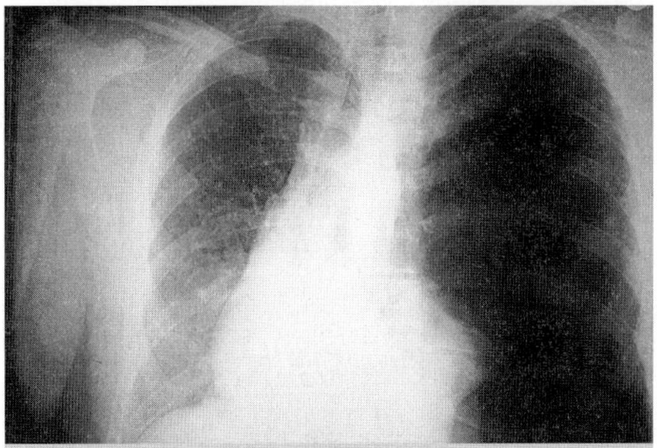

B **Tension pneumothorax.** Note the hyperlucent left lung field with low left hemidiaphragm and rightward mediastinal shift.

▶ RESPIRATORY–PHARMACOLOGY

H_1 blockers	Reversible inhibitors of H_1 histamine receptors.	
1st generation	Diphenhydramine, dimenhydrinate, chlorpheniramine.	Names contain "-en/-ine" or "-en/-ate."
CLINICAL USES	Allergy, motion sickness, sleep aid.	
TOXICITY	Sedation, antimuscarinic, anti-α-adrenergic.	
2nd generation	Loratadine, fexofenadine, desloratadine, cetirizine.	Names usually end in "-adine."
CLINICAL USES	Allergy.	
TOXICITY	Far less sedating than 1st generation because of ↓ entry into CNS.	

Asthma drugs	Bronchoconstriction is mediated by (1) inflammatory processes and (2) parasympathetic tone; therapy is directed at these 2 pathways.
β_2**-agonists**	**Albuterol**—relaxes bronchial smooth muscle (β_2). Use during acute exacerbation.
	Salmeterol, formoterol—long-acting agents for prophylaxis. Adverse effects are tremor and arrhythmia.
Methylxanthines	**Theophylline**—likely causes bronchodilation by inhibiting phosphodiesterase, thereby ↓ cAMP hydrolysis. Usage is limited because of narrow therapeutic index (cardiotoxicity, neurotoxicity); metabolized by P-450. Blocks actions of adenosine.
Muscarinic antagonists	**Ipratropium**—competitive block of muscarinic receptors, preventing bronchoconstriction. Also used for COPD, as is tiotropium, a long-acting muscarinic antagonist.
Corticosteroids	**Beclomethasone, fluticasone**—inhibit the synthesis of virtually all cytokines. Inactivate NF-κB, the transcription factor that induces the production of TNF-α, among other inflammatory agents. 1st-line therapy for chronic asthma.
Antileukotrienes	**Montelukast, zafirlukast**—block leukotriene receptors. Especially good for aspirin-induced asthma. **Zileuton**—a 5-lipoxygenase pathway inhibitor. Blocks conversion of arachidonic acid to leukotrienes.
Omalizumab	Monoclonal anti-IgE antibody. Binds mostly unbound serum IgE. Used in allergic asthma resistant to inhaled steroids and long-acting β_2-agonists.

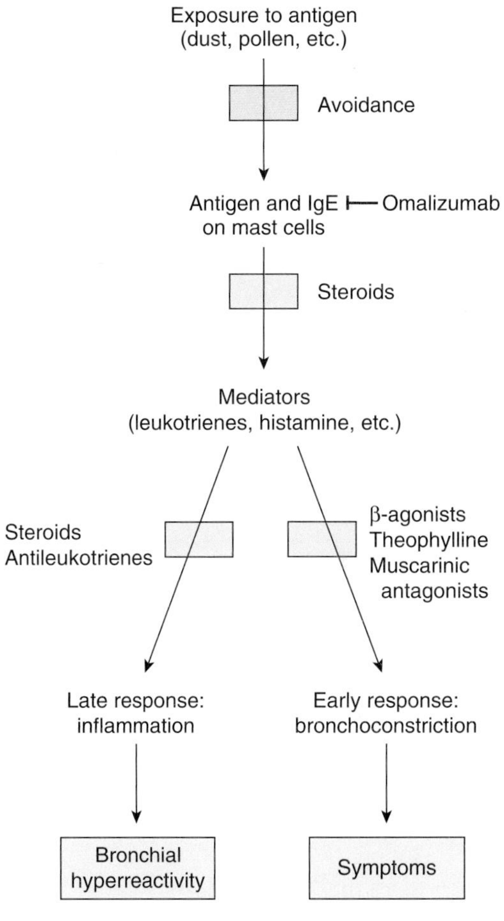

Treatment strategies in asthma

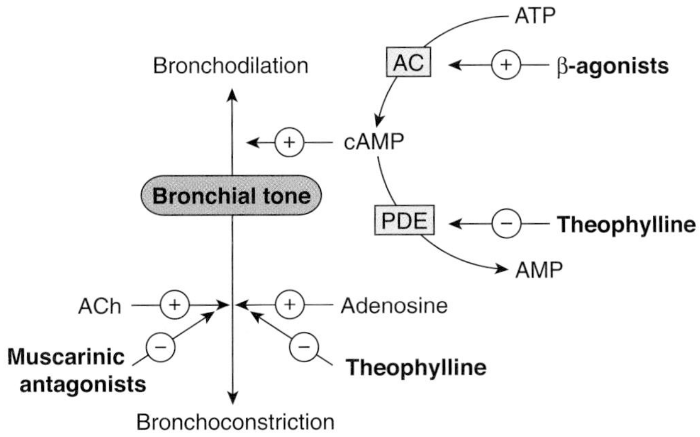

(Adapted, with permission, from Katzung BG, Trevor AJ. *Pharmacology: Examination & Board Review*, 5th ed. Stamford, CT: Appleton & Lange, 1998: 159 and 161.)

Expectorants	
Guaifenesin	Expectorant—thins respiratory secretions; does not suppress cough reflex.
***N*-acetylcysteine**	Mucolytic—can loosen mucous plugs in CF patients. Also used as an antidote for acetaminophen overdose.

Bosentan	Used to treat pulmonary arterial hypertension. Competitively antagonizes endothelin-1 receptors, decreasing pulmonary vascular resistance.

Dextromethorphan	Antitussive (antagonizes NMDA glutamate receptors). Synthetic codeine analog. Has mild opioid effect when used in excess. Naloxone can be given for overdose. Mild abuse potential.

Pseudoephedrine, phenylephrine

MECHANISM	Sympathomimetic α-agonistic nonprescription nasal decongestants.
CLINICAL USE	Reduce hyperemia, edema, and nasal congestion; open obstructed eustachian tubes. Pseudoephedrine also used as a stimulant.
TOXICITY	Hypertension. Can also cause CNS stimulation/anxiety (pseudoephedrine).

Methacholine	Muscarinic receptor agonist. Used in asthma challenge testing.

HIGH-YIELD SYSTEMS

Rapid Review

"Study without thought is vain: thought without study is dangerous."
—Confucius

The following tables represent a collection of high-yield associations of diseases with their clinical findings, treatments, and pathophysiology. They serve as a quick review before the exam to tune your senses to commonly tested cases and "buzzwords."

▶ CLASSIC PRESENTATIONS

CLINICAL PRESENTATION	DIAGNOSIS/DISEASE
Abdominal pain, ascites, hepatomegaly	Budd-Chiari syndrome (posthepatic venous thrombosis)
Achilles tendon xanthoma	Familial hypercholesterolemia (↓ LDL receptor signaling)
Adrenal hemorrhage, hypotension, DIC	Waterhouse-Friderichsen syndrome (meningococcemia)
Arachnodactyly, lens dislocation, aortic dissection, hyperflexible joints	Marfan's syndrome (fibrillin defect)
Athlete with polycythemia	2° to erythropoietin injection
Back pain, fever, night sweats, weight loss	Pott's disease (vertebral tuberculosis)
Bilateral hilar adenopathy, uveitis	Sarcoidosis (noncaseating granulomas)
Blue sclera	Osteogenesis imperfecta (type I collagen defect)
Bluish line on gingiva	Burton's line (lead poisoning)
Bone pain, bone enlargement, arthritis	Paget's disease of bone (↑ osteoblastic and osteoclastic activity)
Bounding pulses, diastolic heart murmur, head bobbing	Aortic regurgitation
"Butterfly" facial rash and Raynaud's phenomenon in a young female	Systemic lupus erythematosus
Café-au-lait spots, Lisch nodules (iris hamartoma)	Neurofibromatosis type I (+ pheochromocytoma, optic gliomas)
Café-au-lait spots, polyostotic fibrous dysplasia, precocious puberty, multiple endocrine abnormalities	McCune-Albright syndrome (mosaic G-protein signaling mutation)
Calf pseudohypertrophy	Muscular dystrophy (most commonly Duchenne's): X-linked recessive deletion of dystrophin gene
"Cherry-red spot" on macula	Tay-Sachs (ganglioside accumulation) or Niemann-Pick (sphingomyelin accumulation), central retinal artery occlusion
Chest pain on exertion	Angina (stable: with moderate exertion; unstable: with minimal exertion)
Chest pain, pericardial effusion/friction rub, persistent fever following MI	Dressler's syndrome (autoimmune-mediated post-MI fibrinous pericarditis, 1–12 weeks after acute episode)
Child uses arms to stand up from squat	Gowers' sign (Duchenne muscular dystrophy)
Child with fever later develops red rash on face that spreads to body	"Slapped cheeks" (erythema infectiosum/fifth disease: parvovirus B19)
Chorea, dementia, caudate degeneration	Huntington's disease (autosomal-dominant CAG repeat expansion)
Chronic exercise intolerance with myalgia, fatigue, painful cramps, myoglobinuria	McArdle's disease (muscle glycogen phosphorylase deficiency)
Cold intolerance	Hypothyroidism
Conjugate lateral gaze palsy, horizontal diplopia	Internuclear ophthalmoplegia (damage to MLF; bilateral [multiple sclerosis], unilateral [stroke])
Continuous "machinery" heart murmur	PDA (close with indomethacin; open or maintain with misoprostol)
Cutaneous/dermal edema due to connective tissue deposition	Myxedema (caused by hypothyroidism, Graves' disease [pretibial])

CLINICAL PRESENTATION	DIAGNOSIS/DISEASE
Dark purple skin/mouth nodules	Kaposi's sarcoma (usually AIDS patients [MSM]: associated with HHV-8)
Deep, labored breathing/hyperventilation	Kussmaul breathing (diabetic ketoacidosis)
Dermatitis, dementia, diarrhea	Pellagra (niacin [vitamin B_3] deficiency)
Dilated cardiomyopathy, edema, alcoholism or malnutrition	Wet beriberi (thiamine [vitamin B_1] deficiency)
Dog or cat bite resulting in infection	*Pasteurella multocida* (cellulitis at inoculation site)
Dry eyes, dry mouth, arthritis	Sjögren's syndrome (autoimmune destruction of exocrine glands)
Dysphagia (esophageal webs), glossitis, iron deficiency anemia	Plummer-Vinson syndrome (may progress to esophageal squamous cell carcinoma)
Elastic skin, hypermobility of joints	Ehlers-Danlos syndrome (type III collagen defect)
Enlarged, hard left supraclavicular node	Virchow's node (abdominal metastasis)
Erythroderma, lymphadenopathy, hepatosplenomegaly, atypical T cells	Sézary syndrome (cutaneous T-cell lymphoma) or mycosis fungoides
Facial muscle spasm upon tapping	Chvostek's sign (hypocalcemia)
Fat, female, forty, and fertile	Cholelithiasis (gallstones)
Fever, chills, headache, myalgia following antibiotic treatment for syphilis	Jarisch-Herxheimer reaction (rapid lysis of spirochetes results in toxin release)
Fever, cough, conjunctivitis, coryza, diffuse rash	Measles (*Morbillivirus*)
Fever, night sweats, weight loss	B symptoms (staging) of lymphoma
Fibrous plaques in soft tissue of penis	Peyronie's disease (connective tissue disorder)
Gout, mental retardation, self-mutilating behavior in a boy	Lesch-Nyhan syndrome (HGPRT deficiency, X-linked recessive)
Green-yellow rings around peripheral cornea	Kayser-Fleischer rings (copper accumulation from Wilson's disease)
Hamartomatous GI polyps, hyperpigmentation of mouth/feet/hands	Peutz-Jeghers syndrome (inherited, benign polyposis can cause bowel obstruction; ↑ cancer risk, mainly GI)
Hepatosplenomegaly, osteoporosis, neurologic symptoms	Gaucher's disease (glucocerebrosidase deficiency)
Hereditary nephritis, sensorineural hearing loss, cataracts	Alport syndrome (mutation in α chain of collagen IV)
Hyperphagia, hypersexuality, hyperorality, hyperdocility	Klüver-Bucy syndrome (bilateral amygdala lesion)
Hyperreflexia, hypertonia, Babinski sign present	UMN damage
Hyporeflexia, hypotonia, atrophy, fasciculations	LMN damage
Hypoxemia, polycythemia, hypercapnia	"Blue bloater" (chronic bronchitis: hyperplasia of mucous cells)
Indurated, ulcerated genital lesion	Nonpainful: chancre (1° syphilis, *Treponema pallidum*) Painful, with exudate: chancroid (*Haemophilus ducreyi*)
Infant with cleft lip/palate, microcephaly or holoprosencephaly, polydactyly, cutis aplasia	Patau's syndrome (trisomy 13)

CLINICAL PRESENTATION	DIAGNOSIS/DISEASE
Infant with failure to thrive, hepatosplenomegaly, and neurodegeneration	Niemann-Pick disease (genetic sphingomyelinase deficiency)
Infant with hypoglycemia, failure to thrive, and hepatomegaly	Cori's disease (debranching enzyme deficiency)
Infant with microcephaly, rocker-bottom feet, clenched hands, and structural heart defect	Edwards' syndrome (trisomy 18)
Jaundice, palpable distended non-tender gallbladder	Courvoisier's sign (distal obstruction of biliary tree)
Large rash with bull's-eye appearance	Erythema chronicum migrans from *Ixodes* tick bite (Lyme disease: *Borrelia*)
Lucid interval after traumatic brain injury	Epidural hematoma (middle meningeal artery rupture)
Male child, recurrent infections, no mature B cells	Bruton's disease (X-linked agammaglobulinemia)
Mucosal bleeding and prolonged bleeding time	Glanzmann's thrombasthenia (defect in platelet aggregation due to lack of GpIIb/IIIa)
Muffled heart sounds, distended neck veins, hypotension	Beck's triad of cardiac tamponade
Multiple colon polyps, osteomas/soft tissue tumors, impacted/supernumerary teeth	Gardner's syndrome (subtype of FAP)
Myopathy (infantile hypertrophic cardiomyopathy), exercise intolerance	Pompe's disease (lysosomal α-1,4-glucosidase deficiency)
Neonate with arm paralysis following difficult birth	Erb-Duchenne palsy (superior trunk [C5–C6] brachial plexus injury: "waiter's tip")
No lactation postpartum, absent menstruation, cold intolerance	Sheehan's syndrome (pituitary infarction)
Nystagmus, intention tremor, scanning speech, bilateral internuclear ophthalmoplegia	Multiple sclerosis
Oscillating slow/fast breathing	Cheyne-Stokes respirations (central apnea in CHF or ↑ intracranial pressure)
Painful blue fingers/toes, hemolytic anemia	Cold agglutinin disease (autoimmune hemolytic anemia caused by *Mycoplasma pneumoniae*, infectious mononucleosis)
Painful, pale, cold fingers/toes	Raynaud's phenomenon (vasospasm in extremities)
Painful, raised red lesions on pad of fingers/toes	Osler's node (infective endocarditis, immune complex deposition)
Painless erythematous lesions on palms and soles	Janeway lesions (infective endocarditis, septic emboli/microabscesses)
Painless jaundice	Cancer of the pancreatic head obstructing bile duct
Palpable purpura on buttocks/legs, joint pain, abdominal pain (child), hematuria	Henoch-Schönlein purpura (IgA vasculitis affecting skin and kidneys)
Pancreatic, pituitary, parathyroid tumors	MEN 1 (autosomal dominant)
Periorbital and/or peripheral edema, proteinuria, hypoalbuminemia, hypercholesterolemia	Nephrotic syndrome
Pink complexion, dyspnea, hyperventilation	"Pink puffer" (emphysema: centriacinar [smoking], panacinar [α_1-antitrypsin deficiency])

CLINICAL PRESENTATION	DIAGNOSIS/DISEASE
Polyuria, renal tubular acidosis type II, growth failure, electrolyte imbalances, hypophosphatemic rickets	Fanconi's syndrome (proximal tubular reabsorption defect)
Positive anterior "drawer sign"	Anterior cruciate ligament injury
Pruritic, purple, polygonal planar papules and plaques (6 P's)	Lichen planus
Ptosis, miosis, anhidrosis	Horner's syndrome (sympathetic chain lesion)
Pupil accommodates but doesn't react	Argyll Robertson pupil (neurosyphilis)
Rapidly progressive leg weakness that ascends following GI/upper respiratory infection	Guillain-Barré syndrome (acute autoimmune inflammatory demyelinating polyneuropathy)
Rash on palms and soles	Coxsackie A, 2° syphilis, Rocky Mountain spotted fever
Recurrent colds, unusual eczema, high serum IgE	Hyper-IgE syndrome (Job's syndrome: neutrophil chemotaxis abnormality)
Red "currant jelly" sputum in alcoholic or diabetic patients	*Klebsiella pneumoniae*
Red "currant jelly" stools	Acute mesenteric ischemia (adults), intussusception (infants)
Red, itchy, swollen rash of nipple/areola	Paget's disease of the breast (represents underlying neoplasm)
Red urine in the morning, fragile RBCs	Paroxysmal nocturnal hemoglobinuria
Renal cell carcinoma (bilateral), hemangioblastomas, angiomatosis, pheochromocytoma	von Hippel–Lindau disease (dominant tumor suppressor gene mutation)
Resting tremor, rigidity, akinesia, postural instability	Parkinson's disease (nigrostriatal dopamine depletion)
Retinal hemorrhages with pale centers	Roth's spots (bacterial endocarditis)
Severe jaundice in neonate	Crigler-Najjar syndrome (congenital unconjugated hyperbilirubinemia)
Severe RLQ pain with palpation of LLQ	Rovsing's sign (acute appendicitis)
Severe RLQ pain with rebound tenderness	McBurney's sign (appendicitis)
Short stature, ↑ incidence of tumors/leukemia, aplastic anemia	Fanconi's anemia (genetic loss of DNA crosslink repair; often progresses to AML)
Single palmar crease	Simian crease (Down syndrome)
Situs inversus, chronic sinusitis, bronchiectasis, infertility	Kartagener's syndrome (dynein arm defect affecting cilia)
Skin hyperpigmentation, hypotension, fatigue	Addison's disease (1° adrenocortical insufficiency causes ↑ ACTH and ↑ α-MSH production)
Slow, progressive muscle weakness in boys	Becker's muscular dystrophy (X-linked missense mutation in dystrophin; less severe than Duchenne's)
Small, irregular red spots on buccal/lingual mucosa with blue-white centers	Koplik spots (measles; rubeola virus)
Smooth, flat, moist, painless white lesions on genitals	Condylomata lata (2° syphilis)
Splinter hemorrhages in fingernails	Bacterial endocarditis
"Strawberry tongue"	Scarlet fever, Kawasaki disease, toxic shock syndrome
Streak ovaries, congenital heart disease, horseshoe kidney, cystic hygroma at birth, short stature, webbed neck, lymphedema	Turner syndrome (45,XO)
Sudden swollen/painful big toe joint, tophi	Gout/podagra (hyperuricemia)
Swollen gums, mucosal bleeding, poor wound healing, spots on skin	Scurvy (vitamin C deficiency: can't hydroxylate proline/lysine for collagen synthesis)

CLINICAL PRESENTATION	DIAGNOSIS/DISEASE
Swollen, hard, painful finger joints	Osteoarthritis (osteophytes on PIP [Bouchard's nodes], DIP [Heberden's nodes])
Systolic ejection murmur (crescendo-decrescendo)	Aortic valve stenosis
Thyroid and parathyroid tumors, pheochromocytoma	MEN 2A (autosomal dominant *ret* mutation)
Thyroid tumors, pheochromocytoma, ganglioneuromatosis	MEN 2B (autosomal dominant *ret* mutation)
Toe extension/fanning upon plantar scrape	Babinski sign (UMN lesion)
Unilateral facial drooping involving forehead	Facial nerve (LMN CN VII palsy)
Urethritis, conjunctivitis, arthritis in a male	Reactive arthritis associated with HLA-B27
Vascular birthmark (port-wine stain)	Hemangioma (benign, but associated with Sturge-Weber syndrome)
Vomiting blood following gastroesophageal lacerations	Mallory-Weiss syndrome (alcoholic and bulimic patients)
Weight loss, diarrhea, arthritis, fever, adenopathy	Whipple's disease (*Tropheryma whipplei*)
"Worst headache of my life"	Subarachnoid hemorrhage

▸ CLASSIC LABS/FINDINGS

LAB/DIAGNOSTIC FINDING	DIAGNOSIS/DISEASE
Anticentromere antibodies	Scleroderma (CREST)
Antidesmoglein (epithelial) antibodies	Pemphigus vulgaris (blistering)
Anti–glomerular basement membrane antibodies	Goodpasture's syndrome (glomerulonephritis and hemoptysis)
Antihistone antibodies	Drug-induced SLE (hydralazine, isoniazid, phenytoin, procainamide)
Anti-IgG antibodies	Rheumatoid arthritis (systemic inflammation, joint pannus, boutonnière deformity)
Antimitochondrial antibodies (AMAs)	1° biliary cirrhosis (female, cholestasis, portal hypertension)
Antineutrophil cytoplasmic antibodies (ANCAs)	Vasculitis (c-ANCA: granulomatosis with polyangiitis [Wegener's]; p-ANCA: microscopic polyangiitis, Churg-Strauss syndrome)
Antinuclear antibodies (ANAs: anti-Smith and anti-dsDNA)	SLE (type III hypersensitivity)
Antiplatelet antibodies	Idiopathic thrombocytopenic purpura
Anti-topoisomerase antibodies	Diffuse systemic scleroderma
Anti-transglutaminase/anti-gliadin/anti-endomysial antibodies	Celiac disease (diarrhea, distention, weight loss)
"Apple core" lesion on abdominal x-ray	Colorectal cancer (usually left-sided)
Azurophilic peroxidase-positive granular inclusions in granulocytes and myeloblasts	Auer rods (acute myelogenous leukemia, especially the promyelocytic [M3] type)
Bacitracin response	Sensitive: *Streptococcus pyogenes* (group A); resistant: *Streptococcus agalactiae* (group B)
"Bamboo spine" on x-ray	Ankylosing spondylitis (chronic inflammatory arthritis: HLA-B27)

LAB/DIAGNOSTIC FINDING	DIAGNOSIS/DISEASE
Basophilic nuclear remnants in RBCs	Howell-Jolly bodies (due to splenectomy or nonfunctional spleen)
Basophilic stippling of RBCs	Lead poisoning or sideroblastic anemia
Bloody tap on LP	Subarachnoid hemorrhage
"Boot shaped" heart on x-ray	Tetralogy of Fallot, RVH
Branching gram-positive rods with sulfur granules	*Actinomyces israelii*
Bronchogenic apical lung tumor on imaging	Pancoast tumor (can compress sympathetic ganglion and cause Horner's syndrome)
"Brown" tumor of bone	Hyperparathyroidism or osteitis fibrosa cystica (deposited hemosiderin from hemorrhage gives brown color)
Cardiomegaly with apical atrophy	Chagas' disease (*Trypanosoma cruzi*)
Cellular crescents in Bowman's capsule	Rapidly progressive crescentic glomerulonephritis
"Chocolate cyst" of ovary	Endometriosis (frequently involves both ovaries)
Circular grouping of dark tumor cells surrounding pale neurofibrils	Homer-Wright rosettes (neuroblastoma, medulloblastoma, retinoblastoma)
Colonies of mucoid *Pseudomonas* in lungs	Cystic fibrosis (autosomal-recessive mutation in *CFTR* resulting in fat-soluble vitamin deficiency and mucous plugs)
Decreased α-fetoprotein in amniotic fluid/maternal serum	Down syndrome or other chromosomal abnormality
Degeneration of dorsal column nerves	Tabes dorsalis (3° syphilis), subacute combined degeneration (dorsal columns and lateral corticospinal tracts affected)
Depigmentation of neurons in substantia nigra	Parkinson's disease (basal ganglia disorder: rigidity, resting tremor, bradykinesia)
Desquamated epithelium casts in sputum	Curschmann's spirals (bronchial asthma; can result in whorled mucous plugs)
Disarrayed granulosa cells in eosinophilic fluid	Call-Exner bodies (granulosa-theca cell tumor of the ovary)
Dysplastic squamous cervical cells with nuclear enlargement and hyperchromasia	Koilocytes (HPV: predisposes to cervical cancer)
Enlarged cells with intranuclear inclusion bodies	"Owl's eye" appearance of CMV
Enlarged thyroid cells with ground-glass nuclei	"Orphan Annie's eyes" nuclei (papillary carcinoma of the thyroid)
Eosinophilic cytoplasmic inclusion in liver cell	Mallory bodies (alcoholic liver disease)
Eosinophilic cytoplasmic inclusion in nerve cell	Lewy body (Parkinson's disease)
Eosinophilic globule in liver	Councilman body (toxic or viral hepatitis, often yellow fever)
Eosinophilic inclusion bodies in cytoplasm of hippocampal nerve cells	Negri bodies of rabies (*Lyssavirus*)
Extracellular amyloid deposition in gray matter of brain	Senile plaques (Alzheimer's disease)
Giant B cells with bilobed nuclei with prominent inclusions ("owl's eye")	Reed-Sternberg cells (Hodgkin's lymphoma)
Glomerulus-like structure surrounding vessel in germ cells	Schiller-Duval bodies (yolk sac tumor)
"Hair on end" (crew-cut) appearance on x-ray	β-thalassemia, sickle cell anemia (marrow expansion)
hCG elevated	Choriocarcinoma, hydatidiform mole (occurs with and without embryo)

LAB/DIAGNOSTIC FINDING	DIAGNOSIS/DISEASE
Heart nodules (granulomatous)	Aschoff bodies (rheumatic fever)
Heterophile antibodies	Infectious mononucleosis (EBV)
Hexagonal, double-pointed, needle-like crystals in bronchial secretions	Bronchial asthma (Charcot-Leyden crystals: eosinophilic granules)
High level of D-dimers	DVT, pulmonary embolism, DIC
Hilar lymphadenopathy, peripheral granulomatous lesion in middle or lower lung lobes (can calcify)	Ghon complex (1° TB: *Mycobacterium* bacilli)
"Honeycomb lung" on x-ray or CT	Interstitial pulmonary fibrosis
Hypercoagulability (leading to migrating DVTs and vasculitis)	Trousseau's syndrome (adenocarcinoma of pancreas or lung)
Hypersegmented neutrophils	Megaloblastic anemia (B_{12} deficiency: neurologic symptoms; folate deficiency: no neurologic symptoms)
Hypertension, hypokalemia, metabolic alkalosis	Conn's syndrome
Hypochromic, microcytic anemia	Iron deficiency anemia, lead poisoning, thalassemia (fetal hemoglobin sometimes present)
Increased α-fetoprotein in amniotic fluid/maternal serum	Dating error, anencephaly, spina bifida (neural tube defects)
Increased uric acid levels	Gout, Lesch-Nyhan syndrome, tumor lysis syndrome, loop and thiazide diuretics
Intranuclear eosinophilic droplet-like bodies	Cowdry type A bodies (HSV or CMV)
Iron-containing nodules in alveolar septum	Ferruginous bodies (asbestosis: ↑ chance of mesothelioma)
Keratin pearls on a skin biopsy	Squamous cell carcinoma
Large lysosomal vesicles in phagocytes, immunodeficiency	Chédiak-Higashi disease (congenital failure of phagolysosome formation)
"Lead pipe" appearance of colon on barium enema x-ray	Ulcerative colitis (loss of haustra)
Linear appearance of IgG deposition on glomerular basement membrane	Goodpasture's syndrome
Low serum ceruloplasmin	Wilson's disease (hepatolenticular degeneration)
"Lumpy bumpy" appearance of glomeruli on immunofluorescence	Poststreptococcal glomerulonephritis (immune complex deposition of IgG and C3b)
Lytic ("hole punched") bone lesions on x-ray	Multiple myeloma
Mammary gland ("blue domed") cyst	Fibrocystic change of the breast
Monoclonal antibody spike	▪ Multiple myeloma (usually IgG or IgA) ▪ Monoclonal gammopathy of undetermined significance (MGUS; normal consequence of aging) ▪ Waldenström's (M protein = IgM) macroglobulinemia ▪ Primary amyloidosis
Mucin-filled cell with peripheral nucleus	Signet ring (gastric carcinoma)
Narrowing of bowel lumen on barium x-ray	"String sign" (Crohn's disease)
Necrotizing vasculitis (lungs) and necrotizing glomerulonephritis	Granulomatosis with polyangiitis (Wegener's; c-ANCA positive) and Goodpasture's syndrome (anti–basement membrane antibodies)
Needle-shaped, negatively birefringent crystals	Gout (monosodium urate crystals)
Nodular hyaline deposits in glomeruli	Kimmelstiel-Wilson nodules (diabetic nephropathy)
Novobiocin response	Sensitive: *Staphylococcus epidermidis*; resistant: *Staphylococcus saprophyticus*

LAB/DIAGNOSTIC FINDING	DIAGNOSIS/DISEASE
"Nutmeg" appearance of liver	Chronic passive congestion of liver due to right heart failure
"Onion skin" periosteal reaction	Ewing's sarcoma (malignant round-cell tumor)
Optochin response	Sensitive: *Streptococcus pneumoniae*; resistant: *Viridans streptococcus*
Periosteum raised from bone, creating triangular area	Codman's triangle on x-ray (osteosarcoma, Ewing's sarcoma, pyogenic osteomyelitis)
Podocyte fusion or "effacement" on electron microscopy	Minimal change disease (child with nephrotic syndrome)
Polished, "ivory like" appearance of bone at cartilage erosion	Eburnation (osteoarthritis resulting in bony sclerosis)
Protein aggregates in neurons from hyperphosphorylation of protein tau	Neurofibrillary tangles (Alzheimer's disease) and Pick's bodies (Pick's disease)
Psammoma bodies	Meningiomas, papillary thyroid carcinoma, mesothelioma, papillary serous carcinoma of the endometrium and ovary
Pseudopalisading tumor cells on brain biopsy	Glioblastoma multiforme
RBC casts in urine	Acute glomerulonephritis
Rectangular, crystal-like, cytoplasmic inclusions in Leydig cells	Reinke crystals (Leydig cell tumor)
Renal epithelial casts in urine	Acute toxic/viral nephrosis
Rhomboid crystals, positively birefringent	Pseudogout (calcium pyrophosphate dihydrate crystals)
Rib notching	Coarctation of the aorta
Ring-enhancing brain lesion in AIDS	*Toxoplasma gondii*, CNS lymphoma
Sheets of medium-sized lymphoid cells with scattered pale, tingible body–laden macrophages ("starry sky" histology)	Burkitt's lymphoma (t[8:14] c-*myc* activation, associated with EBV; "black sky" made up of malignant cells)
Silver-staining spherical aggregation of tau proteins in neurons	Pick bodies (Pick's disease: progressive dementia, changes in personality)
"Soap bubble" in femur or tibia on x-ray	Giant cell tumor of bone (generally benign)
"Spikes" on basement membrane, "dome like" subepithelial deposits	Membranous glomerulonephritis (may progress to nephrotic syndrome)
Stacks of RBCs	Rouleaux formation (high ESR, multiple myeloma)
Stippled vaginal epithelial cells	"Clue cells" (*Gardnerella vaginalis*)
"Tennis racket" shaped cytoplasmic organelles (EM) in Langerhans cells	Birbeck granules (Langerhans cell histiocytosis or histiocytosis X: eosinophilic granuloma)
Thrombi made of white/red layers	Lines of Zahn (arterial thrombus, layers of platelets/RBCs)
"Thumb sign" on lateral x-ray	Epiglottitis (*Haemophilus influenzae*)
Thyroid-like appearance of kidney	Chronic bacterial pyelonephritis
Tram-track appearance of capillary loops of glomerular basement membranes on light microscopy	Membranoproliferative glomerulonephritis
Triglyceride accumulation in liver cell vacuoles	Fatty liver disease (alcoholic or metabolic syndrome)
"Waxy" casts with very low urine flow	Chronic end-stage renal disease
WBC casts in urine	Acute pyelonephritis
WBCs that look "smudged"	CLL (almost always B cell)
"Wire loop" glomerular capillary appearance on light microscopy	Lupus nephropathy
Yellowish CSF	Xanthochromia (e.g., due to subarachnoid hemorrhage)

▶ CLASSIC/RELEVANT TREATMENTS

CONDITION	COMMON TREATMENT(S)
Absence seizures	Ethosuximide
Acute gout attack	NSAIDs, colchicine
Acute promyelocytic leukemia (M3)	All-*trans* retinoic acid
ADHD	Methylphenidate, amphetamines
Alcohol abuse	AA + disulfiram for patient and Al-Anon for family
Alcohol withdrawal	Benzodiazepines
Anorexia	SSRIs
Anticoagulation during pregnancy	Heparin
Arrhythmia in damaged cardiac tissue	Class IB antiarrhythmic (lidocaine, mexiletine, tocainide)
B_{12} deficiency	Vitamin B_{12} supplementation (work up cause with Schilling test)
Benign prostatic hyperplasia	Tamsulosin, finasteride
Bipolar disorder	Lithium, valproate, carbamazepine, lamotrigine (mood stabilizers)
Breast cancer in postmenopausal woman	Aromatase inhibitor (anastrozole)
Buerger's disease	Smoking cessation
Bulimia	SSRIs
Candida albicans	Amphotericin B (systemic), nystatin (oral thrush, esophagitis)
Carcinoid syndrome	Octreotide
Chlamydia trachomatis	Doxycycline (+ ceftriaxone for gonorrhea coinfection), erythromycin eye drops (prophylaxis in infants)
Chronic gout	Probenecid (underexcretor), allopurinol (overproducer)
Chronic hepatitis	IFN-α
Chronic myelogenous leukemia	Imatinib
Clostridium botulinum	Antitoxin
Clostridium difficile	Oral metronidazole; if refractory, oral vancomycin
Clostridium tetani	Antitoxin + vaccine booster + diazepam
Crohn's disease	Corticosteroids, infliximab
Cryptococcus neoformans	Fluconazole (prophylaxis in AIDS patients)
Cyclophosphamide-induced hemorrhagic cystitis	Mesna
Cystic fibrosis	N-acetylcysteine + antipseudomonal prophylaxis (tobramycin/azithromycin)
Cytomegalovirus	Ganciclovir
Depression	SSRIs (first-line)
Diabetes insipidus	Desmopressin (central); hydrochlorothiazide, indomethacin, amiloride (nephrogenic)
Diabetes mellitus type 1	Dietary intervention (low-sugar) + insulin replacement
Diabetes mellitus type 2	Dietary intervention, oral hypoglycemics, and insulin (possible)
Diabetic ketoacidosis	Fluids, insulin, K^+

CONDITION	COMMON TREATMENT(S)
Enterococci	Vancomycin/ampicillin + aminoglycoside
Erectile dysfunction	Sildenafil, vardenafil
ER-positive breast cancer	Tamoxifen
Ethylene glycol/methanol intoxication	Fomepizole (alcohol dehydrogenase inhibitor)
Haemophilus influenzae (B)	Rifampin (prophylaxis)
Generalized anxiety disorder	Buspirone
Heparin toxicity (acute)	Protamine sulfate
HER2/neu-positive breast cancer	Trastuzumab
Hyperaldosteronism	Spironolactone
Hypercholesterolemia	Statin (first-line)
Hypertriglyceridemia	Fibrate
Immediate anticoagulation	Heparin
Infertility	Leuprolide, GnRH (pulsatile)
Influenza	Rimantadine, oseltamivir
Legionella pneumophila	Erythromycin
Long-term anticoagulation	Warfarin
Malaria	Chloroquine/mefloquine (for blood schizont), primaquine (for liver hypnozoite)
Malignant hyperthermia	Dantrolene
Medical abortion	Mifepristone
Migraine	Sumatriptan
MRSA	Vancomycin
Multiple sclerosis	β-interferon, immunosuppression, natalizumab
Mycobacterium tuberculosis	RIPE (rifampin, INH, pyrazinamide, ethambutol)
Neisseria gonorrhoeae	Ceftriaxone (add doxycycline to cover likely concurrent *Chlamydia*)
Neisseria meningitidis	Penicillin/ceftriaxone, rifampin (prophylaxis)
Neural tube defect prevention	Prenatal folic acid
Osteomalacia/rickets	Vitamin D supplementation
Osteoporosis	Bisphosphonates; calcium and vitamin D supplementation
Patent ductus arteriosus	Indomethacin
Pheochromocytoma	α-antagonists (e.g., phenoxybenzamine)
Pneumocystis jirovecii	TMP-SMX (prophylaxis in AIDS patient)
Prolactinoma	Bromocriptine (dopamine agonists)
Prostate cancer/uterine fibroids	Leuprolide, GnRH (continuous)
Prostate carcinoma	Flutamide
Pseudomonas aeruginosa	Antipseudomonal penicillin + aminoglycoside
Pulmonary arterial hypertension (idiopathic)	Sildenafil, bosentan, epoprostenol

CONDITION	COMMON TREATMENT(S)
Rickettsia rickettsii	Doxycycline, chloramphenicol (especially in context of aplastic anemia)
Ringworm infections	Terbinafine, griseofulvin, imidazole
Schizophrenia (negative symptoms)	5-HT_{2A} antagonists (e.g., second-generation antipsychotics)
Schizophrenia (positive symptoms)	D_2 receptor antagonists (e.g., first- and second-generation antipsychotics
SIADH	Demeclocycline, lithium, vasopressin receptor antagonists
Sickle cell anemia	Hydroxyurea (↑ fetal hemoglobin)
Sporothrix schenckii	Oral potassium chloride
Stable angina	Sublingual nitroglycerin
Staphylococcus aureus	MSSA: nafcillin, oxacillin, dicloxacillin (antistaphylococcal penicillins); MRSA: vancomycin
Streptococcus bovis	Penicillin prophylaxis; evaluation for colon cancer if linked to endocarditis
Streptococcus pneumoniae	Penicillin/cephalosporin (systemic infection, pneumonia), vancomycin (meningitis)
Streptococcus pyogenes	Penicillin prophylaxis
Temporal arteritis	High-dose steroids
Tonic-clonic seizures	Phenytoin, valproate, carbamazepine
Toxoplasma gondii	Sulfadiazine + pyrimethamine
Treponema pallidum	Penicillin
Trichomonas vaginalis	Metronidazole (patient and partner)
Ulcerative colitis	5-ASA, infliximab
UTI prophylaxis	TMP-SMX
Warfarin toxicity	Fresh frozen plasma (acute), vitamin K (chronic)
Wegener's granulomatosis with polyangiitis	Cyclophosphamide, corticosteroids

▸ KEY ASSOCIATIONS

DISEASE/FINDING	MOST COMMON/IMPORTANT ASSOCIATIONS
Actinic (solar) keratosis	Precursor to squamous cell carcinoma
Acute gastric ulcer associated with CNS injury	Cushing's ulcer (↑ ICP stimulates vagal gastric secretion)
Acute gastric ulcer associated with severe burns	Curling's ulcer (greatly reduced plasma volume results in sloughing of gastric mucosa)
Alternating areas of transmural inflammation and normal colon	Skip lesions (Crohn's disease)
Aneurysm, dissecting	Hypertension
Aortic aneurysm, abdominal and descending aorta	Atherosclerosis
Aortic aneurysm, arch	Tertiary syphilis (syphilitic aortitis), vasa vasorum destruction
Aortic aneurysm, ascending	Marfan's syndrome (idiopathic cystic medial degeneration)

DISEASE/FINDING	MOST COMMON/IMPORTANT ASSOCIATIONS
Atrophy of the mammillary bodies	Wernicke's encephalopathy (thiamine deficiency causing ataxia, ophthalmoplegia, and confusion)
Autosplenectomy (fibrosis and shrinkage)	Sickle cell anemia (hemoglobin S)
Bacteria associated with gastritis, peptic ulcer disease, and stomach cancer	*H. pylori*
Bacterial meningitis (adults and elderly)	*Streptococcus pneumoniae*
Bacterial meningitis (newborns and kids)	Group B streptococcus (newborns), *S. pneumoniae/Neisseria meningitidis* (kids)
Benign melanocytic nevus	Spitz nevus (most common in first two decades)
Bleeding disorder with GpIb deficiency	Bernard-Soulier syndrome (defect in platelet adhesion to von Willebrand's factor)
Brain tumor (adults)	Supratentorial: metastasis > astrocytoma (including glioblastoma multiforme) > meningioma > schwannoma
Brain tumor (kids)	Infratentorial: medulloblastoma (cerebellum) or supratentorial: craniopharyngioma (cerebrum)
Breast cancer	Infiltrating ductal carcinoma (in the U.S., 1 in 9 women will develop breast cancer)
Breast mass	Fibrocystic change, carcinoma (in postmenopausal women)
Breast tumor (benign)	Fibroadenoma
Cardiac 1° tumor (kids)	Rhabdomyoma, often seen in tuberous sclerosis
Cardiac manifestation of lupus	Libman-Sacks endocarditis (nonbacterial, affecting both sides of mitral valve)
Cardiac tumor (adults)	Metastasis, 1° myxoma (4:1 left to right atrium; "ball and valve")
Cerebellar tonsillar herniation	Chiari malformation (often presents with progressive hydrocephalus or syringomyelia)
Chronic arrhythmia	Atrial fibrillation (associated with high risk of emboli)
Chronic atrophic gastritis (autoimmune)	Predisposition to gastric carcinoma (can also cause pernicious anemia)
Clear cell adenocarcinoma of the vagina	DES exposure in utero
Compression fracture	Osteoporosis (type I: postmenopausal woman; type II: elderly man or woman)
Congenital adrenal hyperplasia, hypotension	21-hydroxylase deficiency
Congenital cardiac anomaly	VSD
Congenital conjugated hyperbilirubinemia (black liver)	Dubin-Johnson syndrome (inability of hepatocytes to secrete conjugated bilirubin into bile)
Constrictive pericarditis	Tuberculosis (developing world); systemic lupus erythematosus (developed world)
Coronary artery involved in thrombosis	LAD > RCA > LCA
Cretinism	Iodine deficit/hypothyroidism

DISEASE/FINDING	MOST COMMON/IMPORTANT ASSOCIATIONS
Cushing's syndrome	▪ Iatrogenic Cushing's (from corticosteroid therapy) ▪ Adrenocortical adenoma (secretes excess cortisol) ▪ ACTH-secreting pituitary adenoma ▪ Paraneoplastic Cushing's (due to ACTH secretion by tumors)
Cyanosis (early; less common)	Tetralogy of Fallot, transposition of great vessels, truncus arteriosus
Cyanosis (late; more common)	VSD, ASD, PDA
Death in CML	Blast crisis
Death in SLE	Lupus nephropathy
Dementia	Alzheimer's disease, multiple infarcts
Demyelinating disease in young women	Multiple sclerosis
DIC	Severe sepsis, obstetric complications, cancer, burns, trauma, major surgery
Dietary deficit	Iron
Diverticulum in pharynx	Zenker's diverticulum (diagnosed by barium swallow)
Ejection click	Aortic/pulmonic stenosis
Esophageal cancer	Squamous cell carcinoma (worldwide); adenocarcinoma (U.S.)
Food poisoning (exotoxin mediated)	*S. aureus*, *B. cereus*
Glomerulonephritis (adults)	Berger's disease (IgA nephropathy)
Gynecologic malignancy	Endometrial carcinoma (most common in U.S.); cervical carcinoma (most common worldwide)
Heart murmur, congenital	Mitral valve prolapse
Heart valve in bacterial endocarditis	Mitral > aortic (rheumatic fever), tricuspid (IV drug abuse)
Helminth infection (U.S.)	*Enterobius vermicularis*, *Ascaris lumbricoides*
Hematoma—epidural	Rupture of middle meningeal artery (trauma; lentiform shaped)
Hematoma—subdural	Rupture of bridging veins (crescent shaped)
Hemochromatosis	Multiple blood transfusions or hereditary *HFE* mutation (can result in CHF, "bronze diabetes," and ↑ risk of hepatocellular carcinoma)
Hepatocellular carcinoma	Cirrhotic liver (associated with hepatitis B and C and with alcoholism)
Hereditary bleeding disorder	von Willebrand's disease
Hereditary harmless jaundice	Gilbert's syndrome (benign congenital unconjugated hyperbilirubinemia)
HLA-B27	Ankylosing spondylitis, Reiter's syndrome, ulcerative colitis, psoriasis
HLA-DR3 or -DR4	Diabetes mellitus type 1, rheumatoid arthritis, SLE

DISEASE/FINDING	MOST COMMON/IMPORTANT ASSOCIATIONS
Holosystolic murmur	VSD, tricuspid regurgitation, mitral regurgitation
Hypercoagulability, endothelial damage, blood stasis	Virchow's triad (results in venous thrombosis)
Hypertension, 2°	Renal disease
Hypoparathyroidism	Accidental excision during thyroidectomy
Hypopituitarism	Pituitary adenoma (usually benign tumor)
Infection 2° to blood transfusion	Hepatitis C
Infections in chronic granulomatous disease	*Staphylococcus aureus*, *E. coli*, *Aspergillus* (catalase positive)
Kidney stones	▪ Calcium = radiopaque ▪ Struvite (ammonium) = radiopaque (formed by urease-positive organisms such as *Proteus vulgaris* or *Staphylococcus*) ▪ Uric acid = radiolucent
Late cyanotic shunt (uncorrected left to right becomes right to left)	Eisenmenger's syndrome (caused by ASD, VSD, PDA; results in pulmonary hypertension/polycythemia)
Liver disease	Alcoholic cirrhosis
Lysosomal storage disease	Gaucher's disease
Male cancer	Prostatic carcinoma
Malignancy associated with noninfectious fever	Hodgkin's lymphoma
Malignancy (kids)	ALL, medulloblastoma (cerebellum)
Mental retardation	Down syndrome, fragile X syndrome
Metastases to bone	Prostate, breast > lung > thyroid, testes
Metastases to brain	Lung > breast > genitourinary > osteosarcoma > melanoma > GI
Metastases to liver	Colon >> stomach, pancreas
Mitochondrial inheritance	Disease occurs in both males and females, inherited through females only
Mitral valve stenosis	Rheumatic heart disease
Mixed (UMN and LMN) motor neuron disease	ALS
Myocarditis	Coxsackie B
Nephrotic syndrome (adults)	Focal segmental glomerulosclerosis
Nephrotic syndrome (kids)	Minimal change disease
Neuron migration failure	Kallmann syndrome (hypogonadotropic hypogonadism and anosmia)
Nosocomial pneumonia	*Klebsiella*, *E. coli*, *Pseudomonas aeruginosa*
Obstruction of male urinary tract	BPH
Opening snap	Mitral stenosis
Opportunistic infection in AIDS	*Pneumocystis jirovecii* (formerly *carinii*) pneumonia
Osteomyelitis	*S. aureus*
Osteomyelitis in sickle cell disease	*Salmonella*
Osteomyelitis with IV drug use	*Pseudomonas*, *S. aureus*

DISEASE/FINDING	MOST COMMON/IMPORTANT ASSOCIATIONS
Ovarian metastasis from gastric carcinoma or breast cancer	Krukenberg tumor (mucin-secreting signet-ring cells)
Ovarian tumor (benign, bilateral)	Serous cystadenoma
Ovarian tumor (malignant)	Serous cystadenocarcinoma
Pancreatitis (acute)	Gallstones, alcohol
Pancreatitis (chronic)	Alcohol (adults), cystic fibrosis (kids)
Patient with ALL /CLL /AML /CML	ALL: child, CLL: adult > 60, AML: adult ~ 65, CML: adult 30–60
Pelvic inflammatory disease	*Chlamydia trachomatis, Neisseria gonorrhoeae*
Philadelphia chromosome t(9;22) (*bcr-abl*)	CML (may sometimes be associated with ALL/AML)
Pituitary tumor	Prolactinoma, somatotropic "acidophilic" adenoma
Primary amenorrhea	Turner syndrome (45,XO)
Primary bone tumor (adults)	Multiple myeloma
Primary hyperaldosteronism	Adenoma of adrenal cortex
Primary hyperparathyroidism	Adenomas, hyperplasia, carcinoma
Primary liver cancer	Hepatocellular carcinoma (chronic hepatitis, cirrhosis, hemochromatosis, α_1 antitrypsin deficiency)
Pulmonary hypertension	COPD
Recurrent inflammation/thrombosis of small/medium vessels in extremities	Buerger's disease (strongly associated with tobacco)
Renal tumor	Renal cell carcinoma: associated with von Hippel–Lindau and cigarette smoking; paraneoplastic syndromes (EPO, renin, PTH, ACTH)
Right heart failure due to a pulmonary cause	Cor pulmonale
S3 (protodiastolic gallop)	↑ ventricular filling (left to right shunt, mitral regurgitation, LV failure [CHF])
S4 (presystolic gallop)	Stiff/hypertrophic ventricle (aortic stenosis, restrictive cardiomyopathy)
Secondary hyperparathyroidism	Hypocalcemia of chronic kidney disease
Sexually transmitted disease	Chlamydia (usually coinfected with gonorrhea)
SIADH	Small cell carcinoma of the lung
Site of diverticula	Sigmoid colon
Sites of atherosclerosis	Abdominal aorta > coronary artery > popliteal artery > carotid artery.
Stomach cancer	Adenocarcinoma
Stomach ulcerations and high gastrin levels	Zollinger-Ellison syndrome (gastrinoma of duodenum or pancreas)
t(14;18)	Follicular lymphomas (*bcl-2* activation)
t(8;14)	Burkitt's lymphoma (c-*myc* activation)
t(9;22)	Philadelphia chromosome, CML (*bcr-abl* fusion)
Temporal arteritis	Risk of ipsilateral blindness due to thrombosis of ophthalmic artery; polymyalgia rheumatica

DISEASE/FINDING	MOST COMMON/IMPORTANT ASSOCIATIONS
Testicular tumor	Seminoma
Thyroid cancer	Papillary carcinoma
Tumor in women	Leiomyoma (estrogen dependent, not precancerous)
Tumor of infancy	Hemangioma (usually regresses spontaneously by childhood)
Tumor of the adrenal medulla (adults)	Pheochromocytoma (usually benign)
Tumor of the adrenal medulla (kids)	Neuroblastoma (malignant)
Type of Hodgkin's	Nodular sclerosis (vs. mixed cellularity, lymphocytic predominance, lymphocytic depletion)
Type of non-Hodgkin's	Diffuse large cell
UTI	*E. coli*, *Staphylococcus saprophyticus* (young women)
Viral encephalitis affecting temporal lobe	HSV-1
Vitamin deficiency (U.S.)	Folate (pregnant women are at high risk; body stores only 3- to 4-month supply; prevents neural tube defects)

▶ EQUATION REVIEW

TOPIC	EQUATION	PAGE
Sensitivity	Sensitivity = TP / (TP + FN)	51
Specificity	Specificity = TN / (TN + FP)	51
Positive predictive value	PPV = TP / (TP + FP)	51
Negative predictive value	NPV = TN / (TN + FN)	51
Odds ratio (for case-control studies)	$\text{Odds ratio} = \frac{a/c}{b/d} = \frac{ad}{bc}$	52
Relative risk	$\text{Relative risk} = \frac{a/(a+b)}{c/(c+d)}$	52
Attributable risk	$\text{Attributable risk} = \frac{a}{a+b} - \frac{c}{c+d}$	52
Number needed to treat	1/absolute risk reduction	52
Number needed to harm	1/attributable risk	52
Body mass index	$\text{BMI} = \frac{\text{weight in kg}}{(\text{height in meters})^2}$	60
Hardy-Weinberg equilibrium	$p^2 + 2pq + q^2 = 1$ $p + q = 1$	83
Volume of distribution	$V_d = \frac{\text{amount of drug in the body}}{\text{plasma drug concentration}}$	227
Half-life	$t_{1/2} = \frac{0.7 \times V_d}{CL}$	227
Drug clearance	$CL = \frac{\text{rate of elimination of drug}}{\text{plasma drug concentration}} = V_d \times K_e$ (elimination constant)	227

TOPIC	EQUATION	PAGE
Loading dose	$LD = C_p \times \frac{V_d}{F}$	227
Maintenance dose	$MD = C_p \times \frac{CL}{F}$	227
Cardiac output	$CO = \frac{\text{rate of } O_2 \text{ consumption}}{\text{arterial } O_2 \text{ content} - \text{venous } O_2 \text{ content}}$	253
	$CO = \text{stroke volume} \times \text{heart rate}$	253
Mean arterial pressure	$MAP = \text{cardiac output} \times \text{total peripheral resistance}$	253
	$MAP = \frac{2}{3}\text{ diastolic} + \frac{1}{3}\text{ systolic}$	253
Stroke volume	$SV = \frac{CO}{HR} = EDV - ESV$	253
Ejection fraction	$EF = \frac{SV}{EDV} = \frac{EDV - ESV}{EDV}$	254
Resistance	$\text{Resistance} = \frac{\text{driving pressure } (\Delta P)}{\text{flow } (Q)} = \frac{8\eta \text{ (viscosity)} \times \text{length}}{\pi r^4}$	255
Net filtration pressure	$P_{net} = [(P_c - P_i) - (\pi_c - \pi_i)]$	265
	$J_v = \text{net fluid flow} = (K_f)(Pnet)$	
Renal clearance	$C_x = U_x V / P_x$	480
Glomerular filtration rate	$GFR = U_{inulin} \times V / P_{inulin} = C_{inulin}$	480
	$GFR = K_f [(P_{GC} - P_{BS}) - (\pi_{GC} - \pi_{BS})]$	480
Effective renal plasma flow	$ERPF = U_{PAH} \times \frac{V}{P_{PAH}} = C_{PAH}$	480
Renal blood flow	$RBF = \frac{RPF}{1 - Hct}$	480
Filtration fraction	$FF = \frac{GFR}{RPF}$	481
Henderson-Hasselbalch equation (for extracellular pH)	$pH = 6.1 + \log \frac{[HCO_3^-]}{0.03\ P_{CO_2}}$	487
Physiologic dead space	$V_D = V_T \times \frac{(Pa_{CO_2}) - Pe_{CO_2}}{Pa_{CO_2}}$	546
Pulmonary vascular resistance	$PVR = \frac{P_{pulm\ artery} - P_{L\ atrium}}{\text{Cardiac output}}$	549
Alveolar gas equation	$PA_{O_2} = PI_{O_2} - \frac{Pa_{CO_2}}{R}$	550

SECTION IV

Top-Rated Review Resources

"Some books are to be tasted, others to be swallowed, and some few to be chewed and digested."

—Sir Francis Bacon

"Always read something that will make you look good if you die in the middle of it."

—P.J. O'Rourke

▶ HOW TO USE THE DATABASE

This section is a database of top-rated basic science review books, sample examination books, software, Web sites, and commercial review courses that have been marketed to medical students studying for the USMLE Step 1. At the end of the section is a list of publishers and independent bookstores with addresses and phone numbers. For each recommended resource, we list (where applicable) the **Title**, the **First Author** (or editor), the **Series Name** (where applicable), the **Current Publisher**, the **Copyright Year**, the **Number of Pages**, the **ISBN**, the **Approximate List Price**, the **Format** of the resource, and the **Number of Test Questions**. We also include **Summary Comments** that describe their style and overall utility for studying. Finally, each recommended resource receives a **Rating**. Within each section, resources are arranged first by Rating and then alphabetically by the first author within each Rating group.

A letter rating scale with six different grades reflects the detailed student evaluations for **Rated Resources.** Each rated resource receives a rating as follows:

A+	Excellent for boards review.
A A–	Very good for boards review; choose among the group.
B+ B	Good, but use only after exhausting better sources.
B–	Fair, but there are many better books in the discipline; or low-yield subject material.

The Rating is meant to reflect the overall usefulness of the resource in helping medical students prepare for the USMLE Step 1. This is based on a number of factors, including:

- The cost
- The readability of the text
- The appropriateness and accuracy of the material
- The quality and number of sample questions
- The quality of written answers to sample questions
- The quality and appropriateness of the illustrations (e.g., graphs, diagrams, photographs)
- The length of the text (longer is not necessarily better)
- The quality and number of other resources available in the same discipline
- The importance of the discipline for the USMLE Step 1

Please note that ratings do not reflect the quality of the resources for purposes other than reviewing for the USMLE Step 1. Many books with lower ratings are well written and informative but are not ideal for boards preparation. We have not listed or commented on general textbooks available in the basic sciences.

Evaluations are based on the cumulative results of formal and informal surveys of thousands of medical students at many medical schools across the country. The summary comments and overall ratings represent a consensus opinion, but there may have been a broad range of opinion or limited student feedback on any particular resource.

Please note that the data listed are subject to change in that:

- Publishers' prices change frequently.
- Bookstores often charge an additional markup.
- New editions come out frequently, and the quality of updating varies.
- The same book may be reissued through another publisher.

We actively encourage medical students and faculty to submit their opinions and ratings of these basic science review materials so that we may update our database. (See p. xvii, How to Contribute.) In addition, we ask that publishers and authors submit for evaluation review copies of basic science review books, including new editions and books not included in our database. We also solicit reviews of new books or suggestions for alternate modes of study that may be useful in preparing for the examination, such as flash cards, computer software, commercial review courses, and Web sites.

Disclaimer/Conflict of Interest Statement

No material in this book, including the ratings, reflects the opinion or influence of the publisher. All errors and omissions will gladly be corrected if brought to the attention of the authors through our blog at **www.firstaidteam.com**. Please note that USMLE-Rx and the entire *First Aid for the USMLE* series are publications by the senior authors of this book; their ratings are based solely on recommendations from the student authors of this book as well as data from the student survey and feedback forms.

▶ QUESTION BANKS

A+

USMLEWorld Qbank **$99–$399** Test/2000 q
USMLEWorld
www.usmleworld.com

An excellent bank of well-constructed questions that closely mirror those found on Step 1. Questions demand multistep reasoning and are often more difficult than those on the actual exam. Offers excellent, detailed explanations with figures and tables. Features a number of test customization and analysis options. Unfortunately, the program does not allow other application windows to be open for reference. Users can see cumulative results both over time and compared to other test takers. Another useful fre is that it gives a percentile score so the user can evaluate his or her performance compared to a large pool of other users who completed the same questions. Can be accessed through iPhone or Androic mobile apps.

A−

Kaplan Qbank **$99–$199** Test/2400 q
Kaplan
www.kaplanmedical.com

A high-quality question bank that covers most content found on Step 1, but sometimes emphasizes recall of overly specific details rather than integrative problem-solving skills. Test content and performance feedback can be organized by both organ system and discipline. Includes detailed explanations of all answer choices. Users can see cumulative results both over time and compared to other test takers. Can be accessed through iPhone or Android mobile apps.

A−

USMLE-Rx Qmax **$99–$199** Test/3000 q
MedIQ Learning
www.usmle-rx.com

A well-priced question bank that offers Step 1–style questions accompanied by thorough explanations. Some obscure material is omitted, making it more straightforward than other question banks. Each explanation includes high-yield facts and references from *First Aid.* However, the proportion of questions covering a given subject area does not always reflect the actual exam's relative emphasis. Question stems occasionally rely on "buzzwords." Most useful to help memorize *First Aid* facts. Provides detailed performance analyses.

B

USMLE Consult **$75–$395** Test/2500 q
Elsevier
www.usmleconsult.com

A solid question bank that can be divided according to discipline and subject area. Questions are more straightforward than those on actual exam. Offers concise explanations with links to Student Consult and First Consult content. Users can see cumulative results both over time and compared to other test takers. Student Consult also offers a Robbins Pathology Test Bank ($35 for 1 month, $65 for 3 months) featuring 500 USMLE-style questions. Purchase of any question bank includes use of the Scorrelator, a tool that predicts your USMLE Step 1 score from your performance on the question bank. Limited student feedback on Student Consult products.

▸ QUESTION BOOKS

A⁻

First Aid Q&A for the USMLE Step 1 **$44.95** Test/1000 q
LE
McGraw-Hill, 2012, 765 pages, ISBN 9780071744027

A great source of approx. 1000 questions drawn from the USMLE-Rx Step 1 Qmax test bank, organized according to subject. Also features one full-length exam of 336 questions. Questions are easier than those found on Step 1, but provide representative coverage of the concepts typically tested. Includes brief but adequate explanations of both correct and incorrect answer choices.

B⁺

Kaplan USMLE Step 1 Qbook **$25.00** Test/850 q
KAPLAN
Kaplan, 2011, 480 pages, ISBN 9781419550478

A resource consisting of seventeen 50-question exams organized by the traditional basic science disciplines. Similar to the Kaplan Qbank, and offers good USMLE-style questions with clear, detailed explanations; however, lacks the classic images typically seen on the exam. Also includes a guide on test-taking strategies.

B⁺

PreTest Clinical Vignettes for the USMLE Step 1 **$29.95** Test/322 q
MCGRAW-HILL
McGraw-Hill, 2010, 311 pages, ISBN 9780071668064

Clinical vignette–style questions with detailed explanations, divided into seven blocks of 46 questions covering basic sciences. In general, questions are representative of the length and complexity of those on Step 1. Images (including pathology slides) are black and white and sometimes difficult to interpret. One of the better books in the PreTest series.

B

Lange Q&A: USMLE Step 1 **$45.95** Test/1200 q
KING
McGraw-Hill, 2008, 528 pages, ISBN 9780071492195

Offers many questions organized by subject area along with three comprehensive practice exams. Questions are often challenging but are not always representative of Step 1 style—difficult concepts are tested, but multistep reasoning is not. Includes detailed explanations of both correct and incorrect answer choices. Black-and-white images only.

B

NMS Review for USMLE Step 1 **$48.95** Test/850 q
LAZO
Lippincott Williams & Wilkins, 2005, 480 pages + CD-ROM, ISBN 9780781779210

A text and CD-ROM that offers 17 practice exams with answers. Some questions are too picky or difficult. Annotated explanations are well written but are sometimes unnecessarily detailed. The six pages of color plates are helpful. The CD-ROM attempts to simulate the computer-based testing format but is disorganized.

▸ INTERNET SITES

A⁻	***WebPath: The Internet Pathology Laboratory*** **http://library.med.utah.edu/WebPath/** Features more than 2000 outstanding gross and microscopic images, clinical vignette questions, and case studies. Includes eight general pathology exams and 11 system-based exams with approximately 1000 questions. Also features 170 questions associated with images. Questions are useful for reviewing boards content but are typically easier and shorter. No multimedia practice questions. Tremendous resource, but in need of an update to retain Step 1 usefulness.	***Free***	Review/Test/1100 q
B⁺	***Lippincott's 350-Question Practice Test for USMLE Step 1*** LIPPINCOTT WILLIAMS & WILKINS **www.lww.com/medstudent/usmle** A free, full-length, seven-block, 350-question practice exam in a format similar to that of the real Step 1. Questions are easier than those on the actual exam, and the explanations provided are sparse. Users can bookmark questions and can choose between taking the test all at once or by section.	***Free***	Test/350 q
B	***The Pathology Guy*** FRIEDLANDER **www.pathguy.com** A free Web site containing extensive but poorly organized information on a variety of fundamental concepts in pathology. A high-yield summary intended for USMLE review can be found at www.pathguy.com/meltdown.txt, but the information given is limited by a lack of images and frequent digressions.	***Free***	Review
B	***Radiopaedia.org*** **www.radiopaedia.org** A user-friendly Web site with thousands of well-organized radiology cases and articles. Encyclopedia entries contain high-yield bullet points of anatomy and pathology. Images contain detailed descriptions but no arrows to demarcate findings. Quiz mode allows students to make a diagnosis based on radiographic findings. Content may be too broad for boards review but is a good complement to classes and clerkships.	***Free***	Cases/Test
B⁻	***The Whole Brain Atlas*** JOHNSON **www.med.harvard.edu/AANLIB/home.html** A collection of high-quality brain MR and CT images with views of normal and diseased brains. The interface is technologically impressive but complex, and many images are without explanations. Subject matter is overly specific, limiting its use as a boards review study tool. Useful adjunct to classes and clerkships.	***Free***	Review
B⁻	***Digital Anatomist Interactive Atlases*** UNIVERSITY OF WASHINGTON **www9.biostr.washington.edu/da.html** A good site containing an interactive neuroanatomy course along with a three-dimensional atlas of the brain, thorax, and knee. Atlases have computer-generated images and cadaver sections. Each atlas also has a quiz in which users identify structures in the slide images; however, questions do not focus on high-yield anatomy for Step 1.	***Free***	Review

▶ COMPREHENSIVE

A+

First Aid Cases for the USMLE Step 1 **$44.95** Review

LE

McGraw-Hill, 2012, 411 pages, ISBN 9780071743976

A series of more than 400 high-yield cases divided into sections by organ system. Each case features a paragraph-long clinical vignette with relevant images, followed by questions and short, high-yield explanations. Offers great coverage of many frequently tested concepts, and integrates subject matter in the discussion of a single vignette. A good source of questions to review material outlined in *First Aid for the USMLE Step 1.*

A−

USMLE Step 1 Secrets **$39.95** Review

BROWN

Elsevier, 2008, 740 pages, ISBN 9780323054393

Clarifies difficult concepts in a concise, easy-to-read manner. Employs a case-based format and integrates information well. Complements other boards study resources, with a focus on understanding preclinical fundamentals rather than on rote memorization. Slightly long for last-minute board cramming.

A−

medEssentials for the USMLE Step 1 **$54.99** Review

MANLEY

Kaplan, 2012, 588 pages, ISBN 9781609780265

A comprehensive review divided into general principles and organ systems, and organized using high-yield tables and figures. Excellent for visual learners, but can be overly detailed and time consuming. Also includes color images in the back along with a monthly subscription to online interactive exercises, although these are of limited value for Step 1 preparation.

A−

Déjà Review: USMLE Step 1 **$24.95** Review

NAHEEDY

McGraw-Hill, 2010, 396 pages, ISBN 9780071627184

A comprehensive resource featuring questions and answers in a two-column, quiz-yourself format similar to that of the Recall series, divided according to discipline. Features a section of high-yield clinical vignettes along with useful mnemonics throughout. Contains a few mistakes, but remains a good alternative to flash cards as a last-minute review before the exam.

B+

Cases & Concepts Step 1: Basic Science Review **$42.95** Review

CAUGHEY

Lippincott Williams & Wilkins, 2009, 400 pages, ISBN 9780781793919

One hundred sixteen clinical cases integrating basic science with clinical data, followed by USMLE-style questions with answers and rationales. Thumbnail and key-concept boxes highlight key facts. Limited student feedback.

B+

Kaplan's USMLE Step 1 Home Study Program **$499.00** Review

KAPLAN

Kaplan, 2008, 1900 pages, ISBN 0S4005C

A resource consisting of two general principle and two organ system review books. All are highly comprehensive, but can be overwhelmingly lengthy if they are not started very early. Although costly, the program can serve as an excellent reference for studying by virtue of its detail. Books can be purchased at www.kaptest.com.

B+ ***First Aid for the Basic Sciences: General Principles*** ***$69.95*** Review
LE
McGraw-Hill, 2012, 560 pages, ISBN 9780071743884

Excellent comprehensive review of the basic sciences covered in year 1 of medical school. Similar to the first part of *First Aid*, organized by discipline, and includes hundreds of full-color images and tables. Best if started with first-year coursework and then used as a reference during boards preparation.

B+ ***First Aid for the Basic Sciences: Organ Systems*** ***$89.95*** Review
LE
McGraw-Hill, 2012, 858 pages, ISBN 9780071743952

A comprehensive review of the basic sciences covered in year 2 of medical school. Similar to the second part of *First Aid*, organized by organ system, and includes hundreds of full-color images and tables. Best if started with second-year coursework and then used as a reference during boards preparation. Each organ system contains discussion of embryology and anatomy, physiology, pathology, pharmacology, and a high-yield rapid review section.

B+ ***Step-Up to USMLE Step 1*** ***$46.95*** Review
MEHTA
Lippincott Williams & Wilkins, 2009, 424 pages, ISBN 9781605474700

An organ system–based review text with clinical vignettes that is useful for integrating the basic sciences covered in Step 1. The text is composed primarily of outlines, charts, tables, and diagrams, making the depth of material covered somewhat limited. Includes access to a sample online question bank.

B+ ***USMLE Step 1 Recall: Buzzwords for the Boards*** ***$46.95*** Review
REINHEIMER
Lippincott Williams & Wilkins, 2007, 480 pages, ISBN 9780781770705

A review of core Step 1 topics presented in a two-column, quiz-yourself format. Best for a quick last-minute review before the exam. Covers many important subjects, but not comprehensive or tightly organized. Sometimes focuses on obscure details. Compare with the Déjà Review series. Includes all questions and answers in downloadable MP3 files so that files can be used on any digital audio playback device.

B+ ***Underground Clinical Vignettes: Step 1 Bundle*** ***$189.95*** Review
SWANSON
Lippincott Williams & Wilkins, 2007, 9 volumes, ISBN 9780781763622

A bundle that includes nine books. Designed for easy quizzing with a group. Case-based vignettes provide a good review supplement. Best when started early with coursework or when used in conjunction with another primary review resource.

B ***USMLE Step 1 Made Ridiculously Simple*** ***$29.95*** Review
CARL
MedMaster, 2010, 400 pages, ISBN 9780940780910

A quick and easy read. Uses a table and chart format organized by subject, but some charts are poorly labeled. Consider as an adjunct to more comprehensive sources.

▶ ANATOMY, EMBRYOLOGY, AND NEUROSCIENCE

Grade	Title / Author / Publisher / Description	Price	Type
A−	***High-Yield Embryology*** DUDEK **Lippincott Williams & Wilkins, 2009, 176 pages, ISBN 9781605473161** A good review of a relatively low-yield subject. Offers excellent organization with clinical correlations. Includes a high-yield list of embryologic origins of tissues.	***$32.95***	Review
A−	***High-Yield Neuroanatomy*** FIX **Lippincott Williams & Wilkins, 2008, 160 pages, ISBN 9780781779463** An easy-to-read, straightforward format with excellent diagrams and illustrations. Features a useful atlas of brain section images, a glossary of important terms, an appendicized table of neurologic lesions, and an expanded index. Overall, a great resource, but more detailed than what is required for Step 1.	***$28.95***	Review/Test/50 Q&A provided online
A−	***Underground Clinical Vignettes: Anatomy*** SWANSON **Lippincott Williams & Wilkins, 2007, 256 pages, ISBN 9780781764759** Concise clinical cases illustrating approximately 100 frequently tested diseases with an anatomic basis. Cardinal signs, symptoms, and buzzwords are highlighted. Also includes 20 additional boards-style questions. A useful source for isolating important anatomy concepts tested on Step 1.	***$27.95***	Review/Test/20 q
A−	***USMLE Road Map: Gross Anatomy*** WHITE **McGraw-Hill, 2006, 258 pages, ISBN 9780071445161** An overview of high-yield gross anatomy with clinical correlations throughout. Also features numerous effective charts and clinical problems with explanations at the end of each chapter. Features good integration of facts, but may be overly detailed and offers few illustrations. Lack of Step 1–related figures limits usefulness. May require an anatomy reference text.	***$31.95***	Review/Test/150 q
B+	***High-Yield Gross Anatomy*** DUDEK **Lippincott Williams & Wilkins, 2010, 320 pages, ISBN 9781605477633** A good review of gross anatomy with some clinical correlations. Contains well-labeled, high-yield radiographic images, but often goes into excessive detail that is beyond the scope of the boards.	***$29.95***	Review
B+	***Atlas of Anatomy*** GILROY **Thieme, 2008, 672 pages, ISBN 9781604060621** A good atlas with more than 2200 high-quality, uncluttered illustrations. Includes clinical correlates and a brief introduction to new topics. Radiographs, MRIs, CT scans, and endoscopic views of the organs also included. Best if used as a reference or during coursework. Access to accompanying Web site with more than 600 illustrations, label on/off function, and timed self-tests also provided.	***$74.95***	Review

B+ ***Clinical Anatomy Made Ridiculously Simple*** ***$29.95*** Review
GOLDBERG
MedMaster, 2010, 175 pages, ISBN 9780940780972

An easy-to-read text offering simple diagrams along with numerous mnemonics and amusing associations. The humorous style has variable appeal for students, so browse before buying. Offers good coverage of selected topics. Best if used during coursework. Includes more detail than typically tested on Step 1.

B+ ***Crash Course: Anatomy*** ***$30.95*** Review
GRANGER
Elsevier, 2007, 264 pages, ISBN 9780323043199

Part of the Crash Course review series for basic sciences, integrating clinical topics. Offers two-color illustrations, handy study tools, and Step 1 review questions. Includes online access. Provides a solid review of anatomy for Step 1. Best if started early.

B+ ***Rapid Review: Gross and Developmental Anatomy*** ***$39.95*** Review/Test/450 q
MOORE
Elsevier, 2010, 284 pages, ISBN 9780323072946

A detailed treatment of basic anatomy and embryology, presented in an outline format similar to that of other books in the series. More detailed than necessary for boards review. Contains high-yield charts and figures throughout, in color. Includes two 50-question tests with extensive explanations, with an additional 350 questions available online.

B+ ***Déjà Review: Neuroscience*** ***$19.95*** Review
TREMBLAY
McGraw-Hill, 2010, 247 pages, ISBN 9780071627276

A resource that features questions and answers in a two-column, quiz-yourself format similar to that of the Recall series. Includes several useful diagrams and CT images. A perfect length for Step 1 neurophysiology and anatomy review.

B+ ***USMLE Road Map: Neuroscience*** ***$31.95*** Review/Test/300 q
WHITE
McGraw-Hill, 2008, 224 pages, ISBN 9780071496230

An outline review of basic neuroanatomy and physiology with clinical correlations throughout. Also features high-yield facts in boldface along with numerous tables and figures. Clinical problems with explanations are given at the end of each chapter. May be overly detailed for Step 1 review, but a good tool to use as a reference.

B ***Elsevier's Integrated Anatomy and Embryology*** ***$37.95*** Review
BOGART
Elsevier, 2007, 448 pages, ISBN 9781416031659

Part of the Integrated series that seeks to link basic science concepts across disciplines. Case-based and Step 1–style questions at the end of each chapter allow readers to gauge their comprehension of the material. Includes online access. Best if used during coursework. Limited student feedback.

B

BRS Embryology **$39.95** Review/Test

Dudek

Lippincott Williams & Wilkins, 2010, 320 pages, ISBN 9781605479019

An outline-based review of embryology that is typical of the BRS series. Offers a good review, but has limited illustrations and includes much more detail than is required for Step 1. A discussion of congenital malformations is included at the end of each chapter along with relevant questions. The comprehensive exam at the end of the book is high yield.

B

Anatomy Flash Cards **$34.95** Flash cards

Gilroy

Thieme, 2009, 376 flash cards, ISBN 9781604060720

High-quality illustrations with numbered labels on one side and answers on the other for self-testing. Occasional radiographic image. Best if used with coursework; too long for boards preparation. Limited student feedback.

B

Clinical Neuroanatomy Made Ridiculously Simple **$22.95** Review/Test/Few q

Goldberg

MedMaster, 2007, 96 pages + CD-ROM, ISBN 9780940780576

An easy-to-read, memorable, and simplified format with clever diagrams. Offers a quick, high-yield review of clinical neuroanatomy, but does not serve as a comprehensive resource for boards review. Places good emphasis on clinically relevant pathways, cranial nerves, and neurologic diseases. Includes a CD-ROM with CT and MR images as well as a tutorial on neurologic localization. Compare with *High-Yield Neuroanatomy.*

B

Netter's Anatomy Flash Cards **$33.25** Flash cards

Hansen

Saunders, 2011, 324 pages, ISBN 9781437716757

Netter's illustrations with numbered labels on one side and answers on the other for self-testing. Each card includes a commentary on the structures and a clinical correlation. Best if used with coursework, but much too detailed for boards preparation. Lack of embryology correlates hurts Step 1 usefulness. Includes online access with additional bonus cards and more than 300 multiple-choice questions. Excellent iPhone app costs approximately the same and has additional functionality.

B

PreTest Neuroscience **$29.95** Test/500 q

Siegel

McGraw-Hill, 2010, 399 pages, ISBN 9780071623476

A high-yield introduction followed by 500 questions with detailed explanations. The question format differs significantly from that typically found on Step 1. Sparse, poor-quality images.

B

Case Files: Gross Anatomy **$33.95** Review

Toy

McGraw-Hill, 2008, 384 pages, ISBN 9780071489805

Review text that includes 53 well-chosen cases with discussion, comprehension questions, and a box of take-home pearls. Tables are good, but schematics are black and white and not representative of Step 1. A reasonable book to work through for those who benefit from problem-based learning.

B

Rapid Review: Neuroscience **$38.95** Review
WEYHENMEYER
Elsevier, 2006, 320 pages, ISBN 9780323022613

A detailed treatment of neuroscience, presented in an outline format similar to that of other books in the series. Should be started early given its extensive treatment of a relatively narrow topic. Contains high-yield charts and figures throughout. Includes two 50-question tests with extensive explanations as well as 250 additional questions online.

B⁻

Gray's Anatomy for Students Flash Cards **$36.95** Flash cards
DRAKE
Elsevier, 2010, 748 pages, ISBN 9780702031784

These flash cards feature renowned Gray's illustrations on the front and labels on the back for self-testing. Notes on clinical importance and reference to accompanying textbook given on back. Much too detailed information on a relatively low-yield subject for effective boards studying. Limited student feedback.

B⁻

BRS Gross Anatomy Flash Cards **$34.95** Flash cards
SWANSON
Lippincott Williams & Wilkins, 2004, 250 pages, ISBN 9780781756549

Clinical anatomy cases presented in flash-card format. Cases are too specific for boards preparation, and anatomy basics and radiographic images are generally excluded. Best suited to students who are already relatively well versed in anatomy.

B⁻

Case Files: Neuroscience **$33.95** Review
TOY
McGraw-Hill, 2008, 408 pages, ISBN 9780071489218

Includes 48 clinical cases with lengthy discussion and 3–5 multiple-choice questions at the end of each case. Cases are well chosen, but the discussion is too lengthy. Questions are not the most representative of those seen on boards.

▶ BEHAVIORAL SCIENCE

A

High-Yield Behavioral Science ***$12.95*** Review

FADEM

Lippincott Williams & Wilkins, 2012, 144 pages, ISBN 9781451130300

An extremely concise yet comprehensive review of behavioral science for Step 1. Offers a logical presentation with charts, graphs, and tables, but lacks questions. Features brief but adequate coverage of statistics. Overall, an excellent, high-yield resource at an unrivaled price.

A⁻

BRS Behavioral Science ***$39.95*** Review/Test/500 q

FADEM

Lippincott Williams & Wilkins, 2008, 216 pages, ISBN 9780781782579

An easy-to-read outline-format review of behavioral science. Offers good, detailed coverage of essential topics, but at a level of depth that often exceeds what is tested on Step 1. Incorporates excellent tables and charts as well as a short but complete statistics chapter. Features high-quality review questions, including a 100-question comprehensive exam.

A⁻

High-Yield Biostatistics ***$28.95*** Review

GLASER

Lippincott Williams & Wilkins, 2005, 128 pages, ISBN 9780781796446

A well-written, easy-to-read text that offers extensive coverage of epidemiology and biostatistics. Includes good review questions and tables, but somewhat lengthy given the low-yield nature of the subject matter on Step 1. New edition expected in 2013.

B⁺

High-Yield Brain & Behavior ***$34.95*** Review

FADEM

Lippincott Williams & Wilkins, 2007, 256 pages, ISBN 9780781792288

Part of the new High-Yield Systems series that covers embryology, gross anatomy, radiology, histology, physiology, microbiology, and pharmacology as they relate to the nervous system. Written by the same author as the *High-Yield Behavioral Science* and *BRS Behavioral Science* texts. Overall, provides a good review of neuroscience and behavioral science but too much detail for most Step 1 takers.

B⁺

Underground Clinical Vignettes: Behavioral Science ***$27.95*** Review/Test/20 q

SWANSON

Lippincott Williams & Wilkins, 2007, 256 pages, ISBN 9780781764643

Concise clinical cases illustrating commonly tested diseases in behavioral science. Cardinal signs, symptoms, and buzzwords are highlighted. Useful for picking out important points in this very broad subject, but requires supplementation from other review sources. Also includes 20 Step 1–style questions.

B

Kaplan USMLE Medical Ethics ***$39.00*** Review

FISCHER

Kaplan, 2009, 216 pages, ISBN 9781419553141

Includes 100 cases, each followed by a single question and a detailed explanation. Also offers guidelines on how Step 1 requires test takers to think about ethics and medicolegal questions. Unfortunately, a lengthy review for such a low-yield subject.

B	***Déjà Review: Behavioral Science*** QUINN **McGraw-Hill, 2010, 226 pages, ISBN 9780071627283** Features questions and answers in a two-column, quiz-yourself format similar to that of the Recall series. Coverage of some topics is too lengthy for Step 1 review purposes, and order of information is nearly opposite that of *First Aid*. Limited student feedback.	***$19.95***	Review
B	***Rapid Review: Behavioral Science*** STEVENS **Elsevier, 2006, 320 pages, ISBN 9780323045711** Similar in style to other books in the Rapid Review series. Provides a good but low-yield review of a broad subject. Includes 100 questions and explanations along with an additional 250 questions online. Limited student feedback.	***$39.95***	Review/ Test/350 q

▸ BIOCHEMISTRY

A

Lange Flash Cards Biochemistry and Genetics **$34.95** Flash cards

BARON

McGraw-Hill Medical, 2005, 300 flash cards, ISBN 9780071447362

Great flash cards featuring a clinical vignette on one side and concise discussion on the other. Each section contains 2–3 cards on biochemistry principles. Excellent resource for boards studying, but no carrying case included.

A⁻

Rapid Review: Biochemistry **$39.95** Review/Test/350 q

PELLEY

Elsevier, 2011, 186 pages, ISBN 9780323068871

A review of basic topics in biochemistry. Presented in outline format, but often goes beyond the level of detail tested on Step 1. High-yield disease correlation boxes are especially useful. Excellent tables and helpful figures are included throughout the text. Best if used as a reference to clarify topics. Offers 350 questions online.

B+

Lippincott's Illustrated Reviews: Biochemistry **$54.95** Review/Test/250 q

CHAMPE

Lippincott Williams & Wilkins, 2010, 544 pages, ISBN 9781608314126

An excellent, integrative, and comprehensive review of biochemistry that includes good clinical correlations and highly effective color diagrams. Extremely detailed and requires significant time commitment, so it should be started with first-year coursework. High-yield summaries at the end of each chapter. Comes with access to the companion Web site with USMLE-style questions.

B+

USMLE Road Map: Biochemistry **$31.95** Review

MACDONALD

McGraw-Hill, 2007, 223 pages, ISBN 9780071442053

A clear, readable outline review of biochemistry with good four-color figures. High-yield references to important diseases of metabolism are scattered throughout, but coverage of clinical correlations is not comprehensive. Includes brief review questions at the end of each chapter. Lacks "big picture" integration of related pathways. Limited student feedback.

B+

Déjà Review: Biochemistry **$19.95** Review

MANZOUL

McGraw-Hill, 2010, 224 pages, ISBN 9780071627177

Features questions and answers in a two-column, quiz-yourself format similar to that of the Recall series. Includes a helpful chapter on molecular biology and many good black-and-white diagrams. More detailed than is usually tested on Step 1.

B+

BRS Biochemistry, Molecular Biology, and Genetics **$42.95** Review/Test

SWANSON

Lippincott Williams & Wilkins, 2009, 432 pages, ISBN 9780781798754

A highly detailed review featuring many excellent figures and clinical correlations highlighted in colored boxes. The biochemistry portion includes much more detail than required for Step 1, but may be useful for students without a strong biochemistry background or as a reference text. The molecular biology section is more focused and high yield. Also offers a chapter on laboratory techniques and a comprehensive, 120-question exam. Questions are clinically oriented.

Grade	Title	Price	Type
B+	***Underground Clinical Vignettes: Biochemistry*** SWANSON **Lippincott Williams & Wilkins, 2007, 256 pages, ISBN 9780781764728** Concise clinical cases illustrating approximately 100 frequently tested diseases with a biochemical basis. Cardinal signs, symptoms, and buzzwords are highlighted. Also includes 20 additional boards-style questions. A nice review of "take-home" points for biochemistry and a useful supplement to other sources of review.	***$27.95***	Review/ Test/20 q
B	***Clinical Biochemistry Made Ridiculously Simple*** GOLDBERG **MedMaster, 2004, 93 pages + foldout, ISBN 9780940780309** A conceptual approach to clinical biochemistry, presented with humor. The casual style does not appeal to all students. Offers a good overview and integration of all metabolic pathways. Includes a 23-page clinical review that is very high yield and crammable. Also contains a unique foldout "road map" of metabolism. For students who already have a solid grasp of biochemistry.	***$22.95***	Review
B	***BRS Biochemistry and Molecular Biology Flash Cards*** SWANSON **Lippincott Williams & Wilkins, 2007, 512 pages, ISBN 9780781779029** Quick-review flash cards covering a range of topics in biochemistry and molecular biology. Inadequate for learning purposes, as cards provide only snippets of isolated information and contain some inaccuracies.	***$39.95***	Flash cards
B	***High-Yield Biochemistry*** WILCOX **Lippincott Williams & Wilkins, 2009, 128 pages, ISBN 9780781799249** A concise and crammable text in outline format with good clinical correlations at the end of each chapter. Features many diagrams and tables. Best used as a supplemental review, as explanations are scarce and details are limited.	***$29.95***	Review
B−	***Case Files: Biochemistry*** TOY **McGraw-Hill, 2008, 488 pages, ISBN 9780071486651** Includes 51 clinical cases with comprehensive discussion and summary box, but too much depth and not enough breadth for boards. Some cases will almost certainly *not* be tested. Questions at the end of each case are not representative of those seen on Step 1.	***$33.95***	Review
B−	***PreTest Biochemistry and Genetics*** WILSON **McGraw-Hill, 2010, 545 pages, ISBN 9780071623483** Difficult questions with detailed, referenced explanations. Features a high-yield appendix, but overall is an overly detailed review of a relatively low-yield subject.	***$29.95***	Test/500 q

▶ CELL BIOLOGY AND HISTOLOGY

A−

High-Yield Cell and Molecular Biology **$29.95** Review
DUDEK
Lippincott Williams & Wilkins, 2010, 272 pages, ISBN 9781609135737

Cellular and molecular biology presented in an outline format, with good diagrams and clinical correlations. Includes USMLE-tested subjects that other review resources do not cover in detail, such as laboratory techniques and second-messenger systems. Not all sections are equally useful; many students skim or read select chapters. Contains no questions or vignettes.

B+

Rapid Review: Histology and Cell Biology **$39.95** Review/Test/350 q
BURNS
Elsevier, 2006, 336 pages, ISBN 9780323044257

A resource whose format is similar to that of other books in the Rapid Review series. Features an outline of basic concepts with numerous charts, but histology images are limited. Two 50-question multiple-choice tests are presented with explanations, along with 250 more questions online.

B+

Déjà Review: Histology and Cell Biology **$19.95** Review
SONG
McGraw-Hill, 2011, 300 pages, ISBN 9780071627269

Features questions and answers in a two-column, quiz-yourself format similar to that of the Recall series. Sections are divided by organ system and vary in quality. Histology images are few and are printed in black and white. Good for a quick review, but some sections are lower-yield than others.

B

Elsevier's Integrated Genetics **$37.95** Review
ADKISON
Elsevier, 2007, 272 pages, ISBN 9780323043298

Part of the Integrated series that seeks to link basic science concepts across disciplines. Case-based and Step 1–style questions at the end of each chapter allow readers to gauge their comprehension of the material. Includes online access. Best if used during coursework; length and comprehensiveness make this less useful as stand-alone Step 1 prep material.

B

High-Yield Genetics **$28.95** Review
DUDEK
Lippincott Williams & Wilkins, 2008, 134 pages, ISBN 9780781768771

A concise, clinically oriented summary of genetics in the popular outline format. Illustrated with schematic line drawings and photographs of the most clinically relevant diseases. By no means an exhaustive resource.

B

High-Yield Histology **$26.95** Review
DUDEK
Lippincott Williams & Wilkins, 2004, 288 pages, ISBN 9780781747639

A quick and easy review of a relatively low-yield subject. Tables include some high-yield information. Contains good pictures. The appendix features classic electron micrographs. Too lengthy for Step 1 review.

B	***BRS Cell Biology and Histology*** GARTNER **Lippincott Williams & Wilkins, 2010, 384 pages, ISBN 9781608313211** Covers concepts in cell biology and histology in an outline format. Can be used alone for cell biology study, but does not include enough histology images to be considered comprehensive on that subject. Includes more detail than is required for Step 1, and information is less high yield than that of other books in the BRS series.	***$39.95***	Review/ Test/500 q
B	***Crash Course: Cell Biology and Genetics*** LAMB **Elsevier, 2006, 224 pages, ISBN 9780323044943** Part of the Crash Course review series for basic sciences, integrating clinical topics. Offers two-color illustrations, handy study tools, and Step 1 review questions. Includes online access. Too much coverage for a low-yield subject.	***$49.95***	Review
B	***USMLE Road Map: Genetics*** SACK **McGraw-Hill, 2008, 224 pages, ISBN 9780071498203** Efficient review of genetics with an emphasis on clinical correlations. Includes a few questions at the end of each chapter that are best suited to test comprehension and are not representative of Step 1. Use only if genetics is a weak subject after reviewing *First Aid*; otherwise, too much depth for a quick review.	***$31.95***	Review
B	***USMLE Road Map: Histology*** SHEEDLO **McGraw-Hill, 2005, 231 pages, ISBN 9780071440127** A concise review book with many clinical correlations. Questions at the end of each chapter are not in clinical vignette format but are suitable for testing comprehension. Black-and-white images. Good for a quick review of a low-yield subject.	***$31.95***	Review
B⁻	***PreTest Anatomy, Histology, and Cell Biology*** KLEIN **McGraw-Hill, 2010, 654 pages, ISBN 9780071623438** A resource containing difficult questions with detailed answers as well as some black-and-white images. Requires extensive time commitment, and much of the material is beyond what is required for Step 1. The most useful part of the book is the high-yield facts section at the beginning, which is divided according to discipline.	***$29.95***	Test/500 q
B⁻	***Wheater's Functional Histology*** YOUNG **Elsevier, 2006, 448 pages, ISBN 9780443068508** A color atlas with illustrations of normal histology with image captions and accompanying text. Far too detailed to use for boards studying given the low-yield nature of the material, but useful as a coursework text or boards reference.	***$79.95***	Review

▶ MICROBIOLOGY AND IMMUNOLOGY

A⁻ ***The Big Picture: Medical Microbiology*** **$49.95** Review

CHAMBERLAIN

McGraw-Hill, 2009, 445 pages, ISBN 9780071476614

Excellent full-color atlas of pathogens and clinical signs of infection. Discussion targets quick boards review. Especially good for visual learners. High-yield appendix. Includes 100 practice questions with discussion.

A⁻ ***Déjà Review: Microbiology & Immunology*** **$19.95** Review

CHEN

McGraw-Hill, 2010, 401 pages, ISBN 9780071627153

Features questions and answers in a two-column, quiz-yourself format similar to that of the Recall series. Provides an excellent review of high-yield facts. Good mnemonics, but only a few images of pathogens in black and white. Good review text on a high-yield topic.

A⁻ ***Clinical Microbiology Made Ridiculously Simple*** **$34.95** Review

GLADWIN

MedMaster, 2011, 400 pages, ISBN 9781935660033

An excellent, easy-to-read, detailed review of microbiology that includes clever and memorable mnemonics. The style of the series does not appeal to everyone. The sections on bacterial disease are most high yield, whereas the pharmacology chapters lack sufficient detail. Recommended to read during coursework and review the concise charts at the end of each chapter during boards review. All images are cartoons; no microscopy images that appear on boards. Requires a supplemental source for immunology.

A⁻ ***Microcards Flash Cards*** **$36.95** Flash cards

HARPAVAT

Lippincott Williams & Wilkins, 2007, 300 pages, ISBN 9780781769242

A well-organized and complete resource for students who like to use flash cards for review. Cards feature the clinical presentation, pathobiology, diagnosis, treatment, and high-yield facts for a particular organism. Some cards also include excellent flow charts organizing important classes of bacteria or viruses. Overall, a good review resource, but at times it is overly detailed, requiring a significant time commitment. Also useful as an aid with coursework.

A⁻ ***High-Yield Microbiology and Infectious Diseases*** **$28.95** Review/Test/200 q

HAWLEY

Lippincott Williams & Wilkins, 2006, 240 pages, ISBN 9780781760324

A very concise review of central concepts and keywords, with chapters organized by microorganism. The last few sections contain brief questions and answers organized by organ system. Also offers a useful chapter on "microbial comparisons" that groups organisms by shared virulence factors, lab results, and the like. Some students may prefer alternative resources with more explanations.

A⁻	***High-Yield Immunology*** JOHNSON **Lippincott Williams & Wilkins, 2006, 112 pages, ISBN 9780781774697** Accurately covers high-yield immunology concepts, although at times it includes more detail than necessary for Step 1 preparation. Good for quick review. The newest edition includes many improvements.	***$28.95***	Review
A⁻	***Review of Medical Microbiology*** MURRAY **Elsevier, 2005, 176 pages, ISBN 9780323033251** A resource that features Step 1–style questions divided into bacteriology, virology, mycology, and parasitology. All questions are accompanied by detailed explanations, and some are paired with high-quality images. Questions are similar to those on Step 1 and provide a nice review. Supplements Murray's *Medical Microbiology*.	***$39.95***	Test/550 q
A⁻	***Medical Microbiology and Immunology Flash Cards*** ROSENTHAL **Elsevier, 2008, 414 pages, ISBN 9780323065337** Flash cards covering the microorganisms most commonly found on Step 1. Each card features full-color microscopic images and clinical presentations on one side and relevant bug information in conjunction with a short case on the other side. Also includes Student Consult online access for extra features. Overemphasizes "trigger words" related to each bug. Not a comprehensive resource.	***$35.95***	Flash cards
A⁻	***Lange Microbiology & Infectious Diseases Flash Cards*** SOMERS **McGraw-Hill, 2010, 200 flash cards, ISBN 9780071628792** Contains a clinical vignette on one side and discussion on the other. Excellent condensed summaries of pathogens, but limited by lack of images that will be tested on boards. Printed on thinner paper than the *Biochemistry & Genetics* component of the series, reducing durability.	***$31.45***	Flash cards
A⁻	***Underground Clinical Vignettes: Microbiology Vol. I: Virology, Immunology, Parasitology, Mycology*** SWANSON **Lippincott Williams & Wilkins, 2007, 256 pages, ISBN 9780781764704** A resource containing 100 concise clinical cases that illustrate frequently tested diseases in microbiology and immunology. Cardinal signs, symptoms, and buzzwords are highlighted. Also includes 20 additional boards-style questions. Best if used as a supplement to other review resources.	***$22.95***	Review/ Test/20 q
A⁻	***Underground Clinical Vignettes: Microbiology Vol. II: Bacteriology*** SWANSON **Lippincott Williams & Wilkins, 2007, 256 pages, ISBN 9780781764711** A resource containing 100 concise clinical cases that illustrate frequently tested diseases in microbiology and immunology. Cardinal signs, symptoms, and buzzwords are highlighted. Also includes 20 additional boards-style questions. Best if used as a supplement to other review resources.	***$22.95***	Review/ Test/20 q

B+	***Basic Immunology*** ABBAS **Elsevier, 2011, 312 pages, ISBN 9781416055693** A useful text that offers clear explanations of complex topics in immunology. Best if used during the year in conjunction with coursework and later skimmed for quick Step 1 review. Includes colorful diagrams, images, tables, and a lengthy glossary for further study. Features online access.	***$64.95***	Review
B+	***Elsevier's Integrated Immunology and Microbiology*** ACTOR **Elsevier, 2006, 192 pages, ISBN 9780323033893** Part of the Integrated series that seeks to link basic science concepts across disciplines. Case-based and Step 1–style questions at the end of each chapter allow users to gauge their comprehension of the material. Includes online access. Best if used during coursework. Limited student feedback.	***$40.95***	Review
B+	***Case Studies in Immunology: Clinical Companion*** GEHA **Garland Science, 2007, 328 pages, ISBN 9780815341451** A text that was originally designed as a clinical companion to *Janeway's Immunobiology*. Provides a great synopsis of the major disorders of immunity in a clinical vignette format. Integrates basic and clinical sciences. Features excellent images and illustrations from Janeway, as well as questions and discussions.	***$49.95***	Review
B+	***Review of Medical Microbiology and Immunology*** LEVINSON **McGraw-Hill, 2012, 710 pages, ISBN 9780071774345** A clear, comprehensive text with outstanding diagrams and tables. Includes an excellent immunology section. The "Summary of Medically Important Organisms" (Part IX) is highly crammable. Can be detailed and dense at points, so best if started early with coursework. Includes practice questions of mixed quality and does not provide detailed explanation of answers. Compare with *Lippincott's Illustrated Reviews: Microbiology*.	***$53.00***	Review/ Test/654 q
B+	***Review of Immunology*** LICHTMAN **Elsevier, 2005, 192 pages, ISBN 9780721603438** Complements Abbas's *Cellular and Molecular Immunology* and *Basic Immunology* textbooks. Contains 500 boards-style questions featuring full-color illustrations along with explanations of all answer choices. A good resource for questions in a lower-yield topic. Limited student feedback.	***$33.95***	Test/500 q
B+	***Rapid Review: Microbiology and Immunology*** ROSENTHAL **Elsevier, 2011, 240 pages, ISBN 9780323069380** A resource presented in a format similar to that of other books in the Rapid Review series. Contains many excellent tables and figures, but requires significant time commitment and is not as high yield as comparable review books. Includes access to companion Web site with more than 400 questions.	***$39.95***	Review/ Test/400 q

B

Lippincott's Illustrated Reviews: Immunology **$54.95** Review/Test/Few q

DOAN

Lippincott Williams & Wilkins, 2007, 384 pages, ISBN 9780781795432

A clearly written, highly detailed review of basic concepts in immunology. Features many useful tables and review questions at the end of each chapter. Offers abbreviated coverage of immune deficiencies and autoimmune disorders. Best if started with initial coursework and used as a reference during Step 1 study.

B

Lippincott's Illustrated Reviews: Microbiology **$54.95** Review/Test/Few q

HARVEY

Lippincott Williams & Wilkins, 2006, 432 pages, ISBN 9780781782159

A comprehensive, highly illustrated review of microbiology that is similar in style to other titles in the Illustrated Reviews series. Includes a 50-page color section with more than 150 clinical and laboratory photographs. Compare with Levinson's *Review of Medical Microbiology and Immunology.*

B

Pretest: Microbiology **$29.95** Review/Test/500 q

KETTERING

McGraw-Hill, 2010, 400 pages, ISBN 97800716233530

Includes a short section on high-yield facts followed by 500 questions in a clinical vignette format. Questions are more difficult than encountered on the boards and some topics discussed are not likely to be tested. A good book to work through with coursework but too low yield for review purposes.

B

Crash Course: Immunology **$49.95** Review

NOVAK

Elsevier, 2006, 144 pages, ISBN 9781416030072

Part of the Crash Course review series for basic sciences, integrating clinical topics. Offers two-color illustrations, handy study tools, and Step 1 review questions. Includes online access. Good length and detail for boards review.

B

USMLE Road Map: Immunology **$31.95** Review

PARMELY

McGraw-Hill, 2006, 223 pages, ISBN 9780071452984

An outline review of immunology with a special focus on molecular mechanisms and laboratory techniques. Features abbreviated coverage of immunologic deficiency and autoimmune diseases that are emphasized on Step 1. Offers a collection of brief review questions at the end of each chapter. Limited student feedback.

B

Case Files: Microbiology **$33.95** Review

TOY

McGraw-Hill, 2008, 382 pages, ISBN 9780071492584

50 clinical microbiology cases followed by a clinical correlation, a discussion with boldfaced buzzwords, and questions. Cases are well chosen, but the text lacks the high-yield charts and tables found in other books in the Case Files series. Images are sparse and of poor black-and-white quality.

▶ PATHOLOGY

Rating	Resource	Price	Type
A+	***Rapid Review: Pathology*** GOLJAN **Elsevier, 2011, 638 pages, ISBN 9780323084383** A comprehensive source for key concepts in pathology, presented in a bulleted outline format with many high-yield tables and color figures. Features detailed explanations of disease mechanisms. Integrates concepts across disciplines with a strong clinical orientation. Lengthy, so best if started early with coursework. Includes access to online Qbank.	***$44.95***	Review/ Test/350 q
A+	***Pathoma*** SATTAR **Pathoma, 218 pages** Novel approach to pathology review, combining a focused textbook with 35 hours of online lectures. Lectures combine "chalk talk" and slide formats to explain pathogenesis in an easy-to-understand manner. Excellent feedback from students.	***$84.99 and up***	Review/Lecture
A	***The Big Picture: Pathology*** KEMP **McGraw-Hill, 2008, 446 pages, ISBN 9780071477482** Excellent full-color atlas of pathologic images with distilled notes on pathophysiology and treatment. Good for quick review and especially good for visual learners. The 130 questions included at the end are more straightforward than those seen on boards, but they emphasize important and tricky concepts.	***$49.95***	Review/ Test/130 q
A	***BRS Pathology*** SCHNEIDER **Lippincott Williams & Wilkins, 2009, 464 pages, ISBN 9780781779418** An excellent, concise review with appropriate content emphasis. Chapters are organized by organ system and feature an outline format with boldfacing of key facts. Includes good questions with explanations at the end of each chapter plus a comprehensive exam at the end of the book. Offers well-organized tables and diagrams as well as photographs representative of classic pathology. Contains a chapter on laboratory testing and "key associations" with each disease. The new edition contains excellent color images and access to an online test and interactive question bank. Most effective if started early in conjunction with coursework, as it does not discuss detailed mechanisms of disease pathology.	***$39.95***	Review/ Test/450 q
A–	***Pathophysiology for the Boards and Wards*** AYALA **Lippincott Williams & Wilkins, 2006, 430 pages, ISBN 9781405105101** A systems-based outline with a focus on pathology. Well organized with glossy color plates of relevant pathology and excellent, concise tables. The appendix includes a helpful overview of neurology, immunology, unusual "zebra" syndromes, and high-yield pearls. Features good integration of Step 1–relevant material from various subject areas. Compare with *Rapid Review: Pathology.*	***$39.95***	Review/ Test/75 q

A⁻ ***Lange Pathology Flash Cards*** ***$34.95*** Flash cards

BARON

McGraw-Hill, 2009, 277 flash cards, ISBN 9780071613057

Flash cards with clinical vignette on one side and discussion including etiology, pathology, clinical manifestations, and treatment on the other. Good tables to help organize diseases, but lack of images limits its utility. Best if used in conjunction with another resource. Printed on thinner paper than the *Biochemistry & Genetics* component of the series, reducing durability.

A⁻ ***Déjà Review: Pathology*** ***$19.95*** Review

DAVIS

McGraw-Hill, 2010, 458 pages, ISBN 9780071627146

Features questions and answers in a two-column, quiz-yourself format similar to that of the Recall series. Integrates pathophysiology and pathology. Includes many vignette-style questions, but only a few images in black and white. Limited student feedback.

A⁻ ***Lippincott's Illustrated Q&A Review of Rubin's Pathology*** ***$48.95*** Review/Test/1100 q

FENDERSON

Lippincott Williams & Wilkins, 2010, 336 pages, ISBN 9781608316403

A review book featuring more than 1100 multiple-choice questions that follow the Step 1 template. Questions frequently require multistep reasoning, probing the student's ability to integrate basic science knowledge in a clinical situation. Detailed rationales are linked to clinical vignettes and address incorrect answer choices. More than 300 full-color images link clinical and pathologic findings, with normal lab values provided for reference. Questions are presented both online and in print. Students can work through the online questions either in "quiz mode," which provides instant feedback, or in "test mode," which simulates the Step 1 experience. Overall, a resource that is similar in quality to *Robbins and Cotran Review of Pathology*.

A⁻ ***Robbins and Cotran Review of Pathology*** ***$49.95*** Review/Test/1100 q

KLATT

Elsevier, 2009, 451 pages, ISBN 9781416049302

A review question book that follows the main Robbins textbooks. Questions are more detailed, difficult, and arcane than those on the actual Step 1 exam, but the text offers a great review of pathology integrated with excellent images. Thorough answer explanations reinforce key points. Requires significant time commitment, so best if started with coursework.

A⁻ ***Underground Clinical Vignettes: Pathophysiology Vol. I: Pulmonary, Ob/Gyn, ENT, Hem/Onc*** ***$27.95*** Review/Test/20 q

SWANSON

Lippincott Williams & Wilkins, 2007, 228 pages, ISBN 9780781764650

Concise clinical cases illustrating 100 frequently tested pathology and physiology concepts. Cardinal signs, symptoms, and buzzwords are highlighted. Also includes 20 additional boards-style questions. Best if used as a supplement to other sources of review.

A−	***Underground Clinical Vignettes: Pathophysiology Vol. II: GI, Neurology, Rheumatology, Endocrinology*** Swanson **Lippincott Williams & Wilkins, 2007, 256 pages, ISBN 9780781764667** Concise clinical cases illustrating 100 frequently tested pathology and physiology concepts. Cardinal signs, symptoms, and buzzwords are highlighted. Also includes 20 additional boards-style questions. Best if used as a supplement to other sources of review.	***$27.95***	Review/Test/20 q
A−	***Underground Clinical Vignettes: Pathophysiology Vol. III: CV, Dermatology, GU, Orthopedics, General Surgery, Peds*** Swanson **Lippincott Williams & Wilkins, 2007, 256 pages, ISBN 9780781764681** Concise clinical cases illustrating 100 frequently tested pathology and physiology concepts. Cardinal signs, symptoms, and buzzwords are highlighted. Also includes 20 additional boards-style questions. Best if used as a supplement to other sources of review.	***$27.95***	Review/Test/20 q
B+	***MedMaps for Pathophysiology*** Agosti **Lippincott Williams & Wilkins, 2007, 259 pages, ISBN 9780781777551** A rapid review that contains 102 concept maps of disease processes and mechanisms organized by organ system, as well as classic diseases. Useful for both coursework and Step 1 preparation. Ample room is provided for notes. A good resource for looking up specific mechanisms, especially when used in conjunction with other primary review sources.	***$39.95***	Review
B+	***Cases & Concepts Step 1: Pathophysiology Review*** Caughey **Lippincott Williams & Wilkins, 2009, 376 pages, ISBN 9780781782548** Eighty-eight clinical cases integrating basic science concepts with clinical data, followed by USMLE-style questions with answers and rationales. Thumbnail and key-concept boxes highlight key facts. Limited student feedback.	***$42.95***	Review/Test/150 q
B+	***Case Files: Pathology*** Toy **McGraw-Hill, 2008, 462 pages, ISBN 9780071486668** Includes 50 clinical cases followed by discussion, comprehension questions, and a pathology pearls box. Cases are well chosen and good for those who prefer problem-based learning; however, utility is limited by scarce and poor-quality black-and-white images.	***$33.95***	Review
B+	***USMLE Road Map: Pathology*** Wettach **McGraw-Hill, 2009, 402 pages, ISBN 9780071482677** A concise yet thorough outline-format review of diseases that are tested on boards. Text is easy to read and includes a glossary of commonly used terms. Questions at the end of each chapter are useful only for testing comprehension. Black-and-white images.	***$31.95***	Test/500 q

B	***PreTest Pathology*** BROWN McGraw-Hill, 2010, 612 pages, ISBN 9780071623490 Difficult questions with detailed, complete answers. High-yield facts at the beginning are useful for concept summaries, but information can easily be obtained in better review books. Features high-quality black-and-white photographs and microscopy slides, making interpretation difficult. Best used as a supplement to other review books.	***$29.95***	Test/500 q
B	***High-Yield Histopathology*** DUDEK Lippincott Williams & Wilkins, 2011, 328 pages, ISBN 9781609130152 A new book that reviews the relationship of basic histology to the pathology, physiology, and pharmacology of clinical conditions that are tested on Step 1. Includes case studies, numerous light and electron micrographs, and pathology photographs. Given its considerable length, should be started with coursework.	***$27.95***	Review
B	***Crash Course: Pathology*** FISHBACK Elsevier, 2005, 384 pages, ISBN 9780323033084 Part of the Crash Course review series for basic sciences, integrating clinical topics. Offers two-color illustrations, handy study tools, and Step 1 review questions. Includes online access. Best if started during coursework.	***$49.95***	Review
B	***Pathophysiology of Disease: Introduction to Clinical Medicine*** MCPHEE McGraw-Hill, 2009, 752 pages, ISBN 9780071621670 An interdisciplinary text useful for understanding the pathophysiology of clinical symptoms. Effectively integrates the basic sciences with mechanisms of disease. Features great graphs, diagrams, and tables. In view of its length, most useful if started during coursework. Includes a few non–boards-style questions. The text's clinical emphasis nicely complements *BRS Pathology*.	***$69.95***	Review/Test/ Few q
B	***Haematology at a Glance*** MEHTA Blackwell Science, 2009, 128 pages, ISBN 9781405179706 A resource that covers common hematologic issues. Includes color illustrations. Presented in a logical sequence that is easy to read. Good for use with coursework.	***$40.95***	Review
B	***Pocket Companion to Robbins and Cotran Pathologic Basis of Disease*** MITCHELL Elsevier, 2012, 774 pages, ISBN 9781416054542 A resource that is good for reviewing keywords associated with most important diseases. Presented in a highly condensed format, but the text is complete and easy to understand. Contains no photographs or illustrations but does include tables. Useful as a quick reference.	***$42.95***	Review

B	***PreTest Pathophysiology*** MUFSON **McGraw-Hill, 2004, 480 pages, ISBN 9780071434928** Includes 500 questions and answers with explanations. Questions are often overly specific, and explanations vary in quality. Features a brief section of high-yield topics. Good economic value.	***$28.95***	Test/500 q
B	***Color Atlas of Physiology*** SILBERNAGL **Thieme, 2009, 456 pages, ISBN 9783135450063** A text containing more than 180 high-quality illustrations of disturbed physiologic processes that lead to dysfunction. An alternative to standard texts, but not high yield for boards review.	***$44.95***	Review

▸ PHARMACOLOGY

A

Kaplan Medical USMLE Pharmacology and Treatment Flashcards ***$44.95*** Flash cards
FISCHER
Kaplan, 2008, 200 flash cards, ISBN 9781427797063

Excellent, easy-to-read flash cards with drug and questions on one side and discussion on the other, offering just the right amount of detail for the boards. Alternative to more traditional pharmacology textbooks.

A

Déjà Review: Pharmacology ***$19.95*** Review
GLEASON
McGraw-Hill, 2010, 219 pages, ISBN 9780071627290

Features questions and answers in a two-column, quiz-yourself format similar to that of the Recall series. Covers most of the drugs needed for Step 1 succinctly. Includes clinical vignettes at the end of chapters for review.

A⁻

Lange Pharmacology Flash Cards ***$34.95*** Flash cards
BARON
McGraw-Hill, 2009, 189 pages, ISBN 9780071622417

A total of 189 pocket-sized flash cards featuring clinical vignettes involving relevant drugs, with high-yield information highlighted in bold. Information content of cards varies—too much information on some, not enough on others. Printed on less durable material.

A⁻

BRS Pharmacology Flash Cards ***$32.95*** Flash cards
KIM
Lippincott Williams & Wilkins, 2004, 640 pages, ISBN 9780781747967

A series of flash cards that facilitate memorization of the appropriate clinical use of drugs rather than describing mechanisms and toxicities in detail. Not a comprehensive review resource, but may be useful for those who find other pharm cards overwhelming. Considered by many to be an excellent resource for quick, last-minute review.

B⁺

Pharmacology for the Boards and Wards ***$39.95*** Review/Test/150 q
AYALA
Lippincott Williams & Wilkins, 2006, 256 pages, ISBN 9781405105118

Like other books in the Boards and Wards series, the pharmacology volume is presented primarily in tabular format with bulleted key points. Review questions are in Step 1 style. At times can be too dense, but does a great job of focusing on the clinical aspects of drugs.

B⁺

Crash Course: Pharmacology ***$49.95*** Review
BARNES
Elsevier, 2006, 248 pages, ISBN 9781416029595

Part of the Crash Course review series for basic sciences, integrating clinical topics. Offers two-color illustrations, handy study tools, and Step 1–style review questions. Includes online access. Gives a solid, easy-to-follow overview of pharmacology. Limited student feedback.

B+ ***Pharmacology Flash Cards*** ***$36.95*** Flash cards
BRENNER
Elsevier, 2009, 640 pages, ISBN 9781437703115

Flash cards for more than 200 of the most commonly tested drugs. Cards include the name of the drug (both generic and brand) on the front and basic drug information on the back. Divided and color coded by class, and comes with a compact carrying case. Lacks figures and clinical vignettes.

B+ ***Lippincott's Illustrated Reviews: Pharmacology*** ***$59.95*** Review/Test/200 q
HARVEY
Lippincott Williams & Wilkins, 2009, 564 pages, ISBN 9780781771559

A resource presented in outline format with practice questions, many excellent illustrations, and comparison tables. Effectively integrates pharmacology and pathophysiology. The new edition has been updated to cover recent changes in pharmacotherapy. Best started with coursework, as it is highly detailed and requires significant time commitment.

B+ ***Pharm Cards: Review Cards for Medical Students*** ***$37.95*** Flash cards
JOHANNSEN
Lippincott Williams & Wilkins, 2010, 240 flash cards, ISBN 9780781787413

A series of flash cards that cover the mechanisms and side effects of major drugs and drug classes. Good for class review, but the level of detail is beyond what is necessary for Step 1. Lacks pharmacokinetics, but features good charts and diagrams. Well liked by students who enjoy flash card–based review. Compare with *BRS Pharmacology Flash Cards.*

B+ ***Elsevier's Integrated Pharmacology*** ***$39.95*** Review
KESTER
Elsevier, 2007, 336 pages, ISBN 9780323034081

Part of the Integrated series that seeks to link basic science concepts across disciplines. Case-based and Step 1–style questions at the end of each chapter allow readers to gauge their comprehension of the material. Includes online access. Best if used during coursework. Limited student feedback.

B+ ***Rapid Review: Pharmacology*** ***$39.95*** Review
PAZDERNIK
Elsevier, 2010, 360 pages, ISBN 9780323068123

A detailed treatment of pharmacology, presented in an outline format similar to that of other books in the series. More detailed than necessary for Step 1 review. Contains high-yield charts and figures. Includes access to the companion Web site with 450 USMLE-style questions.

B+ ***Pharmacology Recall*** ***$42.95*** Review
RAMACHANDRAN
Lippincott Williams & Wilkins, 2008, 592 pages + audio, ISBN 9780781787307

A resource presented in the two-column, question-and-answer format typical of the Recall series. At times questions delve into more clinical detail than required for Step 1, but overall the breadth of coverage is appropriate. Includes a high-yield drug summary. Includes questions and answers that are recorded in MP3 format so that they can be used on any audio player.

B+	***Underground Clinical Vignettes Step 1: Pharmacology*** SWANSON **Lippincott Williams & Wilkins, 2007, 256 pages, ISBN 9780781764858** Concise clinical cases illustrating approximately 100 frequently tested pharmacology concepts. Cardinal signs, symptoms, and buzzwords are highlighted. Also includes 20 additional boards-style questions. Omits some important drugs and lacks detail on mechanisms, so best used as a supplement to other sources of review.	***$27.95***	Review/ Test/20 q
B+	***Katzung & Trevor's Pharmacology: Examination and Board Review*** TREVOR **McGraw-Hill, 2010, 644 pages, ISBN 9780071701586** A well-organized text with concise explanations. Features good charts and tables; the crammable list in Appendix I is especially high yield for Step 1 review. Also good for drug interactions and toxicities. Offers two practice exams but no explanations of the answers. Text includes many low-yield/obscure drugs. Compare with *Lippincott's Illustrated Reviews: Pharmacology*, both of which are better suited to complementing coursework than last-minute studying for boards.	***$49.95***	Review/ Test/1000 q
B	***USMLE Road Map: Pharmacology*** KATZUNG **McGraw-Hill, 2006, 178 pages, ISBN 9780071445818** An outline review of pharmacology divided either by organ system or by disease process. Includes a collection of brief review questions at the end of each chapter. The appendix has useful tables of common side effects and drug classes. Does not contain enough detail to serve as a comprehensive review. Limited student feedback.	***$31.95***	Review
B	***BRS Pharmacology*** ROSENFELD **Lippincott Williams & Wilkins, 2009, 368 pages, ISBN 9780781789134** Features two-color tables and figures that summarize essential information for quick recall. A list of drugs organized by drug family is included in each chapter. Too detailed for boards review; best used as a reference. Also offers end-of-chapter review tests with Step 1–style questions and a comprehensive exam with explanations of answers. An additional question bank is available online.	***$39.95***	Review/ Test/200 q
B	***PreTest Pharmacology*** SHLAFER **McGraw-Hill, 2010, 558 pages, ISBN 9780071623421** Good questions divided into sections by organ system and accompanied by detailed answers. Questions are often more straightforward than Step 1, while others build graph-reading skills and multistep reasoning skills. Sections on general principles and autonomics are especially useful. Best used as a resource for additional questions after other sources have been exhausted.	***$29.95***	Test/500 q

B

Case Files: Pharmacology **$33.95** Review

Toy

McGraw-Hill, 2008, 440 pages, ISBN 9780071488587

Includes 53 cases with detailed discussion, comprehension questions, and a box of clinical pearls. An appealing text for students who prefer problem-based learning, but lacks the level of detail typically tested on Step 1.

B

High-Yield Pharmacology **$27.95** Review

Weiss

Lippincott Williams & Wilkins, 2009, 160 pages, ISBN 9780781792738

A succinct pharmacology review presented in an easy-to-follow outline format. Features a drug index, key points in bold, and summary tables of high-yield facts. Lacks details on mechanisms or drug specifics, so best used with a more comprehensive resource.

▶ PHYSIOLOGY

A

BRS Physiology **$39.95** Review/Test/400 q
COSTANZO
Lippincott Williams & Wilkins, 2010, 384 pages, ISBN 9780781798761

A clear, concise review of physiology that is both comprehensive and efficient, making for fast, easy reading. Includes excellent high-yield charts and tables, but lacks some figures from Costanzo's *Physiology*. Features high-quality practice questions with explanations in each chapter along with a clinically oriented final exam. An excellent boards review resource, but best if started early in combination with coursework. Respiratory and acid-base sections are comparatively weak.

A

Physiology **$59.95** Text
COSTANZO
Saunders, 2010, 493 pages, ISBN 9781416062165

A comprehensive, clearly written text that covers concepts outlined in *BRS Physiology* in greater detail. Offers excellent color diagrams and charts. Each systems-based chapter features a detailed summary of objectives and a Step 1–relevant clinical case. Includes access to online interactive extras. Requires time commitment; best started with coursework.

A⁻

The Big Picture: Medical Physiology **$46.95** Review/Text/108 q
KIBBLE
McGraw-Hill, 2009, 448 pages, ISBN 9780071485678

Well-written text supplemented by 450 illustrations. Chapters conclude with approximately 10 study questions/answers. Consistent organization facilitates relatively quick review. Includes a 108-question practice exam with answers. Best if started early with coursework.

A⁻

BRS Physiology Cases and Problems **$45.95** Review/Test/Many q
COSTANZO
Lippincott Williams & Wilkins, 2012, 368 pages, ISBN 9781451120615

Sixty classic cases presented in vignette format with several questions per case. Includes exceptionally detailed explanations of answers. For students interested in an in-depth discussion of physiology concepts. May be useful for group review.

B⁺

Déjà Review: Physiology **$19.95** Review
GOULD
McGraw-Hill, 2010, 288 pages, ISBN 9780071627252

Features questions and answers in a two-column, quiz-yourself format similar to that of the Recall series. Includes helpful graphs and schematics. Contains clinical vignettes at the end of each organ system similar to those seen on the Step 1 exam.

B⁺

High-Yield Acid-Base Review **$26.95** Review
LONGENECKER
Lippincott Williams & Wilkins, 2006, 128 pages, ISBN 9780781796552

A concise and well-written description of acid-base disorders. Includes chapters discussing differential diagnoses and 12 clinical cases. Introduces a multistep approach to the material. A bookmark with useful factoids is included with the text. No index or questions.

Rating	Resource	Price	Type
B+	***USMLE Road Map: Physiology*** PASLEY **McGraw-Hill, 2006, 219 pages, ISBN 9780071445177** A text in outline format incorporating useful comparison charts and clear diagrams. Provides a concise approach to physiology. Clinical correlations are referenced to the text. Questions build on basic concepts and include detailed explanations. Limited student feedback.	***$26.95***	Review/ Test/50 q
B+	***Appleton & Lange Review: Physiology*** PENNEY **McGraw-Hill, 2005, 224 pages, ISBN 9780071445177** Step 1–style questions divided into subcategories under physiology. Good if subject-specific questions are desired, but may be too detailed for many students. Some diagrams are used to explain answers. A good way to test knowledge after coursework.	***$39.95***	Test/700 q
B	***Rapid Review: Physiology*** BROWN **Elsevier, 2012, 264 pages, ISBN 9780323072601** A resource that offers a good review of physiology in a format typical of the Rapid Review series, albeit with more images. Includes online access to 350 questions along with other extras.	***$39.95***	Review
B	***Elsevier's Integrated Physiology*** CARROLL **Elsevier, 2006, 256 pages, ISBN 9780323043182** Part of the Integrated series that seeks to link basic science concepts across disciplines. A good text for initial coursework, but too long for Step 1 review. Case-based and Step 1–style questions are included at the end of each chapter. Limited student feedback.	***$37.95***	Review
B	***High-Yield Physiology*** DUDEK **Lippincott Williams & Wilkins, 2008, 240 pages, ISBN 9780781745871** An outline review of major concepts written at an appropriate level of depth for Step 1; includes especially detailed coverage of cardiovascular, respiratory, and renal physiology. Features many excellent diagrams and boxes highlighting important equations. Large blocks of dense text make it a slow and disorienting read at times. Limited student feedback.	***$28.95***	Review
B	***PreTest Physiology*** METTING **McGraw-Hill, 2010, 434 pages, ISBN 9780071623506** Contains questions with detailed, well-written explanations. One of the best of the PreTest series. Best for use by the motivated student after extensive review of other sources. Includes a high-yield facts section with useful diagrams and tables.	***$29.95***	Test/500 q

B ***Netter's Physiology Flash Cards*** ***$35.95*** Flash cards

MULRONEY

Saunders, 2010, 200+ flash cards, ISBN 9781416046288

Flash cards contain a high-quality illustration on one side with question and commentary on the other. Good for self-testing, but too fragmented for learning purposes and not comprehensive enough for boards. Limited student feedback.

B ***Acid-Base, Fluids, and Electrolytes Made Ridiculously Simple*** ***$22.95*** Review

PRESTON

MedMaster, 2010, 156 pages, ISBN 9780940780989

A resource that covers major acid-base and renal physiology concepts. Provides information beyond the scope of Step 1, but remains a useful companion for studying kidney function, electrolyte disturbances, and fluid management. Includes scattered diagrams and questions at the end of each chapter. Consider using after exhausting more high-yield physiology review resources.

B ***Case Files: Physiology*** ***$33.95*** Review

TOY

McGraw-Hill, 2009, 456 pages, ISBN 9780071493741

A review text divided into 51 clinical cases followed by clinical correlations, a discussion, and take-home pearls, presented in a format similar to that of other texts in the Case Files series. A few questions accompany each case. Too lengthy for rapid review; best for students who enjoy problem-based learning.

B⁻ ***Vander's Renal Physiology*** ***$39.95*** Text

EATON

McGraw-Hill, 2009, 222 pages, ISBN 9780071613033

Well-written text on renal physiology, with helpful but sparse diagrams and questions at the end of each chapter. Far too detailed for Step 1 review, however. Best if used with organ-based coursework to understand the principles of renal physiology.

B⁻ ***Clinical Physiology Made Ridiculously Simple*** ***$19.95*** Review

GOLDBERG

MedMaster, 2007, 160 pages, ISBN 9780940780217

An easy-to-read text with many amusing associations and memorable mnemonics. The style does not work for everyone. Not as well illustrated as the rest of the series, and lacks some important concepts. Best used as a supplement to other review books.

B⁻ ***Endocrine Physiology*** ***$42.95*** Text

MOLINA

McGraw-Hill, 2010, 303 pages, ISBN 9780071613019

Good but lengthy text on endocrine physiology. Questions at the end of each chapter are helpful to work through, but most are not representative of Step 1 questions. Provides more detailed explanations of endocrine physiology than Costanzo offers but much too lengthy for Step 1 review. May be useful as a coursework adjunct.

B⁻ ***Pulmonary Pathophysiology: The Essentials*** ***$42.95*** Review/Test/50 q

WEST

Lippincott Williams & Wilkins, 2007, 224 pages, ISBN 9780781764148

A volume offering comprehensive coverage of respiratory physiology. Clearly organized with useful charts and diagrams. Review questions at the end of each chapter have letter answers only and no explanations. Best used as a course supplement during the second year.

NOTES

SECTION IV

Commercial Review Courses

▶ COMMERCIAL REVIEW COURSES

Commercial preparation courses can be helpful for some students, but such courses are expensive and may leave limited time for independent study. They are usually an effective tool for students who feel overwhelmed by the volume of material they must review in preparation for the boards. Also note that while some commercial courses are designed for first-time test takers, others are geared toward students who are repeating the examination. Still other courses have been created for IMGs who want to take all three Steps in a limited amount of time. Finally, student experience and satisfaction with review courses are highly variable, and course content and structure can evolve rapidly. We thus suggest that you discuss options with recent graduates of review courses you are considering. Some student opinions can be found in discussion groups on the Internet.

Falcon Physician Reviews

Established in 2002, Falcon Physician Reviews provides intensive and comprehensive live reviews for students preparing for the USMLE and COMLEX. The 7-week Step 1 reviews are held throughout the year with small class sizes in order to increase student involvement and instructor accessibility. Falcon Physician Reviews uses an active learning system that focuses on comprehension, retention, and application of concepts. Falcon Online program components include:

- A full set of color Falcon textbooks
- Hundreds of hours of lectures optimized into high-yield streaming video
- On-screen PowerPoint slides
- A 3-month USMLEWorld or 6-month USMLE Consult Question Bank subscription
- Diagnostic exam
- Available as an iPhone application

Falcon Live programs are currently offered in Dallas, Texas. The fee range is $2599–$6499. The all-inclusive program tuition fee includes:

- Lodging
- Complimentary daily breakfast and lunch
- A full set of color Falcon textbooks
- Daily clinical vignettes
- Daily tutoring
- High-speed Internet service
- Local hotel shuttle service
- A 3-month USMLEWorld or 6-month USMLE Consult Question Bank subscription

For more information, contact:

Falcon Physician Reviews
4800 Regent Boulevard, Suite 204
Irving, TX 75063
Phone: (800) 683-8725
Fax: (214) 292-8568
www.falconreviews.com

Kaplan Medical

Kaplan Medical offers a wide range of options for USMLE preparation, including live lectures, center-based study, and online courses. All of its program offerings focus on providing the most exam-relevant information available.

Live Lectures. Kaplan's LivePrep offers a highly structured, interactive live lecture series led by expert faculty as 7-, 14-, or 16-week courses. This course's advantages include interaction with faculty and peers.

Kaplan also offers LivePrep Retreat, a 6-week course during which students stay and study in high-end hotel accommodations.

Center Study. Kaplan's CenterPrep, a center-based lecture course, is designed for medical students seeking flexibility. Essentially an independent study course, it is offered at Kaplan Centers across the United States for 3-, 6-, or 9-month periods. Students have access to more than 200 hours of video lecture review. CenterPrep features seven volumes of lecture notes and a full-length simulated exam with a complete performance analysis and detailed explanations. The course also includes a Personalized Learning System (PLS), which allows students to create a customized study schedule and track their performance.

Online Programs. Kaplan Medical provides online content- and question-based review. Classroom Anywhere, Kaplan's top-rated course, offers an interactive, online classroom experience with the benefit of live instruction delivered by expert faculty from wherever Internet access is available. Kaplan's OnlinePrep on-demand video lectures and Qbank are included in this course. This course is ideal for students who need a more comprehensive review option, but require a flexible study schedule or are unable to travel to one of Kaplan's live lecture locations.

Kaplan's popular Qbank allows students to create practice tests by discipline and organ system, difficulty, and yield; receive instant onscreen feedback; and track their cumulative performance. Kaplan offers Until Your Test access allowing students to get an immediate edge in school and repeat lectures as often as they like for the next 12 months. Kaplan's Qbank also includes a free integrated mobile app for iPhone and Android devices so students can practice questions on the go. Qbank demos are available at www.kaplanmedical.com.

For more information, call (800) 527-8378 or visit www.kaplanmedical.com.

Northwestern Medical Review

Northwestern Medical Review offers live-lecture review courses, videotaped lectures, and private tutoring in preparation for both the COMLEX Level I and USMLE Step 1 examinations. Two review plans are available for each exam: NBI 200, a 5-day course; and NBI 300, an 8- to 15-day course. All courses are in live-lecture format, and most are taught by the authors of the Northwestern Review Books. In addition to organized lecture notes and books for each subject, courses include Web-based question bank access, audio CDs, and a large pool of practice questions and simulated exams. All plans are available in a customized, onsite format for groups of second-year students from individual U.S. medical schools. Additionally, public sites are frequently offered in East Lansing, MI, and Chicago, IL. Live courses and Center preparations are also globally available at several international sites, including Caribbean Islands (Puerto Rico and select islands), Guadalajara (Mexico), India (several locations), Canada (Ontario), Dubai, and other locations based on demand.

Tuition for each course is $465. Private tutoring, CBT question-bank access, and DVD materials are also available for purchase independent of the live-lecture plans. Northwestern offers a retake option as well as a liberal cancellation policy.

For more information, contact:

Northwestern Medical Review
4800 Collins Rd. #22174
Lansing, MI 48909
Phone: (866) MedPass
Fax: (517) 347-7005
Email: contactus@northwesternmedicalreview.com
www.northwesternmedicalreview.com

PASS Program/PASS Program South

USMLE and COMLEX Review Program. The PASS Program offers a concept-based, clinically integrated curriculum to help students increase board scores, obtain residencies, and broaden their perspective of medicine. Helpful for a wide spectrum of students, including those trying to maximize scores on the first try and those struggling to stay in medical school. PASS accommodates all types of learners: auditory, visual, or kinesthetic, and, with the help of small class sizes, encourages students to interact and to ask questions.

Live Lectures. PASS offers 4-week, 8-week, or extended-stay programs in Champaign, Illinois, and St. Augustine, Florida. Facilities include computer labs, a state-of-the-art lecture hall, student lounges and study areas, and housing. Drill sessions and small study groups take place throughout the week. Tuition (not including housing) for the 4-week program is $2950 and for the 8-week guarantee program is $6000.

One-on-One Tutoring. Included with tuition, students receive one-on-one tutoring from an MD each week they attend the program. Four-week students receive two sessions per week and 8-week students receive four sessions in the first half of the program and five sessions in the second half.

For more information, contact:

PASS Program
2302 Moreland Blvd.
Champaign, IL 61822
Phone: (217) 378-8018
Fax: (217) 378-7809
www.passprogram.net

PASS Program South
120 Sea Grove Main Street
St. Augustine, FL 32080
Phone: (904) 209-3140
www.passprogramsouth.com

The Princeton Review

The Princeton Review offers two flexible preparation options for the USMLE Step 1: the USMLE Online Course and the USMLE Online Workout.

USMLE Online Courses. The USMLE Online Courses offer the following:

- 75 hours of online review, including lessons, vignettes, and drills
- Complete review of all USMLE Step 1 subjects
- Three full-length CBTs
- Seven 1-hour subject-based tests
- Complete set of print materials

- 24/7 access to technical support
- Three months of access to tests, drills, and lessons

More information can be found on The Princeton Review's Web site at www.princetonreview.com.

Youel's™ Prep, Inc.

Youel's Prep, Inc., has specialized in medical board preparation for 30 years. The company provides DVDs, audiotapes, videotapes, a CD (PowerPrep Quick Study), books, live lectures, and tutorials for small groups as well as for individuals (TutorialPrep™). All DVDs, videotapes, audiotapes, live lectures, and tutorials are correlated with a three-book set of Prep Notes© consisting of two textbooks, *Youel's Jewels I*© and *Youel's Jewels II*© (984 pages), and *Case Studies*©, a question-and-answer book (1854 questions, answers, and explanations).

The Comprehensive DVD program consists of 56 hours of lectures by the systems with a three-book set: *Youel's Jewels I and II* and *Case Studies*. Integrated with these programs are pre-tests and post-tests.

All Youel's Prep courses are taught and written by physicians, reflecting the clinical slant of the boards. All programs are systems based. In addition, all programs are updated continuously. Accordingly, books are not printed until the order is received.

Delivery in the United States or overseas is usually within 1 week. Optional express delivery is also available. Youel's Prep Home Study Program™ allows students to own their materials and to use them for repetitive study in the convenience of their homes. Purchasers of any of Youel's Prep materials, programs, or services are enrolled as members of the Youel's Prep Family of Students™, which affords them access to free telephone tutoring at (800) 645-3985. Students may call 24/7. Youel's Prep live lectures are held at select medical schools at the invitation of the school and students.

Programs are custom-designed for content, number of hours, and scheduling to fit students' needs. First-year students are urged to call early to arrange live-lecture programs at their schools for next year.

For more information, contact:

Youel's Prep, Inc.
P.O. Box 31479
Palm Beach Gardens, FL 33420
Phone: (800) 645-3985
Fax: (561) 622-4858
Email: info@youelsprep.com
www.youelsprep.net

Publisher Contacts

ASM Press
1752 N Street, NW
Washington, D.C. 20036-2904
(800) 546-2416
Books@asmusa.org
www.asmpress.org

Elsevier Science
Order Fulfillment
3251 Riverport Lane
Maryland Heights, MO 63043
(800) 545-2522
Fax: (800) 535-9935
www.us.elsevierhealth.com

Exam Master
500 Ethel Court
Middletown, DE 19709-9410
(800) 572-3627
Fax: (302) 283-1222
customer_service@exammaster.com
www.exammaster.com

Garland Science Publishing
711 Third Avenue, 8th Floor
New York, NY 10017
(203) 281-4487
Fax: (212) 947-3027
science@garland.com
www.garlandscience.com

Gold Standard Board Prep
Apollo Audiobooks, LLC
2508 27th Street
Lubbock, TX 79410
(806) 773-3197
info@ApolloAudiobooks.com
www.boardprep.net

John Wiley & Sons
1 Wiley Drive
Somerset, NJ 08875-1272
(800) 225-5945
Fax: (732) 302-2300
custserv@wiley.com
www.wiley.com

Kaplan, Inc.
395 Hudson Street, 4th Floor
New York, NY 10014
kaplanmedical.com

Lippincott Williams & Wilkins
16522 Hunters Green Parkway
Hagerstown, MD 21740
(800) 638-3030
Fax: (301) 223-2398
orders@lww.com
www.lww.com

MedMaster, Inc.
P.O. Box 640028
Miami, FL 33164
(800) 335-3480
Fax: (954) 962-4508
mmbks@aol.com
www.medmaster.net

McGraw-Hill Companies
Order Services
P.O. Box 182604
Columbus, OH 43272-3031
(877) 833-5524
Fax: (614) 759-3749
pbg.ecommerce_custserv@mcgraw-hill.com
www.mhprofessional.com

Parthenon Publishing/CRC Press
Taylor & Francis Group
6000 Broken Sound Parkway, NW, Suite 300
Boca Raton, FL 33487
(800) 272-7737
Fax: (800) 374-3401
orders@taylorandfrancis.com
www.crcpress.com

Princeton Review
2315 Broadway
New York, NY 10024
(866) 877-7737
www.princetonreview.com

Thieme Medical Publishers, Inc.
333 Seventh Avenue
New York, NY 10001
(800) 782-3488
Fax: (212) 947-0108
www.thieme.com
customerservice@thieme.com

SECTION IV

Abbreviations and Symbols

ABBREVIATION	MEANING
1°	primary
2°	secondary
3°	tertiary
A-a	alveolar-arterial [gradient]
AA	Alcoholics Anonymous, amyloid A
AAMC	Association of American Medical Colleges
Ab	antibody
ABP	androgen-binding protein
ACA	anterior cerebral artery
ACC	acetyl-CoA carboxylase
Acetyl-CoA	acetyl coenzyme A
ACD	anemia of chronic disease
ACE	angiotensin-converting enzyme
ACh	acetylcholine
AChE	acetylcholinesterase
ACL	anterior cruciate ligament
AComm	anterior communicating [artery]
ACTH	adrenocorticotropic hormone
ADA	adenosine deaminase, Americans with Disabilities Act
ADH	antidiuretic hormone
ADHD	attention-deficit hyperactivity disorder
ADP	adenosine diphosphate
ADPKD	autosomal-dominant polycystic kidney disease
AFP	α-fetoprotein
Ag	antigen, silver
AICA	anterior inferior cerebellar artery
AIDS	acquired immunodeficiency syndrome
AIHA	autoimmune hemolytic anemia
AL	amyloid light [chain]
ALA	aminolevulinic acid
ALL	acute lymphoblastic (lymphocytic) leukemia
ALP	alkaline phosphatase
α_1, α_2	sympathetic receptors
ALS	amyotrophic lateral sclerosis
ALT	alanine transaminase
AMA	American Medical Association, antimitochondrial antibody
AML	acute myelogenous (myeloid) leukemia
AMP	adenosine monophosphate
ANA	antinuclear antibody
ANCA	antineutrophil cytoplasmic antibody
ANOVA	analysis of variance
ANP	atrial natriuretic peptide
ANS	autonomic nervous system

ABBREVIATION	MEANING
AO×3	alert and oriented to time, place, and person
AOA	American Osteopathic Association
AP	action potential, aorticopulmonary, A & P [ribosomal binding sites]
A & P	ribosomal binding sites
APC	antigen-presenting cell, activated protein C
APP	amyloid precursor protein
APRT	adenine phosphoribosyltransferase
APSAC	anistreplase
aPTT	activated partial thromboplastin time
Apo	apolipoprotein
AR	attributable risk, autosomal recessive, aortic regurgitation
ara-C	arabinofuranosyl cytidine (cytarabine)
ARB	angiotensin receptor blocker
ARDS	acute respiratory distress syndrome
Arg	arginine
ARMD	age-related macular degeneration
ARPKD	autosomal-recessive polycystic kidney disease
AS	aortic stenosis
ASA	acetylsalicylic acid, anterior spinal artery
ASD	atrial septal defect
ASO	anti–streptolysin O
Asp	aspartic acid
AST	aspartate transaminase
AT	angiotensin, antithrombin
ATCase	aspartate transcarbamoylase
ATN	acute tubular necrosis
ATP	adenosine triphosphate
ATPase	adenosine triphosphatase
AV	atrioventricular
AVM	arteriovenous malformation
AZT	azidothymidine
β_1, β_2	sympathetic receptors
BAL	British anti-Lewisite [dimercaprol]
BBB	blood-brain barrier
BCG	bacille Calmette-Guérin
BIMS	Biometric Identity Management System
BM	basement membrane
BMI	body-mass index
BMR	basal metabolic rate
BP	bisphosphate, blood pressure
BPG	biphosphoglycerate
BPH	benign prostatic hyperplasia
BS	Bowman's space

ABBREVIATION	MEANING
BT	bleeding time
BUN	blood urea nitrogen
Ca^{2+}	calcium ion
CAD	coronary artery disease
CAF	common application form
CALLA	common acute lymphoblastic leukemia antigen
cAMP	cyclic adenosine monophosphate
c-ANCA	cytoplasmic antineutrophil cytoplasmic antibody
CBG	corticosteroid-binding globulin
Cbl	cobalamin
CBSSA	Comprehensive Basic Science Self-Assessment
CBT	computer-based test, cognitive-behavioral therapy
CCK	cholecystokinin
CCS	computer-based case simulation
CCT	cortical collecting tubule
CD	cluster of differentiation
CDK	cyclin-dependent kinase
cDNA	complementary deoxyribonucleic acid
CEA	carcinoembryonic antigen
CETP	cholesterol-ester transfer protein
CF	cystic fibrosis
CFTR	cystic fibrosis transmembrane conductance regulator
CFX	circumflex [artery]
CGD	chronic granulomatous disease
cGMP	cyclic guanosine monophosphate
CGN	*cis*-Golgi network
CGRP	calcitonin gene–related peptide
C_H1–C_H3	constant regions, heavy chain [antibody]
ChAT	choline acetyltransferase
CHF	congestive heart failure
χ^2	chi-squared
CI	confidence interval
CIN	candidate identification number, carcinoma in situ, cervical intraepithelial neoplasia
CIS	Communication and Interpersonal Skills
CJD	Creutzfeldt-Jakob disease
CK	clinical knowledge, creatine kinase
CK-MB	creatine kinase, MB fraction
C_L	constant region, light chain [antibody]
CL	clearance
Cl^-	chloride ion
CLL	chronic lymphocytic leukemia
CML	chronic myelogenous (myeloid) leukemia
CMV	cytomegalovirus
CN	cranial nerve
CN^-	cyanide ion
CNS	central nervous system
CO	carbon monoxide, cardiac output
CO_2	carbon dioxide
CoA	coenzyme A
COMLEX-USA	Comprehensive Osteopathic Medical Licensing Examination
COMSAE	Comprehensive Osteopathic Medical Self-Assessment Examination
COMT	catechol-O-methyltransferase
COOH	carboxyl group
COP	coat protein
COPD	chronic obstructive pulmonary disease
CoQ	coenzyme Q
COX	cyclooxygenase
C_p	plasma concentration
CPAP	continuous positive airway pressure
CPK	creatine phosphokinase
CPR	cardiopulmonary resuscitation
Cr	creatinine
CRC	colorectal cancer
CREST	calcinosis, Raynaud's phenomenon, esophageal dysfunction, sclerosis, and teleangiectasias [syndrome]
CRH	corticotropin-releasing hormone
CRP	C-reactive protein
CS	clinical skills
C-section	cesarean section
CSF	cerebrospinal fluid, colony-stimulating factor
CT	computed tomography
CTL	cytotoxic T lymphocyte
CTP	cytidine triphosphate
CV	cardiovascular
CVA	cerebrovascular accident, costovertebral angle
CVID	common variable immunodeficiency
CXR	chest x-ray
Cys	cysteine
DAF	decay-accelerating factor
DAG	diacylglycerol
dATP	deoxyadenosine triphosphate
DCIS	ductal carcinoma in situ
DCT	distal convoluted tubule
ddC	dideoxycytidine [zalcitabine]
ddI	didanosine
DES	diethylstilbestrol
DHAP	dihydroxyacetone phosphate
DHB	dihydrobiopterin
DHEA	dehydroepiandrosterone
DHF	dihydrofolic acid
DHS	Department of Homeland Security
DHT	dihydrotestosterone
DI	diabetes insipidus
DIC	disseminated intravascular coagulation
DIP	distal interphalangeal [joint]
DIT	diiodotyrosine
DKA	diabetic ketoacidosis
DM	diabetes mellitus
DNA	deoxyribonucleic acid
2,4-DNP	2,4-dinitrophenol
dNTP	deoxynucleotide triphosphate
DO	doctor of osteopathy
DPGN	diffuse proliferative glomerulonephritis
DPM	Doctor of Podiatric Medicine
DPP-4	dipeptidyl peptidase-4
DS	double stranded

ABBREVIATION	MEANING
dsDNA	double-stranded deoxyribonucleic acid
dsRNA	double-stranded ribonucleic acid
d4T	didehydrodeoxythymidine [stavudine]
dTMP	deoxythymidine monophosphate
DTR	deep tendon reflex
DTs	delirium tremens
dUDP	deoxyuridine diphosphate
dUMP	deoxyuridine monophosphate
DVT	deep venous thrombosis
EBV	Epstein-Barr virus
EC	ejection click
ECF	extracellular fluid
ECFMG	Educational Commission for Foreign Medical Graduates
ECG	electrocardiogram
ECL	enterochromaffin-like [cell]
ECM	extracellular matrix
ECT	electroconvulsive therapy
ED_{50}	median effective dose
EDRF	endothelium-derived relaxing factor
EDTA	ethylenediamine tetra-acetic acid
EDV	end-diastolic volume
EEG	electroencephalogram
EF	ejection fraction
EGF	epidermal growth factor
EHEC	enterohemorrhagic *E. coli*
eIF	eukaryotic initiation factor
ELISA	enzyme-linked immunosorbent assay
EM	electron micrograph/microscopy
EMB	eosin–methylene blue
EOM	extraocular muscle
Epi	epinephrine
EPO	erythropoietin
EPS	extrapyramidal system
ER	endoplasmic reticulum, estrogen receptor
ERAS	Electronic Residency Application Service
ERCP	endoscopic retrograde cholangiopancreatography
ERP	effective refractory period
ERPF	effective renal plasma flow
ERT	estrogen replacement therapy
ERV	expiratory reserve volume
ESR	erythrocyte sedimentation rate
ESRD	end-stage renal disease
ESV	end-systolic volume
ETEC	enterotoxigenic *E. coli*
EtOH	ethyl alcohol
EV	esophageal vein
F	bioavailability
FA	fatty acid
Fab	fragment, antigen-binding
FAD	flavin adenine dinucleotide
FAD^+	oxidized flavin adenine dinucleotide
$FADH_2$	reduced flavin adenine dinucleotide
FAP	familial adenomatous polyposis
F1,6BP	fructose-1,6-bisphosphate

ABBREVIATION	MEANING
F2,6BP	fructose-2,6-bisphosphate
FBPase	fructose bisphosphatase
Fc	fragment, crystallizable
FcR	Fc receptor
5f-dUMP	5-fluorodeoxyuridine monophosphate
Fe^{2+}	ferrous ion
Fe^{3+}	ferric ion
Fe_{Na}	excreted fraction of filtered sodium
FEV_1	forced expiratory volume in 1 second
FF	filtration fraction
FFA	free fatty acid
FGF	fibroblast growth factor
FGFR	fibroblast growth factor receptor
FISH	fluorescence in situ hybridization
FLAIR	fluid-attenuated inversion recovery
f-met	formylmethionine
FMG	foreign medical graduate
FMN	flavin mononucleotide
FN	false negative
FNHTR	febrile nonhemolytic transfusion reaction
FP	false positive
F1P	fructose-1-phosphate
F6P	fructose-6-phosphate
FRC	functional residual capacity
FSH	follicle-stimulating hormone
FSMB	Federation of State Medical Boards
FTA-ABS	fluorescent treponemal antibody—absorbed
5-FU	5-fluorouracil
FVC	forced vital capacity
GABA	γ-aminobutyric acid
Gal	galactose
GBM	glomerular basement membrane
GC	glomerular capillary
G-CSF	granulocyte colony-stimulating factor
GE	gastroesophageal
GERD	gastroesophageal reflux disease
GFAP	glial fibrillary acid protein
GFR	glomerular filtration rate
GGT	γ-glutamyl transpeptidase
GH	growth hormone
GHB	γ-hydroxybutyrate
GHRH	growth hormone–releasing hormone
G_I	G protein, I polypeptide
GI	gastrointestinal
GIP	gastric inhibitory peptide
GIST	gastrointestinal stromal tumor
Glu	glutamic acid
GLUT	glucose transporter
GM	granulocyte macrophage
GM-CSF	granulocyte-macrophage colony stimulating factor
GMP	guanosine monophosphate
GnRH	gonadotropin-releasing hormone
GP	glycoprotein
G3P	glucose-3-phosphate

ABBREVIATION	MEANING
G6P	glucose-6-phosphate
G6PD	glucose-6-phospate dehydrogenase
GPe	globus pallidus externa
GPi	globus pallidus interna
GPI	glycosyl phosphatidylinositol
GPP	glycogen phosphorylase
GRP	gastrin-releasing peptide
G_S	G protein, S polypeptide
GS	glycogen synthase
GSH	reduced glutathione
GSSG	oxidized glutathione
GTP	guanosine triphosphate
GTPase	guanosine triphosphatase
GU	genitourinary
H^+	hydrogen ion
H_1, H_2	histamine receptors
HAART	highly active antiretroviral therapy
HAV	hepatitis A virus
HAVAb	hepatitis A antibody
Hb	hemoglobin
Hb^+	oxidized hemoglobin
Hb^-	ionized hemoglobin
HBcAb	hepatitis B core antibody
HBcAg	hepatitis B core antigen
HBeAb	hepatitis B early antibody
HBeAg	hepatitis B early antigen
HBsAb	hepatitis B surface antibody
HBsAg	hepatitis B surface antigen
$HbCO_2$	carbaminohemoglobin
HBV	hepatitis B virus
HCC	hepatocellular carcinoma
hCG	human chorionic gonadotropin
HCO_3^-	bicarbonate
Hct	hematocrit
HCTZ	hydrochlorothiazide
HCV	hepatitis C virus
HDL	high-density lipoprotein
HDV	hepatitis D virus
H&E	hematoxylin and eosin
HEV	hepatitis E virus
Hfr	high-frequency recombination [cell]
HGPRT	hypoxanthine-guanine phosphoribosyltransferase
HHb	human hemoglobin
HHV	human herpesvirus
5-HIAA	5-hydroxyindoleacetic acid
HIE	hypoxic ischemic encephalopathy
His	histidine
HIT	heparin-induced thrombocytopenia
HIV	human immunodeficiency virus
HL	hepatic lipase
HLA	human leukocyte antigen
HMG-CoA	hydroxymethylglutaryl-coenzyme A
HMP	hexose monophosphate

ABBREVIATION	MEANING
HMSN	hereditary motor and sensory neuropathy
HMWK	high-molecular-weight kininogen
HNPCC	hereditary nonpolyposis colorectal cancer
hnRNA	heterogeneous nuclear ribonucleic acid
H_2O	water
H_2O_2	hydrogen peroxide
HPA	hypothalamic-pituitary-adrenal [axis]
HPO	hypothalamic-pituitary-ovarian [axis]
HPV	human papillomavirus
HR	heart rate
HRE	hormone receptor element
HRT	hormone replacement therapy
HSV	herpes simplex virus
5-HT	5-hydroxytryptamine (serotonin)
HTLV	human T-cell leukemia virus
HTN	hypertension
HTR	hemolytic transfusion reaction
HUS	hemolytic-uremic syndrome
HVA	homovanillic acid
HZV	herpes zoster virus
IBD	inflammatory bowel disease
IBS	irritable bowel syndrome
IC	inspiratory capacity, immune complex
I_{Ca}	calcium current [heart]
I_f	funny current [heart]
ICA	internal carotid artery
ICAM	intracellular adhesion molecule
ICE	Integrated Clinical Encounter
ICF	intracellular fluid
ICP	intracranial pressure, inferior cerebellar peduncle
ID	identification
ID_{50}	dose at which pathogen produces infection in 50% of population
IDDM	insulin-dependent diabetes mellitus
IDL	intermediate-density lipoprotein
I/E	inspiratory/expiratory [ratio]
IF	immunofluorescence, initiation factor
IFN	interferon
Ig	immunoglobulin
IGF	insulin-like growth factor
I_K	potassium current [heart]
IL	interleukin
Ile	isoleucine
IM	intramuscular
IMA	inferior mesenteric artery
IMED	International Medical Education Directory
IMG	international medical graduate
IMP	inosine monophosphate
IMV	inferior mesenteric vein
I_{Na}	sodium current [heart]
INH	isonicotine hydrazine [isoniazid]
INO	internuclear ophthalmoplegia
INR	International Normalized Ratio

ABBREVIATION	MEANING
IO	inferior orbital [muscle]
IOP	intraocular pressure
IP_3	inositol triphosphate
IPV	inactivated polio vaccine
IR	current × resistance [Ohm's law], inferior rectus [muscle]
IRV	inspiratory reserve volume
ITP	idiopathic thrombocytopenic purpura
IUD	intrauterine device
IUGR	intrauterine growth retardation
IV	intravenous
IVC	inferior vena cava
IVDU	intravenous drug use
JAK/STAT	Janus kinase/signal transducer and activator of transcription [pathway]
JGA	juxtaglomerular apparatus
JVD	jugular venous distention
JVP	jugular venous pulse
K^+	potassium ion
KatG	catalase-peroxidase produced by *M. tuberculosis*
K_e	elimination constant
K_f	filtration constant
KG	ketoglutarate dehydrogenase
K_m	Michaelis-Menten constant
KOH	potassium hydroxide
KSHV	Kaposi's sarcoma–associated herpesvirus
L	left
LA	left atrial, left atrium
LAD	left anterior descending [artery]
LAF	left anterior fascicle
LCA	left coronary artery
LCAT	lecithin-cholesterol acyltransferase
LCFA	long-chain fatty acid
LCL	lateral collateral ligament
LCME	Liaison Committee on Medical Education
LCMV	lymphocytic choriomeningitis virus
LCX	left circumflex artery
LD	loading dose
LD_{50}	median lethal dose
LDH	lactate dehydrogenase
LDL	low-density lipoprotein
LES	lower esophageal sphincter
Leu	leucine
LFA	leukocyte function–associated antigen
LFT	liver function test
LGN	lateral geniculate nucleus
LGV	left gastric vein
LH	luteinizing hormone
LLQ	left lower quadrant
LM	light microscopy
LMN	lower motor neuron
LP	lumbar puncture
LPL	lipoprotein lipase
LPS	lipopolysaccharide
LR	lateral rectus [muscle]

ABBREVIATION	MEANING
LSE	Libman-Sacks endocarditis
LT	labile toxin leukotriene
LV	left ventricle, left ventricular
Lys	lysine
M_1-M_5	muscarinic (parasympathetic) ACh receptors
MAC	membrane attack complex, minimal alveolar concentration
MALT	mucosa-associated lymphoid tissue
MAO	monoamine oxidase
MAOI	monoamine oxidase inhibitor
MAP	mean arterial pressure, mitogen-activated protein
MASP	mannose-binding lectin–associated serine protease
MBL	mannose-binding lectin
MC	midsystolic click
MCA	middle cerebral artery
MCAT	Medical College Admissions Test
MCHC	mean corpuscular hemoglobin concentration
MCL	medial collateral ligament
MCP	metacarpophalangeal [joint]
M-CSF	macrophage colony-stimulating factor
MCV	mean corpuscular volume
MD	macula densa, maintenance dose
MEN	multiple endocrine neoplasia
Met	methionine
Mg^{2+}	magnesium ion
MGN	medial geniculate nucleus
$MgSO_4$	magnesium sulfate
MGUS	monoclonal gammopathy of undetermined significance
MHC	major histocompatibility complex
MI	myocardial infarction
MIF	müllerian inhibiting factor
MIT	monoiodotyrosine
MLCK	myosin light-chain kinase
MLF	medial longitudinal fasciculus
MMC	migrating motor complex
MMR	measles, mumps, rubella [vaccine]
MOPP	mechlorethamine-vincristine (Oncovin)-prednisone-procarbazine [chemotherapy]
6-MP	6-mercaptopurine
MPGN	membranoproliferative glomerulonephritis
MPO	myeloperoxidase
MR	medial rectus [muscle], mitral regurgitation
MRI	magnetic resonance imaging
mRNA	messenger ribonucleic acid
MRSA	methicillin-resistant *S. aureus*
MS	mitral stenosis, multiple sclerosis
MSH	melanocyte-stimulating hormone
MSM	men who have sex with men
mtDNA	mitochondrial DNA
mtRNA	mitochondrial RNA
mTOR	mammalian target of rapamycin
MTP	metatarsophalangeal [joint]
MTX	methotrexate
MUA/P	Medically Underserved Area and Population
MVO_2	myocardial oxygen consumption

ABBREVIATION	MEANING
MVP	mitral valve prolapse
N/A	not applicable
Na^+	sodium ion
NAD	nicotinamide adenine dinucleotide
NAD^+	oxidized nicotinamide adenine dinucleotide
NADH	reduced nicotinamide adenine dinucleotide
$NADP^+$	oxidized nicotinamide adenine dinucleotide phosphate
NADPH	reduced nicotinamide adenine dinucleotide phosphate
NBME	National Board of Medical Examiners
NBOME	National Board of Osteopathic Medical Examiners
NBPME	National Board of Podiatric Medical Examiners
NC	no change
NE	norepinephrine
NEG	nonenzymatic glycosylation
NF	neurofibromatosis
NH_3	ammonia
NH_4^+	ammonium
NHL	non-Hodgkin's lymphoma
NIDDM	non-insulin-dependent diabetes mellitus
NK	natural killer [cells]
N_M	muscarinic ACh receptor in neuromuscular junction
NMDA	N-methyl-D-aspartate
NMJ	neuromuscular junction
NMS	neuroleptic malignant syndrome
N_N	nicotinic ACh receptor in autonomic ganglia
NRMP	National Residency Matching Program
NNRTI	non-nucleoside reverse transcriptase inhibitor
NO	nitric oxide
N_2O	nitrous oxide
NPH	neutral protamine Hagedorn
NPV	negative predictive value
NRI	norepinephrine receptor inhibitor
NRTI	nucleoside reverse transcriptase inhibitor
NSAID	nonsteroidal anti-inflammatory drug
OAA	oxaloacetic acid
OCD	obsessive-compulsive disorder
OCP	oral contraceptive pill
OH	hydroxy
OH_2	dihydroxy
1,25-OH D_3	calcitriol (active form of vitamin D)
25-OH D_3	storage form of vitamin D
3′ OH	hydroxyl
OMT	osteopathic manipulative technique
OPV	oral polio vaccine
OR	odds ratio
OS	opening snap
OTC	ornithine transcarbamoylase
OVLT	organum vasculosum of the lamina terminalis
P-450	cytochrome P-450 family of enzymes
PA	posteroanterior
PABA	para-aminobenzoic acid
$Paco_2$	arterial Po_2
$PAco_2$	alveolar Po_2
PAH	para-aminohippuric acid

ABBREVIATION	MEANING
PALS	periarterial lymphatic sheath
PAN	polyarteritis nodosa
p-ANCA	perinuclear antineutrophil cytoplasmic antibody
Pao_2	partial pressure of oxygen in arterial blood
PAo_2	partial pressure of oxygen in alveolar blood
PAP	Papanicolaou [smear], prostatic acid phosphatase
PAS	periodic acid Schiff
PBP	penicillin-binding protein
PC	plasma colloid osmotic pressure, platelet count, pyruvate carboxylase
PCA	posterior cerebral artery
PCL	posterior cruciate ligament
Pco_2	partial pressure of carbon dioxide
PComm	posterior communicating [artery]
PCOS	polycystic ovarian syndrome
PCP	phencyclidine hydrochloride, *Pneumocystis carinii* (now *jirovecii*) pneumonia
PCR	polymerase chain reaction
PCT	proximal convoluted tubule
PCWP	pulmonary capillary wedge pressure
PD	posterior descending [artery]
PDA	patent ductus arteriosus
PDC	pyruvate dehydrogenase complex
PDE	phosphodiesterase
PDGF	platelet-derived growth factor
PDH	pyruvate dehydrogenase
PE	pulmonary embolism
PECAM	platelet–endothelial cell adhesion molecule
$PEco_2$	expired air Pco_2
PEP	phosphoenolpyruvate
PF	platelet factor
PFK	phosphofructokinase
PFT	pulmonary function test
PG	phosphoglycerate, prostaglandin
Phe	phenylalanine
P_i	plasma interstitial osmotic pressure, inorganic phosphate
PICA	posterior inferior cerebellar artery
PID	pelvic inflammatory disease
PIo_2	Po_2 in inspired air
PIP	proximal interphalangeal [joint]
PIP_2	phosphatidylinositol 4,5-bisphosphate
PK	pyruvate kinase
PKD	polycystic kidney disease
PKU	phenylketonuria
PLP	pyridoxal phosphate
PLS	Personalized Learning System
PML	progressive multifocal leukoencephalopathy
PMN	polymorphonuclear [leukocyte]
P_{net}	net filtration pressure
PNET	primitive neuroectodermal tumor
PNH	paroxysmal nocturnal hemoglobinuria
PNS	peripheral nervous system
Po_2	partial pressure of oxygen
PO_4	salt of phosphoric acid
PO_4^{3-}	phosphate

ABBREVIATION	MEANING
POMC	pro-opiomelanocortin
PPAR	peroxisome proliferator-activated receptor
PPD	purified protein derivative
PPI	proton pump inhibitor
PPRF	paramedian pontine reticular formation
PPV	positive predictive value
PrP	prion protein
PRPP	phosphoribosylpyrophosphate
PSA	prostate-specific antigen
PSS	progressive systemic sclerosis
PT	prothrombin time
PTH	parathyroid hormone
PTHrP	parathyroid hormone–related protein
PTSD	post-traumatic stress disorder
PTT	partial thromboplastin time
PV	plasma volume, venous pressure
PVC	polyvinyl chloride
PVR	pulmonary vascular resistance
R	correlation coefficient, right, R variable [group]
R_3	Registration, Ranking, & Results [system]
RA	rheumatoid arthritis, right atrium
RAAS	renin-angiotensin-aldosterone system
RANK-L	receptor activator of nuclear factor-κ B ligand
RAS	reticular activating system
RBC	red blood cell
RBF	renal blood flow
RCA	right coronary artery
REM	rapid eye movement
RER	rough endoplasmic reticulum
Rh	*rhesus* antigen
RLQ	right lower quadrant
RNA	ribonucleic acid
RNA_i	ribonucleic acid interference
RNP	ribonucleoprotein
ROI	reactive oxygen intermediate
RPF	renal plasma flow
RPGN	rapidly progressive glomerulonephritis
RPR	rapid plasma reagin
RR	relative risk, respiratory rate
rRNA	ribosomal ribonucleic acid
RS	Reed-Sternberg [cells]
RSV	respiratory syncytial virus
RTA	renal tubular acidosis
RUQ	right upper quadrant
RV	residual volume, right ventricle, right ventricular
RVH	right ventricular hypertrophy
Rx	medical prescription
[S]	substrate concentration
SA	sinoatrial
SAA	serum amyloid–associated [protein]
SAM	S-adenosylmethionine
SARS	severe acute respiratory syndrome
SAT	Scholastic Aptitude Test
SC	subcutaneous

ABBREVIATION	MEANING
SCC	squamous cell carcinoma
SCID	severe combined immunodeficiency disease
SCJ	squamocolumnar junction
SCM	sternocleidomastoid muscle
SCN	suprachiasmatic nucleus
SD	standard deviation
SEM	standard error of the mean
SEP	Spoken English Proficiency
SER	smooth endoplasmic reticulum
SERM	selective estrogen receptor modulator
SHBG	sex hormone–binding globulin
SIADH	syndrome of inappropriate [secretion of] antidiuretic hormone
SLE	systemic lupus erythematosus
SLL	small lymphocytic lymphoma
SLT	Shiga-like toxin
SMA	superior mesenteric artery
SMX	sulfamethoxazole
SNc	substantia nigra pars compacta
SNP	single nucleotide polymorphism
SNr	substantia nigra pars reticulata
SNRI	serotonin and norepinephrine receptor inhibitor
snRNP	small nuclear ribonucleoprotein
SO	superior oblique [muscle]
SOAP	Supplemental Offer and Acceptance Program
spp.	species
SR	superior rectus [muscle]
SS	single stranded
ssDNA	single-stranded deoxyribonucleic acid
SSPE	subacute sclerosing panencephalitis
SSRI	selective serotonin reuptake inhibitor
ssRNA	single-stranded ribonucleic acid
SSSS	staphylococcal scalded-skin syndrome
ST	Shiga toxin
STD	sexually transmitted disease
STEMI	ST-segment elevation myocardial infarction
STN	subthalamic nucleus
SV	sinus venosus, splenic vein, stroke volume
SVC	superior vena cava
SVT	supraventricular tachycardia
$t_{1/2}$	half-life
T_3	triiodothyronine
T_4	thyroxine
TA	truncus arteriosus
TAPVR	total anomalous pulmonary venous return
TB	tuberculosis
TBG	thyroxine-binding globulin
3TC	dideoxythiacytidine [lamivudine]
TCA	tricarboxylic acid [cycle], tricyclic antidepressant
Tc cell	cytotoxic T cell
TCR	T-cell receptor
TDF	tenofovir disopeozil fumarate
TdT	terminal deoxynucleotidyl transferase
TFCC	triangular fibrocartilage complex

ABBREVIATION	MEANING
TFT	thyroid function test
TG	triglyceride
6-TG	6-thioguanine
TGA	*trans*-Golgi apparatus
TGF	transforming growth factor
TGN	*trans*-Golgi network
Th cell	helper T cell
THF	tetrahydrofolic acid
Thr	threonine
TI	therapeutic index
TIA	transient ischemic attack
TIBC	total iron-binding capacity
TIPS	transjugular intrahepatic portosystemic shunt
TLC	total lung capacity
T_m	maximum rate of transport
TMP	trimethoprim
TN	trigeminal neuralgia, true negative
TNF	tumor necrosis factor
TNM	tumor, node, metastases [staging]
TOEFL	Test of English as a Foreign Language
ToRCHeS	*Toxoplasma gondii*, rubella, CMV, HIV, HSV-2, syphilis
TP	true positive
tPA	tissue plasminogen activator
TPP	thiamine pyrophosphate
TPR	total peripheral resistance
TR	tricuspid regurgitation
TRAP	tartrate-resistant acid phosphatase
TREC	T-cell recombinant excision circles
TRH	thyrotropin-releasing hormone
tRNA	transfer ribonucleic acid
Trp	tryptophan
TSH	thyroid-stimulating hormone
TSI	thyroid-stimulating immunoglobulin
TSS	toxic shock syndrome
TSST	toxic shock syndrome toxin
TTP	thrombotic thrombocytopenic purpura
TTR	transthyretin
TV	tidal volume
Tx	translation [factor]
TXA_2	thromboxane A_2
UCB	unconjugated bilirubin
UCV	Underground Clinical Vignettes
UDP	uridine diphosphate
UMN	upper motor neuron
UMP	uridine monophosphate
UPD	uniparental disomy
URI	upper respiratory infection
USMLE	United States Medical Licensing Examination
UTI	urinary tract infection
UTP	uridine triphosphate
UV	ultraviolet
V_1, V_2	Vasopressin receptors
VA	Veterans Affairs
Val	valine
VC	vital capacity
V_d	volume of distribution
VD	physiologic dead space
V(D)J	heavy-chain hypervariable region [antibody]
VDRL	Venereal Disease Research Laboratory
VEGF	vascular endothelial growth factor
VF	ventricular fibrillation
V_H	variable region, heavy chain [antibody]
VHL	von Hippel–Lindau [disease]
VIP	vasoactive intestinal peptide
VIPoma	vasoactive intestinal polypeptide-secreting tumor
VJ	light-chain hypervariable region [antibody]
VL	ventral lateral [nucleus]; variable region, light chain [antibody]
VLDL	very low density lipoprotein
VMA	vanillylmandelic acid
VMAT	vesicular monoamine transporter
V_{max}	maximum velocity
VPL	ventral posterior nucleus, lateral
VPM	ventral posterior nucleus, medial
VPN	vancomycin, polymyxin, nystatin [media]
V/Q	ventilation/perfusion [ratio]
VRE	vancomycin-resistant enterococcus
VSD	ventricular septal defect
V_T	tidal volume
vWF	von Willebrand factor
VZV	varicella-zoster virus
WHOML	"worst headache of my life"
WBC	white blood cell
XR	X-linked recessive
XX	normal complement of sex chromosomes for female
XY	normal complement of sex chromosomes for male
ZDV	zidovudine [formerly AZT]

SECTION IV

Photo Acknowledgments

Images marked with [X] are reproduced with permission of USMLE-Rx.com. Images marked with [RU] are reproduced with permission of Dr. Richard P. Usatine and the *Color Atlas of Family Medicine* (www.usatinemedia.com). Images marked with [*] are reproduced with permission of other sources.

Biochemistry

[*] **Osteogenesis imperfecta: Image A.** Osteogenesis imperfecta. Reproduced, with permission, from Wolff K et al. *Fitzpatrick's Dermatology in General Medicine,* 7th ed. New York: McGraw-Hill, 2007: Fig. 139-12.

[*] **Vitamin D: Image A.** Rickets. Reproduced, with permission, from Dr. Michael L. Richardson/Wikimedia Commons.

[*] **Lysosomal storage diseases: Image A.** Gaucher's disease. Reproduced, with permission, from Lichtman MA et al. *Lichtman's Atlas of Hematology*. New York: McGraw-Hill, 2007: Fig. V.H.16.

[*] **Lysosomal storage diseases: Image B.** Niemann-Pick disease. Reproduced, with permission, from Lichtman MA et al. *Lichtman's Atlas of Hematology*. New York: McGraw-Hill, 2007: Fig. V.H.18.

Microbiology

[*] ***Staphylococcus aureus*: Image A.** *Staphylococcus aureus.* Reproduced, with permission, from the Centers for Disease Control and Prevention, Atlanta, GA. Photo credit: Richard Facklam.

[X] **1° and 2° tuberculosis: Image A.** Caseating granuloma. Reproduced, with permission, from USMLE-Rx.com.

[X] **Mycobacteria: Image A.** Acid-fast bacilli. Reproduced, with permission, from USMLE-Rx.com.

[*] **Leprosy (Hansen's disease): Image A.** Leprosy. Reproduced, with permission, from Wolff K et al. *Fitzpatrick's Color Atlas and Synopsis of Clinical Dermatology*, 5th ed. New York: McGraw-Hill, 2005: Fig 22-52.

[*] ***Neisseria:* Image A.** *Neisseria gonorrhoeae*. Reproduced, with permission, from Wolff K, Johnson RA. *Fitzpatrick's Color Atlas and Synopsis of Clinical Dermatology*, 6th ed. New York: McGraw-Hill, 2009: Fig. 24-52.

[*] **Syphilis: Image A.** Painless chancre. Reproduced, with permission, from Wolff K et al. *Fitzpatrick's Dermatology in General Medicine*, 7th ed. New York: McGraw-Hill, 2007: Fig. 200-2.

[*] **Syphilis: Image B.** Syphilis dark-field microscopy. Reproduced, with permission, from the Centers for Disease Control and Prevention, Atlanta, GA. Photo credit: W. F. Schwartz.

[X] ***Gardnerella vaginalis*: Image A.** Bacterial vaginosis. Reproduced, with permission, from USMLE-Rx.com.

[*] **Systemic mycoses: Image A.** *Histoplasma capsulatum*. Reproduced, with permission, from the Centers for Disease Control and Prevention, Atlanta, GA. Photo credit: D. T. McClenan.

[*] **Systemic mycoses: Image B.** *Blastomyces dermatitidis*. Reproduced, with permission, from Brooks GF et al. *Jawetz, Melnick, & Adelberg's Medical Microbiology*, 25th ed. New York: McGraw-Hill, 2010: Fig. 45-18A.

[*] **Systemic mycoses: Image D.** *Paracoccidioides brasiliensis*. Reproduced, with permission, from Wolff K et al. *Fitzpatrick's Dermatology in General Medicine*, 7th ed. New York: McGraw-Hill, 2007: Fig. 190-16.

[*] **Cutaneous mycoses: Image A.** *Malassezia furfur.* Reproduced, with permission, from Wolff K et al. *Fitzpatrick's Dermatology in General Medicine*, 7th ed. New York: McGraw-Hill, 2007: Fig. 189-11.

[*] **Opportunistic fungal infections: Image A (left).** *Candida albicans* pseudohyphae. Adapted, with permission, from Y. Tambe/ Wikimedia Commons.

[*] **Opportunistic fungal infections: Image A (right).** *Candida albicans* germ tubes. Reproduced, with permission, from Brooks GF et al. *Jawetz, Melnick, & Adelberg's Medical Microbiology*, 25th ed. New York: McGraw-Hill, 2010: Fig. 45-21.

[X] **Opportunistic fungal infections: Image B (left).** *Aspergillus fumigatus* septate hyphae. Reproduced, with permission, from USMLE-Rx.com.

Opportunistic fungal infections: Image B (right). *Aspergillus fumigatus* conidiophore. Reproduced, with permission, from Brooks GF et al. *Jawetz, Melnick, & Adelberg's Medical Microbiology*, 25th ed. New York: McGraw-Hill, 2010: Fig. 45-6.

Opportunistic fungal infections: Image C. *Cryptococcus neoformans*. Reproduced, with permission, from the Centers for Disease Control and Prevention, Atlanta, GA.

Opportunistic fungal infections: Image D. *Mucor*. Reproduced, with permission, from Wolff K et al. *Fitzpatrick's Dermatology in General Medicine*, 7th ed. New York: McGraw-Hill, 2007: Fig. 190-19C.

***Pneumocystis jirovecii*: Image A.** *Pneumocystis jirovecii*. Reproduced, with permission, from USMLE-Rx.com.

***Sporothrix schenckii:* Image A.** *Sporothrix schenckii*. Reproduced, with permission, from the Centers for Disease Control and Prevention, Atlanta, GA. Photo credit: Lucille K. Georg.

Protozoa–GI infections: Image B. *Giardia* cyst. Reproduced, with permission, from the Centers for Disease Control and Prevention, Atlanta, GA.

Protozoa–GI infections: Image C. *Entamoeba histolytica*. Reproduced, with permission, from the Centers for Disease Control and Prevention, Atlanta, GA.

Protozoa–GI infections: Image D. *Entamoeba* cyst. Reproduced, with permission, from the Centers for Disease Control and Prevention, Atlanta, GA.

Protozoa–GI infections: Image E. *Cryptosporidium*. Reproduced, with permission, from the Centers for Disease Control and Prevention, Atlanta, GA.

Protozoa–CNS infections: Image A. *Toxoplasma gondii*. Reproduced, with permission, from the Centers for Disease Control and Prevention, Atlanta, GA. Photo credit: L. L. Moore, Jr.

Protozoa–CNS infections: Image B. *Naegleria fowleri*. Reproduced, with permission, from the Centers for Disease Control and Prevention, Atlanta, GA.

Protozoa–CNS infections: Image C. *Trypanosoma gambiense*. Reproduced, with permission, from the Centers for Disease Control and Prevention, Atlanta, GA. Photo credit: Mae Melvin.

Protozoa–Hematologic infections: Image A. *Plasmodium* trophozoite. Reproduced, with permission, from the Centers for Disease Control and Prevention, Atlanta, GA. Photo credit: Steven Glenn.

Protozoa–Hematologic infections: Image B. *Plasmodium* schizont. Reproduced, with permission, from the Centers for Disease Control and Prevention, Atlanta, GA. Photo credit: Steven Glenn.

Protozoa–Hematologic infections: Image C. *Babesia*. Reproduced, with permission, from the Centers for Disease Control and Prevention, Atlanta, GA.

Protozoa–Others: Image A. *Trypanosoma cruzi*. Reproduced, with permission, from the Centers for Disease Control and Prevention, Atlanta, GA. Photo credit: Mae Melvin.

Protozoa–Others: Image B. *Leishmania*. Reproduced, with permission, from the Centers for Disease Control and Prevention, Atlanta, GA. Photo credit: Francis W. Chandler.

Herpesviruses: Image A. Herpes labialis. Reproduced, with permission, from Wolff K et al. *Fitzpatrick's Dermatology in General Medicine*, 7th ed. New York: McGraw-Hill, 2007: Fig. 193-3.

Herpesviruses: Image B. Herpes genitalis. Reproduced, with permission, from Dr. Richard P. Usatine and the *Color Atlas of Family Medicine*.

Herpesviruses: Image C. Herpes zoster. Reproduced, with permission, from Fauci AS et al. *Harrison's Principles of Internal Medicine*, 17th ed. New York: McGraw-Hill, 2008: Fig. 173-3.

Herpesviruses: Image D. CMV. Reproduced, with permission, from USMLE-Rx.com.

EBV: Image A. Atypical lymphocytes in EBV. Reproduced, with permission, from Fauci AS et al. *Harrison's Principles of Internal Medicine*, 17th ed. New York: McGraw-Hill, 2008: Fig. 174-2.

Rotavirus: Image A. Rotavirus. Reproduced, with permission, from the Centers for Disease Control and Prevention, Atlanta, GA. Photo credit: Erskine Palmer.

Measles virus: Image A. Koplik spots. Reproduced, with permission, from Wolff K et al. *Fitzpatrick's Dermatology in General Medicine*, 7th ed. New York: McGraw-Hill, 2007: Fig. 192-1.

Measles virus: Image B. Rash of measles. Adapted, with permission, from Wolff K et al. *Fitzpatrick's Dermatology in General Medicine*, 7th ed. New York: McGraw-Hill, 2007: Fig. 192-3.

Mumps virus: Image A. Mumps. Reproduced, with permission, from the Centers for Disease Control and Prevention, Atlanta, GA.

Rabies virus: Image A. Rabies virus. Reproduced, with permission, from USMLE-Rx.com.

Rabies virus: Image B. Negri bodies. Reproduced, with permission, from the Centers for Disease Control and Prevention, Atlanta, GA. Photo credit: Daniel P. Perl.

ToRCHeS infections: Image A. Congenital syphilis facies. Reproduced, with permission, from Wolff K et al. *Fitzpatrick's Dermatology in General Medicine*, 7th ed. New York: McGraw-Hill, 2007: Fig. 200-28.

ToRCHeS infections: Image B. Hutchinson's teeth. Reproduced, with permission, from Wolff K et al. *Fitzpatrick's Dermatology in General Medicine*, 7th ed. New York: McGraw-Hill, 2007: Fig. 200-31B.

- **Red rashes of childhood: Image A.** Erythema infectiosum. Reproduced, with permission, from Wolff K, Johnson RA. *Fitzpatrick's Color Atlas and Synopsis of Clinical Dermatology*, 6th ed. New York: McGraw-Hill, 2009: Fig. 27-24A.

- **Red rashes of childhood: Image B.** Hand-foot-mouth disease. Reproduced, with permission, from Hurwitz RM et al. *Pathology of the Skin: Atlas of Clinical-Pathological Correlation*, 2nd ed. Stamford CT: Appleton & Lange, 1998.

Pathology

- **Amyloidosis: Image A.** Amyloidosis. Reproduced, with permission, from USMLE-Rx.com.

Cardiovascular

- **Atherosclerosis: Image A.** Atherosclerosis. Reproduced, with permission, from USMLE-Rx.com.

- **Aortic dissection: Image A.** Aortic dissection. Reproduced, with permission, from Brunicardi FC et al. *Schwartz's Principles of Surgery*, 9th ed. New York: McGraw-Hill, 2009: Fig. 22-18.

- **Cardiomyopathies: Image A.** Hypertrophic cardiomyopathy. Reproduced, with permission, from Fuster V et al. *Hurst's The Heart*, 13th ed. New York: McGraw-Hill, 2011: Fig. 82-3.

- **Bacterial endocarditis: Image A.** Splinter hemorrhage. Reproduced, with permission, from USMLE-Rx.com.

- **Rheumatic fever: Image A.** Aschoff body. Adapted, with permission, from Dr. Ed Uthman/Wikimedia Commons.

Endocrine

- **Cushing's syndrome: Image A.** Adrenocortical adenoma. Adapted, with permission, from Chandrasoma P, Taylor CR. *Concise Pathology*, 3rd ed. Stamford, CT: Appleton & Lange, 1998: Fig. 60-3.

- **Pheochromocytoma: Image A.** Pheochromocytoma. Reproduced, with permission, from Kantarjian HM et al. *MD Anderson Manual of Medical Oncology*. New York: McGraw-Hill, 2006: Fig. 31-17.

- **Hyperthyroidism: Image A.** Multinodular goiter. Reproduced, with permission, from USMLE-Rx.com.

- **Hyperthyroidism: Image B.** Graves' disease (exophthalmos). Reproduced, with permission, from USMLE-Rx.com.

- **Thyroid cancer: Image A.** Thyroid papillary carcinoma. Reproduced, with permission, from USMLE-Rx.com; image courtesy of Dr. Stuart Flynn.

- **Diabetes mellitus: Image A.** Diabetic retinopathy. Reproduced, with permission, from McPhee SJ, Papadakis MA. *Current Medical Diagnosis & Treatment 2011*. New York: McGraw-Hill, 2011: Chapter 7.

Gastrointestinal

- **GI embryology: Image A.** Omphalocele. Reproduced, with permission, from USMLE-Rx.com.

- **Peyer's patches: Image A.** Peyer's patches. Reproduced, with permission, from Wikimedia Commons.

- **Achalasia: Image A.** Achalasia. Reproduced, with permission, from Lalwani AK. *Current Diagnosis & Treatment in Otolaryngology—Head & Neck Surgery*, 2nd ed. New York: McGraw-Hill, 2008. Fig 35-3A.

- **Barrett's esophagus: Image A.** Barrett's esophagus. Reproduced, with permission, from USMLE-Rx.com.

- **Stomach cancer: Image A.** Signet ring adenocarcinoma. Reproduced, with permission, from USMLE-Rx.com.

- **Inflammatory bowel disease: Image A.** Crohn's disease. Reproduced, with permission, from Way LW, Doherty GM. *Current Surgical Diagnosis and Treatment*, 11th ed. New York: McGraw-Hill, 2003: 691.

- **Inflammatory bowel disease: Image B.** Ulcerative colitis. Reproduced, with permission, from USMLE-Rx.com.

- **Colorectal cancer: Image A.** "Apple core" lesion. Reproduced, with permission, from USMLE-Rx.com.

- **Cirrhosis and portal hypertension: Image A.** Cirrhosis, gross liver. Reproduced, with permission, from Brunicardi FC et al. *Schwartz's Principles of Surgery*, 9th ed. New York: McGraw-Hill, 2009: Fig. 31-16.

- **Cirrhosis and portal hypertension: Image B.** Cirrhosis, microscopic. Reproduced, with permission, from Brunicardi FC et al. *Schwartz's Principles of Surgery*, 9th ed. New York: McGraw-Hill, 2009: Fig. 31-16.

- **Alcoholic liver disease: Image A.** Macrovesicular steatosis. Reproduced, with permission, from USMLE-Rx.com.

- **Gallstones (cholelithiasis): Image A.** Gallstones. Reproduced, with permission, from Wikimedia Commons.

- **Acute pancreatitis: Image A.** Acute pancreatitis. Reproduced, with permission, from Greenberger NJ et al. *Current Diagnosis & Treatment: Gastroenterology, Hepatology, & Endoscopy*. New York: McGraw-Hill, 2009: Fig. 9-49.

Hematology and Oncology

- **Erythrocyte: Image A.** Erythrocyte. Reproduced, with permission, from Mescher AL. *Junqueira's Basic Histology: Text & Atlas*, 12th ed. New York: McGraw-Hill, 2010: Fig. 12-4A.

- **Platelet (thrombocyte): Image A.** Platelets. Reproduced, with permission, from Mescher AL. *Junqueira's Basic Histology: Text & Atlas*, 12th ed. New York: McGraw-Hill, 2010: Fig. 12-13A.

- **Neutrophil: Image A.** Neutrophil. Reproduced, with permission, from Mescher AL. *Junqueira's Basic Histology: Text & Atlas*, 12th ed. New York: McGraw-Hill, 2010: Fig. 12-7B.

- **Monocyte: Image A.** Monocyte. Reproduced, with permission, from Mescher AL. *Junqueira's Basic Histology: Text & Atlas*, 12th ed. New York: McGraw-Hill, 2010: Fig. 12-12C.

- **Macrophage: Image A.** Macrophage. Reproduced, with permission, from Lichtman MA et al. *Lichtman's Atlas of Hematology*. New York: McGraw-Hill, 2007: Fig. V.H.11.

- **Eosinophil: Image A.** Eosinophil. Reproduced, with permission, from Mescher AL. *Junqueira's Basic Histology: Text & Atlas*, 12th ed. New York: McGraw-Hill, 2010: Fig. 12-9B.

- **Basophil: Image A.** Basophil. Reproduced, with permission, from Mescher AL. *Junqueira's Basic Histology: Text & Atlas*, 12th ed. New York: McGraw-Hill, 2010: Fig. 12-10A.

- **Mast cell: Image A.** Mast cell. Reproduced, with permission, from Mescher AL. *Junqueira's Basic Histology: Text & Atlas*, 12th ed. New York: McGraw-Hill, 2010: Fig. 5-5A.

- **Lymphocyte: Image A.** Lymphocyte. Reproduced, with permission, from Mescher AL. *Junqueira's Basic Histology: Text & Atlas*, 12th ed. New York: McGraw-Hill, 2010: Fig. 12-11C.

- **Plasma cell: Image A.** Plasma cell. Reproduced, with permission, from Mescher AL. *Junqueira's Basic Histology: Text & Atlas*, 12th ed. New York: McGraw-Hill, 2010: Fig. 5-7.

- **Pathologic RBC forms: Image A.** Acanthocyte. Reproduced, with permission, from Fauci AS et al. *Harrison's Principles of Internal Medicine*, 17th ed. New York: McGraw-Hill, 2008: Fig. 58-10.

- **Pathologic RBC forms: Image B.** Basophilic stippling. Reproduced, with permission, from Lichtman MA et al. *Lichtman's Atlas of Hematology*. New York: McGraw-Hill, 2007: Fig. I.B.1.

- **Pathologic RBC forms: Image C.** Bite cell. Reproduced, with permission, from Lichtman MA et al. *Lichtman's Atlas of Hematology*. New York: McGraw-Hill, 2007: Fig. I.C.33.

- **Pathologic RBC forms: Image D.** Elliptocyte. Reproduced, with permission, from Lichtman MA et al. *Lichtman's Atlas of Hematology*. New York: McGraw-Hill, 2007: Fig. I.A.4.

- **Pathologic RBC forms: Image E.** Macro-ovalocyte. Adapted, with permission, from Lichtman MA et al. *Lichtman's Atlas of Hematology*. New York: McGraw-Hill, 2007: Fig. I.C.88.

- **Pathologic RBC forms: Image F.** Ringed sideroblasts. Reproduced, with permission, from Lichtman MA et al. *Lichtman's Atlas of Hematology*. New York: McGraw-Hill, 2007: Fig. V.G.12.

- **Pathologic RBC forms: Image G.** Schistocyte/helmet cell. Reproduced, with permission, from USMLE-Rx.com.

- **Pathologic RBC forms: Image H.** Sickle cell. Reproduced, with permission, from USMLE-Rx.com.

- **Pathologic RBC forms: Image I.** Spherocyte. Reproduced, with permission, from USMLE-Rx.com.

- **Pathologic RBC forms: Image J.** Teardrop cell. Reproduced, with permission, from Fauci AS et al. *Harrison's Principles of Internal Medicine*, 17th ed. New York: McGraw-Hill, 2008: Fig. 58-7.

- **Pathologic RBC forms: Image K.** Target cell. Reproduced, with permission, from USMLE-Rx.com.

- **Other RBC pathologies: Image A.** Heinz bodies. Reproduced, with permission, from Lichtman MA et al. *Lichtman's Atlas of Hematology*. New York: McGraw-Hill, 2007: Fig. I.B.2.

- **Other RBC pathologies: Image B.** Howell-Jolly bodies. Reproduced, with permission, from Lichtman MA et al. *Lichtman's Atlas of Hematology*. New York: McGraw-Hill, 2007: Fig. I.B.3.

- **Microcytic, hypochromic (MCV < 80 fL) anemia: Image B.** β-Thalassemia major. Reproduced, with permission, from USMLE-Rx.com.

- **Intrinsic hemolytic normocytic anemia: Image A.** Sickle cell disease. Reproduced, with permission, from USMLE-Rx.com.

- **Non-Hodgkin's lymphoma: Image A.** Burkitt's lymphoma "starry sky" appearance. Reproduced, with permission, from USMLE-Rx.com.

- **Multiple myeloma: Image A.** Multiple myeloma lytic lesions. Reproduced, with permission, from Kantarjian HM et al. *MD Anderson Manual of Medical Oncology*. New York: McGraw-Hill, 2006: Fig. 8-1.

- **Multiple myeloma: Image B.** Multiple myeloma smear. Reproduced, with permission, from Kantarjian HM et al. *MD Anderson Manual of Medical Oncology*. New York: McGraw-Hill, 2006: Fig. 8-4.

- **Leukemias: Image A.** Acute lymphoblastic leukemia/lymphoma. Reproduced, with permission, from USMLE-Rx.com.

- **Leukemias: Image B.** Small lymphocytic lymphoma/chronic lymphocytic leukemia. Reproduced, with permission, from USMLE-Rx.com.

Leukemias: Image C. Hairy cell leukemia. Reproduced, with permission, from USMLE-Rx.com.

Leukemias: Image D. Acute myelogenous leukemia. Reproduced, with permission, from USMLE-Rx.com.

Leukemias: Image E. Chronic myelogenous leukemia. Reproduced, with permission, from USMLE-Rx.com.

Langerhans cell histiocytosis: Image A. Birbeck granules. Reproduced, with permission, from Lichtman MA et al. *Lichtman's Atlas of Hematology*. New York: McGraw-Hill, 2007: Fig. VI.C.2.

Musculoskeletal and Connective Tissue

Epidermis layers: Image A. Layers of epidermis. Reproduced, with permission, from USMLE-Rx.com; image courtesy of Dr. Kurt Johnson.

Wrist bones: Image A. Wrist bones. Reproduced, with permission, from Brunicardi FC et al. *Schwartz's Principles of Surgery*, 9th ed. New York: McGraw-Hill, 2009: Fig. 44-2B.

Osteoarthritis: Image A. Osteoarthritis. Reproduced, with permission, from USMLE-Rx.com.

Gout: Image A. Tophi in joints. Reproduced, with permission, from USMLE-Rx.com.

Gout: Image B. Gout. Reproduced, with permission, from LeBlond RF et al. *DeGowin's Diagnostic Examination*, 9th ed. New York: McGraw-Hill, 2009: Plate 30.

Sarcoidosis: Image A. Sarcoidosis. Reproduced, with permission, from USMLE-Rx.com.

Polymyositis/dermatomyositis: Image A. Gottron's papules. Reproduced, with permission, from Wolff K et al. *Fitzpatrick's Dermatology in General Medicine*, 7th ed. New York: McGraw-Hill, 2008: Fig. 157-5.

Polymyositis/dermatomyositis: Image B. Heliotrope rash. Reproduced, with permission, from Wolff K, Johnson RA. *Fitzpatrick's Color Atlas and Synopsis of Clinical Dermatology*, 6th ed. New York: McGraw-Hill, 2009: Fig. 14-16.

Myositis ossificans: Image A. Myositis ossificans. Reproduced, with permission, from T. Dvorak/Wikimedia Commons.

Dermatologic macroscopic terms: Image A. Macule. Reproduced, with permission, from Dr. Richard P. Usatine and the *Color Atlas of Family Medicine*.

Dermatologic macroscopic terms: Image B. Patch. Reproduced, with permission, from Dr. Richard P. Usatine and the *Color Atlas of Family Medicine*.

Dermatologic macroscopic terms: Image C. Papule. Reproduced, with permission, from Dr. Richard P. Usatine and the *Color Atlas of Family Medicine*.

Dermatologic macroscopic terms: Image D. Plaque. Reproduced, with permission, from Dr. Richard P. Usatine and the *Color Atlas of Family Medicine*.

Dermatologic macroscopic terms: Image E. Vesicle. Reproduced, with permission, from Dr. Richard P. Usatine and the *Color Atlas of Family Medicine*.

Dermatologic macroscopic terms: Image F. Bulla. Reproduced, with permission, from Dr. Richard P. Usatine and the *Color Atlas of Family Medicine*.

Dermatologic macroscopic terms: Image G. Pustule. Reproduced, with permission, from Dr. Richard P. Usatine and the *Color Atlas of Family Medicine*.

Dermatologic macroscopic terms: Image H. Wheal. Reproduced, with permission, from Dr. Richard P. Usatine and the *Color Atlas of Family Medicine*.

Dermatologic macroscopic terms: Image I. Scale. Reproduced, with permission, from Dr. Richard P. Usatine and the *Color Atlas of Family Medicine*.

Dermatologic macroscopic terms: Image J. Crust. Reproduced, with permission, from Dr. Richard P. Usatine and the *Color Atlas of Family Medicine*.

Pigmented skin disorders: Image A. Albinism. Reproduced, with permission, from Dr. Richard P. Usatine and the *Color Atlas of Family Medicine*.

Pigmented skin disorders: Image B. Melasma. Reproduced, with permission, from Dr. Richard P. Usatine and the *Color Atlas of Family Medicine*.

Pigmented skin disorders: Image C. Vitiligo. Reproduced, with permission, from Dr. Richard P. Usatine and the *Color Atlas of Family Medicine*.

Common skin disorders: Image A. Verrucae. Reproduced, with permission, from Dr. Richard P. Usatine and the *Color Atlas of Family Medicine*.

Common skin disorders: Image B. Condyloma acuminatum. Reproduced, with permission, from Dr. Richard P. Usatine and the *Color Atlas of Family Medicine*.

Common skin disorders: Image C. Intradermal melanocytic nevus. Reproduced, with permission, from Dr. Richard P. Usatine and the *Color Atlas of Family Medicine*.

Common skin disorders: Image D. Junctional melanocytic nevi. Reproduced, with permission, from Dr. Richard P. Usatine and the *Color Atlas of Family Medicine*.

Common skin disorders: Image E. Urticaria. Reproduced, with permission, from Dr. Richard P. Usatine and the *Color Atlas of Family Medicine*.

RU **Common skin disorders: Image F.** Freckles. Reproduced, with permission, from Dr. Richard P. Usatine and the *Color Atlas of Family Medicine*.

RU **Common skin disorders: Image G.** Atopic dermatitis on face. Reproduced, with permission, from Dr. Richard P. Usatine and the *Color Atlas of Family Medicine*.

RU **Common skin disorders: Image H.** Atopic dermatitis in antecubital fossa. Reproduced, with permission, from Dr. Richard P. Usatine and the *Color Atlas of Family Medicine*.

RU **Common skin disorders: Image I.** Allergic contact dermatitis from nickel exposure. Reproduced, with permission, from Dr. Richard P. Usatine and the *Color Atlas of Family Medicine*.

RU **Common skin disorders: Image J.** Allergic contact dermatitis due to neomycin. Reproduced, with permission, from Dr. Richard P. Usatine and the *Color Atlas of Family Medicine*.

RU **Common skin disorders: Image K.** Psoriasis with positive Auspitz sign. Reproduced, with permission, from Dr. Richard P. Usatine and the *Color Atlas of Family Medicine*.

RU **Common skin disorders: Image L.** Psoriatic arthritis. Reproduced, with permission, from Dr. Richard P. Usatine and the *Color Atlas of Family Medicine*.

RU **Common skin disorders: Image M.** Seborrheic keratosis with horn cysts. Reproduced, with permission, from Dr. Richard P. Usatine and the *Color Atlas of Family Medicine*.

RU **Common skin disorders: Image N.** "Stuck on" plaques of seborrheic keratosis. Reproduced, with permission, from Dr. Richard P. Usatine and the *Color Atlas of Family Medicine*.

Rx **Blistering skin disorders: Image A.** Pemphigus vulgaris. Reproduced, with permission, from USMLE-Rx.com.

RU **Blistering skin disorders: Image B.** Bullous pemphigoid. Reproduced, with permission, from Dr. Richard P. Usatine and the *Color Atlas of Family Medicine*.

Blistering skin disorders: Image C. Dermatitis herpetiformis. Reproduced, with permission, from Fauci AS et al. *Harrison's Principles of Internal Medicine*, 17th ed. New York: McGraw-Hill, 2008: Fig. 52-8.

RU **Blistering skin disorders: Image D.** Erythema multiforme. Reproduced, with permission, from Dr. Richard P. Usatine and the *Color Atlas of Family Medicine*.

RU **Blistering skin disorders: Image E (left).** Stevens-Johnson syndrome with eye involvement. Reproduced, with permission, from Dr. Richard P. Usatine and the *Color Atlas of Family Medicine*.

RU **Blistering skin disorders: Image E (right).** Stevens-Johnson syndrome with lip lesions. Reproduced, with permission, from Dr. Richard P. Usatine and the *Color Atlas of Family Medicine*.

RU **Blistering skin disorders: Image F.** Toxic epidermal necrosis with sloughing of skin on face. Reproduced, with permission, from Dr. Richard P. Usatine and the *Color Atlas of Family Medicine*.

RU **Blistering skin disorders: Image G.** Toxic epidermal necrosis with skin sloughing. Reproduced, with permission, from Dr. Richard P. Usatine and the *Color Atlas of Family Medicine*.

RU **Miscellaneous skin disorders: Image A (left).** Acanthosis nigricans with skin tags. Reproduced, with permission, from Dr. Richard P. Usatine and the *Color Atlas of Family Medicine*.

RU **Miscellaneous skin disorders: Image A (right).** Acanthosis nigricans with smooth, velvety appearance. Reproduced, with permission, from Dr. Richard P. Usatine and the *Color Atlas of Family Medicine*.

RU **Miscellaneous skin disorders: Image B (left).** Actinic keratosis on face. Reproduced, with permission, from Dr. Richard P. Usatine and the *Color Atlas of Family Medicine*.

RU **Miscellaneous skin disorders: Image B (right).** Actinic keratoses on hands and forearm. Reproduced, with permission, from Dr. Richard P. Usatine and the *Color Atlas of Family Medicine*.

RU **Miscellaneous skin disorders: Image C (left).** Erythema nodosum in patient with streptococcal infection. Reproduced, with permission, from Dr. Richard P. Usatine and the *Color Atlas of Family Medicine*.

RU **Miscellaneous skin disorders: Image C (right).** Erythema nodosum in patient with leprosy. Reproduced, with permission, from Dr. Richard P. Usatine and the *Color Atlas of Family Medicine*.

RU **Miscellaneous skin disorders: Image D (left).** Lichen planus appearance on light skin. Reproduced, with permission, from Dr. Richard P. Usatine and the *Color Atlas of Family Medicine*.

RU **Miscellaneous skin disorders: Image D (right).** Lichen planus appearance on dark skin. Reproduced, with permission, from Dr. Richard P. Usatine and the *Color Atlas of Family Medicine*.

RU **Miscellaneous skin disorders: Image E (left).** Herald patch of pityriasis rosea. Reproduced, with permission, from Dr. Richard P. Usatine and the *Color Atlas of Family Medicine*.

RU **Miscellaneous skin disorders: Image E (right).** Pityriasis rosea with Christmas tree distribution. Reproduced, with permission, from Dr. Richard P. Usatine and the *Color Atlas of Family Medicine*.

RU **Miscellaneous skin disorders: Image F.** Sunburn and impetigo. Reproduced, with permission, from Dr. Richard P. Usatine and the *Color Atlas of Family Medicine*.

RU **Infectious skin disorders: Image A.** Impetigo. Reproduced, with permission, from Dr. Richard P. Usatine and the *Color Atlas of Family Medicine*.

Infectious skin disorders: Image B. Bullous impetigo. Reproduced, with permission, from Dr. Richard P. Usatine and the *Color Atlas of Family Medicine*.

Infectious skin disorders: Image C. Cellulitis. Reproduced, with permission, from Dr. Richard P. Usatine and the *Color Atlas of Family Medicine*.

Infectious skin disorders: Image D. Necrotizing fasciitis. Reproduced, with permission, from Dr. Richard P. Usatine and the *Color Atlas of Family Medicine*.

Infectious skin disorders: Image E. Staphylococcal scalded skin syndrome. Reproduced, with permission, from Dr. Richard P. Usatine and the *Color Atlas of Family Medicine*.

Infectious skin disorders: Image F. Hairy leukoplakia. Reproduced, with permission, from Dr. Richard P. Usatine and the *Color Atlas of Family Medicine*.

Skin cancer: Image A. Basal cell carcinoma with rolled borders. Reproduced, with permission, from Dr. Richard P. Usatine and the *Color Atlas of Family Medicine*.

Skin cancer: Image B. Basal cell carcinoma with nonhealing ulcer. Reproduced, with permission, from Dr. Richard P. Usatine and the *Color Atlas of Family Medicine*.

Skin cancer: Image C. Basal cell carcinoma with scaling plaque. Reproduced, with permission, from Dr. Richard P. Usatine and the *Color Atlas of Family Medicine*.

Skin cancer: Image D. Basal cell carcinoma histology. Reproduced, with permission, from USMLE-Rx.com.

Skin cancer: Image E. Squamous cell carcinoma on face. Reproduced, with permission, from Dr. Richard P. Usatine and the *Color Atlas of Family Medicine*.

Skin cancer: Image F. Squamous cell carcinoma on lip. Reproduced, with permission, from Dr. Richard P. Usatine and the *Color Atlas of Family Medicine*.

Skin cancer: Image G. Squamous cell carcinoma histology. Reproduced, with permission, from USMLE-Rx.com.

Skin cancer: Image H. Keratoacanthoma. Reproduced, with permission, from Dr. Richard P. Usatine and the *Color Atlas of Family Medicine*.

Skin cancer: Image I. Superficial spreading melanoma. Reproduced, with permission, from Dr. Richard P. Usatine and the *Color Atlas of Family Medicine*.

Skin cancer: Image J. Nodular melanoma. Reproduced, with permission, from Dr. Richard P. Usatine and the *Color Atlas of Family Medicine*.

Skin cancer: Image K. Lentigo maligna melanoma. Reproduced, with permission, from Dr. Richard P. Usatine and the *Color Atlas of Family Medicine*.

Skin cancer: Image L. Acrolentiginous melanoma. Reproduced, with permission, from Dr. Richard P. Usatine and the *Color Atlas of Family Medicine*.

Neurology

Aneurysms: Image A. Berry aneurysm. Reproduced, with permission, from Fauci AS et al. *Harrison's Principles of Internal Medicine*, 17th ed. New York: McGraw-Hill, 2008: Fig. 269-8C.

Intracranial hemorrhage: Image B. Subdural hematoma. Reproduced, with permission, from Chen MY et al. *Basic Radiology*, 1st ed. New York: McGraw-Hill, 2005: Fig. 12-32.

Intracranial hemorrhage: Image D. Hypertensive hemorrhage. Reproduced, with permission, from Waxman SG. *Clinical Neuroanatomy*, 26th ed. New York: McGraw-Hill, 2009: Fig. 25-20.

Hydrocephalus: Image A. Normal pressure hydrocephalus. Reproduced, with permission, from USMLE-Rx.com.

Dementia: Image A. Alzheimer's disease: β-amyloid deposits. Reproduced, with permission, from USMLE-Rx.com.

Multiple sclerosis: Image A. Multiple sclerosis. Reproduced, with permission, from Fauci AS et al. *Harrison's Principles of Internal Medicine*, 17th ed. New York: McGraw-Hill, 2008: Fig. 375-3A.

Adult primary brain tumors: Image A. Glioblastoma multiforme. Reproduced, with permission, from USMLE-Rx.com.

Adult primary brain tumors: Image B. Oligodendroglioma. Reproduced, with permission, from USMLE-Rx.com.

Renal

Nephrotic syndrome: Image A. Focal segmental glomerulosclerosis. Reproduced, with permission, from Lerma EV et al. *Current Diagnosis & Treatment: Nephrology & Hypertension*. New York: McGraw-Hill, 2009: Fig. 25-1B.

Nephrotic syndrome: Image B. Membranous nephropathy. Reproduced, with permission, from USMLE-Rx.com.

Nephrotic syndrome: Image D. Membranoproliferative glomerulonephritis. Reproduced, with permission, from Lerma EV et al. *Current Diagnosis & Treatment: Nephrology & Hypertension*. New York: McGraw-Hill, 2009: Fig. 28-1.

Nephrotic syndrome: Image E. Diabetic glomerulosclerosis. Reproduced, with permission, from USMLE-Rx.com.

- **Nephritic syndrome: Image A.** Rapidly progressive (crescentic) glomerulonephritis. Reproduced, with permission, from USMLE-Rx.com.

- **Kidney stones: Image A.** Staghorn calculus. Reproduced, with permission, from USMLE-Rx.com.

- **Renal cell carcinoma: Image A.** Renal cell carcinoma histology. Reproduced, with permission, from USMLE-Rx.com.

- **Renal cell carcinoma: Image B.** Renal cell carcinoma, gross kidney. Reproduced, with permission, from USMLE-Rx.com.

- **Transitional cell carcinoma: Image A.** Transitional cell carcinoma. Reproduced, with permission, from USMLE-Rx.com.

- **Renal cysts: Image A.** ADPKD. Reproduced, with permission, from USMLE-Rx.com.

Reproductive

- **Hydatidiform mole: Image B.** Molar pregnancy. Reproduced, with permission, from USMLE-Rx.com.

- **Cervical pathology: Image A.** Koilocytes in cervical condyloma. Reproduced, with permission, from USMLE-Rx.com.

- **Polycystic syndrome: Image A.** Polycystic ovary. Reproduced, with permission, from DeCherney AH, Nathan L. *Current Diagnosis & Treatment: Obstetrics & Gynecology*, 10th ed. New York: McGraw-Hill, 2007: Fig. 40-3.

- **Ovarian non–germ cell tumors: Image A.** Mucinous cystadenoma. Reproduced, with permission, from Chandrasoma P, Taylor CR. *Concise Pathology*, 3rd ed. New York: McGraw-Hill, 1997: Fig. 52-10.

- **Malignant breast tumors: Image A.** Comedocarcinoma. Reproduced, with permission, from Schorge JO et al. *Williams Gynecology*. New York: McGraw-Hill, 2008: Fig. 12-11.

- **Prostatic adenocarcinoma: Image A.** Prostatic adenocarcinoma. Reproduced, with permission, from USMLE-Rx.com.

Respiratory

- **Pulmonary emboli: Image A.** Pulmonary embolism. Reproduced, with permission, from USMLE-Rx.com.

- **Pulmonary emboli: Image B.** Pulmonary thromboembolus. Reproduced, with permission, from USMLE-Rx.com.

- **Obstructive lung disease: Image A.** Emphysema. Reproduced, with permission, from USMLE-Rx.com.

- **Pneumoconioses: Image A.** Asbestos bodies. Reproduced, with permission, from Wikimedia Commons.

- **Lung cancer: Image A.** Small cell carcinoma. Reproduced, with permission, from USMLE-Rx.com.

- **Lung cancer: Image B.** Squamous cell carcinoma. Reproduced, with permission, from USMLE-Rx.com.

Index

E

F

G

M

Q

R

▸ NOTES

About the Authors

Tao Le, MD, MHS

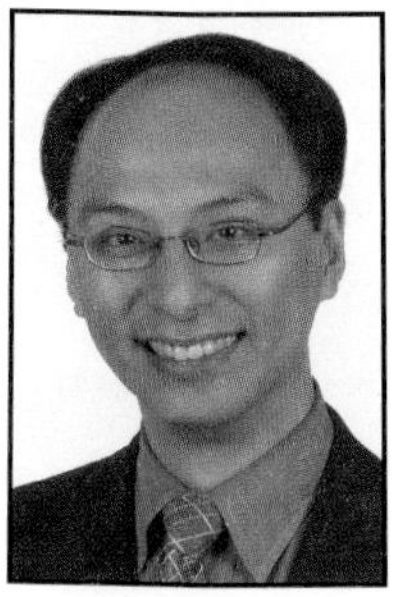

Tao developed a passion for medical education as a medical student. He currently edits more than 15 titles in the *First Aid* series. In addition, he is the founder of the *USMLE-Rx* online video and test bank series as well as a cofounder of the *Underground Clinical Vignettes* series. As a medical student, he was editor-in-chief of the University of California, San Francisco (UCSF) *Synapse,* a university newspaper with a weekly circulation of 9000. Tao earned his medical degree from UCSF in 1996 and completed his residency training in internal medicine at Yale University and fellowship training at Johns Hopkins University. At Yale, he was a regular guest lecturer on the USMLE review courses and an adviser to the Yale University School of Medicine curriculum committee. Tao subsequently went on to cofound Medsn, a medical education technology venture, and served as its chief medical officer. He is currently conducting research in asthma education at the University of Louisville.

Vikas Bhushan, MD

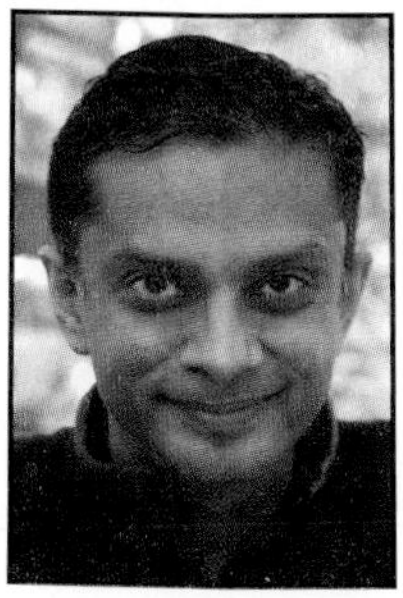

Vikas is a writer, editor, entrepreneur, and teleradiologist. In 1990 he conceived and authored the original *First Aid for the USMLE Step 1*. His entrepreneurial endeavors include a software company, a student-focused medical publisher (S2S), an e-learning company (medschool.com/Medsn), and an ER teleradiology practice (24/7 Radiology). Firmly anchored to the Left Coast, Vikas completed a bachelor's degree in biochemistry at the University of California Berkeley; an MD with thesis at UCSF; and a diagnostic radiology residency at UCLA. His eclectic interests include technology, informatics, independent film, photography, world music, South Asian diasporic culture, and avoiding a day job. Always finding the long shortcut, Vikas is an adventurer, knowledge seeker, and occasional innovator. He enjoys novice status as a kiteboarder and seaplane pilot, and strives to raise his children as global citizens.

Vivek T. Kulkarni

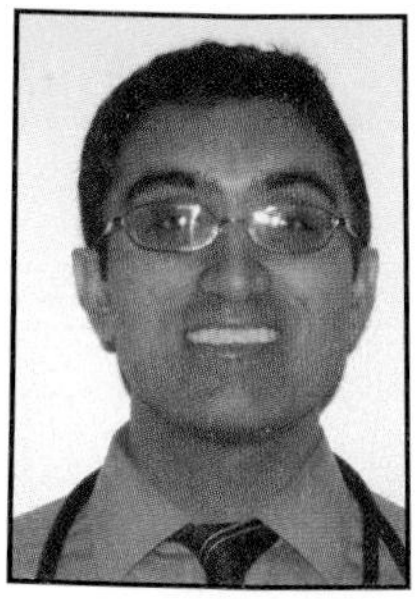

Vivek is currently a fourth-year student at the Yale School of Medicine, where he is pursuing a combined MD/MHS degree. He grew up in the suburbs of Chicago and graduated from Washington University in St. Louis in 2009 with bachelor of arts degrees in mathematics and chemistry. Vivek is doing his master of health sciences research in outcomes evaluation, studying hospital performance and its measurement. His future plans include residency training in internal medicine and a career as a clinician-educator.

Matthew M. Sochat

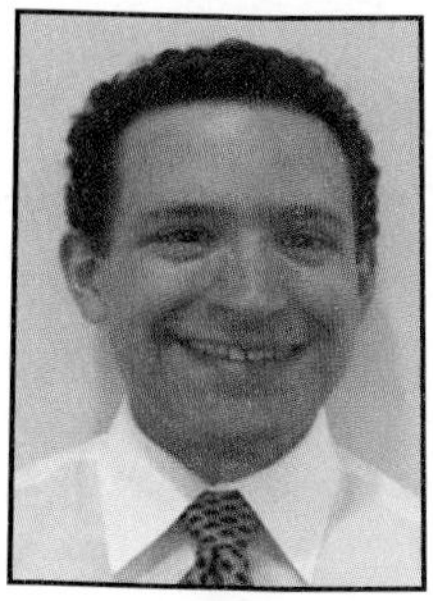

Matthew is currently a fourth-year student at the Warren Alpert Medical School of Brown University. He is a New Englander through and through, growing up in New Hampshire and attending the University of Massachusetts–Amherst, where he earned dual degrees in biochemistry and the classics. This year he is applying to neurology residency programs, planning on becoming a clinician-educator. In his spare time, Matthew enjoys skiing, cooking/baking, traveling, the company of friends/loved ones, and coming up with helpful puns/mnemonics.